Principles of
Oral Diagnosis

Principles of Oral Diagnosis

GARY C. COLEMAN, DDS, MS

Assistant Professor, Department of
Diagnostic Sciences
Baylor College of Dentistry
Dallas, Texas

JOHN F. NELSON, BS, DDS, MEd

Professor, Department of Diagnostic Sciences
Assistant Dean for Clinical Affairs
Baylor College of Dentistry
Dallas, Texas

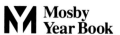

Mosby
Year Book

St. Louis Baltimore Boston Chicago London Philadelphia Sydney Toronto

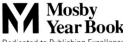
Mosby
Year Book
Dedicated to Publishing Excellence

Editor: Sandy Reinhardt
Developmental Editors: Susie Baxter, Melba Steube
Project Manager: Gayle May Morris
Project Editors: Sheila Walker, Donna L. Walls
Book and Cover Design: Gail Morey Hudson

Printed in the United States of America.

Mosby–Year Book, Inc.
11830 Westline Industrial Drive, St. Louis, Missouri, 63146

Library of Congress Cataloging in Publication Data

Coleman, Gary C.
  Principles of oral diagnosis / Gary C. Coleman and John F. Nelson.
    p.   cm.
  Includes index.
  ISBN 0-8016-1005-2
    1. Teeth— Diseases—Diagnosis. 2. Mouth—Diseases—Diagnosis.
  3. Oral medicine. I. Nelson, John F. II. Title.
    [DNLM: 1. Diagnosis. Differential. 2. Mouth Diseases—diagnosis.
  3. Tooth Diseases—diagnosis.   WU 141 C692p]
  RK308.C66 1992
  617.6'3075—dc20
  DNLM/DLC
  for Library of Congress   92-13124
                                                                  CIP

93 94 95 96 97 CL/WA 9 8 7 6 5 4 3 2 1

Contributors

BYRON W. BENSON, DDS, MS

Associate Professor, Department of Diagnostic Sciences
Baylor College of Dentistry, Dallas, Texas; Consultant, Dental Service
Olin E. Teague Veterans Center, Temple, Texas

MICHAEL W. FINKELSTEIN, DDS, MS

Associate Professor, Oral Pathology, Radiology, and Medicine
University of Iowa College of Dentistry, Iowa City, Iowa

CATHERINE M. FLAITZ, DDS, MS

Associate Professor, Department of Oral Diagnostic Sciences
University of Texas Health Science Center at Houston,
Dental Branch, Houston, Texas

STEVEN D. VINCENT, DDS, MS

Associate Professor, Oral Pathology, Radiology, and Medicine
University of Iowa College of Dentistry, Iowa City, Iowa

To Our Students who Serve as Teachers,

To Our Teachers who are Forever Students, and

To the Patients who Tolerate Our Efforts to Learn.

Preface

Preparing the dental student to formulate diagnostic and treatment planning decisions is the instructional responsibility of the discipline of oral diagnosis. The challenge for the educator is to foster the development of elementary diagnostic skills for the student's early clinical activities and then to gradually prepare the inexperienced clinician for more demanding diagnostic problems. The student's dilemma is the tendency to be overwhelmed by the extensive body of knowledge that must be integrated and applied to evaluate each patient's general and oral health status and then to plan appropriate treatment. Excellent comprehensive volumes are available on subjects that contribute to dental diagnostic decisions such as oral pathology and internal medicine. However, a textbook is not currently in print that provides the dental and dental hygiene student with an introductory correlation of this information as it relates to the clinical diagnostic process. *Principles of Oral Diagnosis* is an attempt to serve this purpose.

The fundamental vocabulary, methods, and factual information of oral diagnosis are presented to the student in the context of describing the diagnostic method. This has effectively determined the organization of the book into three parts.

Part I explains the fundamental nature of the diagnostic method and the techniques of collecting diagnostic information. Included are descriptions of routine diagnostic procedures such as the diagnostic interview, physical examination the patient, and documentation of clinical findings. This is presented initially to prepare the student to perform these procedures relatively early in the course of their training and to appreciate the routine sources of information that contribute to the diagnosis of all patients.

Part II addresses the evaluation and assessment of diagnostic information. The emphasis is on the process of drawing diagnostic data together from different sources that contribute to the evaluation of common clinical conditions and to the formulation of treatment planning decisions.

Part III is concerned with the differential diagnosis of nondental diseases of the oral cavity and associated structures. The strategy of distinguishing these abnormalities on the basis of their clinical features is the focus in these chapters. Decision flow charts and numerous photographs are provided to enhance the student's understanding and application of differential diagnosis to the clinical challenge posed by these conditions.

The selection of the term "principles" for the title reflects the intended scope of *Principles of Oral Diagnosis.* No pretense is made to suggest that this book provides comprehensive coverage of any of the subject areas discussed. Priority is given to presenting the process of identifying the clinical findings that contribute to solving typical diagnostic problems. This is approached by describing and comparing relatively common conditions that are possible explanations for clinical signs and symptoms such as chest pain, abnormal eruption of teeth, pain, and tissue enlargement. Considered another way, this is a book of generalizations that illustrate the systematic approach to dental diagnostic issues. The frequent use of terms such as "often," "usually," and "generally" in the text may become tiresome, but they provide necessary reminders that exceptions exist to most of these generalizations.

This approach to presenting an introduction to oral diagnosis is not without compromises. The scope of the discussion has been limited in several ways to achieve a manageable size for the book. Histopathologic findings, speculation on elusive pathogenic mechanisms, and unusual conditions are excluded because they usually cloud the clinical diagnostic process for the inexperienced clinician. This is most evident in the chapters concerned

with physical assessment and clinical syndromes. A complete discussion of these topics for the dentist is simply not feasible in this context. It is expected that the student clinician will often need to consult more comprehensive sources of information during the evaluation of exceptional patients. The chapters concerning nondental oral lesions excludes many rare and unusual conditions in the interest of demonstrating the differential diagnostic strategy without overloading the student by listing all possibilities. In all sections, the goal is to promote the student's understanding of the decision-making process rather than to specifically address all conceivable diagnostic problems. The assumption is that the student who develops a fundamental understanding of the diagnostic method will then be as well prepared as is possible to manage the exceptional clinical challenges that arise in every dental practice.

An attempt to specifically thank all of the individuals who have contributed to this project would be a lengthy task. For example, numerous students and educators have offered perceptive observations concerning course syllabus materials that served as the basis for the manuscript. However, the efforts of several friends and associates warrant special acknowledgment.

Drs. Benson, Finkelstein, Flaitz, and Vincent were intentionally trapped into agreeing to contribute chapters without a hint of the challenge posed by the relatively short notice, the broad scope of their topics, and the significant space limitations. To further complicate their efforts, the guidance provided by the first author was usually rather nebulous. Nevertheless, these talented individuals promptly produced chapter drafts that were remarkably close to the final manuscript versions. Any deficiencies in these chapters are certainly attributable to factors other than their knowledge, judgment, and diligence.

Dr. Ed Genecov was asked by a total stranger (GCC) to provide photographs illustrating the features of several rare conditions for the chapter covering developmental syndromes. This gentleman not only sorted through the patient records of his busy orthodontic practice to find many of the illustrations in Chapter 20, he also patiently tolerated the ignorance of the authors concerning the diagnosis and treatment of these conditions, which he has specialized in managing for most of his professional career. Unfortunately, space was not available to include examples of the impressive treatment results achieved by this skilled and gracious clinician.

Dr. Joseph Giansanti made a characteristically generous offer to accept the demanding task of reviewing the entire manuscript. He promptly painted early chapter drafts red with comments. His recurring apology for being too critical seemed unusual considering that his observations were consistently appropriate, insightful, and contributory. The knowledge, wisdon, common sense, and effort of this genuine friend have shaped the text of this book. His name is absent from the cover only because he refused the offer.

Whether the critics are harsh or kind, the outcome of *Principles of Oral Diagnosis* would have been far weaker without the benevolence of these busy educators and clinicians. To them and to those who prepared us to accept the demands of this project, we offer more than this simple acknowledgment. We offer the sincere appreciation that it represents.

Gary C. Coleman
John F. Nelson

Contents

PART III

Differential Diagnosis

PART I

Collecting Diagnostic Information

CHAPTER 1

The Diagnostic Method

GARY C. COLEMAN

The role of the healing professions is to apply knowledge and skill toward maintaining and restoring the patient's health. This may not always be completely attainable, but the clinician is expected to strive for optimal results within the limits of the circumstances. The need for treatment and what is the most appropriate treatment are dictated by the health status of the patient. *Diagnosis* is the process of evaluating the patient's health, as well as the resulting opinions formulated by the clinician.

The discipline of dentistry that is specifically concerned with the art and science of health assessment is referred to as *oral diagnosis*. This includes the evaluation of the patient's general health status, which is referred to as *physical assessment*. The discipline of *oral medicine* encompasses all aspects of oral diagnosis with specific attention to the management of patients with compromised general health and the treatment of nondental diseases that affect the oral and perioral tissues. Although these definitions suggest some of the diagnostic responsibilities of the general dentist, the role of diagnostician requires a greater understanding of the methods, terminology, and components of the process. This chapter describes the diagnostic method and its elements and their application in specific clinical situations.

THE DIAGNOSTIC METHOD

Accurate diagnostic decisions rely on a systematic approach to the unique diagnostic challenge posed by every patient. The most effective approach is the application of the scientific method to clinical decisions, which is referred to as the *diagnostic method*. The elements of the scientific method such as data collection and hypothesis testing are referred to by different terms but are conceptually the same in the diagnostic method:

1. *Collection of information*. The initial stage of the diagnostic method is the collection of the available diagnostic information. This includes details verbalized by the patient, features determined by the clinician's examination, and the data derived from adjunc-

tive diagnostic procedures such as laboratory tests. The clinician's obligation while gathering this information is to remain objective. Premature opinions introduce diagnostic bias, which can adversely alter the perception and accuracy of the information collected.

2. *Evaluation of information.* The second step of the process is to organize this information and determine its clinical significance. The clinician mentally compares the findings with basic knowledge, such as anatomy and physiology, and with observations from past clinical experiences. Unusual findings are correlated to identify patterns and relationships that are suggestive of certain diseases. The clinician also assesses the accuracy of the information and attempts to resolve contradictions. This may require repeating some diagnostic procedures or performing additional tests. These comparisons are the basis for preliminary decisions about the significance of the information collected. The clinician must remain objective at this stage or risk biased misinterpretation of the data.

3. *Diagnostic decisions.* The clinician next formulates opinions concerning the nature of unusual findings. Each opinion or diagnosis is the explanation for an element of the patient's status that is most consistent with the available information. This is comparable to formulating a hypothesis in the terminology of the scientific method. The diagnosis in some instances may be somewhat nonspecific, but it should be as specific as the available information justifies.

4. *Reassessment.* The reassessment stage of the diagnostic method is equivalent to hypothesis testing from the scientific method. The diagnosis of an abnormality suggests additional tests or an appropriate treatment. From this the clinician can often predict the response of the abnormality following treatment. Reassessment of the abnormality after treatment essentially tests the diagnosis. Response as predicted confirms the diagnosis to some degree, while an unexpected outcome suggests that the diagnosis may be incorrect.

The diagnostic method as diagrammatically summarized in Fig. 1-1 is never quite this direct in practice. Most patients exhibit dozens of unusual findings that may be related to several different diseases. These diseases often produce overlapping features that complicate the diagnosis. Also, most diagnostic information is associated with some degree of uncertainty. The diagnostic method is effective because the format helps to minimize errors.

COLLECTING DIAGNOSTIC INFORMATION

Several sources of diagnostic information contribute to the assessment of the patient's status. The assembled diagnostic information for a patient is referred to as the *diagnostic database.* This evidence of the patient's initial status also provides a basis for future comparisons to evaluate disease progression, the effectiveness of treatment, and the development of new abnormalities. The diagnostic database consists of the patient history, the physical examination results, and the information obtained from adjunctive diagnostic procedures. The box on p. 6 summarizes the information on the dental diagnostic database and the sequence in which it is typically collected.

Patient History

The patient history (Pt Hx) is the description of past events and related information that contributes to the assessment of the patient's health. This is usually supplied by the patient, but may be provided in some instances by the patient's guardian, previous clinicians, or prior health records. The patient history is organized into the following categories.

Patient identification. The patient's name, age, gender, race, address, phone number, and additional personal data are listed initially. This information is needed primarily for

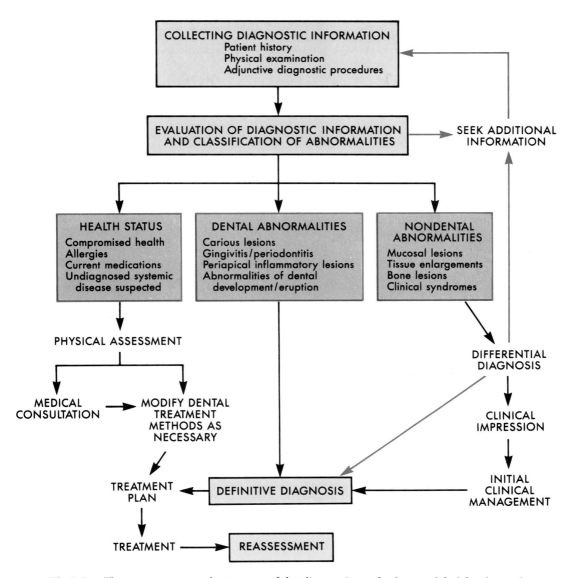

Fig 1-1 The components and sequence of the diagnostic method as modified for the evaluation of the dental patient.

patient identification and administrative purposes. However, the patient's age, gender, and race may contribute to the diagnosis of specific conditions.

Chief complaint. The chief complaint (cc) is a statement of why the patient consulted the dentist. The chief complaint is usually recorded in the patient's words because this may provide insight into the nature of the problem. In some instances the patient's problem is restated by the clinician to ensure clarity.

COMPONENTS OF THE COMPREHENSIVE DENTAL DIAGNOSTIC DATABASE

Patient history

Patient identification
Chief complaint
History of the chief complaint
Medical history
    Past medical conditions
    Infections and immunizations
    Prior hospitalizations
    Known allergies and drug reactions
    Current medical treatment
Family history
Social history
Review of systems
Dental history

Physical examination

General physical appraisal and vital signs
Extraoral examination
Intraoral examination

Adjunctive diagnostic information

Radiographic examination
Clinical laboratory studies
Microscopic examination of tissue samples
Microbiologic studies
Consultations and referrals

History of the chief complaint. The history of the chief complaint (Hx cc) details the patient's awareness of the problem and is occasionally referred to as the *history of present illness.* This includes the duration of the problem, prior occurrences, previous treatment, and the effectiveness of past treatment.

Medical history. The medical history (MH) is a review of health care experiences and medical conditions that have been diagnosed. This information is usually organized into past diseases, immunizations, hospitalizations, known allergies, and current treatment, including medications.

Family history. The family history consists of the health status of family members. This may reveal the possibility of conditions with a genetic tendency such as ischemic heart disease, diabetes, and hemophilia. Communicable infections may also be suspected on the basis of the family history.

Social history. The social history includes marital status, current employment, number of children, level of education, hobbies, and habits. These findings reflect the patient's lifestyle, which can indicate a vulnerability to certain diseases, exposure to specific infections, or dental treatment preferences. The social history also includes the patient's responses to the demands of routine and stressful personal events. These responses reveal the emotional adaptation of patients to their surroundings.

Review of systems. The review of systems (ROS) explores the health and function of the physiologic systems as revealed by the patient's recent experiences and perceptions. This is accomplished by a series of questions concerning specific forms of discomfort, unusual frequency of body functions, difficulty in performing certain tasks, and other experiences often associated with systemic diseases. The review of systems is designed to identify diseases that are undiagnosed and to assess the effectiveness of current treatment in controlling previously diagnosed illnesses.

Dental history. The dental history (Dent Hx) is a summary of past dental care, unusual dental experiences, hygiene practices, and related topics.

Physical Examination

The physical examination provides diagnostic information about the patient that is perceived by the clinician without the use of complex technical devices. This limits the clinician to the primary senses and a few simple diagnostic instruments. The dentist's physical examination is divided into the general patient appraisal, the extraoral examination, and the intraoral examination.

General patient appraisal. The evaluation of the patient's general appearance, gait, posture, speech, and similar observations is referred to as the *general patient appraisal.* This is the impression of the patient's health that could be observed in a nonclinical setting. Measurement of the patient's *vital signs,* which consists of blood pressure, pulse, respiration, and body temperature, is also a part of the general appraisal even though these determinations require techniques beyond simple observation.

Extraoral examination. The extraoral examination (EO Ex) consists of the physical findings beyond the general appraisal that can be perceived without looking in the patient's mouth. The extraoral examination by the dentist is focused on the head and neck, although examination of other regions may yield significant information.

Intraoral examination. The intraoral examination (IO Ex) includes all physical findings within the oral cavity.

Adjunctive Diagnostic Procedures

Adjunctive diagnostic methods rely on "distant" sources of information such as complex diagnostic instruments and other clinicians. These procedures extend and supplement the clinician's primary senses or enhance the accuracy and assessment of past health information. Radiographic examination is an example of a routine adjunctive diagnostic procedure that is essential to the practice of dentistry. Clinical laboratory studies such as blood counts and microscopic examination of tissue samples are examples of adjunctive procedures that are contributory in specific situations. Referrals and consultations that provide diagnostic data and opinions from other clinicians are also considered adjunctive sources of diagnostic information.

EVALUATION OF DIAGNOSTIC INFORMATION

The second stage of the diagnostic method is the evaluation of diagnostic information. The clinician searches for associations and patterns among the data from the health history, physical examination, and adjunctive diagnostic procedures. Related findings are mentally compared with the clinician's knowledge of normal variations among healthy individuals and characteristics indicative of disease. These comparisons support preliminary decisions that eventually provide direction during the diagnosis stage of the process. Comparisons may also reveal that certain findings are inaccurate or inconsistent. This can mean that the preliminary opinion is incorrect, elements of the history and examination should be reevaluated, or additional diagnostic procedures are needed to clarify the situation.

The evaluation of diagnostic information consists of organizing the diagnostic findings obtained during the initial information collection and formulating preliminary opinions concerning the significance of the information. This is simpler to describe in terms of the results than by the actual method. The mental process actually begins during the collection of information with decisions concerning the attention warranted by specific topics of the patient history or atypical physical features. Also, the reliability of specific data may still be under scrutiny later during the diagnosis stage. Specific aspects of evaluating diagnostic information are discussed in Part II of this text.

Organizing Diagnostic Information

The diagnostic data generated by the patient history, the physical examination, and adjunctive diagnostic procedures are generally recorded in the same order in which they are collected. This simplifies the search for specific details in the future or by another clinician, but the findings related to a specific problem are intermixed throughout the patient's diagnostic information. The clinician must mentally reorganize the information by whether it contributes to the evaluation of medical problems, dental conditions, or nondental abnormalities. Some general findings or a specific feature may be related to several problems and appear in more than one category.

Physical assessment. Information related to the patient's medical status is arranged by the physiologic systems. Findings related to a specific system are grouped by their relationship to past conditions, currently diagnosed illnesses, or as unexplained features suggestive of undiagnosed disease. Certain constitutional findings such as recent weight loss or fever are listed as indicative of a general health problem if a relationship to a specific system is not apparent.

Dental conditions. Abnormal dental findings from the chief complaint, dental history, oral examination, and radiographic examination are arranged as primarily affecting either the teeth or the supportive tissues. Further categorization and evaluation of dental conditions are described in Chapter 8. Unusual dental conditions can also contribute to the assessment of systemic conditions. The rapid progression of periodontitis, for example, is a typical consequence of compromised immune function and diabetes mellitus.

Nondental conditions. Abnormalities of the oral cavity and perioral structures that are unrelated to the teeth are generally categorized as mucosal alterations, soft tissue enlargements, abnormalities of bone, and multiple manifestations of a clinical syndrome. The evaluation of diagnostic information related to such conditions is the subject of Chapter 14.

Preliminary Decisions Concerning Diagnostic Information

The patient's unique combination of diagnostic information presents the clinician with several decisions for each diagnostic issue. The relationship, reliability, consistency, and significance of the findings must be determined. From another perspective, preliminary decisions concerning the patient's diagnostic information must be made to identify the patient's diagnostic problems and to determine the approach to their diagnosis.

Relationship of findings. Abnormal features from the patient history and physical examination that are related to a specific physiologic system are grouped during the organization of diagnostic information on the initial assumption that they relate to a single abnormality. In some cases, however, a group of features may be produced by more than one disease. For example, the patient with asthma of chronic duration can develop an acute pulmonary infection. The combination of pulmonary features caused by both conditions could be diagnostically confusing unless the asthmatic features of long duration are considered separately from the recent manifestations of acute infection. Determining the diagnostic features that are related to a single condition can become particularly challenging with older patients who may suffer from several degenerative diseases affecting multiple physiologic systems.

Reliability. The reliability of diagnostic information reflects the diagnostician's opinion of its accuracy. The reliability of information from the patient history is suggested by the patient's confidence in describing the information and by how consistently the patient describes the same facts in response to different questions. The patient's recollection of recent problems is usually more accurate as compared with the memories of a medical problem that developed many years ago.

Reliability may also be affected by the source of the information. A subjective diagnostic feature described verbally by the patient is referred to as a *symptom*. Objective findings observed by the clinician are clinical *signs*. For example, the patient describes the symptom of a toothache, while the dentist attempts to detect the sign of tenderness by applying pressure. Clinical signs are generally more reliable than the patient's symptoms. The clinician's objective observations during the physical examination are often more reliable than the indirect information of adjunctive diagnostic procedures. One reason for this is that adjunctive diagnostic methods such as laboratory tests are vulnerable to technical errors.

Consistency. Consistency refers to the agreement among the available diagnostic data from different sources that relate to a specific topic. Obese body build, a past diagnosis of hypertension, current administration of an antihypertensive medication, and blood pressure measured within the range considered normal are consistent features that mutually support the assessment of controlled hypertension. A medical consultation in which this patient's physician reports the recent diagnosis and treatment of hypertension provides *confirmation* of the dentist's opinion. In the context of this example, measurement of abnormally high blood pressure would be a *contradictory finding* that is inconsistent with the opinion of the physician and patient that the hypertension is controlled.

Consistency of findings supports definitive diagnostic decisions, while inconsistent or contradictory information suggests the need to reevaluate the accuracy of the findings or to obtain additional data. In some instances contradictory findings may represent the effects of more than one disease affecting the same system.

Clinical significance. The clinical significance of most unusual findings can be considered as either an atypical variation of normal or evidence of disease. Most diseases produce both alterations of tissue morphology called *lesions* and compromised function referred to as *dysfunction.* Atypical morphology without evidence of dysfunction may represent an unusual appearance of healthy tissues.

The clinical significance of disease in the context of oral diagnosis depends on the na-

ture and severity of the condition. All dental abnormalities and nondental conditions of the mouth and neighboring structures are clinically significant to the dentist. Diseases affecting the cardiovascular, pulmonary, gastrointestinal, and renal systems may require alteration of dental treatment methods and should be evaluated to the limit of the available information and the dentist's ability. In contrast, many chronic skin diseases and mild arthritis of the lower limbs are examples of diseases with little direct bearing on dental care. Past medical problems that have completely resolved following treatment, such as a surgically repaired hernia, are usually of little importance to the dentist.

Healthy variations of tissue appearance, inconsequential abnormalities, and past medical conditions that have resolved can generally be excluded from additional diagnostic consideration as clinically insignificant. The dentist's confidence in formulating this opinion depends on the reliability and consistency of the diagnostic information. Also, clinicians are usually hesitant to dismiss even the weak evidence of potentially serious condition such as cardiac disease. Any uncertainty justifies consideration of the suspected abnormality as clinically significant. Further evaluation of clinically significant conditions occurs during the diagnosis stage of the diagnostic method.

DIAGNOSIS

The assembly of diagnostic information and its evaluation are directed to achieving a definitive opinion or diagnosis of the patient's condition, which provides the basis for dental treatment decisions. The diagnostic approach for a specific problem depends on whether it involves a systemic disease, a dental condition, or a nondental abnormality of the mouth and adjacent structures.

Systemic Disease

The definitive diagnosis of systemic disease is beyond the scope of dental practice. Few dentists are adequately prepared by training or experience to perform and interpret physical examination procedures, such as the assessment of heart sounds, that are essential to the diagnosis of systemic diseases. The diagnosis of any medical condition suspected following the patient history, physical examination, and evaluation of diagnostic findings must be accomplished by medical consultation. Definitive diagnosis of systemic disease should not be confused with the physical assessment of the patient's health in the context of dental treatment, which is the dentist's responsibility. Chapter 7 is devoted to the physical assessment of the dental patient.

Dental Disease

Dental diseases include dental caries, gingivitis, periodontitis, periapical lesions secondary to pulpal necrosis, developmental dental conditions, and abnormalities of dental eruption. These conditions produce features that are adequately characteristic in most instances that a confident diagnosis can be made. In addition, most dental conditions are so common that dentists rapidly become familiar with the diversity of most common dental diseases. The challenge associated with the diagnosis of dental conditions is generally related to determining the extent of the lesions and other factors that affect treatment decisions, as discussed in Chapters 8, 12, and 13.

Nondental Conditions of the Oral Cavity and Adjacent Structures

The dentist is responsible for the definitive diagnosis and treatment of nondental conditions of the oral cavity and adjacent structures. These abnormalities generally present more challenging diagnostic problems than do dental diseases for two reasons. First, many of these conditions are less common than dental diseases, which limits the opportunities to accumulate experience and confidence in their diagnosis and treatment. Second, the diagnosis of nondental oral conditions based solely on

the appearance of a lesion or signs of dysfunction is less likely to be correct as with dental diseases because similar manifestations may be produced by many different diseases. Therefore the diagnosis of the patient's nondental problem requires the comparison of its features with those of several diseases that are capable of producing the abnormality.

This comparative diagnostic technique is called *differential diagnosis*. The clinician mentally lists the diseases that could explain the general features of the lesion or dysfunction. Specific diagnostic findings of the patient's condition that are contradictory with the typical characteristics of these diseases can be used to exclude them from diagnostic consideration. After eliminating as many diseases from consideration as the information justifies, the remaining possibilities are ranked in the order of diagnostic probability. The most likely diagnosis is referred to as the *working diagnosis,* the *presumptive diagnosis,* or the *clinical impression.* The working diagnosis and the other less likely possibilities determine the need for additional tests and preliminary treatment. Additional procedures such as microscopic examination of surgically removed tissue usually limit the list to a single disease, which is the *definitive diagnosis,* the *final diagnosis,* or just the *diagnosis.* The final diagnosis determines the definitive management of the problem.

Differential diagnosis is a sophisticated approach to challenging diagnostic problems because the decision sequence systematically and logically eliminates unlikely diseases while comparing the remaining possibilities with the patient's condition. This is analogous to hypothesis formulation of the scientific method in that each disease in the differential diagnosis is considered as a hypothetical diagnosis until the condition that most completely and accurately explains the abnormality is identified. The effectiveness of the method depends on the reliability of the diagnostic data, the clinician's experience in evaluating the findings, and the dentist's knowledge of the diagnostic possibilities. The final seven chapters of this text are devoted to the differential diagnosis of nondental disease of oral and perioral tissues.

REASSESSMENT

Reassessment of the abnormality following appropriate management is the final element of the diagnostic method. This usually consists of reevaluating the patient's symptoms and reexamining the affected region at some time interval after treatment. This is the hypothesis testing stage of clinical diagnosis. If the diagnosis is correct, the treatment is appropriate, and the treatment is competently performed, then the response of the condition can be predicted. Curable abnormalities should resolve completely, and incurable diseases should be controlled by the treatment or progress in a manner consistent with the illness. If the reassessment reveals an unexpected result, then the diagnostician must consider whether the treatment was inadequately performed, the treatment was inappropriate, or the diagnosis was incorrect. The essential concept to understanding the diagnostic method is that reassessment is an active diagnostic procedure.

TYPES OF CLINICAL EXAMINATION

The diagnostic method can be modified to most effectively address the needs of the patient. These modifications generally alter the amount of diagnostic information collected initially or the scope of diagnostic decisions made by the clinician.

Comprehensive Dental Diagnosis

The comprehensive dental diagnosis is the dentist's most extensive diagnostic assessment, and it is appropriate for the patient who requests total dental care and has not been evaluated previously. This situation requires the collection of all appropriate diagnostic information and all diagnostic decisions that are within the scope of dental practice. Comprehensive dental diagnosis includes a detailed pa-

tient history, intraoral and extraoral physical examination, typical adjunctive procedures such as dental radiographs, physical assessment, and diagnosis of all oral and perioral conditions.

The value of the comprehensive dental diagnosis extends beyond planning total dental care. These data reflect the patient's initial status, which serves for comparison later in assessing treatment effectiveness. This comprehensive database also protects the clinician by documenting the patient's initial status if treatment complications lead to accusations of substandard care. The comprehensive dental diagnosis requires considerable time, but it reliably provides a sound diagnostic foundation for comprehensive dental care.

Recall Diagnosis

The recall diagnosis is the appropriate approach for a patient who requests total dental care when the results of a prior comprehensive dental diagnosis are available. The assumption is that a portion of this past information is still accurate but other aspects of the patient's medical and dental status may have changed. The goal is to identify the conditions that have changed and supplement the prior database so that it reflects the patient's current status. This can be as simple as asking the patient if there have been any changes since the last appointment, which is always good practice regardless of the time interval, or as complex as repeating most of the comprehensive dental diagnosis. The update refamiliarizes the dentist with the patient's original conditions and provides the new findings for comparison. If a different clinician conducted the original diagnosis, the current dentist must confirm the accuracy of prior data and record current findings prior to diagnostic decisions.

Diagnosis of a Specific Problem

The dentist is frequently asked to provide an opinion concerning a specific problem for a recently evaluated patient. The *SOAP evalua-*

tion is an effective approach to such situations if the available diagnostic database is current and accurate. Consultation requests from other practitioners and reassessment of recent treatment are situations in which the SOAP format is commonly applied. If the diagnostic database is unavailable, then significant portions of the patient history and physical examination must be performed. Clinicians usually review key points of the database to confirm the reliability of the available information. The format of the SOAP evaluation follows:

1. The reason for the evaluation is briefly stated.
2. The 'S' entry is the *s*ubjective information or symptoms of the condition as supplied by the patient.
3. The 'O' entry includes the *o*bjective or physical findings of the clinician.
4. The 'A' entry is the *a*nalysis or clinical impression of the condition by the clinician.
5. The 'P' entry is the *p*lan or recommended management for the problem. This may be a specific treatment, referral to another clinician, or a dismissal of the condition as clinically insignificant.

Emergency Diagnosis

The emergency diagnosis is designed to expeditiously manage a chief complaint such as pain, bleeding, or acute infection that requires immediate attention. The comprehensive diagnostic evaluation is sacrificed in the interest of providing attention to the urgent problem. The scope of the emergency diagnosis depends on the emergency complaint and the clinical situation. The clinician usually explores most aspects of the patient history, but the physical examination is limited in most respects to the chief complaint.

The emergency diagnosis can be demanding because the patient's concern for the chief complaint can interfere with obtaining an adequate patient history. Also, the clinician must determine from the complaint what diagnostic information is needed to adequately evaluate and safely treat the problem.

Screening Diagnosis

The screening diagnosis answers a specific question about the patient. The evaluation is limited to obtaining the information needed to answer this question without accepting comprehensive diagnostic or treatment responsibility for the patient. An example of a screening diagnosis is the oral cancer screening examination that is often conducted at health awareness fairs. The focus is whether or not evidence of oral cancer is present without specific attention to routine dental conditions or physical assessment of the patient. Institutions often rely on a screening diagnosis to determine the patient's general dental treatment needs and to arrange comprehensive dental diagnosis and treatment.

SUMMARY

Oral diagnosis is the dental discipline that is specifically concerned with the assessment of the patient's general and dental health status. This is accomplished by the diagnostic method, which is the process of collecting diagnostic information, evaluating the information, achieving a diagnosis of abnormalities, and reassessing the accuracy of the diagnosis.

The diagnostic information collected by the dentist consists of the patient history, the features identified by physical examination, and the results of adjunctive diagnostic procedures such as radiographs and laboratory tests. The evaluation of diagnostic findings is the organization of this information as it relates to specific topics, the assessment of the reliability and consistency of the information, and the formulation of preliminary opinions concerning the clinical significance of atypical findings. These decisions provide the basis for categorizing conditions as general health problems, dental diseases, or nondental abnormalities in or near the oral cavity.

The diagnosis stage of the diagnostic method includes the physical assessment of the patient's general health as it relates to dental treatment and definitive decisions concerning dental diseases. Nondental diseases affecting the oral and perioral structures are usually evaluated by differential diagnosis, which is the comparison of the features of the patient's condition with the typical features of the diseases capable of causing the abnormality. Differential diagnosis eliminates unlikely causes of the problem on the basis of inconsistent features, which simplifies the further evaluation of more likely illnesses. The diseases that are considered likely explanations of the patient's condition suggest the need for additional diagnostic procedures or preliminary treatment, which in most cases eventually yields a definitive diagnosis. Reassessment of the condition is the final stage of the diagnostic method in which the clinician confirms the accuracy of the diagnosis by evaluating the response of the condition to appropriate management.

The diagnostic method can be modified to accommodate the needs of specific patients.

The comprehensive dental diagnosis is appropriate for the patient who requests complete dental care and has not been previously evaluated. This consists of collecting all of the necessary information to determine the patient's general and dental health status and to plan treatment that will eliminate dental disease. The diagnostic process is less extensive in cases of prior comprehensive evaluation, emergency complaints, specific dental problems, and patient screening. The diagnostic process can be abbreviated in these situations because previous information is available or the scope of the clinical problem is limited.

BIBLIOGRAPHY

DeGowin RL: DeGowin & DeGowin's bedside diagnostic examination, ed 5, New York, 1987, MacMillan.

Harvey AM, Bordley J: Differential diagnosis: the interpretation of clinical evidence, ed 3, Philadelphia, 1979, Saunders.

Wood NK, Goaz PW: Differential diagnosis of oral lesions, ed 4, St Louis, 1991, Mosby-Year Book, Inc.

CHAPTER 2

The Patient History

GARY C. COLEMAN

Dental patients are generally aware of the information that the dentist needs to evaluate their health status and safely provide dental care. The clinician's challenge is to efficiently obtain this information without errors and significant omissions. Historical data can be obtained by the use of a questionnaire, by discussion, or by a combination of the two. A benefit of verbal exchange as compared with the use of a questionnaire is that the factual information is supplemented by nonverbal aspects of the patient's communication such as tone of voice, facial expressions, and "body language." Also, the discussion provides an initial opportunity to establish a positive relationship with the patient. This chapter describes the methods of obtaining the patient history. The interpretation of this information is discussed in Chapter 7.

THE IMPORTANCE OF THE PATIENT HISTORY

The importance of the patient history in the context of dental diagnosis and treatment cannot be overstated. In the past many dentists considered any patient who could physically travel to the dental office as capable of tolerating routine dental procedures. Several reasons suggest why this assumption is currently invalid and why a thorough patient history is important:

1. New diseases and conditions with important implications for the dentist are continually being identified. As an example, AIDS was unknown only a few years ago.
2. The success of new medical treatment methods extends the survival of many patients with significantly compromised health. Before the success of kidney dialysis and transplant procedures for example, patients with renal failure died and therefore never requested dental treatment.
3. The discovery and application of new drugs complicate the diagnosis and treatment decisions for the dental patient. Not only are newer, more power-

ful drugs available to treat many medical conditions, but more people are taking several medications for an extended duration. Many drugs and the interactions of multiple drug regimens have direct implications for the dentist that did not previously exist or were not appreciated.

4. Cost-containment policies of insurance companies have promoted more outpatient medical care. Sick people were unlikely to consult the dentist in the past because they were hospitalized. Now many individuals who are ill or are recovering from acute illness and surgery are seeking routine dental treatment or complaining of dental problems that may be a consequence of their medical problem or its treatment.

5. Relatively few dentists confronted the challenge of treating hospitalized patients prior to the advent of general practice dental residency programs. These programs offer many dental graduates their first unsupervised clinical experience in a hospital setting. Hospital patients typically present a greater diagnostic and therapeutic challenge than the general population.

6. The population in the United States is aging and most older adults suffer from degenerative illnesses. Geriatric patients generally require more insightful and empathetic diagnostic evaluation than do younger, healthier patients.

7. Changing social trends have created more demanding diagnostic responsibilities. One example is the common use of illicit drugs. Another is the current tendency to solve conflicts by litigation. Media publicity about health issues often stimulates unusual or unreasonable patient expectations. Other examples could be cited, but the trend toward increasing diagnostic challenges for the dentist is obvious.

The patient history is the initial mechanism of identifying and evaluating the patient's health status before formulating diagnostic and treatment decisions. Clinical decisions based on an incomplete or inaccurate patient history unnecessarily risks complications.

THE DIAGNOSTIC INTERVIEW

The diagnostic interview is a verbal exchange between the patient and clinician that elicits the patient's knowledge concerning health information. Every diagnostic interview is unique because each fact related by the patient alters the content of the subsequent discussion by revealing the need for clarification and the possibility of related health problems. The goal is to identify all relevant information efficiently. This can be difficult if the patient assumes control of the discussion and wastes time by describing noncontributory topics. Skilled clinicians maintain control by attentively determining the relevant information and provide direction by the use of questions, simple cues, and gestures. Every clinician develops a unique interviewing style that effectively directs the discussion while remaining congenial.

The results of the diagnostic interview may be recorded in several ways. Experienced clinicians often conduct the entire interview and later record the findings from memory to avoid distracting the patient by writing. This fosters better rapport but significant facts can be forgotten. The use of a preprinted form aids in arranging the data, guiding the interview, and avoiding omissions. Regardless of how the clinician prefers to record the data, the interview must remain an active process in which the course of the discussion is determined by the patient's responses.

Methods of Presenting Questions During the Diagnostic Interview

Different methods of phrasing the same question can produce different answers, and variable accuracy, depending on the topic and the patient's personality. In addition, the way in which a question is asked is one of the most useful techniques for maintaining control of the interview. The following approaches illustrate basic options that are available to the clinician in phrasing questions during the diagnostic interview.

Open-ended questions. Open-ended questions prompt the patient into a narrative, which is an effective method of covering a complicated topic. An example is "Can you tell me about your surgery that was performed last year?" This directs the patient to describe the entire topic with the expectation that most of the information will be contributory. The problem that required surgery, the nature of the operation, any complications, the duration of the hospitalization, the response to the surgical stress, and the effectiveness of the procedure in solving the problem may all be significant. Any details omitted by the patient during the narrative can then be elicited by specific questions. The patient should be allowed to respond fully to open-ended questions with few interruptions unless the discussion strays from the topic.

Open-ended questions are perceived as less stressful by most individuals because the doctor cares enough to listen and the patient is given temporary control of the interview. Open-ended questions are most effective with patients who are aware of health issues and can anticipate the information that is contributory. Open-ended questions can also calm anxious patients by providing an opportunity to talk their way through what may be an uncomfortable situation. This approach is less likely to be productive with unresponsive patients and individuals who digress from the topic.

Closed-ended questions. This form of question demands specific information. An example might be, "When did you last see your physician?" The closed-ended question is phrased to limit the patient's answer to a single sentence or less. The clinician should clarify early in the interview that simple answers are

expected for closed-ended questions. This can be conveyed by gestures or by quickly proceeding to the next question after the answer is given. Closed-ended questions are the most specific and efficient method of requesting information but patients may respond too directly without volunteering clarifying information. Also, patients can interpret questions literally, which may lead to misrepresentations. An extreme example of this might follow the question, "How many alcoholic drinks do you have each day?" The patient could answer "three drinks per day" and fail to mention the six drinks consumed each night. The negative impact of numerous closed-ended questions is that the patient perceives the interviewer as cold or remote because the clinician exerts total control.

The direction and control provided by closed-ended questions are most effective with unresponsive patients and those unfamiliar with health issues. Closed-ended questions also abruptly redirect an unproductive conversation. This approach is less effective for responsive and aware patients because they become impatient with the dentist's dominance of the interview.

Leading questions. This technique suggests the answer within the question. The dentist may suspect that recurring morning headaches described by the patient are caused by bruxism and ask, "And I imagine that you also grind your teeth in your sleep, don't you?" A positive response not only confirms the clinician's suspicion about the headache but also promotes the patient's confidence by leaving the favorable impression that the dentist understands the problem. The risk of leading questions is that some patients will respond affirmatively because it is the expected answer rather than the actual situation. Another risk is that the dentist's error in asking a leading question based on an incorrect assumption can cause the patient to lose confidence. A variation of the leading approach is the *option question* in which the patient is provided a limited selection of responses. Asking the patient, "Do you think your headaches are caused by grinding your teeth at night or by stress at your job?" illustrates the technique.

Leading questions are useful in drawing information from unresponsive patients and in winning the confidence of suspicious individuals. Leading questions should be avoided with patients who appear indecisive or are vulnerable to suggestion. Option questions can be effective for sensitive topics and with forgetful patients. Option questions can coax a response from indecisive patients, but the clinician is likely to receive an incorrect response if the actual answer is not provided as an option.

Contradiction questions. The contradiction question states inconsistent information and allows the patient to resolve the contradiction as with this example: "Since you said that you do not have epilepsy, is there another reason for you to be taking a medicine that is usually prescribed to control seizures?" This design forces the patient to face the contradiction by either making another misleading statement or by telling the truth. In this context, an accurate answer is usually easier than another misrepresentation. The same strategy can be presented less aggressively by the clinician accepting blame for the confusion: "I must have written something down wrong. I marked that you have never had epilepsy, but the medication you are taking is usually prescribed for epileptic seizures. Did I make a mistake?" A pause after the question allows the patient to correct the doctor's "mistake," which is more comfortable than admitting the original attempt to hide the condition.

Contradiction questions are effective in obtaining withheld information and when conflicting information has been given. Suspicious, anxious, and more responsive individuals are likely to resent the contradiction approach because of the sense of being trapped.

Indirect questions. Indirect questions often present a topic in such a way that the patient will reveal information beyond what is specifically requested by the question. The question, "Have you had any complications during or after previous dental treatment?" may not be designed to clarify such complications as much as the patient's general attitude toward dental care or the perception of a prior dentist's ability. The *loaded question* is also an indirect approach in which an emotional element is inserted into the phrasing to get the patient's attention. "With the problems you've had in the past, do you think that it might be best to extract all of your teeth?" is a loaded question. Nonverbal responses such as nervous shifting of position or negative facial expressions can be as revealing as the verbal response to an indirect question.

Indirect questions are useful in understanding sensitive or conflicting historical information and in exploring patient attitudes. The primary disadvantage of indirect questions is that the approach can be unproductive and time consuming.

Additional Aspects of Effective Interviewing

Various other interviewing techniques can improve the quality and efficiency of the diagnostic interview beyond the manner in which questions are phrased.

Opening. The dentist's initial contact with the patient should include introductions. The identities of all parties are generally evident from the appointment arrangement. Nevertheless, the dentist's self-introduction projects confidence, and the effort to formally meet the patient is appropriately courteous. Addressing adults by their first name often appears rude unless they specifically request it. Limiting the initial conversation to topics that are unrelated to dentistry helps anxious patients to relax and sets a more personal tone for the diagnostic interview. Neutral topics such as hobbies, common acquaintances, or family activities are best. The dentist can signal the beginning of the diagnostic interview by asking for clarification of the chief complaint.

Choice of questioning method. The initial question concerning the chief complaint should be open-ended such as, "Can you tell me about the problem that brought you in today?" This reinforces the positive atmosphere of the opening conversation because the patient controls the discussion of his or her problem and the dentist cares enough to listen. The dentist can form an initial impression of the patient's awareness of health topics and dentistry, which determines the approach for subsequent topics. Responsive and succinct patients can be given additional open-ended questions. Closed-ended questions can be used to obtain omitted details or to redirect conversational digressions. Less direct questioning methods are reserved until needed to investigate embarrassing topics or if contradictory information becomes apparent. Mixing the form of questions during the course of the interview introduces variety that helps to hold the patient's attention.

Timing. The timing of specific topics during the diagnostic interview helps patients remember specific events. Asking about blood transfusions after discussing hospitalizations prompts the patient to recall what might otherwise have been forgotten. Most patients feel more comfortable answering questions about embarrassing issues such as venereal infections later in the interview.

Choice of words. The clinician should use words that the patient will understand. Most people comprehend the phrase "venereal disease," but others are more familiar with other terms. The patient's health awareness and vocabulary become apparent if open-ended questions are used early in the interview. Emotionally-charged words should be avoided if possible. A patient with features suggestive of AIDS, as an example, might respond negatively to the word "homosexual" but provide a truthful response to the question, "Are there any high-risk factors that would make you vulnerable to AIDS?"

The appropriate use of medical terms by the patient usually indicates that the patient understands the subject. Patients suffering from a chronic disease generally become familiar with the terms and jargon related to that condition. A patient with rheumatoid arthritis who states that the sedimentation rate and rheumatoid factor titer are down since switching to a stronger nonsteroidal antiinflammatory drug must be considered credible. On the other hand, the dentist should be skeptical if the patient's use of medical terms is awkward or the information is inconsistent. This may indicate "self-diagnosis" based on information from popular magazines or similar sources. Many patients who claim "hypoglycemia" or "hypothyroidism" are actually describing that they tire more quickly than when they were younger.

A request for the patient to clarify terms that are vague or confusing is often necessary. A patient who relates an "attack of nerves" could be describing a period of emotional stress or a psychotic episode. The direct approach is usually sufficient: "What do you mean by an 'attack of nerves?'" or "Did your doctor give a specific diagnosis for your problem?" In other cases, the patient may not actually know and questions concerning the treatment or other aspects of the problem may reveal the condition.

Avoid wasting time. Discussing every conceivable medical topic with every patient wastes time. Questioning a 22-year-old patient about diseases that are rare prior to age 50 or exploring the details of an appendectomy performed 20 years ago are unproductive. Most patients become understandably impatient with the discussion of such irrelevancies. This also indicates to the knowledgeable patient that the dentist is following a standard interview format with minimal understanding of the topics.

Gestures and prompts. Gestures and single-word prompts increase the efficiency of the interview. The verbal tone used in saying the word "yes" can either signify agreement and prompt the patient to continue or signal that the response is adequate. Holding up one hand with the palm out can stop noncontributory conversation. The words "why" and "how" quickly redirect the patient to the necessary details. "I understand," said with sincerity often eases the patient through a difficult topic.

Nonverbal communication. Nonverbal communication, such as the patient's "body language" and facial expressions, supplements the verbal information obtained by the attentive clinician. Minimal eye contact, for example, suggests avoidance or insecurity. Rapid glances around the operatory and clenching of the hands reflects fear. Crossed arms, a tilt of the head, hesitation, or squinting of the eyes can suggest skepticism. Numerous other examples could be listed, but those described illustrate the importance of nonverbal expression. Also, most patients are sensitive to the nonverbal expressions of the dentist. For example, avoiding eye contact with the patient makes the clinician appear uncomfortable, insecure, or disinterested.

Humor. Humor during the diagnostic interview can enhance the patient-dentist relationship and help anxious patients to relax. The ability of the dentist to see the humor in daily events and enjoy the clinical setting is appreciated by nearly all patients. Sexual, ethnic, and similar forms humor, however, virtually always have a negative impact that is inappropriate and unprofessional.

Confrontation. As uncomfortable as disagreements can be, situations arise in which confrontation develops during the diagnostic interview. The patient may insist that contradictory elements of the history are correct or disagree with the clinician's opinion. Patients may refuse to discuss sensitive topics with the attitude that the dentist does not need to know such information. A calm explanation of how apparently unrelated problems can affect dental care or why the information is contradictory encourages a more appropriate response in most instances. If the patient argues

or becomes emotional, then the interview should be discontinued and completed at another appointment. The dentist should remain professionally reserved rather than participate in the conflict.

Summarize information and request agreement. An effective technique to confirm accuracy is to summarize the information and request the patient's agreement. This may be done at the end of the interview with simple histories or more frequently for complex medical problems. An example might be, "As I understand it, except for your allergy to penicillin and history of hepatitis, you are in perfect health, is that right?" This moves the interview beyond specific facts and requests the patient to agree with the clinician's conclusions. Often this helps the patient to clear up any misinterpretations or recall omitted details.

Listening. Finally, the dentist should learn to listen. This includes hearing what is said as well as what is not said, not interrupting the patient excessively, and appreciating how the patient verbalizes the information. Patients usually volunteer most relevant information if given the guidance and opportunity.

Sources of the Patient History other than the Patient

The dentist should be somewhat skeptical of medical information that is obtained from anyone other than the patient, but in some cases the patient is unable to provide the history. The most common examples involve children, mentally compromised patients, and those with language problems. The clinician must determine the dependability of the history from any source and should not accept clinical responsibility in cases of unreliable or incomplete information.

A parent or guardian must provide the patient history for a child because a minor cannot be considered a competent source of diagnostic information. Even with older adolescents who are capable of relating the information, the history is considered invalid if legally contested. The dentist should be skeptical of a medical history given by anyone other than a parent or guardian, such as a grandparent who may have brought the child to the appointment.

Mentally compromised patients are typically seen either in an institutional setting or in a private office accompanied by a family member or care provider. The patient's medical records and the staff physician are available in an institution to clarify the patient history. The private office situation is usually uncomplicated because the accompanying family member or care provider is familiar with the patient's history from years of bearing this responsibility.

Language barriers necessitate the presence of an interpreter. A family member usually anticipates the problem and accompanies the patient. This can cause the patient to withhold embarrassing facts from the family member who is interpreting. In addition, the family member may also be weak in English and have difficulty understanding and responding to the clinician's questions. Therefore, the clinician should rely on direct questions that are phrased in simple terms. Many offices located where another language is predominant hire bilingual staff members to improve the reliability of translation.

Occasionally, the only dependable source of the patient history may be the patient's physician. The inconvenience of a medical consultation may be unavoidable to obtain an adequate patient history.

THE HEALTH QUESTIONNAIRE

Most dental and medical offices rely on a health questionnaire to obtain biographical and health information. The health questionnaire functions as a "net" to identify potentially significant topics of the patient history. This is accomplished by nonspecific questions about general health issues and specific questions concerning common diseases. The responses to the questionnaire can then be discussed by the patient and clinician to adequately explore the unique and specific details of the patient's history. This discussion also allows the dentist to clarify misinterpretations and mistaken answers.

Initial evaluation of the patient history with a health questionnaire offers the advantages of saving time and providing documentation of the health history in the patient's handwriting. A significant disadvantage of the questionnaire approach is a greater potential for errors and omissions in comparison to the interview method. For the information from a health questionnaire to be correct and useful, the dentist must assume that the patient:

Can read the questions

Understands the questions

Wants to accurately respond to the questions

Knows or remembers the answers to the questions

Correctly marks or writes the appropriate response

and that the clinician

Identifies the intended responses

Understands the significance of the responses

Evaluates the responses with additional questions

Many of the potential errors in this sequence are less likely if the patient history is obtained entirely by discussion. Also, the shorter interview that follows the questionnaire limits the clinician's evaluation of the patient's nonverbal responses. Finally, reliance on the health questionnaire often appears impersonal and cursory as compared with a comprehensive diagnostic interview conducted by the dentist.

Despite these problems, the health questionnaire method can provide an adequate patient history. Unfortunately, two common practices limit its effectiveness: (1) the busy workload of many practices promotes the tendency to omit the clarification discussion of the questionnaire; and (2) an auxiliary person in many dental offices is given the responsibility of conducting the health questionnaire review with the patient. An individual without training in systemic disease and clinical medicine is unprepared to ask the right questions in the right way to meaningfully evaluate a complex medical history. Also, many patients withhold information from anyone other than the doctor. Both situations compromise the patient history for which the dentist is ultimately responsible.

DISCUSSING SPECIFIC COMPONENTS OF THE PATIENT HISTORY

Specific elements of the patient history require some explanation in the context of collecting the information. The greatest efficiency is achieved by asking general questions within each topic, requesting more specific details for significant positive responses, and dismissing inconsequential issues. The decision about whether or not a positive response is clinically significant relies on factors discussed in Chapter 1 under the heading "Evaluation of Information."

Patient Identification

The simplest method of securing biographic data such as the patient's name, age, address, and the patient's physician is to have the patient write the information on a form. This avoids misspellings, transposition of digits, and other errors that commonly occur when such information is recorded by someone other than the individual. The form used for this information should specify that the patient print the information to avoid errors caused by illegible handwriting.

Chief Complaint

The chief complaint (cc) or reason the patient is seeking treatment is traditionally recorded in the patient's own words to accurately reflect the patient's perception of the problem. Restatement of the problem by the dentist, the *clarification of the chief complaint,*

may be necessary to clearly define the problem. Multiple complaints are listed in the order of importance to the patient.

History of the Chief Complaint

The history of the chief complaint (Hx cc) describes the patient's awareness of the problem from the time it was first noticed and includes all related symptoms. The complexity of the Hx cc depends on the nature of the problem. For example, the Hx cc for a patient requesting a "check-up" consists of the duration since the last dental examination and the information that the patient has no specific dental problems. A complaint of pain requires determination of the location, duration, and nature of the discomfort, as discussed in Chapter 9. A guide to the appropriate content of the Hx cc in various situations is that it should completely reflect the patient's knowledge of the problem.

Medical History

The medical history (MH) is a description of the relevant features of the patient's health status from birth to the moment that the patient enters the dentist's office. This is usually divided into past diseases, characteristic infections and immunizations, hospitalizations, allergies and adverse reactions to drugs, and current medical treatment. This discussion can be initiated with the question, "When did you last see your physician?" This reveals when the patient's health status was last formally evaluated, which can suggest the patient's general attitude toward health care.

Past medical conditions. The patient's known medical conditions are usually explored initially with an open-ended question such as, "Could you tell me about any medical problems that you have had?" An alternative on a health questionnaire is to list a number of common diseases in a check-off format followed by a request to write in any other conditions not listed. Specific questions concerning conditions that are of particular concern to the dentist such as heart murmurs, rheumatic fever, hypertension, diabetes, and bleeding disorders are then appropriate. A negative history for these common diseases should be specifically noted. Positive responses require additional details such as the date of diagnosis, the nature of treatment, if the condition has resolved, and any complications or disabilities caused by the disease.

A question that is often asked to identify medical conditions that still affect the patient is "How would you describe your general health now?" The goal is to identify the illnesses the patient is known to be suffering from and to appreciate the severity of the conditions. Clarification of current medical condition includes the diagnosis, when the diagnosis was made, and the basis of the diagnosis. Current treatment can be identified at this time, but treatment details are recorded separately. Many patients with chronic conditions such as diabetes mellitus can provide exceptionally accurate information. In other situations the problem may have developed recently and a definitive diagnosis has not been reached. Other patients are either unable to comprehend their diseases or refuse to accept them by claiming ignorance. Medical consultation may be necessary in such situations.

Infections and immunizations. The history of characteristic infections and immunizations is generally more contributory to the physician than to the dentist. Past infection or previous immunization can exclude the specific infectious disease from diagnostic consideration of a new infection. The need for immunization may also be suggested by the immunization history. Reimmunization with tetanus toxoid in situations of septic trauma is an example.

Prior hospitalizations. Any condition requiring hospitalization warrants discussion concerning the details listed above. Topics of particular interest include traumatic injuries, surgical procedures, and blood transfusions. This information is often described by patients when asked about prior illnesses, but hospitalizations are recorded separately. Routine procedures such as a tonsillectomy during childhood are likely to be noncontributory except to explain physical findings such as scars of the tonsillar pillars. However, a procedure performed recently without complications demonstrates the patient's ability to tolerate surgical stress. Details concerning uncommon surgical procedures and other hospital treatment can clarify aspects of the patient's past medical conditions. For example, a patient may minimize the significance of a heart condition because he considers himself cured by cardiac surgery that will be described when asked about hospitalizations.

Head and neck trauma is of greatest interest to the dentist. However, indications of trauma to other body parts can suggest the possibility of unappreciated facial injury. Recent injuries are of greater importance from a diagnostic perspective than those that occurred in the distant past. Head injuries that cause a loss of consciousness are of particular concern because associated facial trauma is often overlooked in the urgency of treating more obvious and serious injuries.

Allergies and adverse reactions to medications. Any complication caused by a drug is recorded with the name of the drug, route of delivery, the specific reaction, and when the episode occurred. The nature of the drug reaction is particularly significant because people often mistakenly assume that side effects are allergic reactions. For example, patients often claim to be allergic to tetracycline after experiencing diarrhea, a common nonallergic side effect of the antibiotic. Documentation of a negative history of adverse drug reactions is also necessary, if that is the case. Evidence of a negative drug reaction history can be of medicolegal significance if the initial occurrence of a drug complication results from the dentist's prescription. Allergic reactions to materials other than drugs should also be listed.

Current medical treatment. Current medical treatment may include special diets, limitations of daily activities, and medications.

An adequate description of drug therapy includes the drug, the dosage, the regimen, and the duration of the treatment. The specific therapy including the drug dosage can reveal the physician's opinion of the severity of the patient's condition. Asking the patient to bring the prescription packages for their medications to the diagnosis appointment allows expedient and accurate recording of this information from the label. The dentist should note if noncompliance with the medication regimen is suspected. The routine use of nonprescription or "over-the-counter" (OTC) medications is also listed.

Family History

Questions concerning the family history are directed to genetic conditions and communicable infections. The dentist might suspect, for example, undiagnosed diabetes mellitus, rheumatic heart disease, hemophilia, or tuberculosis if several of the patient's family members are affected. A formal medical history evaluates systemic diseases affecting at least three generations of the patient's family. This information is diagramed as a pedigree in the patient's health record. Such detail is usually not necessary in a dental setting.

Social History

The patient's social history consists of the patient's occupation, hobbies, daily activities, habits, and emotional adaptation. Certain illnesses may be suspected as a consequence of recurring exposure to toxic materials or conditions. Ultraviolet damage from sun exposure associated with an outdoor occupation or hobby is directly related to skin and lip cancer. An intravenous drug habit increases the possibility of viral hepatitis and HIV infection.

The two habits of greatest health significance to the dentist are tobacco and alcohol use. The amount of habitual exposure to these materials roughly corresponds to the probability of oral cancer and other diseases they cause. Cigarette smoking is quantified in *pack-years,* which is the number of packs of cigarettes smoked per day multiplied by the number of years the patient has smoked. Cigar smoking is recorded as number smoked per day and pipe smoking is recorded without specification of the amount. Use of smokeless tobacco is listed with the usual site of placement and the duration of the habit. Alcohol use is specified in average *whiskey equivalents per day.* A whiskey equivalent is defined as one ounce of spirits, four ounces of wine, or twelve ounces of beer. An estimation of the daily alcohol consumption for many drinkers can be obtained by roughly doubling the amount that they will admit to a health professional.

A comprehensive discussion of emotional problems is seldom appropriate in the context of oral diagnosis and few dentists are adequately trained to pursue such issues in any depth. Psychiatric or behavioral information beyond that described by the patient in response to questions concerning past medical conditions should be resolved by consultation with the patient's physician, psychiatrist, or other qualified clinician. However, general questions concerning the demands of work and family situations are appropriate because emotional stress promotes the oral manifestations of several conditions.

The Review of Systems

The review of systems (ROS) is a series of questions that explores the possibility of undiagnosed disease and the effectiveness of current treatment for diagnosed illnesses. These questions attempt to identify symptoms that are commonly associated with organ system dysfunction. Grouping questions by systems encourages an organized approach and minimizes omissions. Positive responses can then be explored as to the frequency, duration, and severity of the symptom. The dentist's obligation is not the definitive diagnosis of systemic illness suggested by such symptoms. The dentist's role is limited to physical assessment in the context of dental care, which implies the need for medical referral when undiagnosed or uncontrolled disease is suspected.

General health. Symptoms associated with decline of the patient's general health include unexplained weight loss, recurring fever, night sweats, lack of energy, and a nonspecific sensation of illness referred to as *malaise.* Suspicion of a disease other than a common, self-limiting illness such as an acute viral infection is warranted if such constitutional symptoms persist more than 1 month. Symptoms indicative of deteriorating general health direct attention to other symptoms affecting specific systems as a possible explanation of the general health effects. The ability to accomplish routine daily activities known as *vital functions* such as eating, sleeping, and mobility provides a reliable indication of good general health in most instances.

Cardiovascular system. Conditions that affect the cardiovascular system are common and most can lead to serious complications during dental treatment. Therefore a large portion of the review of systems by most dentists attempts to identify the cardiovascular symptoms listed in Table 2-1.

Ischemic muscle pain of the legs or chest during exertion and shortness of breath suggest advanced atherosclerosis. The resulting limitation of the blood supply to the heart during increased exertional demand is referred to as *coronary artery disease* or *ischemic heart disease.* Breathing discomfort referred to as *dyspnea* often results from pulmonary edema caused by inefficient cardiac output designated as *congestive heart failure.* Edematous swelling of the extremities also results from congestive heart failure when excessive blood accumulates in the systemic vascular network. Bluish discoloration of nail beds or lips and coldness of the extremities is a consequence of inadequate peripheral circulation or poor oxygenation of the blood related to severe congestive heart failure. Awareness of a pounding heartbeat or irregular heartbeat is a feature of defective control of cardiac function referred to as *arrhythmia.* Any of these symptoms should be clarified in terms of frequency, duration, and severity.

Table 2-1 Common symptoms of cardiovascular disease

Patient complaint	Medical term
Sharp or burning pain of the chest	Angina pectoris
Awareness of a pounding heart beat	Palpitation
Muscle pain of the legs during exertion	Intermittent claudication
Fatigue following minimal exertion	Shortness of breath
Painful breathing	Dyspnea
Swelling of the extremities	Peripheral edema
Difficulty breathing when reclined	Orthopnea
Waking caused by labored breathing	Paroxysmal noctural dyspnea
Irregular heart beat	Arrhythmia
Bluish discoloration of nail beds or lips	Cyanosis
Coldness of the extremities	Atherosclerosis (inadequate peripheral circulation)

Isolated episodes of mild symptoms that are vaguely described by a patient younger than 30 years of age are unlikely to be caused by cardiac disease with the specific exception of congenital heart defects. More frequent occurrence, characteristic description of the symptom, and reference to multiple symptoms by an older patient strongly suggests significantly compromised cardiac function. Even isolated or mild examples of these symptoms in adults past age 30 may represent diminished cardiac efficiency. Many cardiovascular diseases such as hypertension and valvular defects are asymptomatic in their early stages and are only confirmed by medical consultation.

Pulmonary system. Persistent cough, shortness of breath, and labored breathing, known as *dyspnea,* are the usual symptoms of pulmonary disease. The patient should clarify the duration of these symptoms and whether the occurrence is episodic, seasonal, or continuous. Infectious congestion stimulates acute onset of persistent cough that is productive of pus or blood. A chronic cough and dyspnea suggest chronic congestion and the need for medical evaluation. Coughing up blood or *hemoptysis* is an ominous finding, particularly if the patient is an older smoker, because this can be an early symptom of lung cancer. Recurring pulmonary symptoms of mild congestion caused by allergies are indicated by occurrence during certain seasons or following exposure to specific materials.

Gastrointestinal system. Disease of the gastrointestinal (GI) tract can produce a wide variety of symptoms. Vomiting blood called *hematemesis,* persistent vomiting, stabbing epigastric pain, and frequent productive belching, or *gastric reflux,* all reflect upper GI dysfunction. The frequency, severity, duration, and location of symptoms and the effect of ingesting food are usually diagnostically significant. Lower GI abnormalities are typically suspected on the basis of complaints of abdominal pain, excessive GI sounds, fat in the stools, blood in the stools, and constipation or diarrhea. A chronic duration of relatively mild lower GI symptoms aggravated by specific foods or emotional stress should not cause excessive concern unless the severity or frequency of the symptoms has recently increased.

Alcoholics and patients with a history of degenerative liver disease may report liver enlargement or a bleeding tendency related to compromised hepatic production of coagulation proteins. Alteration of the color of the stools referred to as "clay colored stools" and epigastric pain approximately 1 hour after eating fatty foods are the typical symptoms of biliary obstruction.

Immune system. Abnormal immune function can be categorized as immune deficiency, immune hypersensitivity, or autoimmune disease. The symptoms of immune deficiency relate to the uncharacteristic progression or severity of common infections and the development of *opportunistic infections* caused by organisms that do not usually produce disease. The symptoms in both cases are related to the organs or systems infected. The most common locations are portals of entry such as the mouth, vagina, nose, and skin as well as the lungs. Constitutional symptoms such as enlargement of one or more lymph node group, recurring fever, and malaise of extended duration suggest generalized infections that may be related to deficiency of the immune system.

Many patients experience manifestations of hypersensitivity to a variety of materials. A skin rash following contact with jewelry, commercial skin products, and other materials is typical of contact hypersensitivity. This often suggests a greater probability that the patient will develop hypersensitivity to antibiotics and other materials. Nasal congestion, *rhinorrhea* or runny nose, sinus congestion, and dyspnea from episodic bronchial constriction are common complaints indicative of respiratory system hypersensitivity.

Recurring or persistent lesions of the skin and mucous membranes and pain and inflammation of the joints are symptoms produced by several autoimmune diseases. Autoimmune manifestations affecting other systems are less likely to cause symptoms early in the disease course. A characteristic symptom that is frequently associated with autoimmune disease is sharp pain and pallor of the extremities, especially the hands, following exposure to cold; this is known as *Raynaud's phenomenon.*

Endocrine system. Common endocrine disorders are suggested by unusual patterns of growth, changes in energy level, intolerance to mild temperature changes, and unexplained weight changes. *Polyuria* or excessive urination, excessive thirst called *polydipsia,* and *polyphagia* or excessive appetite associated with weight loss is the characteristic presentation of undiagnosed diabetes mellitus. Altered vision, compromised urinary function, and diminished circulation in the extremities are manifestations of advanced vascular sclerosis caused by diabetes of long duration. Alteration of sleep patterns, unusual weight distribution, and changes in secondary sexual characteristics also suggest endocrine dysfunction. Manifestations of endocrine dysfunction often progress gradually and may not be noticed by the patient.

Blood. Symptoms of blood disease relate to deficient function of one or more blood components, which produces constitutional complaints in most instances. *Lassitude* or constant fatigue may be the only symptom of *anemia,* which is the deficiency of red blood cells. Unusual progression of infections such as periodontitis may indicate a functional or numerical inadequacy of white cells. Recent onset of unusual bleeding such as excessive bruising or difficulty controlling the bleeding from a minor cut can result from abnormally low platelet concentration, platelet dysfunction, or a clotting factor deficiency caused by liver disease. Concurrent symptoms of all three categories could indicate bone marrow suppression by toxic materials, certain medications, and malignant neoplasia. In addition, excessive blood loss may produce these symptoms. GI bleeding is the most common form of chronic blood loss. This can be revealed by symptoms of hemorrhoids, bloody stools, polyps, and abdominal pain.

Genitourinary system. Symptoms of renal disease are localized pain and changes in the frequency, volume, or composition of the urine. Painful urination known as *dysuria,* polyuria, minimal urination or *anuria,* cloudy urine indicative of *proteinuria,* and bloody urine called *hematuria* all suggest renal or urinary tract disease. Sharp discomfort in the kidney known as "flank pain" is one of the early symptoms of renal infection or obstruction by kidney stones.

Questions related to symptoms of reproductive system disease usually follow those concerning renal symptoms. Ulcers or warts of the genitalia, discharge from the genitourinary tract, and discomfort are common symptoms of venereal or vaginal mycotic infections. Amenorrhea can indicate pregnancy, menopause, uterine disease, or endocrine dysfunction. Excessive menstrual flow or *menorrhea*

can cause anemia. Painful genital sores may be related to ulcers of the oral cavity in some cases.

Musculoskeletal system. The topic of interest for the dentist in discussing musculoskeletal symptoms is to appreciate conditions that may affect jaw and temporomandibular joint function. An indication of arthritis is evaluated by determining the distribution of affected joints, degree of movement limitation, onset of symptoms, and severity of discomfort. Complaints concerning muscle weakness or pain are approached in a similar manner.

Integumentary system. The patient suffering from a skin disease is usually familiar with the condition because of the superficial location and irritating discomfort of the lesions. Questions should be directed to identifying recurring or recent rashes or *dermatitis,* eruptions, hives called *urticaria,* and *pruritus,* or itching, as indications of inflammatory skin diseases. Abnormalities of the hair and nails are often superficial signs of advanced cardiovascular, renal, hepatic, or GI disease.

Special organs of the head and neck. Abnormalities of the eyes, ears, oropharynx, and nasal structures are of diagnostic interest to the dentist because of the proximity of these structures to the oral cavity. Dryness, itching, excessive tearing, and redness or *erythema* of the eyes indicates inflammation of the mucosal surface known as *conjunctivitis.* Double vision or *diplopia,* loss of visual acuity, and loss of peripheral vision may reflect cranial nerve dysfunction affecting the eyes. Disease of the ears is usually inflammatory and is suggested by earache or *otitis,* discharge, ringing, and dizziness or *vertigo.* Recurring sore throats, pain on swallowing called *dysphagia,* and changes in the voice such as persistent hoarseness indicate disease of the throat or larynx.

Peripheral nervous system. Peripheral nervous system disease produces symptoms of either hyperfunction or functional deficit. Pain located in the distribution of a sensory nerve trunk without apparent cause is an example of sensory hyperfunction. Specific location, frequency, pattern of occurrence, and duration often suggest a specific diagnosis. Loss of sensation or sensory hypofunction may be related to traumatic injury or surgical damage. Examples of motor hyperfunction that the patient may report include "ticks," tremors, and muscle spasms. Motor hypofunction will generally be reported as weakness of the affected part or, rarely, total loss of function. A history of strokes associated with prominent motor dysfunction indicates that the primary defect affects the central nervous system rather than the peripheral nervous system.

Central nervous system. Symptoms suggesting central nervous system (CNS) disease include headache, behavioral changes, and peripheral neural dysfunction. Headaches can be produced by numerous conditions. The pattern of occurrence, location, severity, effectiveness of analgesics, and other features of headache provide direction in their diagnosis as discussed in Chapter 9. Additional symptoms indicating CNS disease include *syncope* or fainting, *vertigo,* insomnia, and loss of muscular coordination called *ataxia.* CNS disease should be suspected as a cause for most peripheral neurologic symptoms unless a history of injury or a similar event explains the abnormality.

The Dental History

The dental history provides insight into the patient's dental hygiene practices, attitude toward dental care, and the nature of past dental treatment. This can supply an impression of the patient's dental treatment expectations and the factors that have produced the patient's current dental condition.

Past dental care for most patients can be summarized as one of three forms: (1) *Routine dental care* implies regular recall appointments and timely treatment of most dental needs. (2) *Episodic dental care* implies less than comprehensive dental care and an irregular pattern of recall examinations. (3) *Symptomatic dental care* indicates that the patient has generally consulted a dentist for relief of pain without regular attention to dental health. The patient's attitude toward dental care is usually revealed by the response to questions such as, "How often do you usually visit the dentist?" or "Are your dental appointments usually for checkups and fillings or for toothaches?"

Affirmative responses to questions concerning negative dental treatment experiences may indicate the need to alter routine dental treatment procedures. Fainting, adverse reaction to anesthetics, excessive bleeding, unusual discomfort, and similar complications should be explored. Negative comments about a previous dentist often reveal potential attitude problems. The patient's perception of a former dentist is likely to become the attitude toward the current dentist unless the patient is carefully managed. Any experiences related to nondental conditions affecting the oral cavity such as recurring ulcers should also be discussed.

The patient should be specifically asked about dental treatment usually provided by dental specialists. Previous periodontal therapy, orthodontic treatment, and removal of third molars can alter both the clinician's perception of the examination findings and his or her judgments concerning treatment and prognosis.

The patient's responses to questions concerning refined sugar ingestion, brushing, flossing, and other habits related to dental health indicates the patient's *perception* of their home care. Whether or not this perception is accurate is revealed during the oral examination. The importance of this perception relates to expectation for improvement following additional oral hygiene instruction. Exceptional dietary habits may explain certain general health problems or indicate limitations imposed by the patient's physician in the treatment of systemic diseases such as hypertension and diabetes.

PRACTICAL ASPECTS OF THE DIAGNOSTIC INTERVIEW

Experience teaches all clinicians that several practical aspects of the diagnostic interview affect the accuracy of the results. The following comments suggest factors that the clinician must consider during the diagnostic interview.

Some patients do not volunteer a complete patient history. Patients who have a personal relationship with the dentist or an office auxiliary, for example, often withhold embarrassing medical information. Certain individuals cannot respond adequately to the dentist's questions, some consider the process a waste of time, and others say whatever they think the dentist wants to hear. The dentist must rely on experience and judgment to reveal contradictory information or inconsistencies with examination findings that indicate an inadequate or inaccurate patient history. Many patients are simply "poor historians," which means they can't remember or they confuse factual information. The clinician may consider objective information such as physical findings or consultations as more reliable in these situations than information from the patient. However, the risk of complications during dental treatment increases dramatically when dental treatment decisions are based on an inadequate or inaccurate patient history. This implies that at times dental care must be delayed until dependable information becomes available.

Some patients lie or attempt to mislead the clinician. This may involve sensitive subjects or the patient may just be trying to "test" the dentist with a contradiction that would be challenged by a knowledgeable clinician. Patients in pain who were refused care by another dentist because of a medical problem often withhold the information in order to receive treatment at the next dental office. Drug abusers often lie to get a prescription for drugs with abuse potential. A typical scenario involves a patient who specifically requests a strong narcotic by telephone for a severe toothache, but the patient refuses to arrange an emergency appointment. Experience, knowledge of common medical conditions, the power of observation, and tempered skepticism are valuable assets in such situations.

The information obtained during the patient history is confidential and the patient's privacy should be maintained. This should be obvious, but the insensitive habit of openly discussing medical topics can develop during professional training in a crowded clinical setting. The patient's right to confidentiality must be respected for two reasons:

1. Discussion of medical information in a way that compromises the patient's privacy is unprofessional. The dentist loses the patient's respect, if not the patient. Consultation with the patient's physician and colleagues should be conducted in a manner that maintains the patient's privacy.
2. The reliability of the information provided by the patient suffers if it becomes apparent that the dentist is unable to respect the confidentiality of personal information. Patients understandably become hesitant to confide in a dentist after overhearing the discussion of another patient's medical problems.

SUMMARY OF THE PATIENT HISTORY

The final step of the patient history is to briefly summarize the significant findings from the diagnostic interview and the clinician's conclusions from this information. This ensures that the significant conclusions from the patient history are obvious and readily available during future clinical events. Medical conditions that require alteration of dental procedures or involve significant risk of complications are clearly stated, while noncontributory data are excluded. An example might be,

"Robert Wilson is an alert 32-year-old male in no distress who requests routine dental care. History includes penicillin hypersensitivity that has caused urticaria and borderline hypertension managed by dietary restriction and weight control. The patient denies other limitations or significant medical conditions."

His childhood infections and the surgical repair of a hernia several years ago are noncontributory in the context of dental treatment and are available in the completed patient history should the need arise. This communicates to another clinician or reminds the original dentist that this healthy young adult male wants comprehensive dental care, is allergic to penicillin, and is prone to hypertension. Otherwise, dental treatment can be planned without specific concern for complications related to his health status.

Definitive conclusions may not be justified following the diagnostic interview, particularly in cases of complex systemic diseases. Medical consultation may be needed to obtain additional information, or the dentist may prefer to delay formulating opinions until after the physical examination. The patient history summary in such instances reflects the conclusions that are justified solely by the history. As an example, a vague history of a heart murmur could be referred to in the summary of the patient history by the entry, "Nonspecific heart murmur identified at age 12 suggests the possibility of valvular defect. Confirmation by medical consultation is required."

SUMMARY

The patient history consists of information that reflects the patient's current and past health status, which may influence the clinician's diagnostic and treatment decisions. The discussion between the dentist and patient that identifies and clarifies this information is referred to as the diagnostic interview. The efficiency of the diagnostic interview and the accuracy of the data produced are both enhanced when the clinician maintains control of the discussion by the effective use of interviewing techniques. The diagnostic interview also provides the opportunity to establish a positive dentist-patient relationship. The health questionnaire is an alternative method of obtaining patient health information. The effectiveness of the approach depends on the den-

tist discussing the written responses with the patient to confirm, explore, and clarify topics identified as potentially significant by the questionnaire.

Every diagnostic interview is unique because the patient's verbal and nonverbal responses to each topic determine the need for additional information and how it can best be obtained. Specific elements of the patient history are discussed in adequate detail to provide the clinician with the necessary information to evaluate problems, conditions, and symptoms. The importance of the chief complaint in motivating the patient to seek treatment warrants discussion of the problem to the limits of the patient's awareness. Past and current medical conditions require specification of the diagnosis, when the diagnosis was made, the treatment, and the effectiveness of the treatment. Previous hospitalizations, current medications, adverse reactions to medications, and related issues are approached in a similar manner. The review of systems is a series of questions concerning symptoms that may be caused by undiagnosed illnesses. Symptoms should be described in terms of frequency, duration, pattern of occurrence, severity, and factors that alter the symptom.

The final element of the patient history is a summary of the contributory information obtained and the conclusions based on this information in the context of oral diagnosis and dental treatment planning. The interpretation of the patient history in conjunction with the findings from the physical examination is referred to as physical assessment, which is discussed in Chapter 7.

BIBLIOGRAPHY

Judge RD, Zuidema GD, Fitzgerald FT, editors: Clinical diagnosis: a physiologic approach, ed 5, Boston, 1988, Little, Brown.

Seidel HM, Ball JW, Dains JE, Benedict GW: Mosby's guide to physical examination, St Louis, 1987, Mosby–Year Book.

Stevenson I: The diagnostic interview, ed 2, New York, 1971, Harper & Row.

CHAPTER 3

Methods of Examination

GARY C. COLEMAN

Physical examination is the diagnostic assessment of the patient's status that relies on the clinician's primary senses with the aid of simple instruments. This specifically excludes adjunctive diagnostic methods that require technically complex devices, such as radiographic examination. The clinician's examination reveals features that supplement and extend the initial impressions of the patient's status gained during the discussion of the patient history. The ability to see a lesion and to feel the texture, consistency, and extent of the abnormality convey objective findings that cannot be obtained in any other way. The perceptions gained during the physical examination by a skillful clinician are in most respects objective and reproducible, which implies that they are often more reliable than information from other sources.

An appreciation of physical examination techniques is necessary to perform the examination and to assess the implications of the information obtained. In addition, understanding the examination methods available to the clinician provides a basis for devising unique examination techniques that may be effective in unusual circumstances.

GENERAL METHODS OF PHYSICAL EXAMINATION

Physical examination methods can be described by the primary sense on which the technique relies. The separate discussion of these methods should not leave the impression that the procedures are performed separately. Most efficient clinicians simultaneously perform visual, palpatory, and functional examinations in one anatomic region before proceeding to the next.

Visual Examination

Passive visual examination referred to as *inspection* is accomplished by the clinician while the patient is in the resting state. Observations made by inspection such as those of general patient appraisal are often more representative if the patient is unaware of the clinician's attention. The more active process of *visualization* is observation after altering the patient's resting status. Opening the mouth, extending the tongue, and removing saliva are all aspects of visualization during the intraoral examination that provide visual access and allow detailed observations. Visualization techniques can make abnormalities appear more prominent or reveal subtle features. For example, removal of saliva may demonstrate the rough superficial texture of a lesion that appeared smooth while wet.

The ability to visually recognize normal variations of color, pattern, contour, symmetry, size, texture, and location of superficial structures is among the clinician's most valuable assets. The inexperienced clinician tends to look for obvious abnormalities during visual examination, while more experienced diagnosticians visually confirm the normal characteristics of anatomic structures. This diagnostic attitude of "confirming normalcy" generally promotes more effective identification of subtle lesions. Also, some diseases are characterized by the features that are not present rather than those that are.

Transillumination is a visual diagnostic method that relies on the passage of light through relatively thin, translucent tissues. The phenomenon can be observed by holding the fingers over a small, intense light source in a darkened room. Transillumination can demonstrate the accumulation of fluid and pus within the maxillary sinus. The patient is placed in a darkened room and an intense light source is placed intraorally with the patient's lips closed around the probe. The tissues overlying the normal maxillary sinus exhibit a dull glow, while congestion or abnormal soft tissue within the sinus blocks the diffusion of light. The frontal sinuses can be similarly evaluated by placing the light source inferior to the supraorbital ridge at the nasal aspect of the orbit.

Examination by Palpation

Palpation is the physical examination method that relies on the sense of touch. Palpation allows the clinician to examine structures deep to the surface and to perceive char-

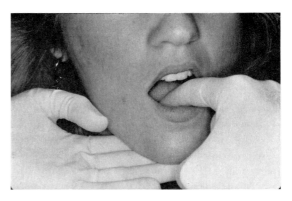

Fig. 3-1   Bimanual palpation of the floor of the mouth.

acteristics such as compressibility, tenderness, and anatomic relationships that are not visually apparent.

Several palpation techniques can be particularly effective during the examination of specific anatomic regions. *Bimanual palpation* is performed with both hands, using one hand to manipulate the tissue while the other hand supports the structures from the opposite side. This provides an appreciation of deep structures by trapping the tissues of interest between the hands in much the same way the inflation of a rubber ball might be judged. Bimanual palpation is the best method for examining the contents of the floor of the mouth as illustrated in Fig. 3-1. *Bidigital palpation* accomplishes the same effect by the use of two fingers for thinner tissues such as the lips. *Bilateral palpation* is simultaneous manipulation of symmetrical structures in an attempt to appreciate a difference from one side to the other. This simultaneous comparison is an effective method of detecting subtle abnormalities of soft tissues such as the parotid glands that vary in firmness and size among individuals.

The response of tissues to pressure can suggest the composition of the structures. Muscle, glandular tissue, and bone all have a characteristic resistance to applied pressure. Perceptions gained by palpation and the implications relative to tissue composition are reflected by the following terms:

Bony hard is the rigid or unyielding sensation of bone tissue and implies that the structure is calcified.

Indurated means hardness but without the rigid sensation associated with calcification. This can be compared with squeezing a dense, solid rubber ball. Induration is a feature of many malignant neoplasms.

Firm masses yield more to pressure than do indurated tissues. However, minimal shape alteration of the structure occurs in contrast to compressible tissues. Many benign neoplastic and hyperplastic enlargements are firm.

Compressible is a relatively nonspecific term indicating that pressure significantly alters the shape of the structure.

Doughy indicates that the structure deforms with a degree of resistance suggesting semisolid contents, then returns slowly to the original shape. Some cysts are characterized by this consistency.

Spongy is the term used when the structure offers minimal resistance to pressure and quickly regains the original contour after the pressure is released. Highly vascular lesions produce this sensation.

A *pitting* response to pressure indicates that the structure offers minimal or moderate resistance and then slowly regains the original contour after the release of the pressure. Edema often produces this response.

Collapsing refers to an easily compressible enlargement that remains deformed after the release of pressure. This implies that the contents of the structure have been displaced. Expression of pus from an abscess is a common example.

Several additional features of an unusual structure should be identified by palpation. The shape, size, and anatomic location of the suspected lesion should be estimated within the limits of the situation. The presence of tenderness usually indicates inflammation and is revealed by the patient's response when pres-

sure is applied. Lesions are considered well-delineated if palpation reveals separation from adjacent tissues or diffuse if this distinction is difficult to discern. Independent lesions are mobile relative to adjacent tissues during manipulation, while resistance to pressure suggests the abnormality is fixed or attached to nearby structures.

Additional diagnostic features of lesions that contain blood can be demonstrated by palpation. The blood that is contained within abnormal vessels can be forced away from the area by palpation. This causes the red lesion to become pale or *blanch* as illustrated by Fig. 16-3. The use of a glass slide to compress the lesion while observing the area is called *diascopy* and may demonstrate this feature. Release of pressure allows refilling of the vessels and a rapid return of the red color. Red lesions produced by extravasation of blood into the connective tissue do not blanch during palpation. A vibrational sensation within tissue called a *thrill* results from blood driven by arterial pressure through large vessels. This is a feature of some vascular malformations.

Examination by Auscultation

Auscultation is the diagnostic process of listening to the sounds made by various body structures. This can be accomplished in some situations without enhancement of the sound. As an example, simply listening to the patient take several deep breaths can reveal wheezing or other sounds suggestive of respiratory obstruction or bronchial constriction. Abnormal temporomandibular joint sounds are often heard by the unaided ear while the patient opens and closes the mouth. Generally, however, enhancement of the clinician's hearing with a stethoscope greatly increases the sensitivity. Auscultation with a stethoscope of the temporomandibular joint during opening can reveal subtle joint sounds during movement that might otherwise be unapparent. The vascular vibration that causes a thrill can also produce a murmur or blowing sound called a *bruit,* which can occasionally be detected by auscultation. Blood pressure measurement also requires auscultation.

A special application of hearing is in the use of *percussion*. Sound is produced by striking the certain structures with short, abrupt blows. An example of the medical application of percussion involves tapping or thumping the patient's back and chest to appreciate the resonance of normal lung tissue.

Examination by Sense of Smell

The sense of smell occasionally contributes diagnostic information. The aroma of alcohol or the fruity scent of acetone associated with uncontrolled diabetes mellitus can provide an immediate understanding of the patient's status. Bacterial infections are characterized by a foul or putrid odor. The professional decorum of the physical examination requires that the clinician pursue the "olfactory examination" discretely. The last primary sense, taste, has no application in physical examination.

Examination by Probing

Probing is the use of a slender device to identify or determine the extent of a narrow tract or cavity. Inflammatory lesions and some developmental defects are occasionally associated with a sinus, which is small epithelium-lined passage to the superficial surface. Gentle probing is the most effective method of convincingly demonstrating these lesions. Probing the major salivary gland ducts can reveal obstructions. Beyond the diagnostic application of the technique, probing can produce the therapeutic release of trapped fluid or pus.

Aspiration is sharp probing with a needle to enter and withdraw material from a tissue structure using negative pressure. The material produced by this technique, the *aspirate,* can reveal the nature of the lesion. Pus produced by aspiration is valuable for microbiologic testing because the chance of contaminating the specimen is minimized. Failure to produce any material by aspiration is equally significant since this indicates that the abnormality is composed of solid tissue. Presurgical aspiration of bone lesions is required to identify lesions containing a dense concentration of vascular structures that could produce uncontrollable hemorrhage without adequate preoperative preparation. The assumption is that the needle puncture site of a vascular mass will be an easier source of hemorrhage to control than a surgical wound.

Aspiration is usually accomplished with a large bore needle of 16 to 20 gauge. This diameter ensures rigidity of the needle while puncturing firm structures such as cortical bone and provides an adequate channel for the passage of gelatinous or semisolid materials. Directing the tip of the needle into a productive site requires considerable skill. Careful movement to several trial sites may be necessary before material can be aspirated. Excessive negative pressure on the syringe plunger can plug the needle with solid tissue and should be avoided.

Evaluation of Function

Many routine clinical tests attempt to demonstrate the normal function of an organ or system. Familiar examples from the medical examination include visual acuity testing and spinal reflex evaluation.

The basis of an effective functional test is to specifically identify the function of interest and to devise a test that isolates that function. The function of interest must often be enhanced or accelerated to allow observation of the response. The dentist, for example, may suspect decreased salivary production from the right parotid gland. The simplest test for this functional deficiency would be to observe if saliva flows from Stensen's duct. Unstimulated salivary flow from the parotid is usually difficult to observe by passive observation. However, visualization of the ductal opening can be enhanced by isolating the area with cotton rolls and drying the surface near the ductal papilla. The flow of saliva can be accelerated by palpating or massaging the parotid gland. The sensory component of salivation can be evaluated by observing saliva production after stimulation with enticing food. The quantity of flow in some instances is diagnostically significant and can be measured volumetrically after collection by expectoration or use of a suction cup device. With all of these results, comparison by testing contralateral function or comparing the results with typical findings from normal patients provides a basis for interpreting the functional test.

Clinical evidence of normal function is usually not an interpretive problem, although the clinician should always consider the possibility of a subtle functional deficiency. Negative results of most functional tests, however, involve interpretive risks because most physiologic functions are too complex for a single test to isolate a single functional component. In the context of the salivation example, the clinician might interpret minimal parotid flow as proof that parotid disease has affected parotid salivary production. That opinion may be incorrect since conditions such as obstruction can also limit saliva flow without deficiency in the production of saliva by the gland. In general, an abnormal functional test result seldom indicates the specific cause of the abnormality. Additional clinical information or a more specific test is usually needed to isolate the dysfunction.

APPLICATION OF PHYSICAL EXAMINATION TECHNIQUES TO DENTISTRY

The dentist relies on general examination methods during nondental portions of the extraoral and intraoral physical examinations. However, specific modifications of these techniques are needed to adequately examination the teeth and supportive structures.

Visual Examination

Patient positioning and the direction of the intraoral light source affect the ability of the dentist to see during the intraoral examination. Optimal orientation becomes second nature with experience, but the inability to see well without straining indicates that either the pa-

tient, the dentist, or the light is incorrectly positioned. Alteration of the patient position and the direction of the intraoral light source to adequately visualize different regions of the mouth is generally necessary several times during the clinical examination. The removal of materials such as food debris and appliances is essential for adequate visualization. The presence of saliva, for example, can obscure the subtle features of many mucosal lesions. The chip air syringe conveniently displaces food, saliva, and other materials. Clearing adherent materials with a cotton gauze may be necessary. Magnifying lenses called "loops" attached to eyeglass frames can enhance visualization.

The intraoral mirror provides indirect visualization of intraoral tissues, which saves the clinician time and effort in viewing maxillary surfaces and recesses of the oral cavity. Obviously, the mirror surface must be cleared frequently to maintain the effectiveness of the viewing surface. The intraoral mirror also serves as a readily available retractor to manipulate soft tissues during the examination. The mirror handle provides a blunt, slender device to probe lesions and percuss teeth.

Transillumination can reveal proximal carious lesions of the anterior teeth. Careful arrangement of the operatory light and intraoral mirror lingual to the teeth allows the clinician to visualize the opalescent glow of the translucent proximal enamel. Carious lesions appear as dark spots in the enamel near the contact points. Transillumination identification of carious lesions is generally less sensitive than radiographs, but situations arise in which the technique is useful. Transillumination is ineffective in revealing proximal lesions of posterior teeth because the thicker proximal surfaces are less translucent.

Examination by Palpation and Percussion

Several modifications of palpation and percussion are especially useful in the examination of teeth and supporting structures. These techniques are used to localize tenderness

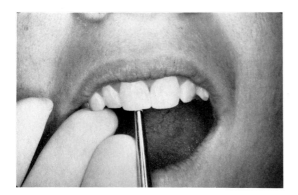

Fig. 3-2   Percussion of the central incisor. Note the direction of the percussive force parallel to the long axis of the tooth and the clinician's use of a finger rest for stabilization.

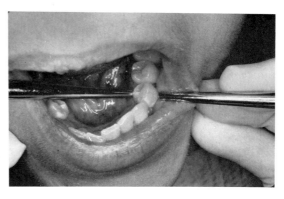

Fig. 3-3   The use of slender instruments to evaluate mobility allows visualization of subtle movement because the clinician's fingers do not cover and obscure tooth surfaces.

and pain and to identify and quantify tooth mobility.

Patients experiencing dental pain can usually indicate exactly which tooth hurts. In some instances, however, the pain is more diffuse and several teeth in the region exhibit lesions such as extensive decay, which suggests more than one possible source of inflammation. Percussion of suspicious teeth in the area with the intraoral mirror handle is a simple and reliable method to identify the source of pain. The clinician lightly taps the occlusal or incisal surfaces of suspected teeth with the impact directed along the long axis of the teeth as shown by Fig. 3-2. The force stretches the periodontal ligament and applies abrupt pressure to the periapical area of the tooth. This instantaneously increases the intensity of the patient's discomfort if inflammation is present. The patient either immediately reacts to the impact or quickly points out that "that's the one." A light tap is usually adequate to elicit the response and care should be taken to avoid excessive force and unnecessary pain. Tapping teeth that appear healthy initially is more likely to elicit an accurate response when the inflamed tooth is percussed because this allows the patient to experience the normal sensation

first. Slightly stronger force may be necessary if the results of light percussion are inconclusive.

The same effect can be achieved by requesting the patient to bite firmly with a wooden stick between the biting surfaces of the suspected tooth and the opposing tooth. Percussion is preferred by most clinicians because the force can be more easily controlled. Percussion is also useful in identifying teeth that are fused or ankylosed to surrounding bone. Percussion of normal teeth produces a dull sound, while ankylosed teeth yield a sharper resonance.

Severe tooth mobility can be demonstrated in most cases by applying light pressure and observing the conspicuous movement. Less dramatic mobility of teeth can be revealed by applying alternating pressure as illustrated in Fig. 3-3. The use of slender instruments keeps the fingertips from obscuring the subtle movement. Another method of detecting mobility is to place the fingertip on the lingual surface of the tooth while gently percussing the facial surface perpendicular to the long axis of the tooth with the mirror handle. Normal teeth are slightly resonant when percussed in this manner, while a dull vibrational sensation called *fremitus* and slight movement can be perceived with mobile teeth. The same effect can be achieved by placing the fingertip on the facial surface of the tooth and requesting the patient to grind the teeth. This often reveals mobile teeth, and identifies the excursive movements that are most traumatic.

As suggested by the methods for detecting tooth mobility, abnormal movement is most evident in facial and lingual directions. Tooth mobility is generally graded subjectively on a scale from zero to three. Zero signifies normal stability, one indicates minimal mobility, two reflects obvious movement, and three means advanced mobility. Vertical movement in the direction of the long axis of the tooth is considered grade three mobility.

Examination by Probing

Much of the intraoral examination consists of probing because this is the most effective method of detecting lesions produced by dental caries and periodontitis. Evidence of these two diseases from other sources such as radiographs is secondary in most instances to the direct results from probing.

Examination for carious lesions. Identification of dental decay is accomplished with a dental probe or explorer. Several different instrument shapes are available, but the shape of the instrument is not as important as the sharpness of the point or tine. Explorer tines become dull with use and must be sharpened or discarded.

Decay is detected by repeatedly pressing and withdrawing the explorer tine at each site of suspected decay. A carious lesion is identified by the sensation known as a "catch" or "stick" when the explorer resists the withdrawal force. This resistance is produced by the penetration of the tine into decalcified dentin (Fig. 3-4, *A*). A definite "stick" is inarguable evidence of decay. However, during the probing of deep fissures the tine may wedge within the gap of a deep fissure (Fig. 3-4, *B*) even though no significant decay is present. These situations can be discerned by the con-

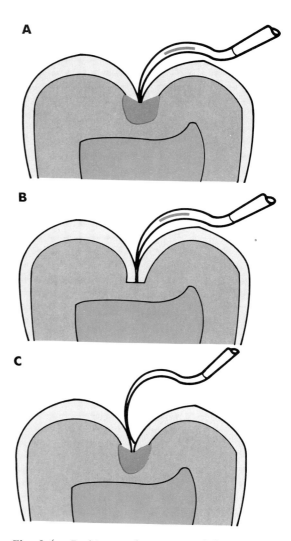

Fig. 3-4   Probing to detect pit and fissure decay. **A,** The tine of the explorer sticks in the decalcified tooth structure of a carious lesion, which yields a "catch" when the explorer is withdrawn. **B,** Wedging of the explorer tine in a narrow fissure yields a false "catch" sensation. **C,** Failure to detect a carious lesion by probing because the angulation of the explorer tine is not directed into the fissure.

trolled application of variable pressure. Light pressure into a noncarious fissure may produce resistance by wedging, but firmer pressure at that point during the second probing results in the same sensation. A carious fissure probed with additional pressure yields an increased sensation of resistance or stronger catch as compared to the initial trial.

Developmental pits and fissures are more prone to decay than smooth tooth surfaces because these recesses retain bacterial plaque to a greater degree. The deepest anatomic pits and grooves are most vulnerable to decay while secondary grooves are less likely sites. Nevertheless, the examination must demonstrate the presence or absence of decay by repeated probing of all susceptible pits and fissures. The probing method used to identify carious lesions of smooth enamel surfaces, interproximal areas, restoration margins, and cemental surfaces is essentially the same as that for pits and fissures. Variations in color, altered contour, evidence of poor hygiene, the patient's symptoms, and the patient's past pattern of carious lesions indicate the likelihood of lesions affecting smooth enamel surfaces.

The identification of early carious lesions is often the source of disagreement among clinicians. The decayed-or-nondecayed decision for each surface of every tooth depends on several variables and the perceptions of the individual dentist. These variables include the sharpness of the explorer tine, the shape of the explorer tine, the amount of pressure applied during probing, the angulation of the probe while pressure is applied (Fig. 3-4, *C*), and the attention of the clinician to probing all vulnerable sites. The opinion as to the presence or absence of decay is, therefore, a matter of professional judgment. This implies that opinions among dentists represent agreement or disagreement rather than issues of right or wrong. In the context of learning to identify decay by probing, an awareness of this problem may help the inexperienced clinician appreciate the variable examination results among dentists.

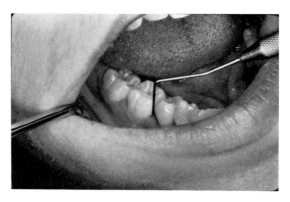

Fig. 3-5 Periodontal probing with the probe directed approximately parallel to the long axis of the tooth and the anticipated contour of the root surface.

Examination of gingival and periodontal tissues. The crevicular pocket depth relative to the gingival margin is generally accepted as indicating the severity of chronic inflammatory damage to the dental supportive tissues. This depth is measured with a slender, blunt periodontal probe by inserting it to the depth of the crevicular pocket and observing the occlusal height of the gingiva against the millimeter markings on the probe. Standard periodontal probing examination of each tooth consists of six probings at the distofacial, mesiofacial, distolingual, and mesiolingual line angles as well as at the midpoints of the facial and lingual surfaces. The probe is aligned roughly parallel to the long axis of the tooth (Fig. 3-5) and the contour of the root surface. Pressure should be adequate to reach the pocket depth without tearing the soft tissue attachment to the root. Bleeding and exudate observed during probing are also significant.

Accurate periodontal probing is necessary in making the initial diagnosis and for future comparisons to assess treatment effectiveness. These comparisons can be misleading and the initial diagnosis is likely to be incorrect if the periodontal probings are inaccurate. The most common technique errors are poor alignment of the probe relative to the teeth and failure to reach the tissue attachment as a consequence of inadequate probing pressure. Probing of patients with pronounced inflammation often causes discomfort, which may produce underestimation of pocket depths because the clinician reduces probing pressure to minimize pain. Prominent calculus ledges can also cause misleading results by obstructing the probe. The problems of tenderness and interference by calculus can be minimized by preliminary debridement and calculus removal followed by definitive probing at a future appointment.

Aspiration. Diagnostic aspiration by the dentist usually is an attempt to remove material from a compressible soft tissue lesion or an abnormality within bone. Aspiration is also a routine part of local anesthetic injections as an indicator that the needle point is located within a blood vessel to avoid intravascular injection of the solution.

Evaluation of Function

The most frequent dental adaptation of functional evaluation is referred to as *pulp testing*. This procedure provides an indication of whether the dental pulp of a tooth is necrotic or vital by assessing sensory nerve responses to irritating stimuli such as temperature extremes and electrical current. Ice and warmed gutta-percha or dental compound applied to the dried facial surface of the tooth provide adequate temperature stimulation. The electrical stimulation is produced by a battery-powered device referred to as a *pulp tester*. The tip of the pulp tester is coated with a conducting material such as toothpaste and placed on the dried tooth surface away from the gingiva. Variations in the strength of the electrical current are set by turning a variable resistor dial. The procedure is to start with a low current setting, touch the tooth, break contact if there is no response, increase the current setting, and touch the tooth again. This sequence continues with increasing current up to the full strength of the battery or until the patient

senses the shock. The process is then repeated on the corresponding contralateral tooth and adjacent teeth for comparison.

Pulp testing is complicated by several practical variables and inherent limitations. Isolation of the tooth to be stimulated and placement of the stimulus on the tooth can be awkward for the posterior teeth in comparison with the anterior teeth. Shorter clinical crowns bring the stimulus closer to the gingiva and increase the likelihood that the patient will sense gingival rather then pulpal stimulation. Extreme differences in the conduction of thermal and electrical stimulation by prosthetic crowns makes comparative responses almost meaningless for crowned teeth. Pulp testing results of molar and premolar teeth are often subject to uncertainty because nerve fibers may be functional in one canal while another canal may be necrotic. In addition, the complex nature of pulpal inflammation affects the reliability of pulp testing. Absolutely necrotic pulp tissue is unreactive to stimulation, while the response of healthy pulp should be similar to that of apparently healthy teeth. However, pulpal inflammation affecting a specific tooth and the response to stimulation can vary between these extremes. The clinical interpretation of pulp testing results is discussed in futher detail in Chapter 8.

Determination of occlusal relationships is another diagnostic technique that is an evaluation of function. The simplest approach to determining occlusal contact points is to place a marking device such as inked tape over the dried occlusal surfaces of the teeth and instruct the patient to bite or grind the teeth in various excursive movements. Marks on atypical occlusal surfaces suggest traumatic functional and parafunctional relationships. This technique is essential during the placement of restorations to ensure that no premature contacts are present before dismissing the patient. Making and mounting diagnostic casts also provides diagnostic information by allowing the dentist to visualize occlusal relationships, alignment, and other features that may be difficult to observe in the mouth.

ADJUNCTIVE DIAGNOSTIC METHODS

The dentist routinely supplements the diagnostic findings obtained from the patient history and physical examination with information from adjunctive procedures. Radiographic examination is the example that contributes to the diagnosis of most dental patients and in certain situations additional procedures may also be justified.

Radiographic Examination

The use of penetrating x-rays to produce images of the teeth and jaws contributes to the diagnosis of carious lesions, periodontitis, periapical inflammation, and nondental jaw lesions. In addition, radiographs provide a detailed record of the patient's dental status at the time of exposure that is valuable for future comparisons.

Several radiographic exposure techniques are available to accomplish different diagnostic goals. *Intraoral radiographs* require placement of the film inside the mouth prior to exposure. This produces radiographs of sharp image resolution, but the area of coverage is limited by the film size that can be comfortably positioned in the mouth. The film for *extraoral radiographs* is positioned outside the patient's mouth during exposure, which offers a larger area of image coverage. The disadvantages of extraoral exposures include poor image resolution and superimposition of the images from cranial and contralateral jaw structures. In general, intraoral exposures are most contributory to the diagnosis of dental lesions and extraoral exposures provide the best information concerning nondental abnormalities.

Bite-wing radiographs (BWs) are intraoral exposures that include the clinical crowns and crestal bone of opposing dental segments. The technique is used almost exclusively in the posterior segments. The sharp image detail of bite-wings generally provides the optimal radiographic demonstration of carious lesions and crestal bone contours for a relative large number of teeth in a single exposure. The clinical disadvantage of bite-wing exposures is that the apices of the teeth are excluded. *Periapical radiographs* (PAs) are intraoral exposures that are designed to show several adjacent teeth entirely including the apices and the surrounding bone. Periapicals effectively reveal periapical inflammatory lesions as well as the size, anatomic contours, and relative position of adjacent teeth. Carious lesions and bone height are also shown but the demonstration of dental decay and periodontal bone loss is somewhat inferior to that of bite-wing views in most instances. Another disadvantage of periapical radiographs compared with bite-wing radiographs is that periapical projections only include a few teeth in a single exposure. A *full mouth series* or survey (FMS) is a combination of between 14 and 21 individual intraoral exposures arranged to achieve periapical visualization of all teeth and bite-wing coverage of posterior teeth. The redundancy of the full mouth series design provides several views of most tooth surfaces to compensate for the practical limitations of exposure technique and malalignment of teeth. This is the most comprehensive radiographic demonstration of the teeth and adjacent bone.

The *occlusal projection* is made by positioning the film on the occlusal surfaces of one arch and requesting the patient to lightly close the teeth for film stabilization. This intraoral technique provides effective visualization of the anterior maxilla and mandible. Different film positions and beam angles allow priority to be given to demonstration of either the teeth or the adjacent tissue. Occlusal radiographs provide high resolution coverage of regions such as the palate that generally cannot be shown by other projections. Also, occlusal exposures can often be achieved when periapical film placement is impractical such as with uncooperative children. The disadvantage of the technique is that the geometry of the pro-

---

CLINICAL FINDINGS THAT JUSTIFY THE EXPOSURE OF RADIOGRAPHS

Historical findings

Previous periodontal or endodontic therapy
History of pain or trauma
Familial history of dental anomalies
Postoperative evaluation of healing
Presence of implants

Clinical signs and symptoms

Clinical evidence of periodontal disease
Large or deep restorations
Deep carious lesions
Malposed or clinically impacted teeth
Swelling
Evidence of facial trauma
Mobility of teeth
Fistula or sinus tract infection
Clinically suspected sinus pathology
Growth abnormalities
Oral involvement in known or suspected systemic
   disease
Positive neurologic findings in the head and neck
Evidence of foreign objects
Pain and/or dysfunction of the temporomandibular
   joint
Facial asymmetry
Abutment teeth for a fixed or removable partial
   prosthesis

Unexplained bleeding
Unexplained sensitivity of teeth
Unusual eruption, spacing, or migration of teeth
Unusual tooth morphology, calcification, or color
Unexplained missing teeth

Patients at high risk for caries may demonstrate any of the following

High level of caries experience
History of recurrent caries
Existing restoration of poor quality
Poor oral hygiene
Inadequate fluoride exposure
Prolonged nursing (bottle or breast)
Diet with high sucrose frequency
Poor family dental health
Developmental enamel defects
Developmental disability
Xerostomia
Genetic abnormality of teeth
Many multisurface restorations
Chemotherapy and/or radiotherapy

Modified from The selection of patients for x-ray examinations: dental radiographic examinations, HHS Pub. FDA 88-8273.

jection usually distorts the shape of the teeth.

Panoramic radiographs are extraoral exposures that demonstrate both the mandible, maxillae, and adjacent structures in a single image. This technique offers the advantages of covering regions of the jaws that are inaccessible for intraoral film placement, and intraoral film positioning is not necessary in cases of limited patient cooperation. In addition, the interpretation of many large jaw lesions is improved because the entire abnormality is shown by a single, continuous radiograph. The greatest disadvantage of panoramic images is that the resolution is poor in comparison to that of intraoral radiographs. This limits the diagnostic sensitivity for carious lesions and peri-

odontal bone loss. A number of additional *extraoral projections of the skull* can contribute to the diagnosis of unusual jaws conditions. The most common example related to dental practice is the cephalometric lateral skull projection used to evaluate cranial and dental development in anticipation of orthodontic treatment. Another example is the Water's skull projection used to demonstrate the maxillary sinus and its contents. Examples of intraoral and extraoral radiographic projections are illustrated in Chapters 8 and 19.

Complex imaging is the general term applied to technically complicated methods of producing diagnostic images. Standard tomography, computerized tomography (CT), magnetic resonance imaging (MRI), sonography or ultrasound imaging, and demonstration of structures by injection of contrast media are examples. Complex imaging techniques are valuable in the diagnosis and presurgical evaluation of soft tissue enlargements, large jaw lesions, and temporomandibular joint disease. These procedures are accomplished by referral and entail considerable expense.

The clinician's responsibility during the information gathering phase of the diagnosis is to determine the most appropriate radiographic evaluation for each patient. The goal is to minimize ionizing radiation exposure without compromising the diagnostic evaluation of the patient. Stated another way, exposure of the patient to potentially harmful radiation should be justified by a reasonable expectation of patient benefit resulting from the diagnosis of potentially harmful diseases. The clinician's suspicion that disease is present is based on findings from the patient history and the physical examination as listed in the box opposite. This is referred to as *ordering radiographs by selection criteria*. Unjustified radiation exposure results from the alternative approach of indiscriminately ordering comprehensive radiographic studies without regard for the individual's dental status. Guidelines for prescribing dental radiographs have been developed under the sponsorship of the Food and Drug Administration (FDA) in consultation with the American Dental Association (ADA) and several organizations representing dental specialty groups. Table 3-1 summarizes these recommendations.

Clinical Laboratory Medicine

Clinical laboratory tests of blood, urine, and other specimens can be a valuable source of diagnostic information concerning the patient's health status. The dentist working in a hospital often has access to screening laboratory studies and in some instances dental treatment decisions may depend on the findings of laboratory tests. Clinical laboratory medicine is considered in Chapter 11.

Pathologic Examination

Pathologic examination of tissue specimens provides the definitive diagnosis for many nondental lesions of the oral cavity. Pathologic examination occurs late in the diagnostic process after the patient history, physical examination, and clinical differential diagnosis of the lesion have been completed, and all or part of the lesion has been removed. The pathologist prepares, examines, and diagnoses the tissue specimen sent by the clinician. Two concepts of this process warrant emphasis:

1. Any tissues other than teeth and some gingival tissues that are worthy of removal must be considered worthy of pathologic examination.
2. The pathologist offers a diagnostic opinion for the tissue specimen. The clinician must make the diagnosis of the patient's condition on the basis of clinical information as well as the opinion provided by the pathologist.

These and other diagnostic issues related to tissue specimens examined by the pathologist are discussed in Chapter 11.

SUMMARY

Physical examination techniques rely on the clinician's primary senses with the aid of simple instruments. Perceptions from visual observation, palpation, auscultation, and probing provide a basis for judgments concerning the possibility that unusual anatomic features may represent the structural effects of disease. Tests of function are designed to reveal physiologic incapacities produced by disease.

Dental modification of physical examination techniques apply the same methods to the unique anatomic demands of the teeth and oral cavity. Probing provides the most direct and reliable method of identifying dental decay and lesions of periodontitis. Intraoral radiographs provide a valuable adjunctive source of information related to these common dental dis-

Table 3-1   Recommended approach to ordering radiographic exposures on the basis of selection criteria

Patient category	Child		Adolescent	Adult	
	Primary dentition (prior to eruption of first permanent tooth)	Transitional dentition (following eruption of first permanent tooth)	Permanent dentition (prior to eruption of third molars)	Dentulous	Edentulous
NEW PATIENT					
All new patients to assess dental diseases and growth and development	Posterior bite-wing examination if proximal surfaces of primary teeth cannot be visualized or probed	Individualized radiographic examination consisting of periapical/occlusal views and posterior bite-wings or panoramic examination and posterior bite-wings	Individualized radiographic examination consisting of posterior bite-wings and selected periapicals; a full mouth intraoral radiographic examination is appropriate when the patient presents with clinical evidence of generalized dental disease or a history of extensive dental treatment		Full mouth intraoral radiographic examination or panoramic examination
RECALL PATIENT					
Clinical caries or high-risk factors for caries	Posterior bite-wing examination at 6-month intervals or until no carious lesions are evident		Posterior bite-wing examination at 6- to 12-month intervals or until no carious lesions are evident	Posterior bite-wing examination at 12- to 18-month intervals	Not applicable
No clinical caries and no high-risk factors for caries	Posterior bite-wing examination at 12- to 24-month intervals if proximal surfaces of primary teeth cannot be visualized or probed	Posterior bite-wing examination at 12- to 24-month intervals	Posterior bite-wing examination at 18- to 36-month intervals	Posterior bite-wing examination at 24- to 36-month intervals	Not applicable

| Periodontal disease or a history of periodontal treatment | Individualized radiographic examination consisting of selected periapical and/or bite-wing radiographs for areas where periodontal disease (other than nonspecific gingivitis) can be demonstrated clinically | Individualized radiographic examination consisting of selected periapical and/or bite-wing radiographs for areas where periodontal disease (other than nonspecific gingivitis) can be demonstrated clinically | | Not applicable |
| Growth and development assessment | Usually not indicated | Individualized radiographic examination consisting of a periapical/occlusal or panoramic examination | Periapical or panoramic examination to assess developing third molars | Usually not indicated |

Modified from The selection of patients for x-ray examinations: dental radiographic examinations, HHS Pub. FDA 88-8273.

eases. Clinical laboratory studies, pathologic examination of tissues, and extraoral radiographs are additional adjunctive procedures that contribute to the diagnosis of nondental conditions.

BIBLIOGRAPHY

Brightman VJ: Rational procedures for diagnosis and medical risk assessment. In Lynch MA, Brightman VJ, Greenberg MS, editors: Burket's oral medicine: diagnosis and treatment, ed 8, Philadelphia, 1984, Lippincott.

DeGowin RL: DeGowin and DeGowin's bedside diagnostic examination, ed 5, New York, 1987, MacMillan.

The Dental Radiographic Patient Selection Criteria Panel: The selection of patients for x-ray examinations: dental radiographic examinations, Public Health Service, Food and Drug Administration Pub No 88-8273, Washington, DC, 1987, US Government Printing Office.

Judge RD, Zuidema GD, Fitzgerald FT, editors: Clinical diagnosis: a physiologic approach, ed 5, Boston, 1988, Little, Brown.

Kerr DA, Ash MM, Millard HD: Oral diagnosis, ed 6, St Louis, 1983, Mosby–Year Book.

Langlais RP, Bricker SL, Cottone JA, Baker BR: Oral diagnosis, oral medicine and treatment planning, Philadelphia, 1984, Saunders.

Seidel HM, Ball JW, Dains JE, Benedict GW: Mosby's guide to physical examination, St Louis, 1987, Mosby–Year Book.

CHAPTER 4

Extraoral Physical Examination

GARY C. COLEMAN

The dentist's physical examination can be divided conceptually and procedurally into extraoral and intraoral portions. The general dentist is primarily interested in the intraoral findings. However, a cursory extraoral examination deprives the clinician of information that contributes to the assessment of general health, some dental conditions, and nondental diseases of the head and neck.

General patient assessment including determination of vital signs typically precedes the extraoral examination, which is then followed by the intraoral examination. This sequence allows the clinician to draw on impressions from general observations while assessing more specific details later in the examination. Also, performing the more intrusive intraoral procedures later in the process is more comfortable for most patients.

GENERAL PATIENT ASSESSMENT

General patient assessment consists of the impressions concerning the patient's health status that can be gained by inspection from a comfortable distance. This process begins during the diagnostic interview and confirms as well as supplements the information obtained during the discussion. The general patient assessment includes observation of the patient's identifying features, mental orientation, emotional status, body size, anatomic proportions, facial form, posture, movements, speech, and determination of the vital signs.

Patient Identification

Patient identification consists of the observation of the patient's apparent age, gender, and race. These demographic features can alert the clinician to the possibility of certain health problems. For example, most 70-year-old men suffer from some degree of compromised cardiovascular function whether or not they are aware of it. Therefore the diagnostic interview for this individual should focus specifically on cardiovascular symptoms, which would not be justified for many other patients. The incidence of hypertension is significantly greater among blacks than other racial groups. Women of child-bearing age may be pregnant or anemic. In other words, the dentist anticipates specific diagnostic issues that require particular attention on the basis of apparent age, gender, and race. These simple observations can also reveal the confusion of previous dental records for patients with the same or similar names.

Mental Orientation and Emotional Status

Essential mental orientation is assessed on the basis of the patient's awareness of person, place, and time. Disorientation usually becomes obvious early in the interview or can be specifically pursued by requesting the patient to name the day of the week or the location of the dental office. Inappropriate responses indicate a degree of mental disorientation that is usually associated with intoxication. Less severe mental disorientation is suggested by inconsistent or inappropriate responses to health questions.

The emotional status of a patient may be described by words such as alert, anxious, fearful, suspicious, confrontational, distressed, and apathetic. The suspicion of an unusual emotional status may originate from both verbal and nonverbal forms of communication. Distress caused by pain and inordinate fear are particularly significant to the dentist.

Suspicion of mental disorientation or abnormal emotional status justifies skepticism concerning the accuracy and completeness of the patient history, which may warrant dismissal of the patient. The dentist assumes considerable responsibility by proceeding with treatment on the basis of unreliable historical information or compromised informed consent. Consultation with a family member or the patient's physician may be an alternative to dismissal if emergency treatment is urgently required.

Habitus, Stature, and Bilateral Symmetry

Stature, habitus, and *bilateral symmetry* are terms that describe the absolute size and relative proportions of body parts. Stature refers to the patient's height and habitus is the term for the patient's body build. Bilateral symmetry refers to the expectation that the midsagittal plane bisects the body into equal parts that normally correspond in form. A broad range of these features can be considered healthy and no absolute measurements define the limits of normal. However, extremes may develop as a consequence of disease.

Stature. Comparing the proportions of body parts can reveal conditions that produce unusual height. The *body ratio* is the upper skeletal segment length divided by that of the lower body segment with the symphysis pubis as the dividing point for measurement. The *stature-to-span ratio* is height divided by the distance from fingertip to fingertip with the arms extended. Both ratios are approximately 1.0 for adolescents and adults. Abnormal ratios may reveal disproportional growth related to developmental conditions or endocrine disorders. For example, markedly small stature or *dwarfism* caused by pituitary dysfunction is characterized by normal body proportions. Body and stature-to-span ratios greater than 1.0 that are associated with dwarfism reflect limited development of the limbs and the relatively normal head-trunk size as results from abnormal epiphyseal bone growth. Similarly, several forms of *gigantism* or large stature are characterized by skeletal and stature-to-span ratios less than 1.0, which indicates excessive limb growth.

Habitus. The diverse body builds among healthy individuals are classified as asthenic, sthenic, hypersthenic, and pyknic habitus. The *asthenic* individual appears slender and underweight as a consequence of less than average bone and muscle mass. The *sthenic* person is well proportioned and athletic in appearance with typical bone and muscular development. The stocky or *hypersthenic* patient exhibits heavy bone and thick muscular proportions. The *pyknic* individual appears heavy, soft, and rounded because of an abundance of body fat in comparison with muscle and bone. *Cachexia* is abnormally decreased tissue mass resulting from malnutrition or chronic debilitation. *Obesity* is an inordinately great fat tissue mass that results in most cases from excessive food intake. The pyknic individual is not necessarily obese but tends to gain weight easily.

Symmetry. The clinician should attempt to determine if asymmetry is a consequence of tissue deficiency, tissue enlargement, or abnormal tissue position. Many tissue deficiencies are explained by injury or degenerative diseases. Localized, unilateral facial swelling caused by infection is the most common asymmetric enlargement that prompts the patient to consult the dentist. *Scoliosis* or lateral curvature of the spine is a congenital malformation that causes asymmetry resulting from abnormal tissue position.

Head and Facial Form

General appraisal of head shape and facial form is based on the same general principles of relative and absolute size, shape, and symmetry used to evaluate body form. Excessive distance between the eyes known as *ocular hypertelorism,* prominent convex contour or *bossing* of the frontal region, a lower than normal position of the ears, and abnormal size or relationship of the jaws are features indicative of abnormal facial development. Any asymmetry is significant. Typical skull shape is described as *normocephalic* or *mesocephalic.* A short, rounded skull shape is referred to as *brachycephalic*, and *dolichocephalic* is the appropriate term for a long, narrow head shape. These abnormalities of cranial and facial form suggest developmental conditions such as those described in Chapter 20.

Posture

Unusual standing or sitting posture may indicate pain caused by certain positions or limitation of movement that prevents the patient from assuming a typical posture. Recent injuries, disability from a past injury, and arthritic disease are the most common causes. The slumping posture that results from inflammatory disease of the spine is another example. Advanced cardiopulmonary disease can force the patient to habitually slump forward to assume a more comfortable breathing position. The clinician should recognize the possibility that fully reclining such patients may hamper breathing.

Gait

Gait is the manner of walking, and most gait abnormalities relate to neuromuscular disability from injury, stroke, or degenerative neuromuscular diseases. The *hemiplegic gait* is characterized by a semicircular lateral swing of the affected leg during stride and is typical of the cerebral damage caused by a stroke. *Ataxic gait* is the staggering, irregular, wide-stanced walk associated with alcohol intoxication or cerebellar dysfunction. *Parkinsonian gait* is characteristic of this degenerative neurologic condition and consists of limited stride, hanging arms, the tendency to surge forward then step back, and rapid or staccato steps. *Tabes dorsalis* refers to neurologic degeneration of tertiary syphilis and results in an ataxic gait with foot slapping and a tendency for the patient to watch the feet to compensate for lost proprioception. *Scissors gait* is characterized by short steps in which one foot crosses over in front of the other. The *foot drop gait* results from weakness of the dorsiflexors of the feet and is identified by the dragging of the toes or excessively high steps to avoid toe dragging called an *equine gait.*

Abnormal Movement

Repetitive or uncontrolled tremors and other abnormal movements can suggest a variety of neurologic disorders. Tremors are categorized as one of three basic types. The *resting tremors* of Parkinson's disease are most evident in the hands and are characterized by rhythmic increases and decreases in muscular tone at rest. A "pill-rolling" movement in which the patient rhythmically cycles the tip of the thumb over the first finger is an example. *Essential tremor* usually involves the head during intentional movement or postural exertion, but not while the muscles are at rest. Muscle tone remains constant during the tremor. The *intentional tremor* of multiple sclerosis is often associated with ataxia and occurs during purposeful movements.

Choreic movements are irregular, involuntary motions that occur spontaneously and involve more than one joint. The movements are without purpose and are similar to the "fidgeting" of children or the restlessness of anxious adults. *Athetoid movements* involve slow, writhing, repetitive movements. Such movements involving the proximal extremities, trunk, and face are a frequent manifestation of cerebral palsy. Similar movements of the lips and tongue are known as *tardive dyskinesia* and can result from the effects of extrapyramidal degeneration or medications such as the phenothiazines.

Speech

Normal speech implies healthy neuromuscular function of the organs that produce the sound, normal cortical function, coherent mental status, and the ability to hear. Obvious speech abnormalities that become apparent during the diagnostic interview are *dysarthria* or slurring of speech and *aphasia,* which is inability to accomplish proper verbal expression. Dysarthria is a nonspecific indication of neuromuscular deficiency or intoxication. Aphasia may be partial or total and implies neuromuscular or cortical defects.

VITAL SIGNS

Determination of the vital signs is the final aspect of the general patient assessment. The vital signs can be quickly determined and provide immediate evidence of the patient's essential physiologic functions. The vital signs consist of the pulse rate, respiration rate, body temperature, and blood pressure.

Some clinicians also include stature, weight, and apparent age versus stated age as vital signs even though these features are less immediate physiologic indicators as compared with the usual four vital signs. Height and weight are useful parameters to evaluate development and growth. Also, weight compared with stature can reflect the nutritional status and the probability of conditions such as cardiovascular disease, diabetes, and endocrine disorders. Qualitative evaluation of these features by observation rather than quantitative measurement is adequate in most instances.

Pulse

The determination of the patient's pulse simultaneously provides evidence of the heart rate, cardiac rhythm, character of cardiac output, and peripheral circulation. The carotid, brachial, radial, and femoral arteries are useful pulse points because of their accessible locations superficial to bone and dense muscle. Radial and brachial pulses are most easily and practically determined in the dental setting, while the carotid pulse indicates blood flow to the brain in a medical emergency or injury. Palpation of the femoral pulse in a dental office is inappropriate, but may occasionally be necessary in a hospital setting. The anatomic locations of the principle pulse points are

Radial pulse: medial-ventral wrist, just proximal to the radial head between flexor carpi radialis and brachioradialis tendons

Brachial pulse: antecubital fossa, medial to biceps tendon

Carotid pulse: inferior and medial to the angle of the mandible, medial to the sternocleidomastoid muscle

Femoral pulse: medial to the anterior superior iliac spine, inferior to the inguinal ligament

The pulse is palpated by placing the tips of the index and middle fingers evenly along the course of the artery at the pulse point. Stabilization with the thumb causes the examiner to sense the pulses of both the patient and the clinician and should be avoided. The pressure necessary to sense the pulse varies in proportion to the amount of tissue overlying the artery but excessive force may obscure the pulse by occluding the artery. Accurate location of the pulse point is more important in palpating the pulse than the amount of pressure. Movement by the clinician or the patient during pulse determination should be minimized to avoid misinterpretation.

Quantitative pulse determination. Counting the pulse surges for 20 or 30 seconds is generally adequate to make the quantitative determination. The count is then multiplied to yield counts per minute. The pulse rate is normally between 60 and 90 surges per minute. Children often have a slightly higher count and athletes usually have a lower count.

Qualitative pulse evaluation. The rhythm, wave form, amplitude, and symmetry of the pulse should also be assessed. *Pulse rhythm* reflects cardiac rhythm and should be regular. Cyclic variations in rhythm corresponding to respiratory inspiration and expiration are normal. Noncyclic abnormalities in rhythm suggest cardiac arrhythmia. The normal *wave form* is a single, even surge. Bigeminal or biphasic surges indicate premature cardiac contractions.

Pulse *amplitude* is interpreted subjectively as the force or pressure of the blood surge. A faint surge with poor distinction between individual pulses is termed weak and if the weak amplitude varies, then the pulse is described as *thready.* This is typical of hypovolemic shock caused by significant hemorrhagic blood loss or dehydration. A *bounding* pulse is easy to find, hard to obliterate with pressure, and does not fade. A bounding pulse is typical of exertion, fever, hyperthyroidism, and advanced atherosclerosis. Pulse amplitude is usually graded on a scale from 0 to 4 with 0 reflecting no palpable pulse, 4 representing a bounding pulse, and 2 as the normal or expected amplitude. *Pulse symmetry* refers to the bilateral compari-

son of the pulse character and rate. For example, a difference in amplitude suggests compromised blood flow within the artery with the weaker pulse.

Respiration Rate

The respiration rate is counted by watching the chest rise and fall for 20 to 30 seconds and recording the adjusted result in counts per minute. A rate of 12 to 20 breaths per minute is considered normal for adults. The rhythm and depth of respiration are often of greater importance in the appraisal of respiratory function than the rate. Functional compromise is indicated by alterations such as *tachypnea* or rapid breathing and *Cheyne-Stokes respiration,* which is shallow breathing with cyclic variation in the respiration rate.

Temperature Measurement

Body temperature measurement is accomplished orally by the dentist and both electronic and mercury thermometers are available. Inaccuracies can result from leaving the thermometer in the mouth for too short a time, mouth breathing, and failure to shake down a mercury thermometer. The cited normal value of 98.6° F (37° C) is for an inactive, hospitalized patient. Active, healthy patients arriving for a dental visit on a warm day may have a temperature over 99° F and readings over 100° F are common among healthy children after strenuous play. Body temperature during sleep can decrease as much as 2° F. Temperatures over 99° F for an inactive individual represents fever.

Blood Pressure Measurement

The blood pressure is an important indication of cardiac function and efficiency. Detection by the dentist of consistently elevated blood pressure or *hypertension* may be a more beneficial health service for certain patients than the dental treatment the dentist provides. Also, blood pressure is monitored as a reflection of circulatory function during episodes of altered physiologic status such as sedation and acute medical emergencies. Automated devices are available that measure the blood pressure, but all clinicians should be able to determine the blood pressure manually.

Physiologic basis of blood pressure measurement. The physiologic mechanisms that form the basis for the blood pressure technique are simple. The goal is to measure the minimum, constant arterial pressure during *diastole* or relaxation of the heart and the maximum pressure during *systole,* contraction of the heart muscle. The *sphygmomanometer* used for blood pressure measurement contains an inflatable bladder within a fabric cuff connected to either a mercury or aneroid pressure indicator. The cuff is wrapped around a limb proximal to a pulse point, which is usually the upper arm superior to the brachial pulse point in the antecubital fossa.

Although somewhat inaccurate, the systolic pressure can be estimated by gradually inflating the cuff until the artery is occluded and the brachial pulse is obscured by cuff pressure that is greater than the systolic pressure. Gradually decreasing the cuff pressure allows the pulse to return when the systolic blood pressure overcomes the lower pressure exerted by the cuff. The pressure at which the pulse fades and reappears is the approximate systolic blood pressure. This is called the *pulse* or *palpatory method* of estimating the systolic pressure. Measurement of diastolic pressure is more difficult and inaccurate by this method, but it can also be estimated.

More accurate results are obtained by using a stethoscope to auscultate the *Korotkoff sounds,* which are resonances produced by blood turbulence within a partially compressed artery. The artery is occluded when the cuff pressure is greater than the systolic pressure and no sound is produced. Cuff pressures less than systolic and greater than diastolic pressure cause partial compression of the

artery and Korotkoff sounds are produced during the pulse surge. Cuff pressure less than diastolic pressure does not distort the artery and no sounds are produced. The systolic and diastolic blood pressures are determined by gradually changing the cuff pressure and noting the pressure at which Korotkoff sounds can and cannot be heard. This is called the *auscultatory method* of blood pressure measurement.

Auscultatory method of blood pressure measurement. The auscultatory technique of blood pressure determination is performed with the patient seated quietly and the arm held at approximately the same level as the heart. The appropriate cuff size for the patient's size should be used because cuffs that are too large yield falsely low values. Cuffs that are too small and cuffs loosely adapted to the arm produce falsely elevated results. Clothing between the arm and the cuff can also cause inaccuracy. The air bladder within the cuff is centered over the brachial artery with the lower cuff edge placed 2 to 3 cm above the antecubital crease. The cuff should be secured around the arm so that it is snug without folds or twists.

The initial step is to estimate the systolic pressure by the pulse method. The brachial or radial pulse is located and the cuff is inflated, and the clinician notes when the pulse disappears, which is the systolic pressure estimate. Inflation continues to between 20 and 30 mm Hg above that point. The cuff is then deflated slowly until the pulse returns to confirm the systolic pressure estimate. The cuff is deflated completely and the patient raises and lowers the arm to clear venous stasis. The bell endpiece of the stethoscope is then placed over the brachial pulse point and the cuff is inflated 20 to 30 mm Hg above the systolic estimate. Slow deflation at the rate of 1 to 2 mm Hg per second allows the first sound to be heard at the systolic blood pressure. Gradual deflation continues at approximately the same rate, which causes changes in the nature of the Ko-

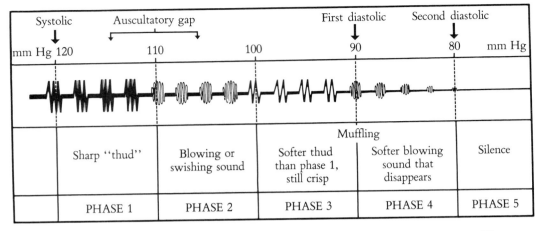

Fig. 4-1   Typical features of Korotkoff sounds during blood pressure measurement. (From Seidel HM and others: Mosby's guide to physical examination, ed 2, St Louis, 1991, Mosby–Year Book.)

rotkoff sounds as illustrated in Fig. 4-1. The pressure at which the sound disappears completely is the diastolic pressure. The process can be repeated if necessary after 1 to 2 minutes with the cuff completely deflated.

The blood turbulence that produces the Korotkoff sounds results from partial compression of the artery in much the same way that compressing the end of a garden hose causes turbulent water flow and noise. The nature of the sound depends on the cuff pressure and degree of arterial distortion. Clinicians inexperienced in blood pressure measurement can misinterpret the phase 1 sounds (Fig. 4-1) as movement, then hear nothing in the auscultatory gap. The first sound is then interpreted at the beginning of phase 3, which yields a falsely low systolic reading. The faint sounds at the end of phase 4 can be missed and lead to a falsely high impression of the diastolic pressure. The interpretation is improved by deflating the cuff slowly at the primary reading points and minimizing movement. As previously described, inaccurate blood pressure measurement can also result from poor cuff placement and incorrect cuff size.

The American Heart Association recommends recording both diastolic readings as 120/90/80 mm Hg. Precise and formal diagnosis of hypertension requires multiple readings on different days from different limbs and in different patient positions. However, recording the systolic and second diastolic pressure or simply the diastolic pressure as 120/80 mm Hg is adequate for hypertension screening and patient care needs in the dental setting. Also, blood pressure determination in the dental operatory using only the right arm in the sitting position is generally adequate.

Normal ranges for adults are a systolic pressure between 100 and 140 mm Hg and diastolic measurement between 60 and 90 mm Hg. The *pulse pressure* is obtained by subtracting the diastolic pressure from the systolic pressure, and it is normally between 30 and 40 mm Hg. The blood pressures of children are usually below the ranges considered healthy for adults. Measurements outside these ranges should be repeated with attention to eliminating technique errors such as poor cuff placement, missed sounds, and incorrect cuff size. Poor technique is indicated by faint or obscure

Korotkoff sounds and an abnormal pulse pressure associated with typical pulse qualities as determined by palpation. An approach to overcoming faint Korotkoff sounds is to have the patient elevate the arm with the cuff in place, inflate the cuff 20 to 30 mm Hg beyond estimated systolic pressure, return the arm to normal position at the level of the heart, and proceed with the auscultatory method as usual. This clears peripheral venous stasis to some degree in patients with congestive heart failure and yields a louder blood surge at the pulse point.

Interpretation of unusual blood pressure readings, assuming technical inaccuracy has been eliminated, should allow for physiologic variation. Anxiety, recent exercise, and advanced age are among the causes of physiologically increased blood pressure. Rapid change in position, shock, and dehydration can cause lower than normal readings.

Comparison of the pulse rate with the blood pressure may aid in interpreting the patient's cardiovascular status. The tendency of the pulse rate to be inversely proportional to the blood pressure as an expression of the baroreceptor influence on heart rate is known as *Marey's law.* Therefore a relatively low pulse rate may suggest that the clinician should anticipate a higher blood pressure reading. Conversely, an abnormally rapid pulse rate is frequently associated with inefficient cardiac function and a low pulse pressure.

A diagnosis of hypertension or hypotension is not within the scope of dental practice. However, routine blood pressure measurement by the dentist is justified for the following reasons:

1. *Patient health screening.* Hypertensive patients are often unaware of their condition and the contribution of hypertension to coronary disease, stroke, and renal disorders is well known. Most patients appreciate a referral to their physician for definitive diagnosis and treatment. The dentist's role is limited to screening and referral. The patient should be informed of the suspicion of high blood pressure rather than offered a diagnosis of hypertension.
2. *Physical status.* Conducting a physical assessment, administering an anesthetic with a vasoconstrictor, and performing dental treatment without determining the vital signs including the blood pressure is poor clinical practice. Complications resulting from high blood pressure such as excessive hemorrhage after surgery can be anticipated or avoided by identifying patients with hypertension.
3. *Baseline data.* Syncope and other medical emergencies that may develop in the dental office can produce dramatic blood pressure changes. Awareness of the patient's resting blood pressure improves the management of the complication by providing a basis for comparison during the emergency.

THE PHYSICAL EXAMINATION OF SPECIFIC EXTRAORAL STRUCTURES

The extraoral examination conducted by the dentist is a detailed anatomic and functional evaluation of the patient that can be performed with the mouth closed and without the use of complex technical devices. Progressing from general to specific observations and following a systematic routine promotes the most thorough appreciation of structural and functional features. The discussion below follows an anatomic and functional sequence for the sake of clarity. However, the specific examination sequence is not as important as the consistency of the clinician's individual approach. Experienced practitioners improve efficiency by concurrently accomplishing several anatomically or functionally unrelated observations.

Facial Form And Symmetry

Facial form is examined by inspection and palpation from frontal, submental, lateral, and supraorbital perspectives. Symmetry, position, and contour of the orbits, pupil alignment, and midline location of the nose can be observed from the frontal perspective. Symmetry and typical contour of the zygomatic arches, ears, mandible, and the resting position of the mouth should also be specifically confirmed. The submental perspective is achieved by asking the patient to hyperextend the head while the clinician is still in the frontal position. This accentuates the visual demonstration of the anatomic triangles of the neck, the shape of the mandible, and the preauricular prominence of the parotid glands.

The lateral perspective reveals the profile contours of the facial bones. This can demonstrate disproportional development of the mandible, maxilla, zygomatic arches, frontal bones, and abnormal ear position. The supraorbital perspective is achieved by looking down the patient's face from above and behind the head. The clinician can visualize the symmetry and relative positions of mandibular, maxillary, and zygomatic structures by slightly adjusting the viewpoint. This is an effective position from which to observe deviation of the mandible during opening.

Skin

The skin of the face and the neck can be inspected concurrently with the examination of facial form. Attention should be directed to unusual variations in integrity, pigmentation, and texture as well as abnormal elevations and depressions. Common conditions that are identifiable by their characteristic appearance such as acne and *nevi,* common "moles," do not warrant additional attention. Inspection and palpation of any other lesions are relied on to determine the specific location, size, surface texture, compressibility, tenderness, delineation of borders, alteration of surface contour, color, and consistency of the lesion. The differential diagnosis of skin lesions relies on these features in addition to the duration and clinical course of the lesion as described by the patient. The terminology and significance of these findings are discussed in Chapter 14.

The facial skin of middle-aged and older patients should be examined carefully for variation in pigmentation, erythema, and roughened thinning that is typical of ultraviolet damage known as *actinic keratosis.* This precancerous condition is caused by years of excessive sun exposure associated with an outdoor hobby or vocation. Fair-skinned patients are particularly vulnerable.

Eyes, Ears, and Nose

Eyes. Abnormalities of the eyes can suggest developmental abnormalities, inflammatory disease, manifestations of systemic disease, and cranial nerve dysfunction. Such conditions may produce related oral manifestations.

Developmental abnormalities involving the eyes suggest the possibility that other facial structures are also affected by disproportional or defective development. *Ocular hypertelorism* refers to excessive space between the eyes and is a feature of several developmental syndromes. A *coloboma* is characterized by a depression or fissurelike malformation of the iris or eyelid margin that is also indicative of developmental conditions. A feature associated with genetic syndromes of defective connective tissue formation is *blue sclera* resulting from thin formation of this structure. A faint bluish tint is commonly observed among healthy children, but darker blue of a child's sclera justifies the suspicion of a connective tissue disorder. *Epicanthal folds* are oblique flaps of skin over the inner canthus of the eye, which is a normal feature for individuals of oriental decent. This observation suggests a developmental abnormality when individuals of other races are affected.

Conjunctivitis, inflammation of the mucous membrane of the eye, is characterized by erythema, excessive tearing, and a sensation of "itchiness." This condition is usually either an allergic reaction or irritation caused by airborne materials. Visualization of the palpebral surface of the lower eyelid as illustrated in Fig. 4-2 is an effective method of distinguishing the

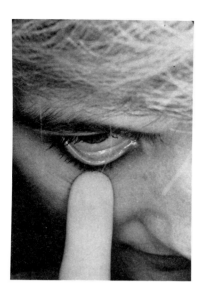

Fig. 4-2 The lower eyelid can be drawn interiorly as shown to reveal the palpebral conjunctiva. Erythema of this surface is a dependable sign of conjunctivitis.

erythema of conjunctivitis from redness of the sclera. Several autoimmune conditions produce oral ulcers as well as subtle ulcers of the conjunctival mucosa that are clinically indistinguishable from conjunctivitis. Matting at the inner canthus or other evidence of an exudate is typical of a bacterial infection.

An early clinical sign of several systemic diseases is altered appearance or function of the eyes. Extensive lysis of red blood cells known as *hemolysis* and liver disease can produce elevated blood concentration of bilirubin. This results in yellowish discoloration of tissues referred to as *jaundice* or *icterus,* which is often initially identified as yellow discoloration of the sclera. Intense aversion to bright light known as *photophobia* is usually associated with inflammation of eye structures but may suggest metabolic conditions such as defective blood pigment metabolism known as *porphyria.* Recent development of bilateral protrusion of the eyeballs referred to as *prop-*

tosis or *exophthalmos* is a sign of hyperthyroidism, while congenital proptosis is produced by developmental deficiency of the middle third of the face. Unilateral exophthalmos usually results from swelling or other enlargement within the orbit that is distorting the position of the eye.

Six of the twelve cranial nerves are involved in sensory or motor functions of the eye. This implies that the eye is the focus of attention during the clinical evaluation of cranial nerve function when intracranial disease is suspected.

Ears. Most conditions affecting the ears that are of diagnostic significance to the dentist are inflammatory or developmental in origin. As with malformations of the eyes, identification of developmental ear conditions suggests the possibility of congenital defects of other facial structures. Congenital malformations of the auricle or external ear include abnormal size, disproportional size of parts of the auricle, or lower than normal position relative to the zygoma. Developmental pits and tissue tags near the tragus are more subtle features of developmental deformity. Congenital defects of the middle and inner ear are often associated with deafness.

Inflammation of the ear can produce symptoms similar to those of temporomandibular dysfunction and inflammatory dental conditions. *Otitis media* is infection of the middle ear that typically follows blockage of the auditory tube by nasopharyngeal congestion. The definitive clinical sign of otitis media is distention of the eardrum as observed by otoscopic examination, although this condition may also be indicated by tenderness when the earlobe is gently pulled. Tenderness elicited by palpation of the mastoid process is characteristic of *mastoiditis.* Temporomandibular joint inflammation is distinguished by the location of tenderness in the preauricular region.

Nose. The dentist's examination of the nose is usually limited to superficial inspection of the surface of the nose and the nares. The

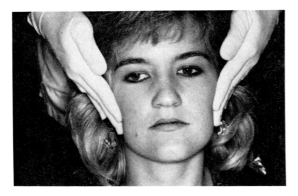

Fig. 4-3   Bilateral palpation of parotid regions.

use of a speculum attached to an otoscope to visualize the floor of the nose is occasionally helpful in determining the superior extent of an anterior maxillary enlargement. Point tenderness elicited by firm palpation of the surface overlying the maxillary, frontal, and ethmoid sinuses is an early and reliable sign of acute bacterial sinusitis. This finding associated with the maxillary sinus can be particularly significant when evaluating the extent of maxillary dental infections.

Parotid Gland and Facial Tissues

Palpation of the facial soft tissues is the principle method of identifying subtle enlargements of the parotid glands, cheeks, lips, and submandibular structures. Bidigital or bimanual palpation is an effective method of assessing tissue composition by compressing the tissues between the clinician's fingertips. Since this involves the placement of the fingers inside the mouth, portions of the evaluation are most conveniently accomplished during the intraoral portion of the examination. In other areas similar compression can be accomplished by palpating the tissues against bone and teeth.

Bilateral palpation of the facial region allows the clinician to compare the relative thickness and compressibility of corresponding soft tissues as illustrated by Fig. 4-3. This can

be accomplished from a frontal position or from behind the patient. The patient is instructed to lightly close the teeth together without clenching. This position produces a relatively uniform contour of bone and teeth with minimal muscular exertion against which to compress the soft tissues. Bilateral palpation of corresponding structures is accomplished by placement of both hands on the skin surface with the fingertips arranged to cover a large surface area. Broad circular movement produces a greater likelihood of "trapping" and identifying abnormalities. An effective sequence is to begin palpating lateral to the orbits and gradually move inferiorly to the temporal fossa, the parotid gland, and the tissue overlying the mandible. The fingers can then be positioned in the infraorbital region and palpation proceeds toward the zygomatic arch and then anteriorly to the tissues overlying the maxilla.

Palpation of the facial soft tissues normally reveals relatively uniform thickness and compressibility. Some variation in different anatomic regions reflects a different proportion of muscle, gland, and other soft tissue components, but the overall impression is of tissue homogeneity rather than heterogeneity. The parotid gland region and the general areas of the preauricular, facial, and parotid lymph nodes (Fig. 4-4) are likely sites for subtle nodal enlargement and should be palpated carefully.

Neck

The neck is most effectively examined from behind the patient with the patient reclined and the head slightly tilted in a hyperextended position. This arrangement aids visualization and palpation by the distention of sternocleidomastoid muscles. Extraoral palpation of the neck can be approached in three anatomic stages: (1) the submental and submandibular regions, (2) anterior and posterior to the sternocleidomastoid muscles, and (3) the midline structures including the larynx, trachea, and thyroid gland.

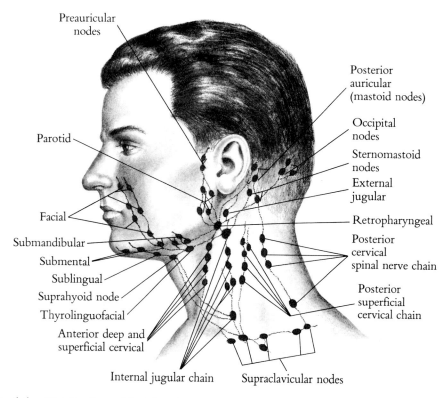

Preauricular nodes

Posterior auricular (mastoid nodes)

Occipital nodes

Sternomastoid nodes

External jugular

Parotid

Retropharyngeal

Facial

Posterior cervical spinal nerve chain

Submandibular

Submental

Sublingual

Suprahyoid node

Posterior superficial cervical chain

Thyrolinguofacial

Anterior deep and superficial cervical

Internal jugular chain

Supraclavicular nodes

Fig. 4-4 Distribution of facial and cervical lymph nodes (From Seidel HM and others: Mosby's guide to physical examination, ed 2, St Louis, 1991, Mosby-Year Book.)

The submental and submandibular triangles are bilaterally palpated by resting the thumbs near the inferior mandibular border and pressing the aligned fingertips inferior and medial to the mandibular border. The fingertips are gradually moved inferiorly to the hyoid bone and then medially and superiorly until the inferior aspect of the submandibular gland can be identified. Further examination of the area is accomplished during the intraoral examination by bimanual palpation of the floor of the mouth. This area contains the submental, submandibular, and suprahyoid lymph node groups (Fig. 4-5).

The sternocleidomastoid muscle region is examined one side at a time with the head hyperextended and turned away from the side

being examined, as shown by Fig. 4-6. This position distends the sternocleidomastoid muscle and allows easier identification of lymph nodes in the posterior and anterior superficial cervical chains (Fig. 4-5). The aligned fingertips are placed along the posterior border of the muscle while the thumb provides counter pressure from the anterior aspect of the muscle. Medial pressure of the fingertips along the posterior muscle border identifies enlarged nodes of the posterior superficial cervical chain. The clinician can gradually move the fingertips inferiorly along the muscle with alternating pressure until the full extent of the region has been palpated. The supraclavicular nodes should also be palpated along the superior clavicular margin. The examination of the anterior cervical

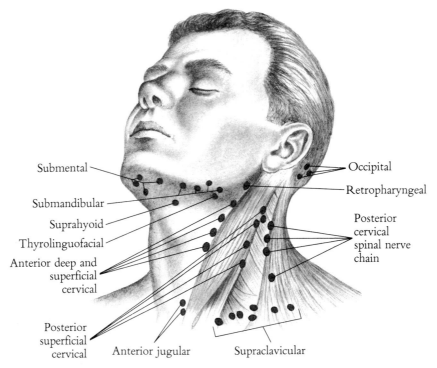

Fig. 4-5   Cervical lymph node groups (From Seidel HM and others: Mosby's guide to physical examination, ed 2, St Louis, 1991, Mosby-Year Book.)

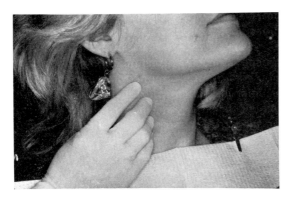

Fig. 4-6   Palpation of the anterior superficial cervical lymph nodes with the patient's head hyperextended and turned to distend the sternocleidomastoid muscle.

chain is accomplished in much the same way with the fingertips aligned medial and anterior to the sternocleidomastoid muscle and the thumb at the posterior border. Medial pressure of the fingertips near the anterior-superior border of the sternocleidomastoid muscle reveals the carotid pulse. The anterior border of the muscle should be thoroughly examined by alternating medial fingertip pressure with incremental movements inferiorly until the the clavicle is reached. The patient should then be instructed to turn the head to assume the same position relative to the opposite side and the examination is repeated for the contralateral structures.

Any lymph node enlargement or *lymphade-*

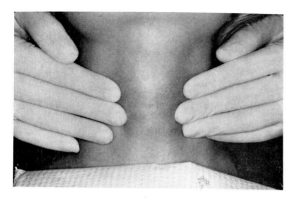

Fig. 4-7   Bilateral palpation of the midline structures of the neck.

nopathy identified by palpation should be assessed for compressibility, tenderness to pressure, and mobility. A firm, nontender, and mobile node that is palpable typically reflects sclerosis that has been caused by a past infection. Multiple tender, mobile, and compressible nodes within a regional group result from an active infection within the tissues drained by that group. Multiple firm and nontender nodes that are fixed or attached to surrounding structures is characteristic of regional metastasis of malignant neoplastic disease.

Palpation of the midline tissues should demonstrate any lateral deviation in the position of the larynx at rest and during swallowing. This is best determined with the fingertips aligned along both sides of the larynx and medial to the sternocleidomastoid muscle as demonstrated in Fig. 4-7. The thyroid gland can also be palpated in this position below the level of the cricoid notch. The thyroid gland is somewhat difficult to identify because of the amorphous compressibility of the tissue and the lateral lobes are located medial and deep to the sternocleidomastoid muscle. The presence of the gland can be perceived by recognizing that the definition of the cartilaginous laryngeal and tracheal rings is obscured by the thyroid tissue during palpation. Normal thyroid tissue is compressible and homogeneous without nodularity or distinct firmness. Any asymmetric mass or nodularity in this region that ascends during swallowing is likely to be associated with the thyroid gland.

By gently moving the larynx laterally a crackling sound or vibration referred to as *crepitus* is normally produced by the rubbing of the cartilaginous structures of the posterior larynx against the cervical spine. Absence of crepitus during this movement suggests abnormal tissue between the larynx and the cervical spine. Placement of the thumb and first finger over the trachea at the midline in the suprasternal notch is the method for identifying *tracheal tugging*, an abnormal pulling sensation synchronized with the patient's pulse. This sign is produced by aortic pressure against the left mainstem bronchus during systole when the vessel is abnormally distended and thinned, which is referred to as an *aneurysm.*

Temporomandibular Joint Function

Routine assessment of jaw function consists of four elements: (1) Palpation of the temporomandibular joint, (2) determination of maximal opening, (3) observation for lateral deviation of the mandible during opening, and (4) palpation to identify tenderness of the muscles of mastication. In addition, auscultation of the temporomandibular joint (TMJ) during movement may reveal joint sounds indicative of degenerative joint disease. The specific degenerative conditions of the TMJ are discussed in Chapter 9.

Pain or tenderness of the TMJ during palpation is one of the most reliable indications of joint inflammation. The preauricular area overlying the TMJ is firmly palpated while the jaws are at rest and during clenching. Bilateral palpation of the joints provides a basis for comparing the amount of discomfort and is more likely to reveal mild tenderness. An alternative approach preferred by some clinicians is insertion of the little finger into the external auditory canal. The patient is then asked to open and close while the examiner exerts pressure on the posterior wall of the joint. Whether the location of palpation is lateral or posterior to the joint, a distinct depression should be felt during opening as the condylar head translates forward. The movement of both joints is normally synchronized. A pop, click, crepitus, or "jump" during opening suggests dysfunction. Auscultation of the joint during jaw movements is generally a more sensitive method for detecting subtle joint sounds. The bell endpiece of the stethoscope usually proves more effective in detecting the high-pitched joint sounds than the diaphragm endpiece.

The measurement of maximal opening is accomplished by requesting the patient to open as wide as possible without pain. The distance from the upper and lower incisor edges is measured at the midline or this distance can be estimated in instances of missing anterior teeth. The patient is then asked to open as far as possible without straining or locking and the measurement is repeated. Normal dentulous adults can open approximately 35 mm or more with no discomfort, although this distance must be adjusted in some instances to allow for extreme patient size. The increase from comfortable opening to maximal opening is generally less than 5 mm. An increase of more than 5 mm associated with joint sounds suggests moderate degeneration of the soft tissue components of the joint. Limited opening with pain suggests more advanced soft tissue degeneration within the joint.

The patient should be observed for lateral deviation on opening by looking down the patient's face from a supraorbital position in the manner illustrated in Fig. 4-8. By watching the tip of the chin relative to the tip of the nose during opening the clinician can identify lateral deviation. Normally no significant deviation occurs. Deviation to one side typically indicates degenerative joint disease on the side toward which the patient deviates. Multiple

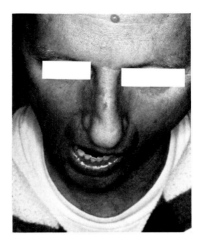

Fig. 4-8   Deviation during opening observed from the supraorbital perspective.

deviations suggest degenerative disease of both joints.

Tenderness of the muscles of mastication results from muscle stress and fatigue, which are characteristic manifestations of jaw dysfunction. The four muscle pairs to be palpated are the temporalis, masseter, medial pterygoid, and lateral pterygoid muscles. The digastric muscles may also be affected in some cases. Both temporalis muscles are palpated simultaneously with the fingertips aligned in a row from the hairline just above the supraorbital ridge to above the ear. The masseter muscles are palpated bilaterally in the area overlying the anterior border of the mandibular ramus. The digastric muscles are palpated with the fingertips aligned roughly parallel to the inferior border of the mandible in the submental and submandibular region.

Palpation of the pterygoid muscles is difficult in most patients, and the results are usually inconclusive because the intraoral position of the examiner's hand does not allow jaw movement during palpation. The medial pterygoid muscle can only be palpated near its insertion by placement of the index finger laterally and posteriorly into the floor of the mouth toward the medial surface of the angle of the mandible. Tenderness of the lateral pterygoid can occasionally be detected by indirect application of pressure. The index finger is positioned distal and posterior to the maxillary tuberosity, and posterior pressure is exerted to compress the interposed tissues against the muscle.

Cranial Nerve Evaluation

Formal clinical evaluation of the function of the cranial nerves is seldom performed during the routine dental examination. One reason is that evidence of a cranial nerve deficiency implies the need to evaluate the patient for central nervous system (CNS) disease, which is beyond the scope of dental practice. Another reason the evaluation is not formally conducted is that the dental examination informally tests the functions of most of the cranial nerves. The procedures described below are methods to more carefully assess cranial nerve function in situations of a suspected neurologic deficiency.

Olfactory nerve. The special sense of smell is conveyed by the the olfactory nerve and is evaluated with strong, characteristic aromas such as onion or garlic. This test is seldom performed to detect neural deficiency because more common peripheral conditions alter the sense of smell and interfere with the sensitivity of the test. *Anosmia* or loss of the sense of smell is usually caused by inflammatory nasal disease. Also, the patient's responses are subjective and many patients with CNS disease effectively sense aromas, but they cannot name or recognize the scent. Older individuals and smokers commonly exhibit diminished olfactory function without neurologic defect.

Optic nerve. The optic nerve conveys the sense of vision and is evaluated by determining visual acuity, extent of visual fields, and by funduscopic examination. Visual acuity can be roughly determined with any printed material or with the Snellen eye chart. Visual fields are determined with one eye covered and the pa

tient's gaze directed forward. The clinician approaches the lateral side of the patient's head with a moving finger and notes when the finger is first visualized. The same approach is used to determine the medial extent of the visual field for that eye and the process is repeated for the other eye. The most sensitive demonstration of optic nerve atrophy is accomplished by visualization of the fundus oculi using an ophthalmoscope, which is beyond the training and experience of most dentists.

The most common gross visual field defect is loss of peripheral vision toward one side in both eyes, which indicates a lesion or defect between the optic chiasma and the visual cortex on the contralateral side. *Bitemporal field defects,* loss of lateral peripheral vision of both eyes, indicates a lesion or defect in the area of the optic chiasma, which is a typical sign of pituitary tumors. Unilateral visual disturbance is usually the consequence of an orbital lesion proximal to the optic chiasma. Pale distention of the fundus oculi known as *papilledema* is demonstrated funduscopically. This feature develops early in the course of intracranial disease affecting the optic nerve. Therefore papilledema is a reliable indication of optic nerve damage in acute cases of increased intracranial pressure such as injury. Visual acuity alone is not a particularly dependable indicator of optic nerve damage.

Oculomotor, trochlear, and abducens nerves. The third, fourth, and sixth cranial nerves supply motor innervation to the muscles of eye movement. The trochlear nerve innervates the superior oblique muscle, the abducens mediates the lateral rectus muscle, and the oculomotor nerve supplies the other ocular muscles. Eye movement is evaluated by asking the patient to follow the examiner's finger with the eyes as the finger is moved throughout the visual field. The movements of each eye should be evaluated individually with the other eye covered and then both are evaluated together. The examiner's finger is then slowly moved from a distance of three feet to within an inch of the nasal bridge to demonstrate the medial rotation of both eyes of *visual convergence* and the constriction of the pupil of *visual accommodation.* A pen light is then used to demonstrate *reactivity to direct light* of the pupil by constriction.

Anisocoria or unequal pupil size is frequently observed among healthy individuals, but it may be caused by several CNS, ciliary, or sympathetic defects. Bilaterally enlarged or diminished pupil size usually suggests either prescription or illicit drug use. Pupils that are dilated and fixed or nonreactive to light reflect cessation of CNS function. *Strabismus,* lack of coordination of the direction of vision of the eyes, results from many conditions, including cranial nerve deficiency. Oculomotor paralysis results in dilated pupil, lateral deviation, and *ptosis* or drooping of the upper eyelid caused by loss of levator palpebrae superioris muscle function. This as well as trochlear and abducens defects and a number of other CNS diseases can produce *binocular diplopia* or double vision. Trochlear paralysis is suggested by inferior, medial gaze of the affected eye from superior oblique muscle weakness and internal rotation, but this subtle defect is rare. Abducens defects present as medial deviation from lateral rectus muscle weakness but this is more often an early feature of increased intracranial pressure. *Nystagmus,* involuntary and cyclic movement of the eyes, of various types is evidence of several CNS and neuromuscular diseases such as multiple sclerosis.

Trigeminal nerve. The ophthalmic, maxillary, and mandibular divisions of the trigeminal nerve convey sensory fibers to these regions and motor innervation of the muscles of mastication, including the temporalis, masseter, lateral pterygoid, medial pterygoid, and anterior belly of the digastric. Other functions of the trigeminal nerve include motor innervation of the tensor palatini, tensor tympani, and mylohyoid muscles as well as autonomic sensory supply to the ciliary, pterygopalatine, submandibular, and otic ganglia. The motor function

of the trigeminal nerve can be tested by observation of jaw movements and biting. The most sensitive trigeminal sensory function, the *corneal reflex,* is tested by brushing the cornea with a wisp of cotton while the patient looks away. Both eyes normally blink simultaneously. The corneal reflex is often absent among stoic individuals or contact lens wearers. Cotton or a pin used to demonstrate skin sensitivity in areas innervated by the three divisions is often more convenient.

Damage from stroke and medullary lesions may cause contralateral sensory defects within the area of one or more divisions of the trigeminal nerve. The deficiency seldom extends all of the way to the midline, however, because sensory fibers crossover at the midline. Unilateral muscle of mastication weakness is seldom identified following a stroke unless other manifestations of the damage are severe and clinically apparent. Most masticatory muscle dysfunction reflects peripheral conditions rather than CNS disease.

Facial nerve. The facial nerve provides motor supply to the muscles of facial expression, the sensory pathway for taste of the anterior two thirds of the tongue, and sensory fibers to a small area of the external auditory meatus and auricle. Secretory parasympathetic innervation to the salivary, lacrimal, and minor nasal mucosa glands are also facial nerve functions. Motor function is evaluated by requesting the patient to smile, elevate the eyebrows, and show the teeth. Asymmetry of facial movement should be carefully observed and evaluated to identify asymmetric facial expression habits. Taste can be evaluated by placing salt and sugar on the lateral borders of the tongue.

The clinician must be alert for abnormalities in the movements of the muscles of facial expression since motor neuropathy of the facial nerve is common. Weakness of the lower muscles of facial expression including the platysma and orbicularis oris usually indicates a CNS defect of the contralateral side. Unilateral weakness of all of the muscles of facial expression often results from a nuclear or peripheral defect known as *Bell's palsy*. Absence of taste on the anterior two thirds of the tongue on the same side as facial weakness indicates the presence of a central lesion, while normal taste with muscle weakness implies a lesion peripheral to the facial canal.

Vestibulocochlear nerve. Hearing and sensory input contributing to balance are supplied by the vestibulocochlear nerve. Normal function is evident by the patient's ability to converse during the diagnostic interview and normal gait. Balance can be assessed by the *Romberg test* in which the patient stands with the eyes closed, arms extended, and the head back. The clinician must be prepared to catch the patient if a balance deficiency exists.

Glossopharyngeal and vagus nerves. The glossopharyngeal nerve conducts taste fibers to the posterior tongue, motor fibers to the stylopharyngeal muscle, parasympathetic fibers to the parotid gland, and sensory fibers to much of the pharynx and structures such as the carotid body. The vagus nerve is responsible for all motor function of smooth muscles, secretory function of all glands, and motor function of most laryngeal, pharyngeal, and soft palate muscles. Afferent supply to the mucosal surfaces of internal organs and inhibitory cardiac innervation are additional vagal functions.

The glossopharyngeal and the vagus nerves provide diverse neural supply but their normal function is rather easily evaluated. The ability to speak clearly demonstrates laryngeal motor function, and the ability to open the mouth and say "ah" with symmetry demonstrates normal muscular function of the oropharynx. Stimulating the gag reflex by brushing the posterior pharynx with the intraoral mirror confirms sensory function of the glossopharyngeal nerves. If a deficient gag reflex is a motor function problem, then the voice is also affected. If the gag reflex is absent and the voice is normal, then the defect is a sensory glossopharyngeal deficiency. Vocal cord paralysis or hoarseness without loss of the gag reflex indicates a laryngeal lesion or a mediastinal disease affecting the recurrent laryngeal branch of the vagus nerve.

Spinal accessory nerve. The eleventh cranial nerve provides motor innervation to the sternocleidomastoid and trapezius muscles. If the patient is able to turn the head to both sides and to shrug the shoulders against pressure, this adequately demonstrates normal function.

Unilateral weakness of the trapezius and the sternocleidomastoid muscles usually reflects deficiency of peripheral origin. Bilateral weakness of both muscles indicates a brain stem lesion or an early sign of primary muscle disease such as muscular dystrophy.

Hypoglossal nerve. The hypoglossal nerves provide the motor supply of the intrinsic and extrinsic muscles of the tongue excluding the palatoglossus muscle. Observation of symmetrical tongue movements during protrusion, elevation, and buccal thrusting of the tongue indicates normal function.

Asymmetry of tongue position or tongue movement suggests unilateral hypoglossal nerve deficiency. At rest the tongue is pulled toward the side of normal muscle strength and away from the side of muscular weakness. On protrusion the tongue deviates toward the weak side, since the stronger muscles essentially push the tongue to this position. Because of cranial nerve crossover, a suspected CNS lesion is contralateral to the side affected by muscular weakness. Therefore a CNS defect would be expected contralateral to the side toward which the tongue deviates on protrusion.

Arms and Hands

The extraoral examination includes assessment of the patient's arms and hands. This can be conveniently accomplished during the blood pressure determination. Three specific features should be observed while examining the arms and hands: (1) skin of the arm, (2) relative size and appearance of the hands, and (3) appearance of the fingernails.

The skin of the arm is examined for lesions in the same manner as the face. Many skin diseases predominantly affect specific anatomic locations and most are likely to affect the skin of either the face or the arms.

Development of the hands and fingers can be altered in several developmental syndromes that also affect the teeth and jaws. Observations of particular interest relative to developmental abnormalities include fused digits known as *syndactyly,* missing fingers, and extra digits referred to as *polydactyly.* Disproportional size or relationships of the fingers and hands is also a feature of several developmental conditions. Generalized inflammatory disease of the joints is often revealed by enlargement, erythema, and tenderness affecting the joints of the hands. The pattern of the joints affected can suggest the type of arthritis. The extent of the manifestations can be a general indicator of the severity of the disease in other joints or the effectiveness of current treatment.

Abnormality of the fingernails can be a manifestation of several systemic diseases. Generalized clubbing of the distal area around the nails is a sign of advanced cardiovascular or cardiopulmonary dysfunction. A dull color and spoon-shaped contour of the nails referred to as *koilonychia* suggests iron deficiency anemia or cardiopulmonary disease. Chalky white or an unusual dark pink color of the nails can result from advanced hepatic or renal disease. Bluish discoloration of the nail bed is an early sign of cyanosis resulting from inadequate blood oxygenation or peripheral circulation. Pitted or linear malformations of several nails may signify a recent severe illness. Abnormality of a single nail usually represents the damage resulting from local injury or infection. Severe malformation of most of the nails or absence of true nail formation suggests a genetic defect affecting the integumentary tissues.

SUMMARY

The extraoral physical examination consists of the general patient assessment, determination of vital signs, and the evaluation of specific extraoral tissues. These observations contribute to physical assessment of the patient and to diagnosis of head and neck abnormalities.

The general patient assessment provides an impression of the person's general health that could be formed during conversation in a nonclinical setting. This consists of visual observation of the patient's apparent age, gender, race, emotional status, anatomic development, posture, movements, and speech. Determination of vital signs is included in general patient assessment as a reflection of essential physiologic functions. Pulse rate, pulse quality, respiration rate and rhythm, blood pressure, and body temperature are the elements of this functional evaluation.

The physical examination of extraoral structures is accomplished by a combination of visualization, palpation, and functional assessment. Head and neck tissues are the focus of the dentist's extraoral examination including the facial form, facial skin, eyes, ears, nose, superficial facial tissues, parotid glands, neck, and temporomandibular function. The need to evaluate the function of specific cranial nerves may be indicated by observations during the head and neck examination, although formal appraisal of the cranial nerves is not a routine part of the dentist's examination. Physical examination of the hands, nails, and arms during the blood pressure determination may reveal additional evidence of skin conditions and systemic disease.

BIBLIOGRAPHY

Brightman VJ: Rational procedures for diagnosis and medical risk assessment. In Lynch MA, Brightman VJ, Greenberg MS, editors: Burket's oral medicine: diagnosis and treatment, ed 8, Philadelphia, 1984, Lippincott.

DeGowin RL: DeGowin and DeGowin's bedside diagnostic examination, ed 5, New York, 1987, MacMillan.

Judge RD, Zuidema GD, Fitzgerald FT, editors: Clinical diagnosis: a physiologic approach, ed 5, Boston, 1988, Little, Brown.

Kerr DA, Ash MM, Millard HD: Oral diagnosis, ed 6, St Louis, 1983, Mosby–Year Book.

Langlais RP and others: Oral diagnosis, oral medicine and treatment planning, Philadelphia, 1984, Saunders.

Seidel HM and others: Mosby's guide to physical examination, St Louis, 1987, Mosby–Year Book.

CHAPTER 5

Intraoral Physical Examination

GARY C. COLEMAN

The mouth by definition is the diagnostic and treatment responsibility of the dentist. The intraoral physical examination always yields essential information that affects the dentist's diagnostic and treatment decisions. Data from the patient history, the extraoral examination, and other sources certainly contribute to the diagnostic evaluation, but information obtained during the intraoral examination exerts the greatest and most direct impact.

Strong intraoral examination skills and an attitude of attention to subtle deviations from typical features are valuable assets to every dentist. The oral examination is most effectively approached with the attitude of confirming normal findings in addition to identifying abnormalities. Omissions or oversights during the examination are less likely if the clinician develops a systematic examination routine. In addition, all intraoral procedures, including physical examination, should be conducted in a manner consistent with infection control recommendations. This specifically includes wearing examination gloves.

EXAMINATION OF THE ORAL SOFT TISSUES

Examination of the oral soft tissues is accomplished by inspection, visualization, and palpation. Oral structures exhibit bilateral symmetry in most respects. Any asymmetric contours or variation in the uniformity of mucosal color or texture within specific anatomic regions suggest the possibility of an abnormality.

Lips

The extraoral surfaces of the lips normally appear pale pink and homogeneous in color with sharp delineation of the mucosal border with the skin. Shallow linear grooves of the lip surface that are aligned perpendicular to the vermilion border are usually present in adults. Common abnormalities involving the external surface of the lip include ulcers, rough surface texture, and patchy, homogeneous white thickening.

The intraoral labial mucosa is visualized by everting the upper and lower lips. The mucosa normally appears deep pink and homogeneous

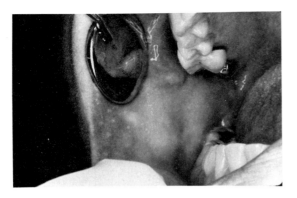

Fig. 5-1 Buccal mucosa. The pale foci near the mirror are Fordyce's granules, and the mild elevation near the maxillary molar is the parotid papilla. The full extent of the buccal vestibule can be visualized when the patient closes the jaws slightly and the clinician retracts the buccal tissues by applying firm pressure on the mirror.

in color near the vermilion surface with a gradual transition to a deeper red and prominent vascularity near the extent of the mucolabial vestibule. Bidigital palpation reveals uniform submucosal consistency and thickness. Firm, submucosal nodules that are less than 1 cm in diameter can be palpated within the lips of many adults. Uniformity in size suggests that these nodules represent fibrosis of the minor salivary glands. The labial frenum normally appears as a slender, midline band or arch of mucosa at the height of the mucolabial vestibule. A small, nodular "tag" of tissue that appears attached to the labial frenum is a healed traumatic tear of the frenum and is a common finding.

Buccal Mucosa

The buccal mucosa is examined visually by having the patient open the mouth to slightly less than maximal opening and then retracting the cheek away from the teeth with a mirror or finger as shown in Fig. 5-1. The buccal mucosa is similar to the labial mucosa in exhibiting a deep, homogeneous pink color at the

level of the occlusal plane and a more red, vascular appearance at the greatest extent of the mucobuccal vestibule. A homogeneous white line, called the *linea alba,* is a common observation at the level of the occlusal plane. This is physiologic thickening of the mucosal epithelium in response to the recurring friction of a cheek-chewing or cheek-sucking habit. The linea alba is usually bilateral when present, and the width varies depending on the nature of the patient's habit. Adjacent to the buccal surface of the maxillary second molar is the parotid papilla (Fig. 5-1) and the associated orifice of the parotid (or Stensen's) duct. The size of the parotid papilla varies among patients, and inexperienced clinicians occasionally mistake a prominent parotid papilla as an abnormal enlargement. Visualization of several drops of saliva flowing from the parotid papilla during extraoral compression of the parotid gland confirms normal function. Most adults exhibit numerous small, yellowish spots on the buccal mucosa, which are ectopic sebaceous glands known as *Fordyce's granules* (Fig. 5-1). These structures are uniformly distributed, are generally less than 1 to 3 mm in diameter, and may appear slightly elevated. As with the lips, bidigital palpation of the buccal mucosa may reveal nodularity attributable to fibrosis of the minor salivary glands.

Buccal Vestibule

The buccal vestibule can be inspected by retracting the cheeks with the fingers while the mouth is open and then asking the patient to bring the teeth nearly together. The buccal and labial vestibules are visualized and palpated to demonstrate their superior and inferior extent and symmetric contours. The facial surfaces of the maxilla and mandible are palpated to identify atypical elevations or depressions in the contour of the bone. The initial signs of many jaw enlargements are partial loss of the buccal vestibular extent and convex expansion of the alveolar bone. The facial surfaces of both the maxilla and the mandible are

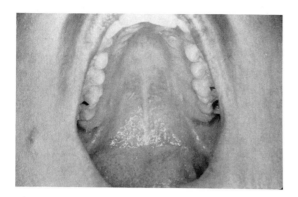

Fig. 5-2. Direct visualization of the hard and soft palates demonstrates the symmetry and contours of these surfaces.

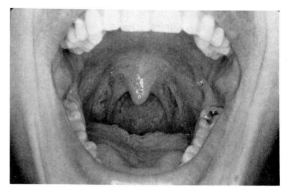

Fig. 5-3. Visualization of the oropharynx while the patient responds to the request to say "ah." The soft palate is symmetrically elevated, revealing the vascular appearance of the posterior pharyngeal wall mucosa. The palatine tonsils are the rough, lobular tissues lateral to the pharyngeal opening between the tonsillar pillars.

firmly palpated by slowly sliding the tip of the finger along the alveolar surfaces at the periapical level to identify the tenderness or enlargement of periapical inflammatory lesions.

Hard Palate

Indirect inspection of the hard palate using the mouth mirror provides a detailed inspection of the surface. Direct vision is accomplished from the submental perspective with the patient's mouth open wide and the head hyperextended. The direct vision approach provides better visualization of the posterior palatal contours in evaluating symmetry of the region, as shown in Fig. 5-2.

The normal palatal mucosa appears pale pink and homogeneous in color. The palatal rugae of the anterior hard palate typically present a folded, corrugated appearance that is symmetric without fissuring between the prominences. The anterior hard palate and the midline of the posterior hard palate are firm to palpation. The lateral aspects of the posterior hard palate and palatal alveolus are slightly more compressible. The palatal alveolus is palpated at the periapical level for tender foci in the same manner as the facial alveolus. A common abnormality of the hard palate in adults is

a bony hard enlargement at the midline, called a *maxillary torus*.

Soft Palate

The soft palate is easily inspected during direct visualization of the hard palate. Depression of the tongue with a mouth mirror is often necessary to fully demonstrate the soft palate. Functional elevation of the soft palate is illustrated by requesting the patient to say "ah," and muscular depression is revealed by asking the patient to blow air through the nose while the nostrils are compressed. Palpation of the soft palate causes gagging and is not routinely performed unless an abnormality is observed visually. Palpation can then be accomplished by using a single finger to quickly stroke laterally from the midline. The normal soft palate is spongy and homogeneous to palpation without nodularity.

The mucosa of the soft palate typically appears reddish pink with prominence of the underlying vascularity (Fig. 5-3). The soft palate of older individuals may appear somewhat yellow as a consequence of an increased proportion of submucosal fat tissue. The soft palate normally appears loose and mobile with symmetric changes in contour during function.

Oropharynx

The oropharynx is visualized directly while the tongue is depressed with the mouth mirror and the patient says "ah." The nodular tissues shown in Fig. 5-3 between the tonsillar pillars are the palatine tonsils. Palpation of the oropharynx also causes gagging and is not routinely performed unless an abnormality is visually apparent. Palpation of the tonsillar pillar is most effectively accomplished with a stroking motion over the suspicious area using a single finger. Application of blunt pressure with the mirror handle may reveal additional features without causing excessive patient discomfort. The tonsillar pillar area and tonsillar bed are normally spongy to palpation if the underlying muscles are relaxed. These muscles usually contract in response to the pressure of palpation, resulting in a firmer, more muscular resistance.

Children often exhibit prominence of the "tonsils," which may be pronounced enough to suggest obstruction of the pharyngeal opening. This condition is not considered abnormal unless it is associated with signs of inflammation or obstruction, such as difficulty swallowing and mouth breathing. In adults the tonsils are often atrophic and difficult to visualize. Surgical removal produces pale scarring of the tonsillar bed and pillars. This is characterized by a radial or stellate pattern of distinct, pale, flat white lines in this area (see Fig. 15-17). Occasionally the tonsillectomy may have been incomplete, resulting in the retention of several lymphoid nodules. Conspicuous surface crypts are occasionally observed on the tonsillar surface, which is normal unless they exhibit erythema and exudate.

The posterior pharyngeal wall normally appears richly vascular with a variable number of discrete gelatinous-appearing surface promi-

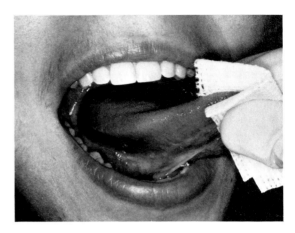

Fig. 5-4. Visualization of the lateral border of the tongue.

nences that are coral pink and homogeneous in color. These are lymphoid aggregates that are separate from the palatine, lingual, and pharyngeal tonsils. Erythema of the tonsillar pillars and oropharynx without discomfort is commonly associated with smoking and nasal congestion. Erythema associated with complaints of pain on swallowing is typical of pharyngitis.

Tongue

The dorsum of the tongue is best visualized by requesting the patient to protrude the tongue while the mouth is open. The ventral surface is most effectively examined visually by requesting the patient to touch the palate with the tip of the tongue while the mouth is open. The lateral borders and posterior surfaces of the tongue are demonstrated by wrapping the tip of the tongue with a cotton gauze and gently drawing the tongue out of the mouth and laterally (Fig. 5-4). Bidigital palpation of the tongue reveals its muscular consistency.

The dorsal tongue surface normally exhibits a relatively uniform pale pink color and a uniformly rough surface texture consisting of numerous filiform papillae with a scattering of the larger fungiform papillae. Approximately 10 to 14 larger circumvallate papillae are responsible for the nodular, irregular contours in the posterior region of the dorsal tongue surface. The median groove or fissure varies in prominence and may be unapparent. The presence of numerous deep fissures on the dorsal surface is referred to as *fissured tongue* and is a common anatomic variation. The ventral surface appears vascular and smooth with the exception of the lingual frenum and the thin, webbed projections of the plica fimbriata lateral to the frenum. Large, bluish vessels called *lingual varicosities* are dilated veins that are often seen in a symmetric pattern on the ventral surface of the tongue and floor of the mouth. These distended vessels are of no clinical significance.

Floor of the Mouth

The floor of the mouth can be visualized at the same time the ventral surface and lateral borders of the tongue are examined. Bimanual palpation of the floor of the mouth as shown in Fig. 3-1 is the most effective palpation technique for this region.

The floor of the mouth exhibits a rolling contour that changes with different tongue positions and the degree of contraction of the extrinsic tongue muscles. The sublingual caruncles are demonstrated in Fig. 5-5 as nodular elevations immediately lateral to the lingual frenum midway between the alveolus and the base of the tongue. They contain the orifices of the submandibular (or Wharton's) ducts. Salivary flow from these structures can normally be produced by compression of the submandibular glands. These glands are normally mobile, well delineated, slightly compressible, and located in the posterior aspect of the lateral floor of the mouth. The sublingual glands are located in the anterior, lateral floor of the mouth. The sublingual glands are more compressible, less distinctly delineated, and somewhat more difficult to identify by palpation as compared with the submandibular glands.

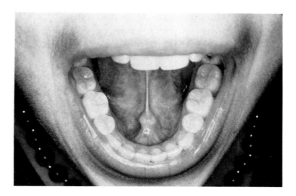

Fig. 5-5. Visualization of the floor of the mouth and the ventral surface of the tongue by requesting the patient to touch the palate with the tip of the tongue. The lingual frenum and sublingual caruncles are apparent.

The primary purpose of palpating this area is to identify enlarged submandibular or submental lymph nodes, salivary stones (known as *sialoliths*) along the course of Wharton's duct, and asymmetric, nodular enlargement of the salivary glands. The lingual contour of the mandible is examined visually and by palpation for typical contour, mucosal lesions, and periapical tenderness. Bony hard, typically bilateral prominences of the lingual alveolar process in the mandibular canine region are called *mandibular tori* and are a common observation among adults.

EXAMINATION OF THE TEETH

Examination of the teeth generally follows the intraoral soft tissue examination. The dental examination can be approached as a two-stage process: (1) dental orientation examination of the teeth by visual inspection and (2) comprehensive examination of each tooth by visualization and probing. This approach enhances diagnostic accuracy by familiarizing the clinician with the general nature of the patient's dental status before the examination of more specific features.

Dental Orientation Examination

The orientation portion of the dental examination is accomplished by most clinicians during the soft tissue examination. This visual inspection of the teeth is accomplished using the mouth mirror without specific efforts to remove saliva and food debris from the teeth. Initial determinations include the teeth present, the quality of oral hygiene, and the general extent of calculus. The presence of generalized dental conditions such as extensive decay, dental malformations, discoloration, and malalignment is also observed. The quality, extent, and types of past dental treatment also contribute to the general dental assessment.

Indications of poor oral hygiene include accumulations of food debris, bacterial plaque, gingival inflammation, and fetid breath. Poor oral hygiene contributes significantly to the development and progression of dental caries and periodontitis. However, numerous other factors affect this cause-and-effect relationship for each individual. Predictably, many patients with poor oral hygiene suffer from extensive dental decay and periodontitis. However, other patients with poor oral hygiene exhibit little decay and minimal periodontitis. Poor oral hygiene should promote the suspicion that dental decay and periodontitis are present, but the suspicion must be confirmed by examination.

The presence of numerous carious lesions and restorations that reflect past decay regardless of oral hygiene effectiveness should prompt the dentist to evaluate other contributory factors, such as diet. Cavities of typically decay-resistant surfaces should be suspected. Numerous cavities may reflect the absence of routine dental treatment in recent years, increased vulnerability to decay, or both. This may be clarified by additional questions about recent dental care, diet, and oral hygiene habits. Exceptional vulnerability to decay indicates that careful examination for easily overlooked lesions such as cervical cavities is necessary.

The orientation examination reveals the number of erupted teeth in the mouth. The patient history and additional findings from the dental orientation may suggest why certain teeth are absent. The extraction of numerous teeth because of decay or periodontal destruction not only indicates vulnerability to these diseases, but also suggests a patient priority limited to symptomatic dental care. An absent premolar in each quadrant usually indicates past orthodontic treatment and the need to specifically examine for abnormalities that are occasional complications of orthodontic correction. Several missing teeth in one area and good general dental health otherwise may indicate that the teeth were lost as a result of traumatic injury and the need to examine for additional traumatic damage in the area. A generalized pattern of teeth that did not form or formation of extra teeth may suggest a developmental syndrome. Radiographs are essential to determining the presence of teeth because many clinically absent teeth have not erupted.

Generalized abnormal color of the teeth may result from incorporation of pigmented materials during dental development or from a genetic defect of dental tissues. Symmetric color abnormality limited to teeth that form simultaneously and normal appearance of teeth that calcify at other times suggest severe illness during development. Discoloration of a single tooth usually reflects pulpal necrosis. A small tooth, particularly if it appears slightly yellow or whiter in color as compared with the other teeth, is often a retained deciduous tooth associated with a missing or impacted succedaneous tooth.

Excessive wear can result from a diet consisting primarily of coarse foods or from *bruxism,* which is habitual grinding of the teeth. Excessive wear can cause overclosure of the jaws and may be associated with muscular or temporomandibular joint pain. Supereruption of unopposed teeth often leads to a more rapid progression of periodontitis and complex restorative considerations. Malalignment can cause greater focal vulnerability to periodontitis and may suggest the need for orthodontic evaluation. Jaw relationships, identification of crossbites, and other unusual occlusal relationships should be determined.

Observation of coronal tooth fractures supports the suspicion that additional, less obvious damage caused by a traumatic episode, such as pulpal necrosis, root fractures, or tooth mobility, may be present. Multiple fractures or traumatic injuries may be an indication of physical abuse or a seizure disorder.

The nature and extent of past dental treatment become apparent during the orientation inspection of the patient's mouth. The presence of numerous restorations that appear technically sound and well planned suggests that the patient is decay prone and has received regular care by a skilled dentist. A concerted effort to identify recurrent decay is appropriate in such cases. Conspicuous examples of technically poor restorative care should prompt skepticism about the general quality of other seemingly satisfactory dental restorations in the same mouth. Indications of treatment for a chief complaint without definitive care, such as pulpal access openings without completion of the endodontic procedure, suggest a poor patient attitude toward complying with dental treatment recommendations.

Comprehensive Physical Examination of Teeth

The comprehensive dental examination is a detailed diagnosis of each tooth for evidence of decay, malformation, and other abnormalities. The difference from the visual orientation examination is that the comprehensive examination also includes palpation and probing. The clinician's attitude should be that this examination will serve as the primary basis for diagnostic and treatment decisions and that information from other sources, such as radiographs, will be supplemental.

All tooth surfaces should be examined in detail visually and by probing for evidence of decay. Occlusal surfaces must be examined by probing all decay-prone pits and fissures. Lesions may be suggested visually by chalky white or dark discoloration or cavitation, but a catch by decalcified sites during probing is definitive evidence of decay. Facial and lingual surfaces are usually adequately examined visually, with the exception of exposed root surfaces and developmental irregularities such as buccal pits. Both of these conditions require probing of the vulnerable sites in essentially the same manner as for the occlusal pits and fissures.

Access to the interproximal surfaces for probing is limited in many situations by narrow embrasure spaces and enlarged gingival tissues. Most small interproximal cavities of posterior teeth must be identified radiographically because their location immediately apical to the contact point is usually inaccessible to the probe. Unfortunately, this situation leads many dentists to rely entirely on radiographs to diagnose all interproximal cavities and defects. This causes interproximal cavities to be overlooked when radiographic demonstration of decay is inconclusive as a consequence of conditions such as malalignment and restorations. Positioning the explorer tine interproximally and directing pressure axially as illustrated in Fig. 5-6 is often an effective method to complement radiographic detection of interproximal decay.

Existing restorations are usually documented during the comprehensive dental examination. From a diagnostic perspective, the pattern of past dental care indicates the nature of the patient's dental caries experience. In addition, the pattern of existing restorations is an important consideration during dental treatment planning. Metallic restorative materials are visually obvious. Some porcelain and composite restorations may not be apparent even to experienced clinicians. Probing with an explorer for margins or gently sliding the explorer tip across the surface to detect the grainy or glossy surface texture of composite

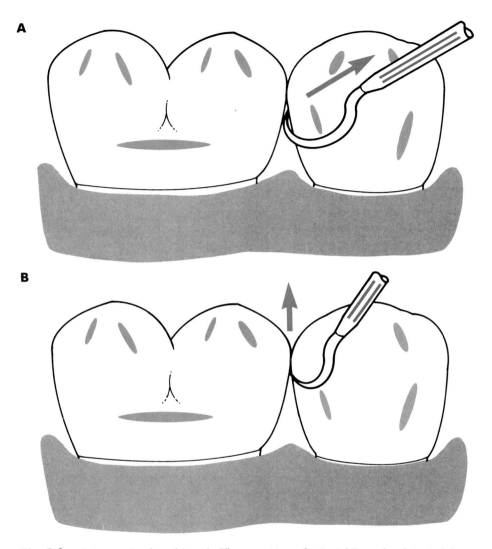

Fig. 5-6. Interproximal probing. **A,** The sensation of a "catch" can be detected for many interproximal carious lesions by placement of the explorer tine immediately apical to the contact point in such a way that pressure can be directed axially and slightly superiorly. **B,** Angulation of the explorer so that the probing pressure is directed superiorly results in a false "catch" sensation from wedging within the embrasure.

materials usually reveals these esthetic restorations. All margins of dental restorations are decay-prone sites and must be probed.

In addition to examination by visualization and probing, each tooth should be examined by palpation and percussion for signs of mobility, tenderness, and fracture. Additional methods of examination are selectively employed by most dentists. For example, electrical and thermal pulp testing is normally undertaken only if pulpitis or pulpal necrosis is suspected on the basis of other findings. Transillumination to detect interproximal decay affecting incisors is not generally used unless more consistently definitive methods, such as probing and radiographic examination, are inconclusive.

EXAMINATION OF THE PERIODONTIUM

The goal of the periodontal examination is to identify evidence of destructive inflammatory disease of the dental supportive tissues. Visual examination of healthy gingiva reveals uniform, noncompressible contours with typical, homogeneous pink color and stippling. Signs of gingival inflammation include erythema, edema, exudate expressed by palpation, and pain. Areas of gingival enlargement, recession, or cleft formation require particular attention during the probing portion of the periodontal examination.

Periodontal probing of gingival sulcus depth by the six-point-per-tooth format is usually performed after the comprehensive dental examination. Healthy gingival sulcus depth is normally expected to be in the range of 1 to 2 mm without bleeding or exudate during probing. Greater depth suggests deterioration and apical displacement of the gingival attachment to the root surface. Determination of periodontal pocket depth not only provides one of the best diagnostic indications of the patient's periodontal status, but is also vital for later comparisons in determining treatment effectiveness. Possible causes of inaccurate periodontal probing results are described in Chapter 3.

Several additional diagnostic findings can be of considerable importance in the periodontal evaluation. The vertical width of the attached gingiva is normally at least 3 mm. Teeth with less attached gingiva are vulnerable to loss of attachment and the eventual formation of clefts. Excessive frenum pressure can produce similar defects. Tooth mobility can result from conditions such as lateral occlusal forces, habits, and loss of alveolar bone sup-

port. Unless the causes of mobility can be corrected, the nonphysiologic stretching of the periodontal apparatus usually leads to gradual deterioration of the dental attachment. Periodontal pocket formation between the roots of a multirooted tooth is referred to as a *furcation defect* or *furcation involvement.* These defects are generally difficult to treat and indicate a relatively poor periodontal prognosis. The severity of the furcation defect is usually graded subjectively by the clinician as early, moderate, or advanced, based on the depth of the defect and the contours of the furcation. Additional local conditions, such as malalignment of teeth and poor adaptation of dental restorations, that directly affect periodontal health should also be identified.

PRACTICAL ASPECTS OF INTRAORAL EXAMINATION

Skilled dentists rely on several general examination methods to efficiently achieve consistently accurate results. The importance of these examination principles justifies repeating them:

1. Performing different portions of the examination in a routine, systematic sequence minimizes oversights and omissions. The specific sequence is not as important as the consistency of the dentist's approach.

2. Visual findings are optimized by favorable patient positioning, good lighting, a clean mirror, and elimination of oral materials with the air syringe. Inability to see clearly by either direct or indirect visualization implies the need to change one of these factors.

3. Accurate probing results require the use of appropriate instruments that are in good condition. A sharp explorer is necessary to detect subtle carious lesions.

4. Accuracy and efficiency are enhanced when the clinician relies on general observations to guide specific, detailed portions of the examination.

5. Accuracy is promoted by frequent compari-

sons of the findings from different diagnostic sources to confirm consistency. Contradictions reveal errors, oversights, and conditions that require additional evaluation. For example, radiographic and probing evidence of decay and periodontitis should be mutually confirmational in most cases.

SUMMARY

Physical examination of the oral cavity can be divided conceptually into assessment of soft tissues, examination of the teeth, and periodontal evaluation. Procedurally, however, the efficient clinician often pursues elements of all three portions of the examination simultaneously.

The examination of oral soft tissues relies on visualization and palpation. The lips, buccal mucosa, vestibular contours, hard palate, soft palate, oropharynx, tongue, and floor of the mouth are all characterized in health by specific features that can be determined by these methods. Palpation of the alveolar processes during the soft tissue examination may reveal features, such as periapical tenderness or expansion, that are indicative of bone disease.

The examination of the teeth is conducted in two stages. The orientation dental examination is primarily visual and is usually accomplished during the soft tissue examination. This inspection provides the clinician with a general impression of the patient's dental status, which aids in making the detailed diagnostic determinations for each tooth during the comprehensive dental examination. The comprehensive assessment includes examination of each tooth by visualization, probing, and palpation for the presence of abnormalities such as carious lesions and developmental defects.

The periodontal examination seeks to identify inflammation of the supportive tissues and the periodontal tissue destruction that it causes. Gingival inflammation is indicated by erythema, edematous enlargement, and exudate or bleeding from these tissues during palpation. Inflammatory damage to the supportive structures produces apical migration of the gingival attachment to the tooth root. This is demonstrated by probing the crevicular space to identify periodontal pocket formation. Additional effects of periodontal destruction, such as tooth mobility, furcation involvement, and absence of attached gingiva, suggest more advanced inflammatory disease.

BIBLIOGRAPHY

Brightman VJ: Rational procedures for diagnosis and medical risk assessment. In Lynch MA, Brightman VJ, Greenberg MS, editors: Burket's oral medicine: diagnosis and treatment, ed 8, Philadelphia, 1984, Lippincott.

Kerr DA, Ash MM, Millard HD: Oral diagnosis, ed 6, St Louis, 1983, Mosby–Year Book.

Langlais RP and others: Oral diagnosis, oral medicine and treatment planning, Philadelphia, 1984, Saunders.

CHAPTER 6

Documentation

GARY C. COLEMAN

Documentation in the context of health care refers to the production of a physical record that contains the pertinent information related to the diagnosis and treatment of the patient. More commonly used phrases such as "patient records" or "patient charting" essentially reflect aspects of this process.

The importance of patient documentation is revealed by listing several functions of the record. Patient documentation compensates for the limitations of the clinician's memory. Diligent efforts to identify and gather diagnostic data are wasted if essential facts are forgotten or misplaced by the time clinical decisions must be made. A comprehensive patient documentation format also minimizes omissions by reminding the clinician of the diagnostic information needed to complete the patient database. Adequate records are vital in institutions and group practices where several clinicians may eventually treat the patient. The documented information from the previous clinician saves the new clinician and the patient the time of repeating diagnostic procedures. Finally, in an era of frequent litigation, the patient documentation serves as a legitimate record of the clinician's perspective of information and events related to the diagnosis and treatment of an accusatory patient. This may be the dentist's only defense against complaints of inappropriate or substandard care.

Nearly as many patient documentation formats exist as there are dentists and all approaches offer advantages and are limited by disadvantages. Learning documentation procedures, adapting to a new record approach, and eventually devising an individualized patient record scheme are facilitated by an understanding of the features of an ideal patient documentation system.

FEATURES OF THE IDEAL PATIENT DOCUMENTATION SYSTEM

The perfect dental record system does not exist. Each record system is strong in some aspects and weak in others. If a perfect system did exist, however, it would achieve the following goals:

1. It would allow *quick and easy data entry.*
   For example, materials would be arranged

in the order that patient history and examination results are routinely gathered by the clinician.

2. It would allow *quick and easy data retrieval.* Information referred to frequently such as the patient's treatment plan and medical status would be located in an obvious or easily accessible part of the record. A consent form for a past surgical procedure, on the other hand, would rarely be needed and would be stored away from materials that are referred to more often.

3. It would be *comprehensive* by accommodating the complex information associated with complicated clinical situations.

4. It would be *brief* without redundancy.

5. It would be *clear* in demonstrating data even to someone other than the clinician who assembled and recorded the information. The design of the record would eliminate inconsistencies in the location of facts, ambiguous terms, and obscure abbreviations.

6. It would make using the data *convenient.* For example, the recording of dental decay would not be on the reverse side of the page on which the treatment plan is listed because the dentist would need to flip the page back and forth while planning treatment.

7. It would be *easily expandable* so that patient treatment over a period of years would retain the original findings as well as incorporate new information in a logical sequence.

8. It would be *versatile.* This can be considered from two perspectives. First, the documentation should be compatible with the clinical approach of all clinicians who use it and, second, it should accommodate the diversity of dental patients routinely treated. This also requires that different clinical departments in an institution must accept the approach as consistent with their perspective.

9. It would be *efficient* by quickly conveying complex information. As an example, the record design would provide a summary of the patient's medical status that can orient an experienced clinician in a few moments of study.

10. It would be *economical.* This consideration extends beyond the cost of materials for individual records to concerns such as long-term storage.

11. In training institutions the record system must also be *educational* by reinforcing diagnostic, treatment planning, and patient management principles.

As previously indicated, a perfect record system that achieves all of these goals is not possible. A versatile and comprehensive record system is unlikely to be brief, efficient, or economical. Therefore all patient documentation approaches are compromises of these goals and the compromise that serves best for one dentist is unlikely to work as well for another. As an example, the most effective system for the periodontist would probably be awkward and inefficient for the oral surgeon or restorative dentist.

A blank sheet of paper could be considered as the simplest patient documentation approach. It is certainly economical, versatile, and brief in design. Few clinicians would accept the approach, however, because of the time needed to repeatedly write procedural or identifying phrases such as "patient name" or "chief complaint" for every patient. Also, the lack of standardization in format from one clinical visit to the next would eventually make finding prior information difficult. The solution to these problems is the use of printed, standardized forms to record routine clinical information.

Operation of a dental office or clinic without relying on standardized forms to document information is hard to imagine. Fill-in-the-blank forms can be easily customized to the individual clinician's preferences and methods. Variable topics can be accommodated by a series of blank lines and noncommittal labels such as "Additional Comments" or "Additional Information." These standard forms can then be arranged in the most effective sequence to produce a patient record scheme that fits the dentist's methods and is the best compromise of the documentation goals for that practitioner.

As many options as the dentist has in formulating a patient documentation format, certain basic functions must be accomplished by all health record systems. A general approach to the recording of health care information known as the *problem-oriented patient record* has gained wide acceptance because it effectively accomplishes these essential functions.

PROBLEM-ORIENTED PATIENT RECORD

Most health care record systems are in one sense or another a modification of the problem-oriented documentation method. The concept underlying this approach is easier to understand if an alternative record scheme is briefly described for comparison.

The dentist of the nineteenth century typically provided dental care to a limited number of people who usually lived their entire lives within a few miles of their birth place. Treatment generally consisted of procedures to solve specific complaints. The dentist's memory was adequate to recall diagnostic information because it was limited to a brief patient history and simple physical findings. For these reasons, the dentist needed to document little more than the treatments provided for various complaints, the fee charged, and whether or not the patient paid the bill. Such information from several episodes of treatment for an individual or family was listed chronologically as the events occurred. This simple format of chronologically listing care as it is provided is referred to as the *treatment-oriented patient record*. Medical records of this era were somewhat more complex, but the chronological listing of procedures and results was essentially the same.

The problem-oriented patient record focuses not on treatments and results, but on the perceived health problems of the patient. In a sense, the problem-oriented format approaches clinical documentation from the diagnostic or patient perspective rather than from the treatment or clinician's viewpoint. The problem-oriented approach organizes clinical information into sections by the function that the information serves toward solving the patient problems. The dental application of this approach can be considered by describing the organization of the problem-oriented dental record.

ORGANIZATION OF THE PROBLEM-ORIENTED DENTAL RECORD

The problem-oriented patient record organizes information into baseline diagnostic data, identification of problems or the diagnosis of abnormalities, the plan for solving the problems, the actual problem-solving or treatment, and the outcome or reevaluation of the treatment. Other materials are also included to accomplish the administrative and legal functions of the record.

Administrative Documentation

This section functions to record information needed to interact with the patient on nonclinical matters. For example, the information needed for billing or insurance claims are in this section. The patient's name, address, telephone number, insurance carrier, place of work, and physician's name are examples of information that relate primarily to patient identification and administration. Documentation of the patient's informed consent for dental care is also included in the administrative section.

The complexity of the administrative section of the record typically increases with the patient volume of the dental care facility. A single practitioner's office may effectively record this information in a small section of the health history form, while a large dental clinic may require several pages to manage these issues. Administrative information is usually located near the front of the patient record for easy access by auxiliary personnel. Administrative information is usually duplicated on patient billing or ledger forms that are filed separately from the patient's clinical chart in most dental offices.

Diagnostic Database

The diagnostic database documents the patient's status at the initial diagnostic evaluation. This consists of the patient's chief complaint, past medical history, review of systems, physical examination findings, and results of adjunctive diagnostic procedures. The diagnostic database is the basis for the clinician's diagnostic and treatment planning decisions.

The patient history is usually accomplished by a combination of health questionnaire completed by the patient and additional discussion of responses, although some dentists prefer to conduct the entire patient history by interview. Numerous health questionnaires and patient history forms are commercially available. Two important features from a documentation perspective that all patient history forms should contain are (1) a specific space to succinctly summarize the patient's medical status and (2) a mechanism to record changes in the patient's medical status.

Many medical conditions and the use of certain medications by the patient necessitate modification of routine dental procedures to minimize the risk of complications. For example, penicillin is the antibiotic of choice for most dental infections, but its use is contraindicated for the patient with known allergy to the drug. The patient record should provide a conspicuous reminder to the clinician that the typical antibiotic therapy method must be altered for this patient. This notation is often referred to as a *medical alert* and is located in a portion of the record such as the treatment plan that the clinician is likely to consult at the beginning of each appointment. Some practitioners prefer color codes on the chart cover as a reminder. The important points in the use of medical alerts are (1) The medical alert should made in such a way that it will explicitly convey the medical warning without risk of misinterpretation. (2) The medical alert should be located where it will be noticed every time the clinician refers to the record. (3) Sensitive medical information should not be recorded on the cover of the record where it poses a potential breach of confidentiality.

The simplest documentation approach for the findings from the extraoral and nondental intraoral examinations is to simply provide space on the examination form for a written description of any lesions. This is ideal for patients with few abnormalities, but recording numerous findings for other patients can become tedious. An alternative is to list anatomic sites and common lesions with a corresponding column of "Normal" or "Abnormal" check-off boxes with space for more specific notes. This provides a "checklist" to document that routine aspects of the examination were performed without significant findings. Fig. 6-1 illustrates the combination of this approach and the use of anatomic diagrams on which to graphically represent abnormalities. Diagrammatic depiction of lesions with additional narrative comments more accurately conveys the nature of most conditions than a written description alone.

The documentation of the extraoral examination probably represents the greatest variation in content from one dental setting to another. Greater complexity of the extraoral examination forms is typically found in dental school records to reinforce examination skills and in oral surgeons' offices as needed to accommodate the extraoral aspects of these practices. In contrast, the periodontist, endodontist, and general dentist are less likely to invest a large amount of record space to record findings that seldom directly affect their practice. This should not imply that extraoral find-

BAYLOR COLLEGE OF DENTISTRY
Department of Oral Diagnosis
Examination Record

DATE ____________________

PATIENT'S NAME ____ REGISTRATION NO. ______________

COMPLETED BY ____________________________________ APPROVED BY ______________________________

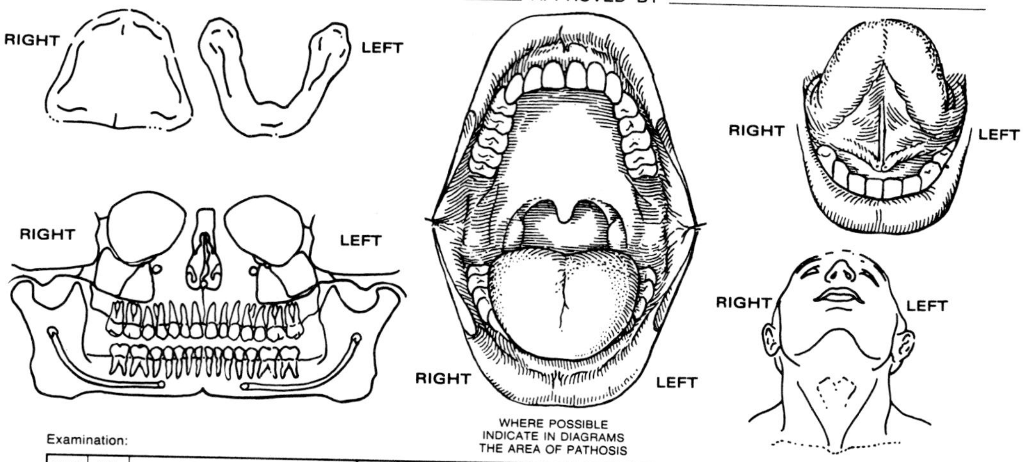
RIGHT
LEFT
RIGHT
LEFT
RIGHT
LEFT
RIGHT
LEFT
RIGHT
LEFT
WHERE POSSIBLE
INDICATE IN DIAGRAMS
THE AREA OF PATHOSIS

Examination:

YES	NO	HEAD AND NECK	YES	NO	TONGUE	YES	NO	TEETH
		1. Abnormalities			15. Abnormal size			26. Excessive wear
		2. Facial Asymmetry			16. Abnormal surface			27. Discoloration
		3. Lymphadenopathy			17. Lesions			28. Rampant decay
		4. Lesions			FLOOR OF MOUTH			29. Abnormal number
		FACE AND LIPS			18. Abnormalities			30. Demineralization
		5. Abnormalities			19. Lesions			31. Abnormal morphology
		6. Lesions			OROPHARYNX			OCCLUSION
		TEMPRO-MAND. JOINT			20. Palatine tonsils			32. Class I
		7. Limited Opening			21. Lesions			33. Class II
		8. Pain			GINGIVA			34. Class III
		9. Clicking, Popping, Crepitus			22. Abnormalities			35. Crossbite-r-l-ant-post
		10. Evidence-Bruxism			23. Lesions			36. Ant. open-bite
		PALATE			EDENTULOUS RIDGES			37. Centric intrf.
		11. Abnormal size/shape			24. Mand. abnormalities			38. Primary dent.
		12. Lesions			25. Max. abnormalities			39. Protrusive intrf.
		CHEEKS						40. Working intrf.
		13. Abnormalities						41. Balancing intrf.
		14. Lesions						

REMARKS: ____

____

____

____

Fig. 6-1 This examination form is designed to accommodate the findings from the physical and radiographic examinations excluding the comprehensive assessment of individual teeth. The anatomic diagrams allow the clinician to draw in unusual features and the "Remarks" section provides space to describe abnormalities in additional detail. The check-off format of the center section reminds the clinician of the specific elements of the physical examination to be completed. Checking off the "No" box for each element documents that examination was performed and that no abnormality was identified. A "Yes" response requires additional clarification in the "Remarks" section. Generalized abnormalities of the teeth including excessive wear, developmental defects, and occlusal relationships can also be indicated and described.

ings are not relevant to them, but the priority of extensive documentation for such findings is not as great.

Dental practitioners regardless of specialty or practice setting need to allocate sufficient documentation space for the description of nondental lesions of the oral cavity. The clinical management of such lesions requires comparison of the original features with changes following treatment or a reevaluation period. These comparisons are compromised if essential features such as lesion size were not recorded when the lesion was first identified. A common error in documenting nondental lesions is to record a diagnosis rather than the physical findings. This leaves the clinician with nothing for future comparison and introduces diagnostic bias. The diagnosis is appropriately recorded in the "Problem List" of the diagnosis section.

The anatomic diagrams illustrated in Fig. 6-1 allow efficient diagrammatic recording of features such as the location, shape, and extent of soft tissue lesions. Descriptive information such as the color, surface texture, and delineation of borders can then be recorded in addition to the graphic depiction to achieve a brief yet complete reflection of the abnormality. Photographs provide another effective method of documenting soft tissue lesions for future comparison. This does not replace the need to record diagnostic features in the patient database, but nothing serves better for later comparison than high-quality photographs. Documentation of the physical examination of the teeth and periodontal tissues is described later in this chapter.

Problem List

The problem list of the problem-oriented patient record is a summary listing of the patient's complaints, lesions, and conditions that warrant additional diagnostic evaluation or treatment. In addition, the tentative or definitive diagnosis is recorded for each problem. Considered from the treatment planning per-

spective, all additional diagnostic and treatment procedures must be justified by a listed patient problem. The problem list is organized by the priority of the problems in the judgment of the clinician. This is usually in the sequence of the chief complaint, current medical conditions, general dental problems, and specific dental lesions.

The diagnosis is preliminary in the problem list of medical records because the clinical evaluation of most medical problems will not yield a definitive diagnosis. Additional diagnostic tests are usually necessary to confirm clinical opinions or reach a definitive diagnosis. In contrast, the dentist can confidently reach a definitive diagnosis of most dental conditions on the basis of the diagnostic database. For this reason, most experienced dentists do not formally record a list of patient problems. Instead, they mentally organize the problems from the patient database and proceed directly to treatment planning. Although this is feasible for the experienced dentist, inexperienced clinicians find treatment planning simplified if patient problems are listed as part of the diagnostic process as described in Chapter 12.

Treatment Plan

The treatment plan is a listing of the diagnostic, preventive, therapeutic, and reevaluation procedures that are indicated in the clinician's judgment to solve the patient's problems. This listing is in the sequence in which the treatment will be performed. Accurate listing of the patient's problems provides a direct format for generation of the treatment plan. A large part of the treatment planning process can be accomplished by simply deciding the best approach for solving each listed problem in sequence of priority.

The documentation of the patient treatment plan provides space to list the procedures and for additional information about each specific treatment such as the anticipated fee, treatment completion date, and dental procedure code. Recording this information together aids in presenting the treatment proposal to the patient, tracking the course of treatment, and guiding auxiliary personnel in the completion of insurance claim forms. The treatment plan form should also provide space to record any necessary changes that become apparent as treatment progresses.

Progress Notes

The progress notes are the chronologic description of the events that are related to the patient's dental care as they occur. The progress notes can also be used to record administrative actions such as telephone conversations and payment of insurance claims. The patient record is designed so that a blank form can be inserted following a filled form to maintain the chronologic sequence of entries.

The progress notes serve two essential functions in the patient record. The first is to aid the clinician's memory in recalling the details of patient interactions during the course of patient care. This includes clarifying past events for any other dentist involved in treating the patient. Vital information for any progress note includes the date, the nature of the event, method of anesthesia, the result of the event, and the signature of the responsible clinician. This includes the student's signature and the countersignature of the supervising dentist in a teaching clinic. The function of the progress note is compromised if any of these items are omitted.

The second function of the progress note is to reflect the nature of the event as it occurred if questions about the event should ever arise. Entries should be permanent and unaltered as much as possible. All entries in the progress notes should, therefore, be made in ink. Any corrections are made by drawing a single line through the error and making the correction above or after the error. Alterations such as erasures and the use of "white-out" are avoided because they suggest record falsification after the fact in a situation involving accusation or litigation.

The progress notes section can become lengthy in the course of numerous patient visits. For this reason, the entries should be brief but adequate to inform a knowledgeable individual at a future date of the actions and events. Progress note content is analogous to the "who, what, when, where, why" of the news reporter. This essential information must always be recorded or questions concerning who performed the procedure or where the restoration was placed will eventually arise. A helpful indicator of the detail required in a progress notes entry for a particular event is that more detailed entries are needed for more significant events. A major treatment complication such as a drug reaction demands explanation in considerable detail, while more routine procedures such as border molding and final impressions for dentures can be limited to little more than that description. The clinician must remember while writing each progress note that it may provide the only description of the event from the clinician's perspective if a conflict or problem develops later.

Critically important information such as a change in the patient's medical status should not be "buried" in the progress notes where it will be difficult for another clinician to find. If, for example, a patient reports the recent development of an allergy to penicillin, a progress note to that effect is less likely to inform another clinician of the problem than updating the medical summary section and adding a medical alert to the patient record.

CHARTING DENTAL FINDINGS

Diagrammatic representation of dental findings or *dental charting* is a quick, efficient, and accurate method of recording the large volume of detailed information that is needed to reflect the patient's dental status. The experienced clinician can scan the dental chart and quickly learn or recall a great deal concerning the dental status of the patient.

Dental findings are recorded diagrammatically rather than in a narrative format. Any attempt to record dental diagnostic findings without graphic representation of the teeth fails as a consequence of the large volume of detailed information. The comprehensive dental examination can produce as many as ten to twenty items of information for each tooth. This makes a written description of the dental data impractical. The dentist's selection from among different dental charting schemes is based more on clinician's personal preference than inherent superiority of one approach compared with another.

Orientation

Several aspects of the clinician's preference for orientation of the dental charting are usually labeled to avoid confusion. This is particularly helpful when referring to the dental charts from another office or clinic. The example shown by Fig. 6-2 on pp. 82-83 demonstrates the diagram of the teeth oriented as if facing the patient with the patient's left to the right of the page. The alternative is a chart designed with the patient's right to the right of the page as if the clinician assumed a lingual perspective. This lingual orientation is favored by some dentists, but the generally accepted orientation is as if facing the patient. Both methods are commonly used and the same orientation preference affects how intraoral radiographs are viewed. Confusion can also arise over which aspect of the diagram represents the facial or lingual surfaces of the teeth, although the orientations is usually apparent by the design of the diagram. Nevertheless, labels to clarify the orientation minimize confusion. The primary teeth are usually represented by a separate diagram. This allows the same form to be used for adults and children.

Another aspect of orientation applies to the designation of teeth. Constantly repeating the anatomic terms for each tooth verbally and in written narrative is awkward and time consuming. Several abbreviation schemes for designating teeth have been developed to solve this problem. The most commonly used method in

North America is the Universal Numbering System. This approach assigns the maxillary right third molar the number "1" and the rest of the maxillary teeth are numbered in sequence toward the left third molar, which is "16." The mandibular left third molar is assigned "17" and the mandibular teeth are numbered in sequence around the arch toward the right to number "32," the mandibular right third molar. The primary teeth are designated by the capital letters "A" through "T" in the same sequence from maxillary right most posterior to the most distal mandibular right primary tooth. An alternative system of designating the primary teeth assigns the maxillary right second primary molar the abbreviation "1d" and the same sequence as the Universal System is followed to abbreviate the remaining primary teeth.

At least five other abbreviation schemes for the normal complement of teeth are in use. Most dental schools and insurance carriers rely on the Universal System. The approach used by many orthodontists, however, abbreviates the mandibular right first molar as "46" because it is the sixth tooth from the midline in the fourth quadrant. The symbol "$\underline{8}$" in another system indicates the eighth tooth in the upper left quadrant, the maxillary left third molar. The common use of different dental abbreviation systems requires the specification of the system or use of the full anatomic designations in all communications with other dentists to avoid confusion. This is particularly important with referrals for irreversible procedures such as extractions.

Charting Existing Dental Conditions

Dental charting relies on a diagram of the teeth on which to draw representations of existing restorations, carious lesions, and other significant findings. Symbols and abbreviations allow the clinician to record additional features such as missing teeth, impactions, and malalignments within the compact charting format. Space is usually provided adjacent to the anatomic diagram for recording periodontal probing depths, tooth mobility, and other findings related to periodontal health.

A detailed discussion of dental charting is impractical because the combination of symbols, abbreviations, and diagraming techniques are unique for each dental charting scheme. An example of the dental charting for a hypothetical patient is shown in Fig. 6-2 to illustrate one approach. Existing restorations are drawn as shaded shapes, which allows distinction from the carious lesions that can be shown as open outlines or in a different color. Periapical lesions, endodontic obturations, and other features identified radiographically can also be recorded on the anatomic diagram.

Periodontal probing depths are recorded in spaces adjacent to the anatomic diagram. The scaled horizontal lines of the example allow prominent periodontal defects to be represented quantitatively by being drawn on the anatomic diagram. Additional features of periodontitis such as mobility, clefts, and gingival bleeding are documented in this example by the use of symbols in spaces designated for each tooth adjacent to the diagram.

Conditions that affect all or most of the teeth are most efficiently recorded by written description. Narrative description of excessive wear or generalized toothbrush abrasion adequately documents these conditions without the clutter of graphically representing each site of lost tooth structure on the anatomic diagram. A short narration concerning the general features of the patient's periodontal health is also appropriate in most instances.

In contrast to other portions of the patient record, dental findings may be recorded graphically in pencil. Although this point could be argued by many clinicians, the practical justification is too compelling. Errors nearly always occur during dental charting. Incorrect entries made in pencil can easily be erased and corrected, while errors in ink present difficulties in clarifying the correct information in the limited space of a graphic chart.

PRACTICAL ASPECTS OF CLINICAL DOCUMENTATION

New dental examination results from a recall examination should be recorded on a new dental chart to avoid confusion by intermixing new findings with the original diagnostic information. Maintaining consistency in the use of symbols, abbreviations, and diagraming techniques also minimizes misinterpretations of the dental charting.

Several aspects of documentation in general are appropriately repeated for emphasis:

1. All entries must be signed and dated. This is particularly important in clinical situations involving more than one clinician.

2. All entries must be clearly stated and in adequate detail to provide the significant information or to describe the event. Obscure abbreviations, illegible handwriting, and omission of essential details produce meaningless entries.

3. All entries with the exception of dental charting should be made in ink to counter claims of alteration. Mistaken entries should have a single line drawn through them and the correction entered above or after the error. The clinician should then initial and date the change.

4. All elements of the patient record including original forms, radiographs, supplemental forms, and consultation letters should be identified with the patient's name, the date, and the patient's assigned identification number, if applicable. The assumption must be that any item can and eventually will become separated from the record.

5. Patient records should be protected from loss and damage. The value of a patient record in one sense is determined by the time invested in determining and recording the clinical information. From another perspective, materials such as radiographs and the progress notes are irreplaceable.

6. Unfortunate situations develop daily in which patients are upset or disappointed with dental treatment regardless of the

Light Blue: Existing
Dark Blue: Carious - Abnormal

EXAMINATION CHART

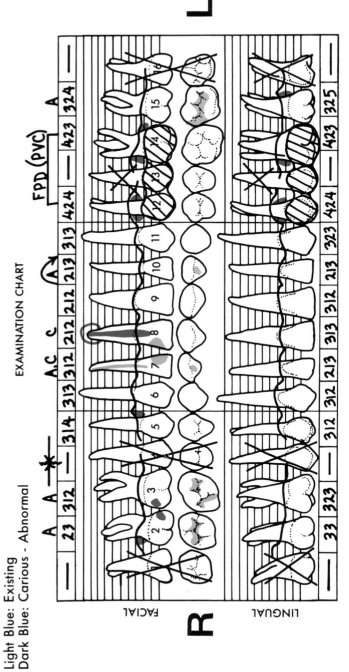

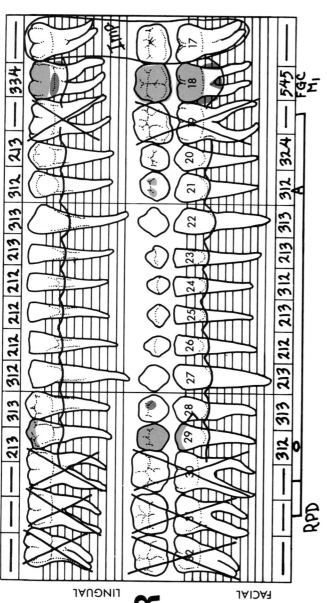

Fig. 6-2 This examination form is designed to record the physical findings from the comprehensive dental examination. The dental condition of a hypothetical patient is represented to illustrate one approach to dental charting. The light blue shaded areas represent existing restorations. The black lines that parallel the cervical levels of the teeth signify the estimated crestal bone contours based on radiographic and clinical findings. Dark blue shading on the teeth indicates dental decay and dark blue shading adjacent to root surfaces reflects periodontal defects. *Arrows* indicate shifting and rotation of teeth. Abbreviations reflect the nature of existing restorations as amalgam (*A*), composite (*C*), fixed partial denture (*FPD*), full gold crown (*FGC*), onlay (*O*), and removable partial denture (*RPD*). The symbol *M* represents grade one mobility of the mandibular left second molar.

quality of the procedures. This is an inherent aspect of providing health care. The patient record is the only documentation of the clinician's perception of an event that results in a conflict. Sloppy, incomplete records reflect negatively on the clinician during peer or legal reviews initiated because of problems. A clear and comprehensive patient record reflects positively on the clinician and implies that the diagnostic decisions and treatment procedures have also been accomplished in an appropriate and professional manner.

7. Few busy professionals enjoy paperwork. Patient documentation can be substantially reduced in the setting of a private office as compared with an institution and still function adequately. A priority for brevity and simplicity do not, however, justify abbreviating the patient record to the point that it fails to serve as adequate documentation of clinical information and events.

SUMMARY

Patient documentation is the physical record of the pertinent information related to the diagnosis and care of the patient. All patient documentation formats represent compromises among ideal characteristics and necessary functions of the patient record. These compromises are designed to be most consistent with the priorities, practice setting, and preferences of the clinician who uses the record.

The problem-oriented patient record organizes patient data by the function that the information serves in solving the patient's problems. Administrative materials consist of information needed for nonclinical activities. The patient database includes the diagnostic findings from the patient history, physical examination, and adjunctive diagnostic procedures. The problem list summarizes the patient's abnormalities and conditions that require additional diagnostic evaluation and treatment. The treatment plan lists the procedures necessary to solve the patient's problems in the sequence in which the treatment will be provided. The progress notes section of the patient record allows the clinician to maintain a chronologic description of clinical events that represent progress in solving the patient's problems.

The diagnostic findings from the dental examination are documented with a combination of an anatomic diagram of the teeth and narrative descriptions of generalized dental conditions. The large amount of detailed information necessary to reflect the patient's dental status can be recorded in a efficient, condensed form by drawing existing decay and restorations on the diagram and using abbreviations and symbols to indicate other significant findings.

BIBLIOGRAPHY

Barsh LS: Dental treatment planning for the adult patient, Philadelphia, 1981, Saunders.

Feinstein AR: The problems of the "problem oriented medical record," Ann Intern Med 78:751, 1973.

Judge RD, Zuidema GD, Fitzgerald FT, editors: Clinical diagnosis: a physiologic approach, ed 5, Boston, 1988, Little, Brown.

PART II

Patient Evaluation and Treatment Planning

CHAPTER 7

Physical Assessment

GARY C. COLEMAN

Dentists rely on the patient history and clinical examination to evaluate the patient's medical status and to determine if there is a need for additional diagnostic information. This is referred to as *physical assessment* and consists of three areas of responsibility:

1. The evaluation of the patient's known medical conditions
2. The identification of signs or symptoms that might suggest the possibility of an undiagnosed medical condition
3. The identification of potential complications that may develop during dental treatment because of a patient's compromised health

Physical assessment by the dentist is most effectively approached by focusing on conditions that are relatively common and that usually require modification of dental treatment.

Relatively obvious clinical signs and symptoms that appear during the course of most diseases are referred to as *cardinal indicators of disease*. Pain, abnormal vital signs, compromised organ function, unexplained weight loss, and changes in physical appearance are among the most evident and reliable indicators of systemic illness. Identifying these signs and symptoms may provide direction in determining the organ systems affected and narrow the clinician's search for the cause. Cardinal disease indicators are also helpful in evaluating the progression or severity of previously diagnosed diseases. The following sections suggest the important clinical features of common diseases that should be considered during the physical assessment of the dental patient. This discussion is intended to illustrate the assessment process rather than provide comprehensive coverage of all possible medical conditions. The dentist should expect clinical situations to frequently arise in which medical reference materials and the patient's physician must be consulted to fully appreciate the nature and implications of the patient's medical condition.

CARDIOVASCULAR DISEASES

Cardiovascular diseases include abnormalities of the heart and blood vessels. The most common symptoms associated with cardiovascular disease are shortness of breath, or *dyspnea*; difficulty breathing when reclined, or *orthopnea*; fatigue; chest pain; and palpitations.

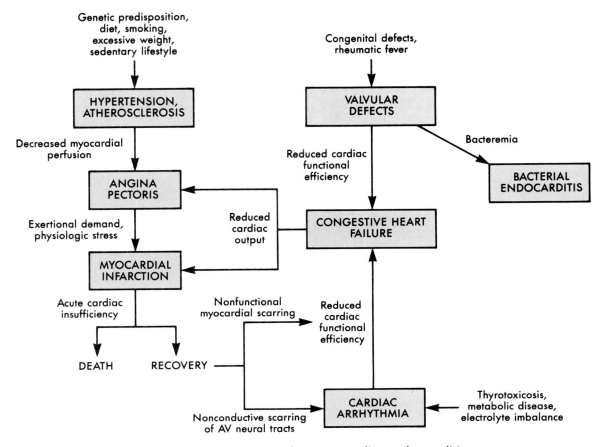

Fig. 7-1. Interrelationships of common cardiovascular conditions.

Clinical signs include elevated blood pressure, abnormal pulse, edema, cardiac murmurs, and peripheral cyanosis. Hypertension, atherosclerosis, angina pectoris, myocardial infarction (MI), congestive heart failure (CHF), cardiac arrhythmias, and valvular defects are the most common conditions affecting the cardiovascular system. Patients suffering from one cardiovascular disease often develop symptoms of other forms of cardiac insufficiency, as illustrated in Fig. 7-1.

Hypertension

Hypertension is episodic or consistent elevation of blood pressure beyond what is con-sidered normal. The accepted range of healthy blood pressure must be adjusted for age and gender, but general limits for adults are as follows. Diastolic pressure:

Less than 85 mm Hg is considered nor-motensive

Between 85 and 89 mm Hg is high normal

From 90 to 104 mm Hg indicates mild hypertension

From 105 to 114 mm Hg indicates moderate hypertension

Greater than 115 mm Hg indicates severe hypertension

If the diastolic pressure is below 90 mm Hg, then systolic pressure:

Below 140 mm Hg is considered normotensive

Between 140 and 159 mm Hg indicates borderline isolated systolic hypertension

Greater than 160 mm Hg indicates isolated systolic hypertension

Blood pressure greater than 200/140 is considered *malignant hypertension* and is usually accompanied by spontaneous hemorrhage of the retina and other vulnerable sites. Use of the designation *accelerated hypertension* indicates progressive increase in blood pressure and implies progression to malignant hypertension if immediate treatment is not instituted.

No direct cause can be identified for over 90% of all cases of hypertension, which are referred to as *essential hypertension.* The condition is usually asymptomatic, and blood pressure measurement is the only dependable method of identification. Factors that contribute to the development and severity of hypertension include diet, obesity, smoking, sedentary lifestyle, race, gender, and heredity. Renal disease, endocrine dysfunction, toxemia of pregnancy, and certain cardiovascular disorders are the direct cause of most of the remaining 10% of cases. Hypertension contributes to the development of atherosclerosis, cardiac disease, renal degeneration, and cerebrovascular conditions. The severity of previously diagnosed hypertension is suggested by the complexity of the treatment regimen and the effectiveness of control. Potential complications of severe hypertension during dental treatment include difficulty in establishing hemostasis and the remote possibility of cerebrovascular rupture and stroke.

Valvular Heart Disease

The most common and functionally significant anatomic heart abnormalities that affect adults are valvular defects. Narrowing, or *stenosis,* of a heart valve restricts outflow of blood during contraction, whereas valvular insufficiency, or *regurgitation,* allows backflow during myocardial relaxation. Both conditions are functionally inefficient and require greater than normal myocardial exertion to maintain cardiac output. The heart's functional potential, referred to as *cardiac reserve,* generally overcomes this valvular inefficiency at rest in younger patients. With age, however, cardiac reserve decreases, which typically limits the ability of the heart to compensate during peak exertional demand. Valve defects may be congenital malformations or acquired damage. The majority of acquired heart valve defects are caused by rheumatic fever. Valvular heart defects are summarized in Table 7-1.

Heart valve defects are initially identified by auscultation of abnormal heart sounds, referred to as *murmurs.* The affected valve and the severity of the defect can usually be determined by the timing of the murmur relative to normal heart sounds and the anatomic location of greatest murmur intensity. Some murmurs are recognized as functional, or "innocent," on the basis of additional tests that demonstrate normal cardiac output. Functional murmurs are commonly identified in children, and the murmur often disappears during adolescence. Functional murmurs are typically produced by pulmonic valve dysfunction and require no clinical consideration beyond recognition.

The dentist must be concerned with two potential complications for patients reporting a history of a heart murmur or specific valvular defect. First, most defective heart valves are vulnerable to infective endocarditis during most dental procedures, as described below. The prophylactic antibiotic treatment recommended to minimize the possibility of this infection is detailed in Chapter 13. Second, stressful dental procedures may precipitate acute cardiac insufficiency by stimulating cardiac demand that exceeds the diminished cardiac reserve associated with valvular dysfunction. Indications of limited cardiac reserve are blood pressure abnormalities, signs of CHF, and *cardiomegaly,* or enlargement of the heart. Medical consultation is often necessary to safely treat the patient with valvular heart disease.

Table 7-1   Summary of the features associated with specific forms of valvular heart disease

Valvular defect	Consequence	Signs and symptoms	Clinical course
Mitral stenosis	Limited left atrial outflow leads to increased left atrial and pulmonary venous pressures	Often mild and exertional dyspnea and cough may not develop until fourth decade; progresses to pulmonary edema, atrial arrhythmia, cardiac ischemia	Chronic pulmonary hypertension eventually produces right-sided congestive heart failure and increasing limitation of cardiac reserve and activity
Mitral regurgitation (includes mitral valve prolapse with regurgitation)	Normal output maintained by greater ventricular contraction; with greater severity the left atrium enlarges and cardiac output is compromised	Only severely affected patients suffer symptoms of dyspnea, fatigue, and orthopnea	Condition tends to be progressive in severely affected individuals; may eventually cause pulmonary hypertension and progress to right-sided congestive heart failure
Mitral valve prolapse without regurgitation	Cardiac function is not compromised unless mitral regurgitation develops	Most patients are asymptomatic for life; consider as mitral regurgitation if abnormal cardiac function develops	Considered as a function defect in most instances, but regurgitation may develop in some cases
Aortic stenosis	Obstruction of left ventricular outflow compensated for by left ventricular hypertrophy; pulmonary pressure eventually increases	Can be asymptomatic for years; progressive fatigue, exertional dyspnea, angina, and syncope develop with age as compensation becomes inadequate	Increased pulmonary pressure, dyspnea, and orthopnea develop as a reflection of left-sided congestive heart failure; right-sided congestive heart failure is eventually observed in advanced cases
Aortic regurgitation	Backflow of cardiac output is compensated for by greater left ventricular contraction; this is adequate at rest, but not during exertion	Palpitation, tachycardia, and angina develop because backflow adversely affects coronary blood supply; elevated systolic pressure and wide pulse pressure are typical signs	Angina with other myocardial ischemia symptoms and weakness are the predominant and progressive features; signs of congestive heart failure often develop

Modified from Wilson JD and others, editors: Harrison's principles of internal medicine, ed 12, New York, 1991, McGraw-Hill.

Table 7-1 Summary of the features associated with specific forms of valvular heart disease

Valvular defect	Consequence	Signs and symptoms	Clinical course
Tricuspid stenosis	Limited blood flow into the right ventricle produces systemic venous congestion	Uncommon valvular defect and usually associated with mitral stenosis or other defects; symptoms of other valve dysfunction are predominant	Portal hypertension, ascites, and systemic venous congestion may be more severe or refractory to treatment than expected based on the signs of mitral dysfunction
Tricuspid regurgitation	Usually functional and secondary to right ventricular dilation; may complicate the effects of associated insufficiencies of other valves	Peripheral edema and portal hypertension may develop if pulmonary hypertension from other conditions further limits right ventricular output	Usually well tolerated unless complicated by other conditions
Pulmonic valve defects	Typically functional defects without alteration of cardiac efficiency	Asymptomatic	Clinically insignificant unless severe pulmonary hypertension develops

Infective Endocarditis

Infective endocarditis is typically a streptococcal infection that is initially confined to the surface of the heart valves. Heart valves deformed by rheumatic fever, congenitally malformed valves, and prosthetic heart valves are vulnerable to the infection, whereas normal heart valves are unlikely to be affected. Bacteria typically gain access to the heart during a *transient bacteremia*, or episode of bacteria in the circulating blood. This can result from blood contact with skin and mucosal surfaces contaminated by bacteria during dental procedures.

Infective endocarditis may be acute and rapidly progressive or chronic and insidious. Fever, malaise, and a history of an anatomic heart defect or murmur are the most consistent findings. Recent history may reveal a surgical procedure, localized infection, or injury suggesting the possibility of bacteremia. Additional valvular damage, *septicemia* (bacteria growing in the blood), and abscesses of major

organs caused by septic emboli are among the potentially life-threatening sequelae of infective endocarditis. The American Heart Association recommends prophylactic antibiotic protection for patients vulnerable to bacterial endocarditis during dental procedures likely to cause bacteremia, as described in Chapter 13.

Angina Pectoris

The cardinal clinical feature of angina pectoris is episodic chest pain. Atherosclerotic narrowing of coronary arteries compromises the myocardial blood supply and results in cardiac ischemia and episodic pain during periods of increased functional demand. The term *stable angina* indicates cardiac ischemia only during exceptional exertion, with rapid recovery following cessation of activity. *Unstable angina* is characterized by more frequent occurrence of spontaneous chest pain that persists with rest. Stable angina may persist for years without additional manifestations of cardiac ischemia, whereas patients with unstable angina are considered to represent a continual risk for MI. Etiologic factors of cardiac ischemia include hypertension, obesity, diet, smoking, stress, gender, and genetic predisposition. Additional factors such as compromised cardiac output of CHF, decreased oxygen-transport capability of anemia, and inadequate blood oxygenation of primary pulmonary diseases are contributory in many instances.

The most dependable indicators of the severity of ischemic heart disease are the amount of exertion that precipitates angina and the frequency, duration, and intensity of the chest pain. Stable angina can generally be managed by stress reduction methods during routine dental procedures. Evidence of unstable angina warrants medical consultation. The physician may alter the patient's medication, recommend dental treatment in a hospital setting, or require delay of dental treatment until the patient's condition improves.

Myocardial Infarction

MI, or a "heart attack," is ischemic necrosis of a portion of the myocardium. The MI may be the initial manifestation of ischemic heart disease, but patients typically experience anginal episodes before an acute MI. The clinical features of MI vary from mild, transient anginal symptoms without actual diagnosis of the infarction to massive myocardial necrosis and death. Three sequelae are significant concerns for all MI survivors: (1) additional MIs are likely; (2) myocardial scarring decreases myocardial reserve; and (3) myocardial scarring can interfere with nodal impulses and cause cardiac arrhythmias (Fig. 7-1). The cardiac reserve of the recovered heart attack survivor is generally indicated by the amount of physical exertion that elicits anginal pain and its intensity following recovery.

Congestive Heart Failure

CHF is compromised efficiency of cardiac function relative to the metabolic requirements of the body. In other words, the heart cannot pump enough blood to meet physio-

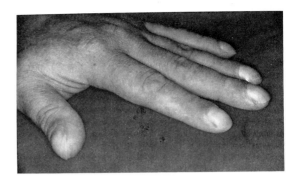

Fig. 7-2. The characteristic enlargement and rounded contour of the nails referred to as clubbing of the digits.

logic demands. Functional compromise may result from valvular insufficiency or MI affecting primarily the right or left ventricle, although in most cases both are deficient to some degree. The typical course is gradual development and chronic progression of CHF, but the acute onset of CHF can result from infectious cardiomyopathy, toxic conditions, or cardiac insufficiency following infarction.

Most clinical signs of CHF result from venous congestion and edema. Ankle swelling is usually the first sign indicating the systemic venous congestion of right ventricular deficiency. More severe right ventricular inadequacy is suggested by *pitting edema,* demonstrated by palpation of the ankles, and edematous distention of the wrists, the abdomen, and periorbital tissues. Inadequate tissue perfusion can yield additional effects such as cyanosis, clubbing of the digits (Fig. 7-2), anginal pain, decreased urine output, congestive hepatomegaly, and syncope from inadequate cerebral perfusion, known as *Stokes-Adams syndrome.* Left ventricle failure produces pulmonary hypertension and edema expressed clinically as *dyspnea,* or shortness of breath. *Orthopnea* (labored breathing when reclined) and *paroxysmal nocturnal dyspnea,* indicated by waking from sound sleep because of breathing distress, both suggest more advanced left ventricular impairment. Limited myocardial perfusion re-

Table 7-2 Summary of cardiac arrhythmias

Term	Features	Clinical significance
Sinus bradycardia	Resting heart rate <60 beats/min	Normal for athletes, can indicate sinus node dysfunction among elderly patients; extrinsic causes include increased intracranial pressure, myxedema, and hypothermia
Sinus tachycardia	Resting heart rate >100 beats/min (rarely exceeds 200 beats/min)	Response to anxiety, exercise, thyrotoxicosis, hypoxemia, hypotension, fever, depleted blood volume, or congestive heart failure
AV dissociation	Atrial and ventricular contractions are not coordinated	Atrial and ventricular premature complexes (contractions) indicative of nodal conduction defects (AV blocks) of variable severity
Atrial tachycardia*	Atrial contraction rate between 120 and 250 beats/min	AV block may be present, also caused by digitalis intoxication and hypokalemia
Atrial flutter*	Atrial contraction rate between 250 and 350 beats/min	AV block almost always present with persistent forms, paroxysmal episodes may be caused by stress, such as that of infection or respiratory failure
Atrial fibrillation*	Disorganized atrial contractions at rates >350 beats/min	Both paroxysmal and persistent forms, associated with severe myocardial ischemia, compromised cardiac function, sepsis
Ventricular tachycardia†	Resting rate >100 beats/min	Usually secondary to cardiac ischemia, infarction, myocarditis, cardiomyopathies, or drug toxicity; serious if sustained because of the risk of progression to fibrillation
Ventricular flutter and fibrillation†	Disorganized ventricular contractions at rates >150 beats/min	Usually caused by ischemic heart disease; cardiac output is severely compromised

Modified from Wilson JD and others, editors: Harrison's principles of internal medicine, ed 12, New York, 1991, McGraw-Hill.

*Loss of booster pump function during periods of atrial arrhythmia usually does not lower resting cardiac output in patients with otherwise healthy cardiac function. However, the loss of atrial function during exertion can lower peak demand output as much as 40% with potential critical implications. This is particularly significant if other conditions, such as valvular defects, myocardial ischemia, or ventricular hypertrophy, limit ventricular function.

†Optimal ventricular function depends on synchronous contraction. When normal contraction sequence is lost, then cardiac output drops dramatically. Output may still be adequate if other factors such as valve function and coronary artery perfusion are not compromised. However, the combination of several compromising conditions or exertion usually leads to inadequate cardiac output relative to demand.

sulting in MI is the most significant risk during dental treatment of patients with severe CHF.

Cardiac Arrhythmia

Cardiac arrhythmia is defined as abnormality in the rate, regularity, or sequence of myo-cardial contraction. Terms used to refer to common cardiac arrhythmias are listed in Table 7-2. Extrinsic causes include infection, potassium imbalance, abnormal serum calcium concentration, numerous drugs, caffeine, alcohol, thyrotoxicosis, and anxiety. The most common intrinsic causes of chronic cardiac arrhythmia are myocardial ischemia and scarring of atrioventricular neural tracts, referred to as *AV blocks,* which develop following infarction. Reduced cardiac output and the resulting inadequate perfusion of vital organs such as the brain, heart, and kidneys are the most serious sequelae of cardiac arrhythmia.

The clinical signs of cardiac arrhythmia include palpitation, pulse irregularity, heart rate below 40 beats/min or above 140 beats/min, and abnormal blood pressure. Evidence of CHF, syncope, angina, or decreased urine output in addition to pulse or blood pressure abnormalities suggests advanced compromise of cardiac function. The electrocardiograph (ECG) provides the definitive diagnosis of cardiac arrhythmias. The primary concern of the dentist is the possibility that stressful dental procedures or excessive absorption of epinephrine from anesthetic injections could precipitate or worsen cardiac arrhythmia.

PULMONARY DISEASES

Persistent coughing is the most common single feature of chronic respiratory disease and should be categorized as productive or nonproductive. *Dyspnea,* or breathing distress, during exertion typically occurs with pulmonary disease, whereas dyspnea at rest is more often associated with CHF. Fatigue with mild exertion, an abnormal respiratory rate, and peripheral cyanosis indicate impaired blood oxygenation. Fever and malaise in addition to a productive cough suggest pulmonary infection. Hemoptysis, or coughing up blood, is an early feature of parenchymal destruction by infection, a malignant neoplasm, or vascular rupture. The symptoms of left-sided CHF and chronic pulmonary conditions are similar and may cause diagnostic difficulty. Generally, the clinical features, course of the disease, and diagnostic aids such as chest radiographs are effective in establishing the diagnosis. Chronic pulmonary conditions the dentist must fre-

quently evaluate are asthma and chronic obstructive pulmonary disease (COPD).

Asthma

Asthma produces paroxysmal attacks of reversible, generalized airway obstruction caused by mucosal edema, contraction of bronchial smooth muscles, and production of thick secretions. Asthma is categorized as *atopic* when the underlying hyperirritability appears mediated by the immune system and as *nonatopic* when physical irritation or other factors are the primary cause. Approximately 50% of asthmatic persons are classified as atopic and react to specific allergens, such as dust, animal dander, and pollens. Nonatopic asthmatic persons react primarily to the physical irritation of environmental pollution, dust, cigarette smoke, infection, exercise, and emotional stress.

Asthmatic attacks are characterized by the abrupt onset of dyspnea, coughing, and wheezing accompanied by watery, itchy eyes and rhinorrhea. Severe attacks can result in hypoxia and peripheral cyanosis. Although CHF and diffuse pulmonary infections can produce similar symptoms, both are much less acute in onset. Administration of a bronchodilator produces immediate relief for asthmatic distress but is ineffective for other conditions. The asthmatic patient who requires systemic medications such as corticosteroids in addition to a bronchodilator for control must be considered to be severely affected.

Chronic Obstructive Pulmonary Diseases

COPDs are categorized as chronic bronchitis or emphysema on the basis of whether obstruction occurs predominantly in the bronchi or near the alveoli, respectively. The obstruction is caused by a mucous coagulum containing particulate debris from smoking or chronic exposure to airborne material. Both conditions produce chronic distention of lung parenchyma caused by decades of forced inspiration past these obstructing materials and partially blocked expiration. The effects of distention and chronic inflammation cause tissue scarring and a progressive decrease in alveolar surface area that eventually compromises effective gaseous exchange.

A nonproductive, hacking cough is the only clinical sign of early COPD. The patient history reveals cigarette smoking or chronic exposure to airborne irritants, as well as frequent respiratory infections. With time, dyspnea, exertional shortness of breath, and high-pitched breathing sounds called *rhonchi* develop. A feature of advanced COPD is thoracic enlargement yielding a "barrel-chested" appearance. The emphysemic patient commonly exhibits asthenic habitus, flushed facial skin, and labored breathing collectively described as a "pink puffer" appearance. In contrast, chronic bronchitis is usually characterized by the combination of excessive weight, edema caused by CHF, and cyanosis from limited pulmonary function, which is referred to as the "blue bloater" presentation.

Patients with advanced COPD are at risk for cardiac ischemia secondary to compromised pulmonary function during stressful dental treatment. Severe exertional dyspnea, dyspnea at rest, and evidence of CHF all indicate an increased likelihood of this complication and the need for medical consultation before dental treatment.

GASTROINTESTINAL DISEASES

Gastrointestinal (GI) conditions involve fewer direct implications for the dentist as compared with cardiovascular or pulmonary diseases, but potential clinical complications do exist. Several symptom groups should direct the dentist's attention to the possibility of undiagnosed GI disease. Abdominal pain is often the initial symptom during the early stage of many GI conditions. Nausea, vomiting, diarrhea, cramping pain, and bloody stools reflect disruption of function by infection, obstruction, or other conditions. Unexplained weight loss and pain indicate the possibility of malabsorption, and jaundice indicates liver disease by the accumulation of bilirubin in the blood.

Peptic Ulcerative Disease

Peptic ulcers are believed to be caused by excessive gastric acid secretion as a consequence of emotional stress, specific foods, and other sources of irritation. Most peptic ulcers respond to symptomatic treatment, but complications can develop, including excessive bleeding, anemia, and perforation. An additional clinical concern is that gastric carcinoma and peptic ulcers produce similar clinical symptoms.

Recurrent epigastric pain that is relieved by ingestion of food and antacids is the most consistent symptom of peptic ulcers. Gastric perforation should be suspected if epigastric pain becomes constant and is associated with *hematemesis,* or vomiting of blood. Gastritis also produces epigastric pain, but the discomfort generally occurs immediately after ingestion of aspirin, alcoholic beverages, and other materials that are irritating to the gastric mucosa.

Increasing severity of pain, constant pain, vomiting, hematemesis, and ineffective control of symptoms by food intake and antacids indicate severe peptic ulcerative disease or gastric carcinoma. Medical referral is indicated. The dentist should be concerned in such situations that blood loss may cause anemia and that an acquired bleeding tendency may develop from depletion of coagulation proteins and platelets. Analgesics such as aspirin, ibuprofen, and codeine cause gastric irritation and should not be recommended for patients prone to gastritis and peptic ulcers.

Malabsorption Diseases

Malabsorption is defined as the limited ability to absorb nutrients from an adequate diet. Acquired malabsorption affecting adult pa-

Table 7-3 Classification of malabsorption disorders

Category	Conditions
1. Inadequate digestion	Gastrectomy, pancreatitis, pancreatic carcinoma, cystic fibrosis, pancreatic resection
2. Abnormal bile salt concentration	Hepatic disease, cholestasis, bacterial proliferation caused by hypomobility or obstruction, interference with bile function by drugs
3. Inadequate absorptive surface	Intestinal resection
4. Lymphatic obstruction	Lymphoma, metastatic neoplasia, intestinal lymphangiectasia
5. Vascular compromise	Congestive heart failure (portal hypertension), constrictive pericarditis, mesenteric vascular deficiency, vasculitis
6. GI mucosal alteration	Regional enteritis, tropical sprue, collagenous sprue, amyloidosis, radiation enteritis, infectious enteritis (salmonellosis, giardiasis), eosinophilic enteritis, celiac sprue (gluten-induced enteropathy), other less common genetic conditions of biochemical deficiency
7. Endocrine disorders	Hypoparathyroidism, adrenal insufficiency, hyperthyroidism
8. Conditions that cause multiple effects	Diabetes mellitus, Zollinger-Ellision syndrome (ulcerogenic tumor), systemic sclerosis, Whipple's disease

Modified from Wilson JD and others, editors: Harrison's principles of internal medicine, ed 12, New York, 1991, McGraw-Hill.

tients can be caused by the underlying conditions listed in Table 7-3. Malabsorption should not be confused with similar clinical manifestations attributable to the inadequate nutritional intake of starvation and psychiatric eating disorders.

Malabsorption results in a gradual, unexplained weight loss over several months and the production of bulky, oily stools, referred to as *steatorrhea.* Epigastric pain similar to that caused by peptic ulcers may also occur. Signs of specific dietary deficiencies often develop, including anemia, glossitis, scurvy, and a bleeding tendency. The findings listed in Table 7-4 and the results of endoscopy with gastric or duodenal biopsy usually yield the specific diagnosis.

The primary diagnostic concern for the dentist is identification of the undiagnosed individual suffering from limited nutritional absorption, resulting anemia, and vitamin deficiency. The possibility of malabsorption should be considered in cases of concurrent glossitis and unexplained weight loss.

Intestinal Disease

Chronic lower GI conditions are categorized as focal or diffuse. Small hernial pouchings through the serosal wall (called *diverticula*), enlargements extending into the luminal space (called *polyps),* and vascular enlargements in the anal region (referred to as *hemorrhoids*) are the most common focal lesions. *Irritable bowel syndrome, regional enteritis,* and *ulcerative colitis* are examples of diffuse intestinal diseases. Irritable bowel syndrome consists of emotionally related GI muscle spasms, often aggravated by certain foods. Both regional enteritis, also referred to as *Crohn's disease,* and ulcerative colitis are idiopathic, inflammatory conditions that cause ulceration of GI mucosa.

Intestinal conditions cause cramping pain resulting from abnormal motility and blood in the stools from mucosal ulcers. Polyps and diverticula are vulnerable to mechanical injury by luminal contents, which causes episodic bleeding and cramps. Irritable bowel syndrome is suggested by a chronic course of in-

Table 7-4   Signs and symptoms associated with disorders of malabsorption

Sign or symptom	Mechanism
Unexplained weight loss	Malabsorption of proteins, carbohydrates, and fats leading to catabolism of body tissue components to maintain essential metabolic functions
Weakness	Anemia, electrolyte depletion (hypokalemia), hypoglycemia
Diarrhea	Impaired absorption of water and electrolytes, especially in large bowel
Steatorrhea	Impaired absorption of fat
Glossitis, cheilitis, stomatitis	Deficiency of iron, folate, vitamin B_{12}, and other vitamins
Anemia	Deficiency of iron, folate, vitamin B_{12}, and other vitamins
Ecchymosis, petechiae	Vitamin K deficiency causes hypoprothrombinemia; impaired platelet production and increased capillary fragility results from vitamin deficiencies
Amenorrhea, decreased libido	Protein and caloric starvation
Bone pain	Protein depletion causes osteoporosis; calcium malabsorption causes osteomalacia
Tetany	Hypocalcemia
Patchy dermatitis	Deficiency of zinc, fatty acids, vitamin A, and other vitamins

Modified from Wilson JD and others, editors: Harrison's principles of internal medicine, ed 12, New York, 1991, McGraw-Hill.

termittent constipation, diarrhea, and cramping pain relieved by antispasmodic drugs. Bleeding is unusual because the mucosa is intact.

Both regional enteritis and ulcerative colitis are characterized by a chronic clinical course of periods of cramping pain, mild fever, fatigue, GI bleeding, diarrhea, and weight loss intermixed with periods of remission. Regional enteritis produces ulcers of any portion of the alimentary mucosa, including the mouth, although lesions limited to the small bowel make up the most common clinical presentation. Ulcerative colitis affects only the large bowel and rectum. Treatment includes supportive care and corticosteroid administration. Surgical removal of the colon is reserved for severe cases of ulcerative colitis.

The dentist's diagnostic interest in intestinal conditions relates to possible malabsorption and chronic blood loss, which may cause anemia, diminished host resistance, and a bleeding tendency. Rarely the patient with regional enteritis may exhibit oral lesions. Long-term corticosteroid treatment of regional enteritis and ulcerative colitis can cause increased vulnerability to infection and adrenal suppression.

Hepatitis

Hepatitis is the general term for inflammation of the liver. Causes of hepatitis include viral infection, certain drugs, alcohol, and exposure to organic solvents such as carbon tetrachloride. Viral hepatitis can be caused by at least five different viruses as summarized in Table 7-5.

Clinical features of hepatitis include upper right quadrant abdominal enlargement and tenderness, as well as general findings such as fever, anorexia, nausea, malaise, and headache. Identification of intracellular hepatic enzymes such as transaminases by blood serum analysis, as discussed in Chapter 11, indicates hepatic necrosis.

Disruption of metabolic functions of the liver produces several significant features of hepatitis. Yellowish discoloration of the skin

Table 7-5 Comparison of the features associated with different forms of viral hepatitis

Feature	Hepatitis A	Hepatitis B*	Hepatitis C	Hepatitis E
Colloquial designation	Infectious hepatitis	Serum hepatitis	Non-A, non-B hepatitis	Non-A, non-B hepatitis
Incubation	15-45 days	30-180 days	15-160 days	14-60 days
Onset	Acute	Often insidious	Insidious	Acute
Typical age of occurrence	Children, young adults	Any age	Any age, usually adults	Young adults
Transmission route:				
Fecal-oral	Typical route	Not considered possible	Unknown	Typical route
Percutaneous	Unusual	Typical route	Typical route	Not considered possible
Nonpercutaneous†	Possible, but unlikely	Possible, often likely	Possible, often likely	Possible, but unlikely
Severity	Mild	Often severe	Moderate	Mild
Prognosis	Generally good	Worse with age, debility	Moderate	Good
Progression	Not considered possible	Occasional (>10%)*	Common (10%-50%)	Not considered possible
Prophylaxis	IG‡	Hepatitis B vaccine, IG	None currently	None currently
Carrier (US gen. pop.)	Not considered possible	Less than 1%	Approximately 1%	Not considered possible

Modified from Wilson JD and others, editors: Harrison's principles of internal medicine, ed 12, New York, 1991, McGraw-Hill.

*Delta hepatitis must be associated with hepatitis B infection, and the combination infection is often clinically indistinguishable from hepatitis B. However, the combined infections are more likely to cause progression to severe, chronic forms of hepatitis.

†Sexual and perinatal contacts represent the most clinically significant situations of viral hepatitis transmission by nonpercutaneous means, although other examples of intimate contact can occasionally produce infection.

‡IG, specific antiviral (A or B) immune globulin preparations.

and mucous membranes, referred to as *jaundice* or *icterus,* indicates inadequate bilirubin metabolism. Severe hepatic necrosis may interfere with production of blood proteins such as albumin and coagulation factors. Impaired metabolism of hormones, medications, and toxic exogenous materials may also become clinically apparent.

Acute hepatitis resulting from drugs or other toxic materials can usually be clarified by the patient history. Exposure to most exogenous toxins occurs by deliberate ingestion as an attempted suicide, ingestion of near-lethal amounts of ethanol, or exposure to organic solvent fumes. The patient history may reveal use of medications or illicit drugs known to cause hepatic injury. A history of travel or of drinking untreated water may suggest exposure to hepatitis A or E, whereas a history of blood-to-blood contact, such as a recent transfusion or intravenous (IV) drug abuse, suggests hepatitis B or C infection. Laboratory tests including serum enzymes, bilirubin, and serologic demonstration of viral antigens or antibodies are invaluable in the diagnosis of hepatitis.

Acute hepatitis, particularly if icteric, requires immediate medical referral. Any medications known to cause hepatic toxicity that have been recently prescribed by the dentist should be discontinued. Hepatitis can cause altered liver metabolism of many drugs, which produces unusual pharmacologic effects. This must be considered before any medications are administered. Coagulation function should be tested before any surgical procedures are done. The patient with a history of or who currently has hepatitis must be considered infectious until proved otherwise.

Hepatic Cirrhosis

Hepatic cirrhosis is defined as diffuse replacement of the liver parenchyma with scar tissue following chronic, recurring hepatic necrosis. Cirrhosis may result from toxic accumulation of endogenous substances, as occurs with several rare, metabolic diseases, or from exogenous toxins such as drugs. Chronic viral hepatitis and functional conditions such as portal congestion produced by CHF and biliary obstruction can also lead to cirrhosis. Cirrhosis associated with alcoholism, which is the most common cause, is also referred to as *Laënnec's, micronodular, portal,* and *fatty cirrhosis.* Genetic disease or chronic alcoholism as the source of cirrhotic injury is usually clarified by the patient history. However, historical information is less likely to explain cirrhosis produced by insidious conditions such as chronic viral hepatitis and drug toxicity.

Clinical features of cirrhosis are produced by insufficient liver function and portal hypertension caused by fibrotic blockage of hepatic vascular channels. Alcoholic patients are usually asymptomatic until the fourth or fifth decade, when liver enlargement and firmness to palpation become apparent. Malnutrition seems to promote alcoholic cirrhosis, which explains the typical asthenic habitus. Gastritis and peptic ulcers are also common in alcoholic persons. Portal hypertension produces edema, ascites, and varicose distention of esophageal, rectal, and periumbilical veins as collateral pathways for portal blood. Such varicosities can be a source of life-threatening hemorrhage. Weakness, weight loss, anorexia, nausea, vomiting, and icterus may appear during extended drinking bouts. *Gynecomastia* (spontaneous breast enlargement), testicular atrophy in men, and amenorrhea in women are features of advanced cirrhosis produced by ineffective hepatic metabolism of normal steroidal hormones. Skin abnormalities include rhinophyma, nonspecific hyperpigmentation, and spider angiomas. Diminished coagulation protein production is demonstrated by purpura, petechial hemorrhage, and GI hemorrhage.

Routine dental treatment of patients with cirrhosis rarely involves complications unless hepatic damage is severe, as indicated by icterus, a bleeding tendency, and manifestations of portal hypertension. Observation of these features implies the need for medical consultation before dental treatment, particularly if the origin of hepatic necrosis is not clarified by the patient history. Drugs should be prescribed for cirrhotic patients with the expectation of compromised hepatic metabolism.

ENDOCRINE DISEASES

Endocrine abnormalities are diverse in their clinical manifestations and are difficult to diagnose because of the insidious onset of clinical manifestations. One positive aspect in the diagnosis of endocrine abnormalities is that laboratory blood analysis generally provides a definitive diagnosis.

Diabetes Mellitus

Diabetes mellitus is a carbohydrate metabolism disorder characterized by hyperglycemia and glycosuria resulting from inadequate insulin synthesis. The disease is classified as either type 1 or type 2, although individuals may exhibit intermediate features of the disease.

Type 1 diabetes mellitus is characterized by relatively abrupt cessation of insulin production affecting patients before the age of 40. The diagnosis of type 1 diabetes is generally based on the characteristic findings in one of two clinical situations. The first involves the triad of *polyuria, polydipsia,* and *polyphagia* with unexplained weight loss of several months' duration, which implies a progressive decrease in insulin production. The second is known as a *diabetic ketoacidotic crisis* and is characterized by the acute onset of nausea, vomiting, stupor, and eventual coma following physiologic stress. This results from inadequate insulin reserve during a dramatic increase in insulin demand and the toxic increase in blood concentration of ketones and acids generated by compensatory fat and protein metabolism. Administration of insulin is the only effective treatment for type 1 diabetes. Secondary effects of diabetes such as retinopathy, nephropathy, neuropathy, and gangrene of the feet often become apparent 2 to 3 decades after diagnosis and appear to be caused by sclerosis of small blood vessels.

Type 2 diabetes usually affects overweight individuals past the age of 40. In contrast to type 1 diabetes, few clinical signs or symptoms develop early in the disease course, because the decline in insulin production is gradual. The condition is usually first suspected on the basis of abnormal results from screening laboratory tests. Treatment initially consists of dietary control of carbohydrate intake and weight reduction. Antihyperglycemic sulfonyl urea therapy may be added to stimulate islet cell insulin production. If diet and antihyperglycemic medication fail to maintain control, then treatment with insulin becomes necessary. Small-vessel sclerosis and resulting conditions also occur in type 2 diabetes, but the patient is usually older when symptoms develop. The laboratory diagnosis of diabetes is discussed in Chapter 11.

The type of diabetes and the degree of therapeutic control are the two most significant factors in the assessment of the disease. Type 1 diabetes is typically more severe because the only available insulin is exogenous, which makes control among the variables of dietary sugar intake, metabolic demand, and in-sulin administration difficult. Therefore the type 1 diabetic patient is more likely to be "brittle," or poorly controlled, and the disease is more likely to progress to acute *diabetic coma* caused by hyperglycemia or *hypoglycemic insulin shock.* The dentist must also expect both type 1 and type 2 diabetic patients to be more vulnerable to infection and to heal more slowly in comparison with healthy patients.

Hypothyroidism

Hypothyroidism is characterized by abnormally low blood concentrations of iodothyronine (T_3) and tetraiodothyronine (T_4), decreased oxygen consumption, and a low basal metabolic rate. Possible causes include low dietary iodine intake, resulting in *nontoxic goiter;* low level of thyroid-stimulating hormone caused by pituitary deficiency; infection known as *thyroiditis;* and autoimmune damage from *Hashimoto's thyroiditis.*

If hypothyroidism develops during growth, then short stature, mental retardation, and other effects collectively known as *cretinism* result. *Myxedema* is caused by the onset of hypothyroidism after physical development. Mild hypothyroidism is characterized by complaints of lethargy, constipation, and cold intolerance. More advanced myxedema produces slowed mental and motor activity, anorexia, weight gain, dry skin, muscle pain, and altered voice. Severe edema and coma can develop without treatment. Additional features such as thyromegaly suggest the possibility of hypothyroidism, but the definitive diagnosis usually relies on laboratory testing. Management is by hormone replacement therapy in addition to treatment of the primary disease process.

Thyroid deficiency without treatment can be roughly estimated based on the clinical features described above. The replacement hormone dosage for treated patients reflects the functional compromise. Direct complications during dental treatment are rarely related to hypothyroidism.

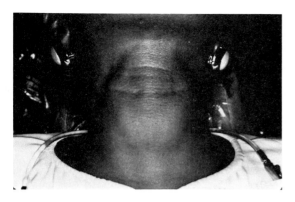

Fig. 7-3. Goiter demonstrated by hyperextension of the head. This 33-year-old woman was unaware of this diffuse, firm, symmetric enlargement in the region of the larynx. An abnormal pulse pressure (138/68 mm Hg) was determined, which is a common feature of Graves' disease.

Thyrotoxicosis

Thyrotoxicosis, or *hyperthyroidism,* is produced by an excessive amount of endogenous or exogenous thyroid hormone, which elevates the basal metabolic rate. Specific conditions that produce thyrotoxicosis include *Graves' disease* caused by autoimmune mechanisms, *toxic multinodular goiter* resulting from a regulatory defect, and functional thyroid neoplasms. *Thyrotoxic crisis,* also known as *thyroid storm,* is an acute, fulminating increase in the severity of thyrotoxicosis affecting hyperthyroid patients during surgical or septic stress. It results from a sudden release of thyroid hormone, which may be related to acute adrenocortical insufficiency.

Mild clinical features of thyrotoxicosis include nervousness suggestive of anxiety, blood pressure abnormalities, tremor, weakness, sweating, heat intolerance, emotional instability, and warm, moist skin. Enlargement of the thyroid, referred to as *goiter,* is a frequent feature and is illustrated in Fig. 7-3. Decreased muscle mass, weight loss, nausea, vomiting, diarrhea, cardiac arrhythmia, tachycardia, and macular skin pigmentation suggest advanced disease. Exophthalmos with infrequent blinking is often seen with functional thyroid adenomas and Graves' disease but is uncommon with toxic multinodular goiter. The acute onset of high fever, irritability, delirium, tachycardia, hypertension, vomiting, and diarrhea associated with surgery or sepsis are typical of thyrotoxic crisis. The initial treatment of nonneoplastic hyperthyroidism is by inhibition with antithyroid drugs, such as propylthiouracil and methimazole. If normal thyroid function cannot be achieved with antithyroid drugs, thyroid function is usually reduced by either partial or total surgical removal or by the administration of radioactive iodine.

Because of the possibility of thyrotoxic crisis, medical evaluation of patients reporting a history of elevated thyroid function may be indicated before any surgical procedures are done. Thyrotoxic crisis should be considered when a patient exhibits rapid deterioration in status associated with a surgical procedure or sepsis.

Adrenocortical Insufficiency

The most significant manifestations of adrenocortical insufficiency reflect deficient secretion of glucocorticoids, such as cortisol, although the secretion of mineralocorticoids and androgens may also be affected. Primary adrenocortical insufficiency, also known as *Addison's disease,* is rare and results from destruction of the adrenal cortices by infection or other causes. Secondary adrenocortical insufficiency is more common and is produced by inadequate pituitary production of adrenocorticotropic hormone (ACTH). ACTH secretion may be limited by degenerative conditions of the pituitary gland or by overload of the feedback inhibition of ACTH synthesis by excessive corticosteroid concentration in the blood. The latter mechanism explains the iatrogenic adrenal suppression after discontinuation of corticosteroid therapy.

Chronic adrenocortical insufficiency is suggested by the insidious onset of progressive fatigue, anorexia, weight loss, nausea, vomiting, hypotension, and patchy hyperpigmentation of skin and mucous membranes. This is most commonly observed following abrupt discontinuation of corticosteroid therapy. Most cases of acute adrenocortical insufficiency, known as *Waterhouse-Friderichsen syndrome,* are caused by hemorrhagic necrosis of the adrenal glands during overwhelming sepsis. The clinical features of this condition are similar to those of chronic adrenal suppression but are more severe.

Some degree of adrenocortical insufficiency should be suspected in patients who have taken systemic corticosteroids within the preceding 12 months. Episodes of physiologic stress such as dental treatment can create an abrupt increase in glucocorticoid demand beyond the depressed secretory potential of the patient's adrenal glands. This is managed by corticosteroid supplementation as discussed in Chapter 13. Medical consultation is justified if the patient history fails to adequately clarify the treatment regimen of recently or currently administered systemic corticosteroids.

Adrenal Cortex Hyperfunction

Excessive blood concentration of cortisol or other glucocorticoids and the resulting effects are known as *Cushing's syndrome.* The pathophysiologic causes include excessive ACTH secretion in response to hypothalamic abnormality, excessive ACTH production by functional neoplasms, and excessive cortisol production by functional neoplasms. The source of elevated corticosteroids, however, for the majority of patients who exhibit features of Cushing's syndrome, is chronic administration of steroid medications in the treatment of inflammatory or autoimmune diseases. In other words, most cases of Cushing's syndrome are iatrogenic, although this is usually an unavoidable consequence of the antiinflammatory therapy.

Cushing's syndrome is characterized by

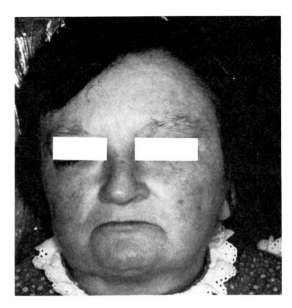

Fig. 7-4. The round or moon face appearance of Cushing's syndrome.

truncal obesity with slender extremities, "moon face" (Fig. 7-4), hypertension, peripheral edema, weakness, and abdominal striae. Advanced features include osteoporosis, ecchymosis, glucose intolerance, and adipose enlargement in the posterior cervical region, known as a "buffalo hump." Diagnostic evaluation for possible endogenous causes of increased glucocorticoid synthesis is necessary if cushingoid features are not explained by corticosteroid therapy of long duration.

Medical consultation for dental patients taking steroid medications is often justified by concern for either possible sequelae of chronic steroid therapy or the underlying disease being treated. Systemic steroid therapy of long duration causes suppression of the immune system in addition to causing iatrogenic Cushing's syndrome. Therefore progressive dental infections often require aggressive treatment to compensate for inhibited immune system function. Suppression of endogenous glucocorticoid synthesis requires an increase in corticosteroid dosage to compensate for the increased demand during stressful dental procedures, as discussed in Chapter 13.

Other Endocrine Abnormalities

Endocrine disorders such as acromegaly and multiple endocrine neoplasia syndromes are rare disorders and are beyond the scope of this discussion. Excellent summaries are available in the listed references. Secondary hyperparathyroidism is a relatively common endocrine abnormality but is nearly always a sequela of degenerative renal disease and is discussed in the following section.

GENITOURINARY DISEASES

Clinical symptoms are usually reliable in directing the attention of both the patient and the clinician to genitourinary (GU) conditions. Flank pain suggests kidney disease, whereas abnormalities of the lower GU tract produce bladder or urethral discomfort during voiding. Patients are usually aware of abnormal frequency of urination and altered urine appearance. The increase in blood concentration of nitrogenous metabolic wastes readily reveals advanced renal insufficiency, which can be confirmed by laboratory tests.

The renal conditions are grouped as either acute or chronic in onset. The discussion of reproductive system disease is limited to sexually transmitted infections, since other conditions seldom directly affect dental treatment.

Acute Renal Disease

Renal function can be rapidly compromised by bacterial infections, renal hypoperfusion, deposition of endogenous proteins, exogenous nephrotoxins, or acute obstruction by kidney stones, referred to as *nephroliths*. Regardless of the cause, symptoms increase in severity within hours or days of onset. Acute nephritis is potentially reversible without permanent damage, depending on the effectiveness of early treatment.

Acute renal insufficiency is characterized by abnormality in volume and frequency of urine production, abnormal character of the urine produced, and increased blood concentration of nitrogenous wastes, referred to as *azotemia.* Acute nephritis and acute renal failure are both characterized by decreased urine output and progressive azotemia. Infection is suspected on the basis of bacteriuria, pyuria, and tenderness of the infected region. Renal tubule toxicity is indicated by polyuria, nocturia, electrolyte imbalance, and metabolic acidosis. Nephrolithiasis is easily identified by severe cramping pain of the flank, referred to as *renal colic.*

Uremia, the clinical condition resulting from azotemia, is characterized by the scent of ammonia, nausea, hypertension, vomiting, altered vision, convulsions, and coma. The onset of uremia demonstrates that renal deterioration has exceeded the renal functional reserve and that irreversible renal damage is likely if the condition is not quickly controlled. Uremia also degrades hepatic, pulmonary, and cardiac efficiency, which can be of critical significance if the function of any of these organs is already marginal. The definitive diagnosis of renal disease relies heavily on the laboratory studies described in Chapter 11.

Immediate medical referral of any patient suspected of acute renal disease is warranted, although the dentist is more likely to confront similar symptoms caused by chronic renal diseases. Aspirin and acetaminophen are known to cause tubular toxicity and should be avoided in patients with renal compromise. Tetracycline and phenobarbital are primarily excreted by the kidneys and may accumulate in the blood if serum creatinine, an indicator of renal clearance, is elevated. Such drugs should only be prescribed after consideration of possible complications. In addition, patients with marginal cardiac or cirrhotic conditions and a recent onset of uremia can be affected by additional reduction in heart and liver function, which must be considered if emergency dental treatment is necessary.

Chronic Renal Disease

A progressive, irreversible decline in renal function is the unifying feature of chronic renal disease irrespective of the specific cause. Progression of acute renal failure to irreversible parenchymal damage is generally clinically apparent on the basis of the features of the acute illness. Chronic degenerative renal diseases may progress insidiously until azotemia develops. Diabetes mellitus, hypertension, and glomerulonephritis resulting from deposition of abnormal blood proteins are the most common causes of chronic renal failure.

Persistence of azotemia for over 3 months defines chronic renal failure. Hypertension and anemia are usually present to some degree and may be accompanied by hematuria, proteinuria, electrolyte imbalance, and edema. Polyuria is typical of primary damage to the renal tubules, whereas oliguria usually indicates glomerular damage.

The *nephrotic syndrome,* which is characterized by proteinuria and the associated loss of blood proteins, is one of the serious consequences of diabetes and autoimmune diseases such as systemic lupus erythematosus (SLE). Hypoalbuminemia develops with persistent proteinuria, which leads to compensatory elevation of serum lipid concentration or hyperlipidemia to maintain osmotic balance of the blood. Eventually the loss of other blood proteins and smaller molecules, including coagulation factors and calcium, contribute significantly to the clinical picture. *Hypertensive nephropathy* is characterized by chronic hypertension, a gradual onset of mild proteinuria, and azotemia. Marked renal insufficiency is uncommon with hypertensive nephropathy, but a gradual, progressive deterioration in renal reserve is typical. Urinary tract obstruction by urethral strictures, tumors, nephroliths, and prostatic hypertrophy can also produce chronic renal symptoms such as pain, oliguria, and urine retention.

A consequence of many chronic renal diseases is excessive urinary loss of calcium, which produces the clinical condition known as *renal osteodystrophy* or *secondary hyperparathyroidism.* Even a slight decrease in serum calcium concentration can adversely affect numerous physiologic processes, including muscle function and blood coagulation. Therefore a decrease in serum calcium stimulates a rapid increase in parathyroid hormone (PTH) secretion, which promotes calcium release from bone. Abnormal radiographic trabecular and cortical bone morphology suggestive of osteomalacia eventually develops as calcium is drained from bone if urinary calcium loss persists. In advanced cases medullary bone may be replaced by soft tissue, or "brown tumors," a condition referred to as *osteitis fibrosa cystica.* Calcium metabolism is further compromised in chronic renal disease by impaired renal metabolism of vitamin D, which diminishes calcium absorption from the gut, and increased phosphate retention, which promotes abnormal calcium deposition in bone. This is demonstrated by focal sclerotic bone deposition, as well as by the metastatic calcification in soft tissue that is often observed in advanced renal osteodystrophy. Similar findings can be caused by *primary hyperparathyroidism,* which is a rare condition of excessive PTH secretion by a functional adenoma. Radiographic findings of renal osteodystrophy, as described in Chapter 19, seldom contribute to the diagnosis of chronic renal disease but may reflect the severity of the condition.

Treatment of chronic renal disease attempts to arrest the primary disease process, maintain residual kidney function, and control the electrolyte imbalance, acidosis, anemia, and other metabolic effects. Renal failure eventually demands either renal dialysis or a kidney transplant. Dialysis is the artificial filtration of the patient's blood or peritoneal fluid. The required frequency of dialysis depends on the degree of residual renal function. Dialysis is usually employed until a suitable donor kidney becomes available or indefinitely for patients considered poor risks for transplantation. Renal transplantation is the treatment goal of most patients with renal failure, but the surgery and antirejection drug regimen are contraindicated in some cases.

Chronic renal failure treated by dialysis and chronic renal failure treated by transplantation are two clinical situations that can lead to complications during dental treatment. Dental treatment of hemodialysis patients is optimally timed, as described in Chapter 13, to avoid the anticoagulant effect of heparin immediately after dialysis and the azotemia present immediately before dialysis. Also, dialysis patients are at high risk for blood-borne infections because of the necessity for repeated venous punctures. The renal transplant patient is typically receiving antirejection drugs, including cyclosporine and corticosteroids. This entails immunosuppression, development of cushingoid features, hypertension, and generalized gingival hyperplasia. Analgesics and drugs primarily excreted by the kidneys should be avoided, if possible, in all cases of chronic renal insufficiency.

Sexually Transmitted Infections

Most venereal diseases are localized infections that are easily treated with minimal impact on the patient's general health. However, the sexual practices of some individuals entail increased risk of exposure to more serious infections such as hepatitis B and human immunodeficiency virus (HIV). This warrants concern for the welfare of the patient and the risk of nonsexual infection in the dental setting. Table 7-6 lists the variety of organisms spread by sexual contact and the resulting infections. In general, these organisms die quickly outside the host, which implies that infection by casual contact is improbable or impossible. Also, an individual's probability of infection by most of these organisms increases with sexual contact frequency and partner diversity.

Venereal infections are assessed clinically by categorization of symptoms, history of contact, and laboratory studies, which are briefly discussed in Chapter 11. Urethritis and vaginitis usually represent relatively localized gonococcal, chlamydial, or trichomonal infections. *Vaginal candidiasis* is the most common nonvenereal infection that must be considered with complaints of vaginal discomfort. An isolated, painless, raised ulcer is typical of a primary *syphilitic chancre*. Multiple, recurring ulcers that are preceded by vesicles suggest *herpes simplex infection*. Multiple wartlike lesions affecting both partners are typical of *condyloma acuminatum*. Symmetric, nonpruritic skin rash, lymphadenopathy, malaise, and painless mucosal ulcers called *mucous patches* are observed with *secondary syphilis*. Degenerative central nervous system (CNS) and cardiovascular disease can be serious consequences of *tertiary syphilis*.

Antimicrobial medications generally cure gonococcal, treponemal, chlamydial, and trichomonal infections. Eradication of condyloma lesions requires removal by surgical excision, cryosurgery, chemical cautery, or laser cautery. Treatment of herpes simplex virus is symptomatic and supportive, since no cure is available.

Certain oral lesions, as discussed in Chapters 16, 17, and 18, may suggest the possibility of oral venereal infections, particularly in patients who are considered high risk by historical or clinical findings. Treatment of oral venereal infections could be considered within the dentist's prerogative, but the frequent coexistence of genital infection with oral lesions indicates medical referral as the approach for more comprehensive management. A history of effectively treated past venereal infection may indicate a greater likelihood of reinfection but specifically requires no alteration of dental management.

Patients with active venereal infections must be considered to present an infectious risk in the dental setting to dental personnel, as well as to other patients. However, because the patient history often fails to reveal venereal and other infections, treating all patients as be-

Table 7-6 Summary of sexually transmitted infections

Organism	Disease	Manifestations
BACTERIA		
Neisseria gonorrhoeae	Gonorrhea	Urethritis, cervicitis, endometritis, pharyngitis, pelvic inflammatory disease, conjunctivitis, disseminated infection
Treponema pallidum	Syphilis	Chancre, disseminated manifestations of secondary syphilis, degenerative organ disease of tertiary syphilis
Chlamydia trachomatis	Chlamydia infection	Cervicitis, vulvovaginitis, urethritis, epididymitis, trachoma, lymphogranuloma venereum, pharyngitis (unusual)
Calymmatobacterium granulomatis	Granuloma inguinale	Genital ulcers, granulomatous tissue damage
Mycoplasma hominis	Postpartum fever	Fever, sepsis following delivery
Haemophilus ducreyi	Chancroid	Genital ulcers
Ureaplasma urealiyticum		Nonspecific urethritis
Haemophilus vaginalis		Nonspecific vaginitis
Group B streptococcus species		Neonatal sepsis, meningitis
Shigella species*	Shigellosis	Enterocolitis
Campylobacter species*		Enterocolitis
VIRUSES		
Herpes simplex virus, type 2 (HSV-2) (HSV-1 less common)	Herpes	Vesicles, ulcers
Human immunodeficiency viruses (HIV-1 and HIV-2)	AIDS	Compromised immune function, opportunistic infections, Kaposi's sarcoma
Human papilloma viruses (various types)	Condyloma acuminatum	Genital and oral venereal warts, cervical carcinoma
Hepatitis B virus (HBV)	Hepatitis B	Acute viral hepatitis, may become chronic
Hepatitis C virus (HCV)	Hepatitis C	Acute viral hepatitis, may become chronic
Molluscum contagiosum virus	Molluscum contagiosum	Numerous papules with soft central material
Cytomegalovirus	Mononucleosis, glandular fever	Fever, malaise, lymphadenopathy
PROTOZOA		
Trichomonas vaginalis	Trichomonal infection	Vulvovaginitis, pharyngitis possible
*Giardia lamblia**	Giardiasis	Enteritis, malabsorption, diarrhea
*Entamoeba histolytica**		Enterocolitis
ECTOPARASITES		
Phthirus pubis	Pubic lice	
Sarcoptes scabiei	Scabies	
FUNGUS		
Candida albicans		Nonspecific vaginitis

Modified from Wilson JD and others, editors: Harrison's principles of internal medicine, ed 12, New York, 1991, McGraw-Hill.
*Represents primarily oral-fecal exposure in the context of sexual activity.

ing potentially infectious is more effective than selective infection control for patients known to be infected.

AIDS

Acquired immunodeficiency syndrome (AIDS) is caused by at least two lymphotrophic retroviruses that are designated HIV-1 and HIV-2. The sexual spread of HIV probably represents incidental blood-to-blood contact during intimacy, although the virus is present in semen and other body fluids of infected individuals.

HIV infection is categorized clinically into four distinct stages. Stage I infection is characterized by nonspecific features of an acute viral infection, such as mild fever and malaise, of several weeks' duration. This prodromal episode occurs within several weeks of the infectious contact. Stage II is the asymptomatic latent period of several years that generally follows the prodromal symptoms. Serologic tests during stage II, as described in Chapter 11, indicate that the patient is HIV seropositive and infectious. Stage III HIV infection is indicated by relatively nonspecific clinical features such as fatigue, mild fever, night sweats, malaise, weight loss, and generalized nontender lymphadenopathy; these were collectively referred to at one time as AIDS-related complex (ARC). Stage III may last for months or years. Stage IV is characterized by opportunistic infections that develop because a significant proportion of the T_4-helper lymphocyte population has been destroyed by HIV infection, which results in diminished effectiveness of the cellular immune response. Common examples include rapidly progressive periodontitis, oral candidiasis, other fungal infections, pneumonia caused by *Pneumocystis carinii*, and hairy leukoplakia of the tongue caused by unsuppressed viral stimulation of the oral epithelium. Multiple, nodular surface lesions of Kaposi's sarcoma and other neoplasms often develop in the terminal stage of the disease, apparently representing deficient lymphocyte suppression of the neoplasms.

Antibodies to HIV can usually be detected within 6 months of infection, but clinical evidence of stage III or IV disease usually does not appear for years. During this latent period the individual is infectious but asymptomatic, which partially explains the dramatic spread of the illness. AIDS is considered fatal, although drugs such as zidovudine (azidothymidine, AZT) appear to slow the progression. At this time the only effective approach is prevention by the use of condoms or by avoidance of sexual and blood-to-blood contact with infected individuals.

CONDITIONS AFFECTING THE NERVOUS SYSTEM

Neurologic conditions are categorized as regional or generalized and are further divided on the basis of acute versus chronic onset. The initial goal of neurologic evaluation is to determine if the defect is central (CNS) or peripheral (peripheral nervous system, PNS). A regional loss of peripheral sensory or motor function implies a focal lesion resulting from injury or compression by a tumor. The cardinal features of acute central neurologic conditions are alteration of consciousness, vertigo, and confusion. Gradual loss of memory and other cortical functions suggest chronic degenerative conditions. Common neurologic abnormalities that the dentist must evaluate are categorized as cerebrovascular conditions, seizure disorders, and generalized neuromuscular deficiencies. Conditions characterized by pain of the head and neck are considered in Chapter 9.

Cerebrovascular Disease

Cerebrovascular disorders are conditions of abnormal brain function caused by blood vessel disease. The initiating event may involve short lapses of blood supply, vessel rupture, or vessel blockage by emboli or thrombosis. Various terms such as stroke, apoplexy, shock, and cerebrovascular accident (CVA) reflect the typically dramatic onset. The severity and extent of the neurologic deficit depends on the duration of ischemia and the extent of brain tissue affected. A *transient ischemic attack* (TIA) produces temporary neurologic symptoms that resolve when the blood supply improves. *Cerebral infarction,* or ischemic necrosis caused by inadequate blood supply, results in permanent neurologic damage. Patients prone to stroke are usually elderly and hypertensive, and exhibit evidence of atherosclerosis, such as intermittent claudication and angina pectoris. Intracranial hemorrhage entails interruption of blood supply, as well as the urgent danger posed by a rapid increase in intracranial pressure. Intracranial hemorrhage usually results from vascular injury or rupture of aneurysms following relatively mild traumatic injury.

Acute ischemia produces regional neurologic deficiency that may be virtually instantaneous or progress within several minutes to a few hours. The resulting neurologic abnormality depends on the affected artery. Recurring episodes of neural dysfunction lasting from a few seconds to as long as 30 minutes without permanent neurologic defect characterize TIAs. Dizziness and lapses in attention commonly occur, but unconsciousness or convulsions are unusual. The manifestations of CVA range from sudden hemiplegia and unconsciousness in severe instances to the sudden appearance of an inconsequential neural defect without additional findings. TIAs commonly precede CVAs. Permanent motor deficits often result from strokes because the middle cerebral artery blood supply to motor regions is most commonly affected. Additional manifestations of stroke can include numbness, blindness, diplopia, and speech disorders. The clinical features of intracranial hemorrhage are similar to those of a CVA with the added features of violent headache, collapse, absence of hemiplegia, and absence of prodromal TIAs. An additional differentiating feature of intracranial hemorrhage is that the neurologic deficiency gradually progresses as pooling blood compresses brain tissue, as compared with the initial maximal

severity of neural defects caused by ischemia.

Clinical evidence of recent TIAs or the sudden onset of a neural deficit requires medical referral to clarify the condition before routine dental care is undertaken. Medical consultation is also warranted for recovering stroke patients. Six months is often recommended as a minimum stabilization period following a CVA, during which time dental care should be delayed, but consultation provides more specific direction in individual cases. Anticoagulant therapy during this recovery period can cause hemostasis difficulties during dental treatment. This must also be considered if dental treatment cannot be delayed. Following control of hypertension and other contributory conditions, the stabilized stoke patient generally presents no greater stroke risk during routine dental care than do patients of similar age and general health. Neural defects can make oral hygiene practices and handling of dental appliances difficult. Devices such as electric toothbrushes and prosthetically redesigned appliances may be helpful.

Seizure Disorders

Seizure disorders, also referred to generally as *epilepsy,* are defined as chronic conditions of episodic brain dysfunction caused by excessive neuronal discharge. Although many forms of CNS injury can cause seizure disorders, most patients are affected by idiopathic epilepsy. Idiopathic epilepsy is associated with no demonstrable morphologic defects and is genetically determined by undefined mechanisms. Symptoms develop before early adulthood. Organic brain diseases resulting from stroke, injury, and other conditions producing morphologically detectable lesions can also cause convulsive dysfunction. Physiologic imbalances such as uremia, hypoglycemia, and hypocalcemia can also induce seizures, although the symptoms resolve following effective treatment of the cause unless organic brain injury occurs.

The history of seizures is characterized by abrupt onset of attacks, short duration, and recurrence. *Grand mal* and *petit mal* are the most common types, and numerous other patterns have been described. Grand mal seizures are characterized by an aura or "odd sensation" that is followed by loss of consciousness, muscular convulsions, and a recovery period of mild confusion and deep sleep. Petit mal seizures are identified by a sudden vacant facial expression and loss of muscle tone without convulsions, followed by an abrupt return to normal. Most seizure disorders can be controlled by medications such as phenobarbitol, phenytoin, and primidone.

Prevention of seizures during dental treatment, minimization of injury if a seizure occurs, and management of gingival hyperplasia caused by phenytoin (discussed in Chapter 18) are the principal considerations in treating epileptic patients. Seizure in the dental setting is unlikely if the condition is well controlled by medication. Relatively poor control as indicated by recent seizures or past episodes related to anxiety may require alteration of the medication as directed by the physician. Management during a convulsive seizure includes limb restraints to minimize injury, evacuation of vomit to avoid aspiration, and breathing support if apnea develops.

Degenerative Neural and Neuromuscular Disorders

Degenerative neural and neuromuscular diseases include conditions of generalized muscular dysfunction caused by a wide variety of pathologic processes. *Multiple sclerosis* and *Parkinson's disease* are caused by CNS degeneration. *Progressive muscular dystrophy* is genetically determined skeletal muscle degeneration, and *myasthenia gravis* results from degeneration of the neuromuscular junction. Generalized, chronic, progressive abnormalities of movement, such as tremors, weakness, abnormality of gait, and altered speech, are general features of these conditions.

Multiple sclerosis becomes apparent early in life with the onset of slurred speech, tremor during movement, sensory disturbances, and impaired vision. Periods of remission and exacerbation are typical. Parkinsonism affects older patients and produces chronic, progressively severe resting tremors, rigidity, fixed facial expression, gait abnormality, and "pill rolling" movement of the fingers. Muscular dystrophy typically affects children, producing progressive muscle weakness, and familial occurrence is usually noted. Myasthenia gravis usually affects young adult women, producing muscular weakness and fatigue involving the eyes, chewing, speaking, and swallowing.

Tremors can complicate routine dental treatment for some patients. Sedation or other alternative treatment approaches may be required. Oral hygiene aids such as electric toothbrushes may be beneficial.

CONNECTIVE TISSUE DISEASES

The nonspecific nature of the phrase "connective tissue diseases" implies the diversity of the conditions grouped in this category. All of these conditions, also referred to as "collagen diseases" or "collagen-vascular diseases," are caused by development of a humoral or cellular autoimmune response directed against connective tissue components. General features include gradual onset, sclerosing vasculitis, progressive deterioration, and improvement with antiinflammatory medications. The broad range of clinical features is attributable to the variety of cellular, subcellular, and tissue components for which autoimmune sensitivity can develop in different patients. In addition, many patients exhibit signs and symptoms representing considerable overlap or blurring of distinctions among these diseases, which explains "mixed connective tissue disease" as a diagnosis applied in some situations. Most affected patients are young to middle-aged adults, and women are afflicted more often than men. Connective tissue disorders caused by immune mechanisms are summarized in Table 7-7.

Table 7-7 Summary of common immune system disorders affecting connective tissues and joints

Condition	Typical clinical features
Rheumatoid arthritis (RA)	Chronic polyarthritis in a symmetrical distribution; Raynaud's phenomenon; joint enlargement, tenderness, and deformity are common features; periarticular rheumatoid nodules and vasculitis may develop
Sjögren's syndrome (SjS)	Affects 15%-20% of RA patients; mucosal and conjunctival dryness (sicca syndrome) in addition to other autoimmune manifestations; this is usually RA, although some patients exhibit features more suggestive of SSc or SLE; bilateral parotid enlargement is common; more than one third of SjS patients develop renal abnormalities
Systemic sclerosis (SSc; scleroderma)	Raynaud's phenomenon; fibrosis of skin causing stiffness, limitation of movement, and flexion contractures of hands (sclerodactyly); variable pattern of arthralgia and limited movement may develop; manifestations of organ system fibrosis can include renal failure, dyspnea, and GI hypomobility leading to esophageal pain and/or malabsorption
Systemic lupus erythematosus (SLE)	Arthralgia, myalgia, light sensitive malar ("butterfly") rash, skin nodules and ulcers with scarring and depigmentation; renal deterioration is the most consistent and significant systemic manifestation, but CNS, cardiopulmonary, hemopoietic, and GI damage with resulting symptoms may also develop
Mixed connective tissue disease (MCTD)	Raynaud's phenomenon, polyarthritis, swollen hands or sclerodactyly, esophageal dysfunction, and pulmonary damage are the most typical features, but most of the features described in this table are possible manifestations of MCTD
Ankylosing spondylitis (AS)	Lower spinal pain develops during late adolescence or early adulthood; additional sites of bone pain may develop in an asymmetric distribution; constitutional signs such as fatigue, fever, weight loss, or night sweats may also be observed; severe cases progress to spinal deformity, ankylosis, degeneration, and fracture

Modified from Wilson JD and others, editors: Harrison's principles of internal medicine, ed 12, New York, 1991, McGraw-Hill.

Rheumatoid Arthritis

The underlying lesion of rheumatoid arthritis is chronic inflammation of the synovial lining. Numerous theories regarding the precise mechanism to explain the interaction of possible antigenic stimulants and immune responses have been proposed, but none has been fully confirmed. Central to the disease is the presence of a group of circulating IgM antibodies collectively known as *rheumatoid factor.*

Chronic, degenerative arthritis affecting multiple synovial joints in a symmetric distribution is the characteristic presentation of rheumatoid arthritis. Swelling, warmth, and tenderness of the proximal interphalangeal and metacarpophalangeal joints are usually the earliest manifestations, in contrast to the enlargement of distal interphalangeal joints that is typical of osteoarthritis (Fig. 7-5). The rate of progression and the severity of joint deterioration vary considerably among patients and are roughly proportional to the rheumatoid factor titer. The development of round, rubbery masses at sites of external pressure, called *rheumatoid nodules,* results from rheumatoid vasculitis and indicates a poor prognosis. Additional systemic complications may include malaise, anemia, lung nodules, and cardiac le-

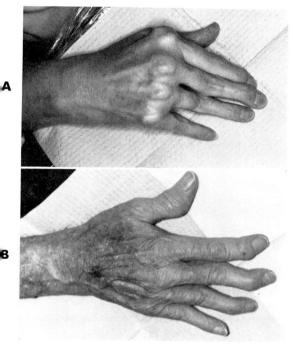

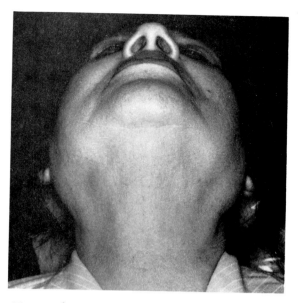

Fig. 7-6. Bilateral parotid enlargement of Sjögren's syndrome as demonstrated from the submental perspective with the patient's head in a hyperextended position.

Fig. 7-5. **A,** The hand of a 62-year-old woman suffering from rheumatoid arthritis. Diagnostic features include enlargement of the metacarpophalangeal joints and ulnar deviation deformity of the fingers. **B,** The hand of a 74-year-old man with osteoarthritis. In contrast to the damage of rheumatoid arthritis, the distal interphalangeal joints are usually most severely affected by osteoarthritis.

sions. Approximately 15% of patients with rheumatoid arthritis also exhibit dry eyes, xerostomia, and bilateral parotid enlargement (Fig. 7-6), which are collectively referred to as *Sjögren's syndrome.*

Treatment of rheumatoid arthritis is usually by aspirin, corticosteroids, or nonsteroidal antiinflammatory drugs. Combinations of several drugs may be necessary to achieve control. The dentist must consider the possibility of a bleeding tendency caused by these medications, as well as possible analgesic masking of symptoms caused by dental disease. Chronic corticosteroid administration may cause adre-

nocortical insufficiency and the development of cushingoid features. Oral hygiene aids may be helpful in cases of severe deformities of the hands.

Systemic Lupus Erythematosus

SLE is an autoimmune disease resulting from the development of antinuclear antibodies (ANAs) to endogenous DNA and nuclear proteins. A broad variety of lesions can develop, and most organs can be affected, but the clinical effects all relate to either small-vessel sclerosis or inflammation of serosal membranes. The term *discoid lupus erythematosus* distinguishes those patients with skin lesions only, whereas SLE indicates that at least one additional organ system is affected.

The most consistent clinical feature is photosensitive skin atrophy and erythema located in the midface region, known as a "butterfly rash." Other sun-exposed skin surfaces may also be affected. Nearly 50% of SLE patients experience signs of renal disease ranging from mild proteinuria to renal failure. Sterile serosal inflammation of the pleura, pericardium, peritoneum, or joints can develop and is manifested by pain and tenderness at these sites. Vascular deterioration can also cause neuropathy and seizures in as many as one half of affected individuals. A positive serum ANA test confirms the diagnosis.

Oral ulcers may develop in severely affected individuals, particularly following prolonged sun exposure or physiologic stress. Chronic corticosteroid administration is the treatment of choice, and adverse effects of the medication may require alteration of dental treatment. Consultation with the patient's physician may be indicated, depending on the extent of systemic disease.

Systemic Sclerosis

Systemic sclerosis (SSc) is a chronic debilitating disease characterized by vasculitis and fibrosis of connective tissues. SSc is also referred to as *scleroderma* because of the predominant sclerosis of dermal connective tissues. The autoimmune mechanism of the disease is poorly understood, but ANA reactivity with the nucleolus is seen almost exclusively in SSc.

Dermal sclerosis of the digits is particularly noticeable, producing enlargement and limitation of movement of the digits, known as *sclerodactyly*. Facial changes characterized by loss of skin folds and limited mobility are referred to as a "masked face" appearance. Additional skin abnormalities that occasionally develop include calcinosis and telangiectasias. Trismus and degeneration of the temporomandibular joints may develop in severe cases. *Raynaud's phenomenon* is vasospasm of the hand leading to blanching, cyanosis, and erythema following exposure to cold. The reaction affects 90% of SSc patients and may be the earliest manifestation of SSc or other connective tissue disease. Additional features of SSc include GI hypomobility, esophageal reflux, malabsorption, pulmonary fibrosis, myocardial sclerosis, and polyarthritis.

The dentist must be concerned with the multisystemic implications of this disease and its treatment, including chronic corticosteroid administration. In addition, trismus and related jaw dysfunction can cause discomfort and limited access during dental treatment.

MALIGNANT NEOPLASTIC DISEASE

Malignant neoplasia, or *cancer,* is a term given to a group of diseases that are characterized by abnormal cell proliferation resulting in invasion and destruction of adjacent tissues and in metastatic spread to distant sites. The clinical manifestations of cancer usually reflect pressure effects of local tumor enlargement and compromised function of organs infiltrated by tumor. Advanced malignancy may also produce constitutional signs such as weight loss, anemia, and weakness. Occasionally symptoms may result from the secondary features of the lesion, such as hormone production by a glandular neoplasm. More than 100 distinct forms of malignant neoplasia are recognized and can be broadly classified on the basis of initial growth pattern as either solid tumors or neoplasms of hemopoietic and immune system origin. Solid malignant neoplasms initially form a primary mass or enlargement. Hemopoietic and immune system neoplasms originate from cell populations that exist normally as isolated cells and include the leukemias, lymphomas, and multiple myeloma.

Solid Malignant Neoplasms

Microscopic characteristics of the neoplastic cells generally indicate the cell type of origin, which forms the basis for diagnosis. Lesions composed of cells that display epithelial characteristics are classified as *carcinomas,* whereas neoplasms with predominantly cellular features of connective tissues are designated as *sarcomas.* Carcinomas can usually be categorized as either squamous cell carcinoma if features of lining epithelium are present or adenocarcinoma if the morphology suggests a glandular origin. Descriptive terms such as "well differentiated" or "poorly differentiated" are attempts to correlate the cellular morphology of the malignancy with the expected clinical course. In addition, clinical findings such as tumor size, evidence of lymph node spread, and distant metastasis determine *staging,* which is the assessment of the clinical progression or extent of the disease. Staging guidelines for different malignant diseases attempt to relate clinical and pathologic findings at the time of diagnosis with the prognosis and optimal treatment of the cancer. Staging criteria, therefore, are specific for each form of malignancy and for each site of occurrence.

Clinical features of solid malignant neoplasms are generally attributable to either mass effects of the enlargement or alteration of the affected organ's function. Signs of mass effect include clinically apparent enlargement, neuropathy caused by compression, pain, limitation of movement, surface ulceration, and obstruction. Loss of function reflects destruction of normal tissues. The onset and gradual progression of these symptoms within weeks or months suggest the possibility of malignant neoplasia. Superficial malignant neoplasms usually appear heterogeneous with poorly delineated borders. Induration, absence of tenderness, enlargement of regional lymph nodes, and fixation to surrounding structures also suggest malignant neoplasia.

Early diagnosis and treatment are positive prognostic factors for nearly all malignant neoplasms. Referral for diagnosis and treatment should not be delayed when clinical signs and symptoms suggest a malignancy.

Patterns of Metastasis

Solid malignant neoplasms progress by three mechanisms: (1) direct extension or local invasion, (2) hematogenous spread, and (3) spread to regional lymph nodes via lymphatic drainage. Hematogenous distribution of tumor to distant sites and lymphatic spread to regional lymph nodes are defined as metastasis, and the resulting lesions are referred to as *secondary* or *metastatic tumors.* Specific malignancies exhibit the tendency to metastasize by either the hematogenous or lymphatic route, although either route is possible with most cancers. The progression of a localized malignant neoplasm into a regional or generalized disease usually entails a dramatic decline in prognosis and the need for more aggressive treatment methods.

Hematogenous metastasis involves distribution of isolated cells or small cellular clumps in the bloodstream from the primary tumor to a distant site. Sarcomas and prostatic adenocarcinoma usually metastasize hematogenously. Highly vascular organs, such as the lung, liver, and brain, are the most likely sites. The factors that determine whether or not tumor cells hematogenously deposited at a specific site will form a metastatic lesion are poorly understood.

Carcinomas typically metastasize initially by infiltration of tumor cells into afferent lymphatic channels, resulting in transport to the regional lymph nodes. Many cancers of deep structures, such as the maxillary sinus, are first suspected when metastatic enlargement of regional lymph nodes is identified. This emphasizes the importance of palpating regional lymph nodes during routine clinical examinations. The regional spread of malignancy is a negative prognostic indicator in cancer staging, but less so in most instances as compared with distant, hematogenous metastasis.

Neoplasia of Hemopoietic and Immune System Origin

Disseminated cancers are characterized by neoplastic proliferation of hemopoietic and immune system cells. The neoplastic cells mimic their cells of origin during initial progression by spreading as individual cells or small cell groups rather than forming a primary tumor mass. Table 7-8 summarizes the classification of common malignancies that develop from

Table 7-8   Summary of common neoplasms of hemopoietic and immune system origin

Origin/disease	Occurrence	Clinical features
HEMOPOIETIC ORIGIN		
Acute lymphocytic leukemia (ALL)	Most common among infants and children	Anemia, thrombocytopenia and bleeding, weakness, vulnerability to infection, bone pain; rapidly progressive without therapy
Acute myelogenous leukemia (AML)	More common with advancing age	Similar to ALL; rapidly progressive without therapy
Chronic lymphocytic leukemia (CLL)	Unusual before middle age, increased incidence with age	May be discovered incidentally, most signs are related to organs affected by leukemic cell infiltration; anemia and thrombocytopenia eventually develop; slowly progressive course of several years despite available therapy
Chronic myelogenous leukemia (CML)	Broad age range, incidence increases with age	Similar clinically to CLL during chronic stage; acute or "blast" stage similar to ALL and AML
Hairy cell leukemia	Patients usually beyond age 40	Splenomegaly, impaired host resistance, or vasculitis in addition to moderate pancytopenia; clinical course may be chronic and insidious, but many examples are more rapidly progressive; infection is the usual cause of death
Polycythemia vera	Late middle age or older	Splenomegaly and increased production of myeloid elements, but dominant feature is elevated hemoglobin and red cell count; symptoms may relate to increased blood viscosity; chronic, indolent course; most patients die of vascular complications
IMMUNE SYSTEM ORIGIN		
Hodgkin's lymphoma	Bimodal occurrence between ages 15 and 35 and past age 50	Localized nontender enlargement of lymphoid tissues and spread to contiguous nodes; many patients experience no other symptoms, although fever, night sweats, weight loss, or other constitutional symptoms affect approximately one third of patients; course depends on pathologic subtype and disease staging

Table 7-8 Summary of common neoplasms of hemopoietic and immune system origin

Origin/disease	Occurrence	Clinical features
IMMUNE SYSTEM ORIGIN—cont'd		
Non-Hodgkin's lymphoma	Most common between ages 20 and 40	Persistent painless peripheral lymphadenopathy affecting multiple node groups; other lymphoid tissues, such as the palatine tonsils, may also be enlarged; cough, chest pain, GI symptoms, and other symptoms of visceral obstruction may develop; course depends on pathologic subtype and disease staging
Multiple myeloma	Older adults, unusual before age 40	Bone pain, multiple radiolucencies of bone, susceptibility to bacterial infection, renal disease, Bence Jones protein in urine, anemia; course is unpredictable and varies from rapidly progressive to chronic and indolent

the hemopoietic and immune system tissues.

Leukemia originates from hemopoietic tissue and is classified by the cell of origin as *myelogenous* or *lymphocytic*. Both myelogenous and lymphocytic leukemias are further classified as acute or chronic on the basis of cellular features and clinical disease course. The diagnosis of leukemia is based on the identification of morphologically abnormal, immature white cells in the peripheral blood and bone marrow. Symptoms related to anemia and deficiency in platelet production are often associated with leukemia and result from the replacement of normal hemopoietic tissues by neoplastic cells. The total white blood cell count is usually elevated, and immature cells predominate. Gingival enlargement is a common feature of leukemia.

Lymphoma originates from the lymphatic and reticuloendothelial organs and produces multiple enlargements of these tissues. Pathologic and clinical findings allow further classification as *Hodgkin's* or *non-Hodgkin's lymphoma*. Lymphoma initially presents as multiple, rubbery, nontender enlargements of lymphoid structures. Cervical lymph nodes are enlarged in more than one half of affected patients. In addition, Hodgkin's lymphomas often produce unexplained weight loss, night sweats, and mild fever.

Multiple myeloma originates from plasma cells and most often affects middle-aged to elderly patients. Clinical features of multiple myeloma include multiple "punched out" radiolucencies of bone, pain of affected bones, anemia, and a bleeding tendency. Myeloma cells release abnormal immunoglobulins into the serum, producing a *monoclonal gammopathy* that can be detected by laboratory methods. Increasing serum concentration of monoclonal immunoglobulins referred to as *Bence Jones proteins* leads to their excretion in the urine in over 50% of patients with multiple myeloma.

Principles of Cancer Treatment

The most dependable primary treatment for most solid malignant neoplasms is total surgical excision. If any portion of the lesion remains after surgery, the residual neoplastic cells continue to grow and spread. Therefore total surgical excision of the malignancy is not feasible in many cases involving distant metastases and tumor infiltration into vital structures. In general, small and superficial malignancies can be cured surgically, whereas larger, deeper lesions are less likely to be cured by surgery alone.

Soon after the discovery of x-rays in 1895, ionizing radiation exposure was observed to produce shrinkage or total disappearance of many malignancies with only minor injury to surrounding normal tissues. Clinicians also observed that spacing the radiation dosage over time in multiple exposures called *fractions* damaged tumors as much as a single dose with the benefit of decreased injury to normal tissues. The underlying strategy of all radiotherapy soon emerged: (1) minimize injury to normal tissues by employing fractionation, limiting the field of exposure, and delivering the radiation to deep tumors from different beam directions called *portals* and then (2) deliver the maximum ionizing radiation dosage that the normal tissues can tolerate to maximize tumor cell killing. Radiation can also be delivered to solid malignancies through implantation of radioactive rods or seeds into the tumor, which is referred to as *interstitial radiotherapy.*

The sensitivity to radiation varies among different neoplasms. Carcinomas typically exhibit greater radiosensitivity, whereas most sarcomas are relatively radioresistant. Unfortunately, most cancers cannot be totally eradicated within the dosage tolerance of adjacent normal tissues. The combination of radiotherapy and surgical removal of solid malignant neoplasms was eventually shown to increase the likelihood of successful tumor eradication in most cases beyond the expected success rate for either treatment alone.

Surgery and radiotherapy offer little in the treatment of most disseminated malignancies, such as leukemias and lymphomas. This pro-

moted the search for effective anticancer drugs. Chemotherapeutic agents are classified as antimetabolites and cytotoxic alkylating agents. Chemotherapy strategy generally uses combinations of agents from both classes administered in a series of dosages near the toxicity tolerance of the patient to kill all mitotically active malignant cells. Chemotherapy is the primary treatment method for malignancies of hemopoietic and immune system origin. It is also useful as adjunctive therapy for solid tumors treated at the primary and regional sites by surgery and radiotherapy.

An emerging approach in the treatment of disseminated malignancies called *bone marrow transplantation* relies on killing all bone marrow and immune system cells with radiation and chemotherapeutic agents. The patient's immune and hemopoietic cell populations are then replaced by infusion of bone marrow tissue from an antigenically similar donor. Immunosuppressive drugs are often required following the transplantation to control *graft-versus-host disease,* which results from attack by the immunologically active lymphocytes from the donor against the tissues of the host.

Treatment of the cancer patient varies depending on the specific tumor, its location, and the staging of the disease. In general, curative cancer therapy for solid tumors entails the combination of surgery to remove the primary tumor; radiotherapy to kill cancer cells in the primary area, including regional lymphatic metastasis; and chemotherapy to kill distant, hematogenous metastasis. This combination represents the greatest probability of total eradication of all malignant cells. Clinical observation is then directed to surveillance for the appearance of any tumor regrowth. The therapeutic goal in advanced cases may be *palliation,* which means that surgery, radiotherapy, and chemotherapy are used to control symptoms when the prognosis is believed to be terminal. Refinements in drug combinations, discovery of new antineoplastic drugs, and development of immunologically specific tumor-killing mechanisms represent the current forefront of cancer therapy.

Oral Complications of Cancer Treatment

Treatment methods that effectively kill cancer cells also injure normal cell populations. This often causes adverse side effects and complications affecting the oral cavity during and after treatment. The tissues most vulnerable to injury from radiation and antitumor drugs during therapy are composed of actively dividing cell populations, such as hemopoietic and basal epithelial cells. Therefore bone marrow suppression and mucosal ulceration produce the most common and dramatic clinical complications as treatment progresses. Chronic and permanent injuries to the oral tissues as a consequence of cancer therapy usually result from direct tumoricidal radiation exposure of the oral tissues and major salivary glands. Also, tissue defects can be produced by surgical attempts to totally excise large primary tumors of the head and neck.

Complications during cancer treatment. The adverse oral effects of cancer therapy are difficult to predict and are highly dependent on the specific features of the treatment regimen, the resistance of the host tissues to injury, and the patient's tolerance. Direct radiation exposure causes *oral mucositis* in most patients by the second week of the treatment course. Initial mucosal inflammation and atrophy soon progress to painful ulceration that persists for 2 to 3 weeks after completion of radiotherapy. Similar mucosal lesions are produced by anticancer drugs in approximately 20% to 50% of patients undergoing chemotherapy. Because mastication is painful and increases the severity of the ulcers, anorexia and poor nutritional intake often result. Treatment of oral mucositis is limited to symptomatic care relying on analgesics and topical anesthetics for pain control, as well as coating suspensions to provide superficial protection.

Chemotherapeutic drugs suppress bone marrow production of blood cell precursors, which eventually causes a decrease in circulating blood cells. The resulting leukopenia deprives the patient of a primary mechanism for resisting infection. In addition, the oral mucosal barrier to microbes is often compromised by mucositis. This allows development of unusual infections and exceptionally severe manifestations of common infections. Opportunistic infections such as candidiasis frequently develop during the course of chemotherapy. Primary herpes simplex infections or emergence of secondary herpetic lesions can be particularly severe as compared with those affecting healthy patients. In addition, chronic oral infections, such as periodontitis and periapical lesions, are frequently exacerbated by cancer chemotherapy. Anemia and bleeding diathesis caused by thrombocytopenia are less common consequences of bone marrow suppression.

Complications that develop subsequent to cancer therapy. Oral complications that appear following cancer treatment are caused by direct radiation exposure of the jaws and the major salivary glands. The radiation dosage required for effective primary or adjuvant therapy of most head and neck cancers is 40 to 65 Gy (4000 to 6500 rad). The radiation damage to normal tissue in this tumoricidal dosage range is produced by a combination of initial cell necrosis, fibrosis, and irreversible vascular sclerosis.

Radiation injury of the major salivary glands produces a dramatic decrease in salivary flow within the first 2 weeks of the radiotherapy course. The resulting oral dryness, called *xerostomia,* is progressive and persistent during radiotherapy, and the salivary tissue damage is irreversible in most cases, leaving the patient permanently xerostomic. Xerostomia may be less severe if the tumor location allows direction of the primary radiation beams to spare one or more of the major salivary glands. The relative absence of lubricating saliva during radiotherapy contributes to the severity of the oral mucositis, loss of taste sensitivity, and mastication difficulties.

Two additional consequences of xerostomia develop after completion of radiotherapy. Xerostomia deprives the teeth of a primary defense against carious decalcification. A rampant increase in dental decay, referred to as *radiation caries,* often develops unless exceptional measures to control decay can be maintained. Radiation-induced carious lesions characteristically affect root surfaces, although the incidence of decay of other tooth surfaces is also increased. Minimal salivary flow causes decreased host resistance to superficial oral infections. Recurrent oral candidiasis frequently develops in xerostomic patients. Rapid progression of periodontitis in the absence of saliva is also common.

Treatment of xerostomia and the direct consequences of diminished salivary flow for the patient receiving head and neck radiotherapy rely on the use of artificial saliva preparations, the maintenance of superb oral hygiene, and the scheduling of frequent dental recall examinations. Most patients report symptomatic improvement through increased daily fluid intake and the use of artificial saliva. Sialogogues such as pilocarpine may provide beneficial stimulation of salivary flow. A common response of the xerostomic patient that should be specifically avoided is the tendency to drink sucrose-rich beverages, which promotes radiation caries beyond any control measures. Daily home fluoride applications in addition to effective plaque control increase decay resistance. The fluoride preparation prescribed should be nonacidic to prevent dental erosion. Frequent dental visits allow early identification of oral infections such as candidiasis, reinforcement of effective oral hygiene practices, early identification of carious lesions, and periodic periodontal scaling.

The most significant consequence of radiation-induced vascular sclerosis and the resulting diminished blood supply following tumoricidal radiation exposure is the increased vulnerability of bone to a severe form of osteomyelitis known as *osteoradionecrosis.* The mandible is much more likely to be affected than the maxilla because of the anatomic differences in vascularity between the two jaws. Osteoradionecrosis typically occurs within 2 years of tumoricidal radiation exposure to bone totaling at least 40 Gy and usually more than 50 Gy. Loss of mucosal integrity through minor injury, chronic trauma from an ill-fitting prosthesis, or simple tooth extraction allows bacterial entry into the alveolar bone. Chronic, painful progression of infection, necrosis, and sequestration of necrotic bone occurs despite normally effective infection control treatments such as antibiotic therapy, irrigation, and drainage. Aggressive surgical and hyperbaric oxygen treatments in addition to high-dose antibiotic therapy may control progression of osteoradionecrosis, but the infection usually persists.

The most effective management of osteoradionecrosis is prevention. Extraction of hopeless and compromised teeth before radiotherapy decreases the likelihood that extractions will be necessary after radiotherapy. Aggressive treatment to control radiation caries and periodontitis are justified to decrease the need for future extractions. Finally, if extractions become unavoidably necessary, an atraumatic surgical approach, closure by primary intention, and attentive care following surgery are essential.

Surgical excision of malignant neoplasms can produce significant tissue defects and deformities. The two treatment options available for these conditions are plastic surgery repair and prosthetic replacement. Plastic tissue repair is generally preferable; however, compromised vascularity of adjacent tissues caused by adjunctive radiotherapy may not allow extensive surgical procedures. Cooperation of the oncologist, plastic surgeon, and maxillofacial prosthodontist is essential in achieving optimal rehabilitation of patients recovering from treatment of head and neck cancer.

SUMMARY

The dentist's goal in assessing the patient's health status is to apply the information obtained toward providing safe dental care. This requires an understanding of common systemic diseases, their treatment, and the appropriate modifications of dental treatment methods to minimize potential risks of complications. The dentist may also suspect undiagnosed disease and consult the patient's physician as necessary to arrange definitive diagnosis and treatment.

The systemic conditions described briefly in this chapter are routinely encountered by the practicing dentist, but they are by no means the limit of the dentist's clinical responsibility. Rare conditions, unusual features of common diseases, and unfamiliar medications often require the dentist to consult reference materials and the patient's physician for information and guidance.

BIBLIOGRAPHY

Ariyan S: Cancer of the head and neck, St Louis, 1987, Mosby–Year Book.

Greenspan D and others: AIDS and the mouth: diagnosis and management of oral lesions, Copenhagen, 1990, Munksgaard.

Judge RD, Zuidema GD, Fitzgerald FT, editors: Clinical diagnosis: a physiologic approach, ed 5, Boston, 1988, Little, Brown.

Langlais RP and others: Oral diagnosis, oral medicine and treatment planning, Philadelphia, 1984, Saunders.

Little JW, Falace DA: Therapeutic considerations in special patients, Dent Clin North Am 28:455-469, 1984.

Lynch MA, Brightman VJ, Greenberg MS, editors: Burket's oral medicine: diagnosis and treatment, ed 8, Philadelphia, 1984, Lippincott.

Rose LF, Kaye D, editors: Internal medicine for dentistry, St Louis, ed 2, 1990, Mosby–Year Book.

Seidel HM and others: Mosby's guide to physical examination, St Louis, 1987, Mosby–Year Book.

Wilson JD and others, editors: Harrison's principles of internal medicine, ed 12, New York, 1991, McGraw-Hill.

CHAPTER 8

Clinical Evaluation of Dental Conditions

GARY C. COLEMAN

The diagnosis of most dental abnormalities is uncomplicated because their clinical and radiographic features are characteristic. However, experienced clinicians appreciate that many unusual dental conditions and atypical presentations of common lesions can complicate the diagnosis. The challenge for the dentist is to accurately assess the severity and extent of dental lesions as a prerequisite of treatment planning.

To simplify the diagnostic process and provide a logical format for discussion, dental abnormalities are categorized by the following designations according to both the cause of the condition and the tissues affected:

1. Developmental dental abnormalities
2. Abnormalities of eruption
3. Regressive alterations of teeth
4. Carious lesions
5. Pulpal inflammation
6. Periapical inflammatory lesions secondary to pulpal necrosis
7. Inflammatory conditions of the supportive tissues

Most dental abnormalities can be diagnosed within one of these disease categories.

DEVELOPMENTAL DENTAL ABNORMALITIES

Developmental dental abnormalities are characterized clinically by abnormal appearance of tooth shape, color, or size. Isolated teeth, several teeth, or the entire dentition may be affected. Many genetically determined dental malformations that affect one tooth also affect the corresponding tooth on the contralateral side. In general, the presence of one dental developmental abnormality suggests the presence of others.

Gemination

Gemination is abnormal tooth form resulting from cleavage of a tooth germ during early development. The resulting structure appears larger than the normal tooth and often exhibits a groove or cleft parallel to the long axis, suggesting the union of two tooth crowns. A single root and pulp chamber can be demonstrated radiographically. By definition, the geminated tooth must represent one tooth in the normal complement of teeth. This rare anomaly usually occurs in the anterior segments and can affect either primary or permanent teeth.

Macrodontia, fusion, and concrescence are other diagnostic possibilities to be considered in situations of suspected gemination. The isolated macrodont exhibits large crown size but no evidence of cleavage or other indication of the union of two tooth forms. Absence of an adjacent tooth or the radiographic appearance of two separate pulp chambers indicates the anomaly to be fusion or concrescence rather than gemination. Gemination requires no specific treatment, although placement of a crown may provide esthetic improvement.

Fusion

Fusion results from the merging of two separate tooth buds during development. The resulting structure appears abnormally large clinically as shown in Fig. 8-1, and radiographs reveal continuity of enamel and dentin at the joined surface. The crowns and pulps may appear separate or completely merged, depending on the stage at which the fusion occurred. Anterior teeth are usually affected. Fusion may involve two teeth of the normal dental complement or a normal tooth and a supernumerary tooth. Therefore the fused structure may represent one or two teeth in the normal complement of teeth.

Macrodontia, gemination, and fusion are possible explanations of a large tooth in place of a single tooth. A definitive diagnosis of fusion can be made if the anomaly must be considered as two teeth to account for the normal number of teeth and if separate pulp chambers are present. If the anomaly represents a single tooth and a single pulp chamber is present, then the distinction between fusion and gemination usually cannot be made. No treatment is specifically required.

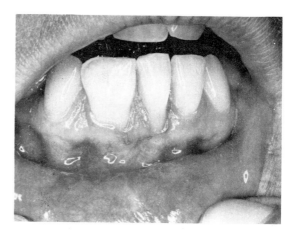

Fig. 8-1   Fusion of mandibular lateral and central incisors.

Concrescence

Concrescence is the union of two teeth by merger of cementum. This can be considered as a special form of fusion, although the anomalies are considered separately because concrescence generally occurs after coronal development. At least one tooth is unerupted in most cases. Radiographic findings include two fully formed teeth attached along root surfaces with distinctly separate pulp chambers as illustrated in Fig. 8-2. The dentin-cementum thick-

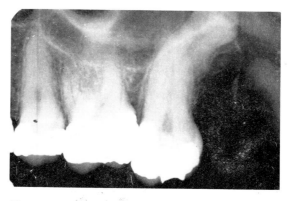

Fig. 8-2   Concrescence of maxillary second and third molars.

ness between the pulp canals at the site of junction is often greater than the normal radicular thickness of two separate teeth. Careful examination of the radiograph reveals absence of the periodontal ligament space separating the two roots.

Concrescence is unlikely to be confused with other examples of abnormal tooth morphology. The primary clinical complication of concrescence results during efforts to remove the joined teeth.

Dilaceration

Dilaceration is a common dental malformation characterized by abrupt angular bends of the root or roots relative to the long axis of the crown. Many examples are identified radiographically in situations that suggest an altered path of eruption. Dilaceration may also distort the crown of the tooth, but this is much less commonly observed.

Radiographic features are usually adequate to make a definitive diagnosis. Dilaceration should not be confused with the normal, gradual, distal curvature of the apical one half to one third of most roots. Dilaceration can cause complications during extraction and endodontic procedures.

Dens in Dente

Dens in dente, also known as *dens invaginatus,* is a common dental anomaly resulting from prominent axial invagination of the stratum intermedium into the dental papilla during development. Radiographs reveal a thin rim suggestive of enamel, with an ovoid shape that projects apically from the lingual pit area (Fig. 8-3). Maxillary lateral incisor teeth are most commonly affected, and a prominent lingual pit may be the only clinical indication of the defect. The magnitude of the defect ranges from little more than a pronounced lingual pit to an invagination that approaches the apex. Dens in dente of both maxillary lateral incisors is often present if one incisor is affected.

The radiographic appearance of dens in dente is characteristic. The clinical significance

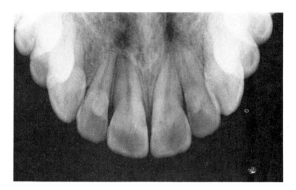

Fig. 8-3   Dens in dente of both maxillary lateral incisors.

of dens invaginatus relates to the close approximation of the pulp tissue to the enamel and dentin pouch. Continuity of the defect with the oral cavity allows collection of oral fluid and bacterial plaque that often leads to decay and pulpal necrosis soon after eruption. Placement of a restoration or sealant may prevent this complication.

Dens Evaginatus

Dens evaginatus is a developmental dental anomaly analogous to dens invaginatus, except that the altered enamel contour is directed away from the pulp rather than axially. A small, ovoid lobule of enamel is typically located in an occlusal pit area of a mandibular premolar. The prominence often contains a small pulpal extension that can easily be exposed during operative procedures. This complication may be avoided by placement of a sealant over the occlusal pits and fissures soon after eruption.

Taurodontia

Taurodontia is a developmental anomaly affecting molar teeth characterized by a disproportionally prominent apical extension of the pulp chamber. The teeth appear normal in all respects clinically, but radiographs reveal the abnormally large pulp chamber and the more apical location of the furcation (Fig. 8-4). This may affect a single molar or several molars.

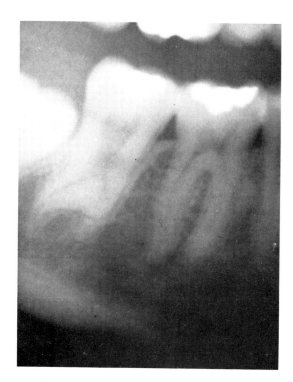

Fig. 8-4 Taurodontia affecting the mandibular second molar.

Few other conditions can be confused with the characteristic radiographic appearance of taurodontia. Taurodontia requires no treatment, but modification of endodontic techniques is required if such treatment becomes necessary.

Turner's Malformation

Turner's malformation results from damage to a permanent tooth during development from inflammation or traumatic injury affecting the adjacent deciduous tooth. This malformation usually affects incisors and second premolars. The damage or injury to the deciduous tooth must occur while the crown of the permanent tooth is developing to result in Turner's malformation. Incisor malformation usually results from traumatic intrusion of the deciduous incisors before age 3. Damage to develop-

ing second premolars is typically caused by pulpal necrosis and periapical inflammation affecting the deciduous second molars before age 8. The malformed succedaneous tooth exhibits morphologic defects such as enamel hypocalcification, enamel pitting, distortion of coronal shape, and abnormal root formation.

In many situations the diagnosis of Turner's malformation is speculative because of the lengthy time lapse between injury and eruption. The presence of normal teeth that formed at the same time as the malformed tooth supports the diagnosis of Turner's tooth. Altered appearance of several teeth that develop simultaneously is more typical of enamel hypocalcification caused by physiologic stress. Teeth affected by Turner's malformation often require coronal restoration.

Enamel Pearl

The enamel pearl, also known as *enameloma,* is an isolated, globular enamel prominence located near the cementoenamel junction of molar teeth. This rare anomaly often occurs bilaterally, and familial occurrence is common. An enamel pearl is usually identified clinically during periodontal probing as a smooth, rounded, subgingival prominence of the root surface near furcations. Its presence can be confirmed radiographically by identification of a round, sharply delineated radiopacity near the cervical region (Fig. 8-5).

Enamel pearls may be confused with calculus accumulations until the smooth surface is appreciated during scaling. They often promote the progression of periodontitis by retaining plaque, which may justify removal. However, endodontic treatment may become necessary because enamel pearls often contain pulp tissue extensions.

Dental Malformations Associated with Congenital Syphilis

Identification of the clinical features referred to as Hutchinson's triad and serologic demonstration of antitreponemal antibodies as discussed in Chapter 11 are required for the

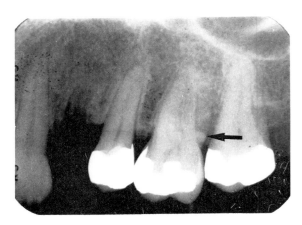

Fig. 8-5   Enamel pearl *(arrow)* located in distal furcation of the maxillary first molar. Note the tertiary dentin formation associated with the large restorations.

diagnosis of congenital syphilis. *Hutchinson's triad* consists of interstitial keratitis of the eye, deafness, and malformations of permanent teeth. The association of all three features may not be appreciated until the permanent teeth erupt. The dental anomalies caused by congenital syphilis are referred to as *Hutchinson's incisors* and *mulberry molars*. Hutchinson's incisors are narrow at the incisal edge compared to the cervical width, with notching of the incisal edges. Several or all of the incisors are usually affected. Mulberry molars are usually first molars that exhibit numerous small, poorly formed cusps yielding a pebbly appearance. Additional findings may include depression of the nasal bridge referred to as *saddle nose deformity,* frontal bossing, and a defect of the hard palate.

Observation of Hutchinson's triad warrants medical referral for serologic diagnosis and antibiotic treatment if not previously administered. Restoration provides esthetic improvement of the incisors.

Anomalous Tooth Anatomy

Dental anatomic variations such as anomalous cusps are commonly observed by the dentist. Prominent lingual cusps of maxillary incisor teeth have been given the special name of *talon cusps.* Anomalous cusps may occasionally cause functional interferences or require modification of restorative preparations. Anomalous roots may complicate endodontic procedures and extractions.

Abnormalities of Tooth Size

Microdontia is abnormally small teeth. A single tooth is usually affected, but rarely the entire dentition may be microdontic. The most common example of microdontia is the *peg lateral incisor,* which is a maxillary lateral incisor that exhibits a narrow mesial-distal width and conical convergence of the crown. Supernumerary teeth are usually microdontic. *Macrodontia* is defined as abnormally large teeth. Macrodontia usually affects a single tooth. It typically exhibits no cleavage furrow or lobulations indicative of the merger of two distinct dental formations such as in both fusion and gemination. Restorative treatment of peg lateral incisors and other abnormalities of teeth size may provide esthetic and functional improvement.

Anodontia

Anodontia means failure of teeth to develop, although clinical usage of the term implies that the majority of permanent teeth have not formed. Anodontia is rare and is usually a manifestation of *hypohydrotic ectodermal dysplasia* as described in Chapter 20. *Partial anodontia* and *hypodontia* describe failure of several or many teeth to form, and the phrase *congenitally missing teeth* is commonly used in reference to one or a few teeth that have not developed. The third molars, maxillary lateral incisors, and second premolars most frequently fail to form.

Radiographs are essential to the diagnosis because many clinically absent teeth are unerupted. In some cases the patient may recall extraction during childhood as an explanation of a missing tooth. Establishing normal function and esthetics in cases of anodontia or

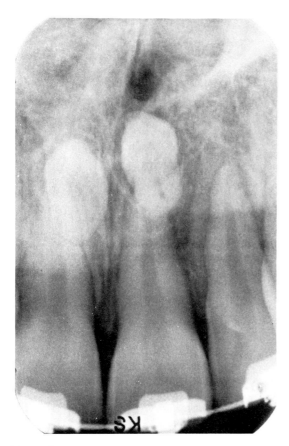

Fig. 8-6   Two mesiodens located in the periapical area of maxillary central incisors.

partial anodontia requires prosthetic replacement.

Supernumerary Teeth

Teeth formed in addition to the normal dental complement are referred to as supernumerary teeth. Supernumerary teeth are usually impacted, microdontic, and morphologically primitive compared to normal teeth. Supernumerary teeth most commonly occur near the midline of the maxilla (Fig. 8-6) and are referred to as *mesiodens* in this location. The terms *distodens* or *fourth molar* refers to a supernumerary tooth located distal to the third

molar. *Paramolar* describes a microdontic supernumerary tooth located buccal or lingual to the molars.

Unerupted supernumerary teeth are usually asymptomatic and are discovered incidentally during radiographic examination. Numerous impacted supernumerary teeth can be a diagnostic feature of Gardner's syndrome and cleidocranial dysplasia as discussed in Chapter 20. Removal of supernumerary teeth is not justified unless malalignment, cystic enlargement, interference with the eruption of other teeth, or similar complications are identified or anticipated.

Amelogenesis Imperfecta

Amelogenesis imperfecta refers to a several closely related, genetically determined conditions of generalized enamel malformation. Distinctions among different forms are based on the inheritance pattern and characteristics of the defective enamel. Since more similarities than differences exist among the various forms, clinicians generally refer to all cases of generalized, genetic enamel malformation as amelogenesis imperfecta. The enamel may be totally absent or thinned, or normal coronal contours may develop. The surface texture of the enamel, when present, is usually rough, globular, pitted, or wrinkled. Tooth color may appear relatively normal, or it can vary from brown to a pale yellow. The defective enamel is usually brittle or soft and in severe cases can be removed with a dental instrument. The radiographic features of dentin and pulp tissues are normal, whereas the enamel often appears atypically radiolucent (Fig. 8-7) or is absent. Vulnerability to severe attrition and dental caries becomes apparent soon after eruption.

The differential diagnosis of amelogenesis imperfecta includes consideration of other forms of generalized dental malformation. Radiographic findings can be relied on to exclude dentinogenesis imperfecta and dentin dysplasia because these conditions produce generalized calcification of the pulp chambers. The malformations of odontodysplasia and enamel hypo-

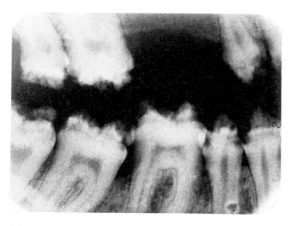

Fig. 8-7   Generalized globular, radiolucent appearance of enamel that is characteristic of amelogenesis imperfecta. The dentin and pulp tissues appear unaffected.

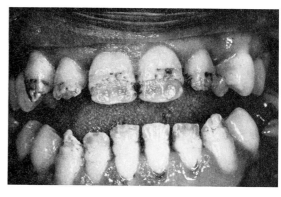

Fig. 8-8   Enamel hypocalcification resulting from physiologic stress. This particularly severe example was caused by a serious illness shortly after birth. Note the normal formation of enamel of the cervical areas of the incisors and the normal appearance of the premolars.

calcification caused by physiologic stress generally affect characteristic groups of teeth rather than the entire dentition. Dental fluorosis may cause surface irregularity and discoloration of the enamel surface, but the teeth are not vulnerable to excessive attrition or dental decay in contrast to amelogenesis imperfecta. Optimal treatment is coronal restoration of all erupted teeth at an early age to minimize the effects of attrition and dental caries. The prognosis of teeth affected by amelogenesis imperfecta without such treatment is poor.

Enamel Hypocalcification Resulting from Physiologic Stress

Physically stressful conditions such as severe illness, dietary deficiency, radiotherapy, and some medications can disrupt dental development. These conditions produce distinct bands of enamel malformation, compared to the normal appearance of adjacent enamel and other teeth that calcified before or after the stressful episode, as illustrated in Fig. 8-8. The patient history often reveals a severe illness at the age corresponding to the formation of the defective enamel. Enamel hypocalcification has been attributed to exanthematous fevers such as measles and scarlet fever, although the severity of the stress is probably more significant in producing these malformations than the presence of exanthem. The extent and severity of enamel hypoplastic defects are roughly proportional to the seriousness and duration of the condition. Therefore a variety of hypoplastic enamel defects can be observed among affected patients, but the defects exhibited by an individual generally appear similar. Arrested root development, bands of enamel pitting, chalky white enamel hypocalcification, and furrowlike depressions extending to the dentin are typical features of enamel malformation caused by physiologic stress. A common pattern of enamel malformation produced by stressful illness involves the incisors and first molars, which suggests stress during or soon after the neonatal period.

A definitive diagnosis of enamel hypoplasia caused by physiologic stress can be made

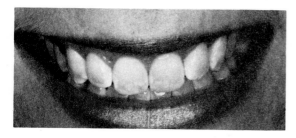

Fig. 8-9 Dental fluorosis. The generalized intermixture of dark and chalky white discoloration is characteristic of this form of intrinsic staining.

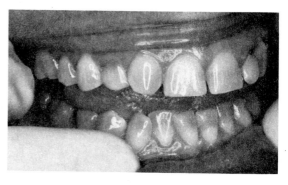

Fig. 8-10 Dark, bandlike pattern of intrinsic staining of incisors caused by administration of tetracycline during infancy. Note the transposition of the maxillary canine and the lateral incisor.

when the locations of malformation correspond to the sequence of dental development and when history confirms a corresponding stressful condition. Mild defects may not require treatment, whereas severe malformations often justify crowns to achieve normal esthetics and function.

Intrinsic Staining

Significant serum concentrations of certain materials during dental development can cause staining by their incorporation into the calcified dental tissues. This is referred to as intrinsic staining and should not be confused with *extrinsic staining* that results from exposure of erupted teeth to materials such as coffee and tobacco. Public drinking water with a fluoride concentration significantly greater than 1 ppm predictably causes a dose-dependent malformation referred to as *mottled enamel* or *dental fluorosis.* Mild examples appear as flecks, spots, or bands of pale white, opaque enamel. Splotchy brown and white enamel discoloration as shown in Fig. 8-9 is typical of moderate mottling. More severe fluorosis appears dark brown in color, with pitting or other surface irregularities. Teeth affected by fluorosis are predictably resistant to dental caries. *Tetracycline staining* results when the drug is administered during dental calcification. Bands of yellow or brownish-grey discoloration, with-

out pitting or other surface defects, as illustrated in Fig. 8-10, are localized in a pattern corresponding to dental development at the time of administration. Blood pigment staining of deciduous teeth resulting from the neonatal hemolysis of *erythroblastosis fetalis*, Rh factor incompatibility, is another example of intrinsic staining.

The diagnosis of intrinsic staining relies on the patient history and the pattern of discoloration. Removal of stains by polishing indicates extrinsic staining. Dental fluorosis is produced by high natural fluoride concentration of the public water supply and predictably affects individuals who grow up in these communities. Tetracycline staining can usually be identified by the distinct banding of characteristic colors and history. The history is definitive in cases of erythroblastosis fetalis, and the permanent dentition is minimally affected.

Dentinogenesis Imperfecta

Dentinogenesis imperfecta, also known as *hereditary opalescent dentin,* is a genetically determined malformation affecting the dentin. Both the primary and permanent dentitions are uniformly greyish-blue to yellowish-brown in

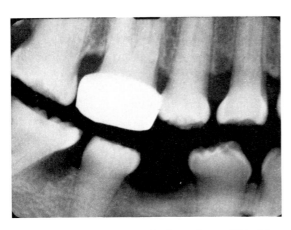

Fig. 8-11 Dentinogenesis imperfecta. This bitewing radiograph demonstrates the generalized radiopacity of the pulp chambers, the prominent cervical constriction, and vulnerability to attrition that are features of this condition.

color with a unique opalescent appearance. Radiographic features (Fig. 8-11) include calcification of the pulp chambers and canals soon after eruption, prominent cervical constriction, and relatively short roots. The normal enamel often cleaves away from the occlusal and incisal surfaces during function, which promotes rapid attrition.

The characteristic color abnormality of all teeth, in addition to their radiographic features, leaves little doubt about the diagnosis. Teeth affected by dentin dysplasia can be distinguished by the normal clinical appearance. Amelogenesis imperfecta affects enamel, and pulpal calcification is less prominent. Dentinogenesis imperfecta may be concurrent with a related developmental defect in bone formation referred to as *osteogenesis imperfecta,* which is discussed in Chapter 20. Crowning of all teeth at a relatively early age to prevent excessive attrition is optimal treatment.

Dentin Dysplasia

Dentin dysplasia is a genetic condition in which abnormal dentin synthesis obliterates the pulp chamber and canals of all primary and permanent teeth. Affected teeth appear normal clinically in contrast to dentinogenesis imperfecta. At least two forms of the condition are recognized. Type I dentin dysplasia is the more severe form, in which pulpal obliteration progresses before eruption. This produces abortion of root formation that results in short roots (Fig. 8-12, *A),* mobility, and premature loss of teeth. In addition, multiple periapical inflammatory lesions develop without evidence of the typical causes of pulpal necrosis. Type II dentin dysplasia is characterized by normal root development and extensive pulpal calcification demonstrated radiographically after eruption. Abnormal dentin formation in the pulp chamber often produces a characteristic *thistle-shaped* radiographic appearance (Fig. 8-12, *B).*

The combination of normal clinical appearance and generalized pulpal calcification demonstrated radiographically is characteristic of dentin dysplasia. The prognosis for type I dentin dysplasia is poor, considering the unfavorable root support of the teeth. The prognosis for type II dentin dysplasia is essentially normal, except that, if endodontic treatment becomes necessary, it may be complicated by abnormal dentin formation.

Odontodysplasia

Teeth affected by odontodysplasia, also known as *ghost teeth,* exhibit prominent pulp spaces, thin calcified dental tissues, and delayed eruption. This condition typically affects several adjacent teeth while all other teeth appear normal. Unilateral, segmental deformity of the maxillary incisors and canine teeth is the most common distribution, although more generalized malformation is possible. The cause of the condition is unknown.

The segmental occurrence of severely malformed teeth with normal development of all other teeth is characteristic of odontodysplasia. The possibility that such dental defects could represent multiple Turner's malforma-

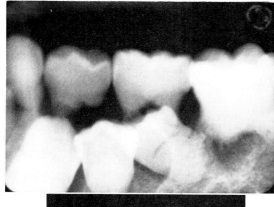

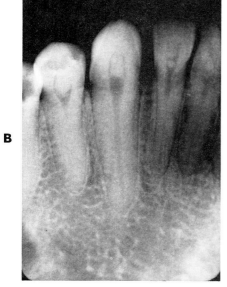

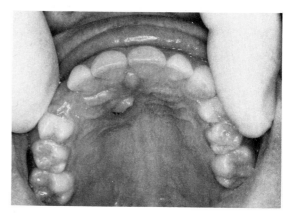

Fig. 8-13 Ectopic eruption of maxillary canine palatal to the incisors.

ABNORMALITIES OF ERUPTION

The category of eruption abnormalities includes complications resulting from failure of teeth to achieve optimal position in the dental arch. The initial suspicion is usually based on the absence of a tooth after the expected age of eruption. Frequently associated findings are discomfort, jaw enlargement, and malalignment of adjacent teeth. Abnormalities of eruption are common and are generally clarified by radiographic evaluation. Failure of numerous teeth to erupt may suggest unusual developmental or systemic conditions.

Ectopic Eruption

Ectopic eruption is misdirection of eruption that results in an abnormal position of the tooth as shown in Fig. 8-13. The relatively rapid movement of both normal and ectopic eruption that occurs during root formation is referred to as *active eruption.* Radiographic demonstration of apical closure of the tooth root indicates the end of active eruption. The more gradual movement of *passive eruption* follows apical closure.

The eruption of a developing tooth proceeds in the general direction of the functional surface and parallel to the long axis of the

Fig. 8-12 Dentin dysplasia. **A,** Radiographic features of type I dentin dysplasia, including extensive pulpal calcification, short roots, and a periapical radiolucency of the first molar without a typical reason for pulpal necrosis. In contrast, **B** illustrates the normal root development and the large pulpal calcifications that produce the characteristic *thistle-shaped* pulp chamber appearance of type II dentin dysplasia.

tions may be clarified by history or histologic examination of the teeth. Prosthetic replacement is indicated following removal of the malformed teeth.

tooth. Normal eruption and eventual positioning of the tooth in the arch are likely if the path of eruption is generally directed toward the appropriate position for the tooth and no obstructions are present. Misdirection of the eruption path relative to the normal tooth position or interposed structures such as adjacent teeth or lesions suggest that ectopic eruption will occur. A limitation of radiographs in the assessment of eruption is that facial or lingual misdirection is often not apparent.

Several complications can result from ectopic eruption and obstruction of eruption. Failure of the tooth to fully emerge into the oral cavity by the end of active eruption is *impaction*. Ectopic eruption that results in complete eruption but abnormal tooth position produces *malalignment.* Inadequate arch space often contributes to this problem. *Transposition* is an unusual reversal of the positions of two teeth. Most transpositions involve ectopic eruption of the maxillary canine either distal to the maxillary first premolar or mesial to the maxillary lateral incisor (see Fig. 8-10). Additional possible complications include external resorption of adjacent teeth and interference with the eruption of other teeth.

Early recognition of ectopic eruption can allow redirection by interceptive orthodontic treatment in some cases. Active orthodontic treatment may be required to correct malalignment after active eruption is complete. Complications such as external resorption, impaction, and loss of arch space may require extraction of teeth in addition to orthodontic treatment.

Impaction

Impaction is defined as failure of teeth to erupt fully into the oral cavity by the end of active eruption. Most isolated impactions can be attributed to ectopic eruption or obstruction of the path of eruption by an adjacent tooth. The third molars and the maxillary canine teeth are most commonly affected. Less common causes of isolated impactions include obstruction by cysts or other lesions within bone.

Multiple impactions can be a manifestation of several developmental and systemic conditions. Developmental syndromes such as cleidocranial dysplasia and Gardener's syndrome include multiple unerupted teeth as a diagnostic feature. Other developmental syndromes produce hypoplasia of the mandible or the maxillae, which can cause multiple impactions by limitation of available space. Systemic conditions that affect development in general such as cretinism, abnormal calcium and phosphate metabolism, and severe dietary deficiency also interfere with dental development and eruption. Radiotherapy and chemotherapy during development can also arrest tooth formation.

Impacted teeth are categorized by the degree of eruption and position relative to adjacent teeth as demonstrated radiographically. These factors affect the complexity of the surgical procedure necessary to accomplish removal. The designations *full bony-, partial bony-,* and *soft tissue impaction* refer to the radiographic relationship of the crown of the impacted tooth to the crest of the alveolar ridge. Similarly, the terms *mesioangular-, distoangular-, vertical-,* and *horizontal impaction* indicate the orientation of the long axis of the impacted tooth relative to an adjacent tooth. These relationships influence the amount of tissue that must be reflected and the surgical approach in establishing access for tooth removal without damaging adjacent teeth.

Surgical removal of impacted teeth may be justified to eliminate pain, recurring infection, external resorption of adjacent teeth, and other complications. Periodic radiographic reevaluation of impactions may be adequate management if no symptoms or complications are present.

Unexplained Loss of Teeth

Loss of teeth can be explained in most instances by exfoliation, traumatic injury, or advanced degenerative dental diseases such as

Table 8-1 Conditions that cause loss of teeth

ISOLATED TOOTH LOSS	
Explained tooth loss	Extensive carious lesions, advanced periodontitis, periapical inflammatory lesions secondary to pulpal necrosis, traumatic injury, typical exfoliation of deciduous teeth, dental malformations such as type I dentin dysplasia
Unexplained tooth loss	External resorption, localized destructive lesions of bone such as cysts and neoplasms
LOSS OF MULTIPLE TEETH	
Systemic diseases	Hypophosphatasia, pseudohypophosphatasia, rickets, vitamin D−resistant rickets, renal osteodystrophy, idiopathic histiocytosis, disseminated malignancy, advanced systemic disease such as renal failure (uremia)
Conditions that promote destructive forms of periodontitis	Severe nutritional deficiencies, hemopoietic disorders, immune system deficiencies such as AIDS and corticosteroid therapy, cyclic neutropenia, diabetes mellitus, juvenile periodontitis, Papillon-Lefèvre syndrome

periodontitis and dental caries. Occasionally, however, unexplained mobility develops, and teeth are extruded or must be extracted in the absence of these conditions. Such unexplained tooth loss presents a diagnostic problem that can be considered as an isolated or multifocal phenomenon.

Isolated examples of unexplained tooth loss are usually caused by destruction of supportive bone by the enlargement of a lesion that originated within the adjacent bone. Radiographic evaluation generally demonstrates such lesions, and clinical features such as jaw expansion may also be present. Cysts, benign neoplasms, and other slow-growing lesions typically produce gradual shifting of teeth. Patients may complain about increasing size of a diastema or the teeth "feeling high" as a consequence of a nonfunctional occlusal relationship after shifting. External root resorption is also possible and typically progresses without symptoms until minimal root support produces mobility and tenderness. Malignant neoplasms and some vascular lesions progress more rapidly and often extrude rather than shift teeth. Discomfort is generally present, although not as severe as would be expected with dental infections.

Developmental and systemic conditions may cause unexplained loss affecting several teeth from different segments as a consequence of poor formation or noninflammatory destruction of supportive structures. The examples listed in Table 8-1 are characterized clinically by mobility and tenderness affecting multiple teeth, without evidence of jaw enlargement or acute inflammation. Other diseases promote rapidly destructive periodontitis by decreasing the host resistance to the infectious process. Generalized mobility, pain, disproportionately severe gingival inflammation, and progression despite conventional treatment methods suggest such diseases.

The prognosis for the affected teeth is poor in most instances by the time symptoms reveal the problem. Treatment of the causative condition is the priority to prevent progression of the condition and to minimize the damage to additional teeth. Extraction of hopelessly mobile teeth and prosthetic replacement of missing teeth are indicated if the condition can be controlled.

Follicular Enlargement

The normal radiographic width of the follicular space of unerupted teeth is between 2 and 3 mm. Width of the pericoronal radiolucency beyond 3 to 4 mm is the initial feature of abnormal increase in follicular soft tissue. This common abnormality in the absence of symptoms usually represents early development of a follicular cyst or idiopathic hyperplasia of the follicular tissue. Follicular cysts are divided into eruption cysts and dentigerous cysts, depending on whether or not tooth eruption appears likely. A variety of odontogenic tumors and other odontogenic cysts less commonly appear radiographically as pericoronal radiolucent enlargements.

The differential diagnosis of pericoronal radiolucent enlargements includes odontogenic cysts and tumors as discussed in Chapter 19, but most enlargements are follicular cysts or follicular hyperplasia. The less concentric the radiolucency is around the crown of the tooth, the more likely it is that the lesion is one of the less common odontogenic lesions. Surgical removal and histopathologic evaluation is indicated unless eruption appears imminent.

Pericoronitis

Pericoronitis is inflammation of the soft tissue surrounding the crown of a partially erupted tooth. The mandibular third molars are most frequently affected. The follicular epithelium of the tooth merges with the mucosal epithelium of the oral cavity at the mesial aspect of the tooth, but a flap or *operculum* of follicular and alveolar tissue partially covers a portion of the crown as shown in Fig. 8-14. The space between the pericoronal soft tissue and the tooth is difficult to clean and traps food, bacteria, and plaque. The resulting inflammation is characterized by a chronic course of soreness and foul taste from the area. Acute exacerbations eventually develop and are marked by sudden onset of mild fever, pain, purulent discharge, edema, and trismus. Clinical examination and exposure of intraoral

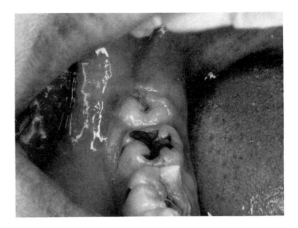

Fig. 8-14 Pericoronitis. Soft tissue operculum associated with partially erupted mandibular third molar. The patient described a recurring course of episodic acute infections associated with the tooth.

radiographs can be difficult in cases of severe trismus. The acute episodes resolve following infection control treatment but predictably recur at variable intervals. Trauma by the opposing teeth often aggravates the inflammation.

The patient's description of the clinical course and identification of a partially erupted tooth in the region of pain allows a definitive diagnosis. Treatment consists of aggressive saline lavage of the infected follicular space by the dentist and providing the patient with an irrigation syringe to continue periodic irrigation. Antibiotic therapy and pain medication are beneficial in the presence of evidence of disseminated infection such as fever. Dramatic improvement is expected within 24 hours. If complete eruption of the tooth appears likely, then the patient is instructed to continue irrigation of the pericoronal tissue until eruption can be confirmed. Removal of partially impacted teeth after resolution of the acute infection prevents recurrence of the pericoronitis.

Supereruption and Mesial Drift

Chronic absence of a tooth causes dental complications that result from the tendency of

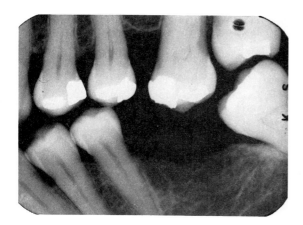

Fig. 8-15 Supereruption and mesial drift. The maxillary second molar has supererupted into the gap, and the mandibular third molar has tipped mesially. This has produced traumatic occlusal relationships and sites between the maxillary molars and mesial to the mandibular molar that are prone to periodontitis. Note the prominent radiopaque pulp stones within the pulp chambers of the maxillary second molar and the mandibular molar.

adjacent and opposing teeth to shift into the edentulous gap. Supereruption, also referred to as *hypereruption,* describes the gradual extrusion of unopposed teeth into edentulous spaces. Supereruption occurs by passive eruption, which is associated with the formation of cellular cementum and a slow rate of progression versus active eruption. Teeth distal to edentulous spaces tend to gradually drift mesially into the space, with some degree of tilting or tipping in most instances. Distal drift of the tooth mesial to a gap also occurs in some cases but is usually much less pronounced than mesial drift. Fig. 8-15 illustrates the consequences of supereruption and mesial tipping such as irregularity of the occlusal plane, traumatic functional relationships, and sites prone to periodontitis. The extended prognosis for supererupted and mesially tipped teeth is poor because the combination of dysfunctional relationships and the unfavorable increase in the crown-to-root ratio usually culminates in mobility and tenderness. In addition, many patients with evidence of periodontal bone loss and supereruption of a multirooted tooth are likely to develop periodontal inflammation within furcations earlier than otherwise expected.

The diagnosis of supereruption and mesial drift is usually apparent. Many teeth affected by advanced supereruption also exhibit pronounced cementum thickness referred to as *hypercementosis* that accumulates during passive eruption of long duration. Reduction and coronal restoration of a supererupted tooth may be necessary to reestablish a level occlusal relationship before prosthetic restoration of the opposing edentulous space. Orthodontic uprighting of mesially tipped teeth is often necessary for optimal results of a fixed or removable prosthesis. Prevention by the prompt replacement of missing teeth is the most effective management of supereruption and mesial tipping.

REGRESSIVE ALTERATIONS OF TEETH

This category consists of conditions that produce gradual, potentially detrimental alterations of teeth, with the specific exclusion of dental caries and periodontitis. All of these conditions, excluding fractures of teeth, are characterized by slow, gradual progression without dramatic symptoms.

Reactive Alterations of Dentin

One of the few available adaptive mechanisms of teeth in response to stimuli of the oral environment is the formation of additional dentin to further insulate the sensitive pulpal tissue. This process is demonstrated radiographically as a smaller-than-expected pulp chamber size relative to the size and coronal contours of the tooth. The phrase *secondary dentin formation* implies that this additional dentin formation occurs gradually in response to routine functional and thermal stimulation. Secondary dentin is characterized radiographically by a uniform increase in coronal dentin thickness. Most adults exhibit evidence of the process, and the extent varies among individuals.

The presence of secondary dentin increases the distance and the time required for carious lesions to progress from the tooth surface to the pulp. Therefore the clinician effectively has less time to identify and treat decay in children before the pulp is affected than in adults. Also, the formation of additional dentin replaces superficial pulpal tissues such as pulp horns within several years of eruption. This decreases the probability of mechanical pulp exposures during restorative procedures for adults in comparison to the recently erupted teeth of children. Extensive secondary dentin formation tends to decrease pulpal sensitivity to stimulation and must be considered during pulp testing and the diagnosis of dental discomfort.

Tertiary dentin formation is dentin produced in response to a specific stimulus such as a deep carious lesion, tooth fracture, advanced attrition, or restorative treatment. Radiographs reveal a focal increase in dentin thickness corresponding to the site of abnormal stimulation (see Fig. 8-5). Sequential radiographs demonstrate that the tertiary dentin formation occurs relatively rapidly when compared to the gradual, uniform thickening of secondary dentin formation. Tertiary dentin formation explains in part the gradual decrease in thermal sensitivity following placement of metallic restorations.

A third response of dentin to stimulation is gradual calcification of dentinal tubules, which is called *dentinal sclerosis*. This process affects dentin chronically exposed to the oral environment by decay, attrition, or cervical abrasion. Dentinal sclerosis is suggested by a glazed, glassy surface texture of exposed dentin. Dentinal sclerosis effectively insulates the pulp from thermal, chemical, and tactile stimulation of exposed dentin.

Reactive alterations of dentin are appropriately considered as physiologic responses rather than pathologic processes. An important diagnostic implication in clinical situations of suspected pulpal necrosis, however, is that evidence of additional dentin formation implies pulpal vitality. Conversely, a tooth exhibiting a uniformly large pulp chamber compared to that of adjacent teeth should be suspected of pulpal necrosis (see Fig. 8-29).

Generalized radiographic evidence of secondary dentin formation may appear to be similar to the extensive pulpal calcification of dentinogenesis imperfecta and dentin dysplasia. However, the extensive pulpal calcification of both dentinogenesis imperfecta and dentin dysplasia occurs soon after eruption, whereas extensive secondary dentin formation is associated with advanced age. The sensitivity of exposed dentin to external stimulation is minimized by dentinal sclerosis. The use of various "desensitization" products and procedures relieves sensitivity by promoting dentinal sclerosis.

Pulp Calcification

Pulp calcification occurs in two forms: pulp stone formation within vital pulps and dystrophic calcification of necrotic pulp tissue. *Pulp stones,* also referred to as *denticles,* are small, globular, radiopaque bodies incidentally identified radiographically within the outline of the pulp chamber. Pulp stone formation is common, and multiple teeth are usually affected (see Fig. 8-15). *Dystrophic pulp calcification* is typically identified radiographically as the absence of a substantial proportion of the pulp chamber radiolucency of a single tooth as illustrated in Fig. 8-16. The tooth is usually asymptomatic, but the patient history, clinical features, or radiographic findings often suggest a cause of pulpal necrosis. Blunt trauma prior to complete apexification of the tooth is the situation most likely to produce dystrophic pulp calcification because the open apex allows vascular diffusion and calcification of necrotic tissue. Dystrophic pulp calcification is less likely

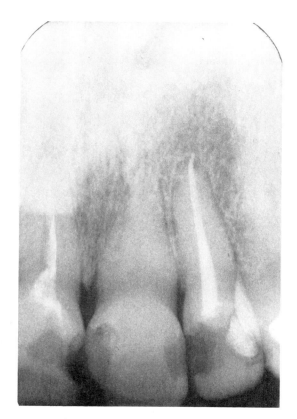

Fig. 8-16 Dystrophic pulp calcification of the maxillary central incisor.

following similar injury to teeth after apexification because of the limited vascular diffusion to the necrotic pulp.

Both pulp stones and pulpal calcification are relatively characteristic radiographically and are not likely to be confused with other conditions. Pulp stones are inconsequential and require no treatment, although their presence may complicate endodontic treatment if it becomes necessary. Endodontic treatment of teeth with dystrophic pulp calcification is indicated if pain, periapical radiolucency, or other evidence of inflammation suggests that remnants of necrotic pulp tissue are still present within the tooth. Endodontic treatment is not justified in the absence of indications of active inflammation. Esthetic restoration may be beneficial if the tooth appears darkened.

Attrition

Attrition is the gradual loss of incisal and occlusal tooth structure resulting from functional and parafunctional contact with opposing teeth. Factors directly affecting the rate of attrition include age, diet, gender, exposure to abrasive materials, and parafunctional habits such as bruxism and clenching. Uniformly flat, evenly worn functional surfaces of all teeth are characteristic of advanced attrition. Flat, shiny, smooth spots on the enamel surfaces called *wear facets* indicate early attrition and often reveal dysfunctional occlusal relationships.

The diagnostic features of attrition are characteristic and unlikely to be confused with other conditions. Excessive attrition at a relatively early age suggests an intrinsic dental defect such as dentinogenesis imperfecta or amelogenesis imperfecta. Unglazed porcelain restorations can produce dramatic localized attrition. Excessive dental attrition produced by habits like bruxism can be minimized by fabrication of an acrylic bite appliance.

Abrasion

Abrasion is the gradual loss of tooth structure caused by nonfunctional habits involving contact with objects other than the opposing teeth. Cervical wear of exposed root surfaces by habitual horizontal scrubbing with a stiff toothbrush and incisal wear of a pipe smoker's teeth from grasping the pipe stem are common examples. The defects produced by cervical toothbrush abrasion are angular notches bordered occlusally by the cementoenamel junction. This is often associated with apical displacement of the gingival tissue, which is attributable in part to the abrasive brushing habit. The internal surfaces are glassy smooth and usually exhibit no evidence of carious decalcification. The maxillary canine and maxillary premolar teeth are most prominently affected in most cases.

Location, history, and the appearance of angular defects without carious decalcification provide a definitive diagnosis of abrasion. Initial treatment is elimination of the causative habit, which is usually adequate management for mild defects. Restoration of severe cervical abrasion is occasionally necessary to control pulpitis and to prevent pulpal necrosis.

Erosion

Erosion is the gradual loss of tooth structure caused by chemical dissolution by acids that are either of gastric or dietary origin. Repeated or habitual regurgitation can produce dramatic dental erosion proportional to frequency, duration, and volume. *Chronic gastric reflux* related to abnormal esophageal-gastric function such as a hiatal hernia can produce recurring exposure of the teeth to gastric acid. *Bulemia* and *anorexia* are psychiatric eating disorders that most commonly affect young adult women and feature habitual, intentional regurgitation after eating as a method of weight control. Anorexics appear asthenic, whereas bulemics exhibit normal habitus or slightly excessive weight. Some patients describe habitual exposure to acidic foods such as sucking on lemons or sipping citric juices as a cause of erosion. In other cases, mints or candies eaten habitually are the source of acid.

The enamel of eroded teeth appears uniformly thinned, and in severe cases the dentin is exposed. A characteristic feature of advanced erosion is the appearance of amalgam restoration margins that extend uniformly beyond the contour of the eroded tooth surfaces. The most prominent erosion is limited to a specific region in most cases, which may suggest the source of acid. Erosion resulting from regurgitation most severely affects the lingual surfaces of the maxillary anterior teeth, whereas erosion from lemon sucking is most pronounced on labial or buccal surfaces as shown by Fig. 8-17.

The clinical features of erosion are adequately characteristic to make the diagnosis. Identifying the acid source and minimizing ad-

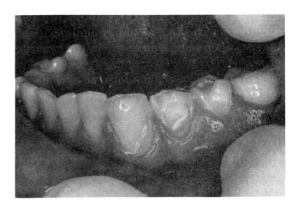

Fig. 8-17 Erosion of the mandibular canine and premolars caused by a lemon sucking habit.

ditional exposures are the initial treatment goals. Chronic gastric reflux is revealed by frequent productive belching and a sour taste following sleep or while in a reclined position. Elevation of the head and shoulders often limits the regurgitation. Citrus habits are easily identified and discontinued by discussing the consequences with the patient. Erosion caused by the habitual regurgitation of eating disorders is more difficult to confirm because denial of the behavior is typical. An eating disorder is suspected on the basis of excluding other possibilities. Referral of the eating disorder patient for counseling is appropriate, but the referral is often rejected. Restoration of eroded teeth may be necessary after the erosion is controlled.

Hypercementosis

Hypercementosis is the formation of excessive cementum and is a common incidental radiographic finding. The apical one third to one half of the root exhibits a smooth, bulbous widening as contrasted with the occlusal one third of the root (Fig. 8-18). The arrangement of the periodontal ligament space and lamina dura surrounds the bulbous enlargement and is otherwise normal in appearance. Hypercementosis is often associated with prominent supereruption and represents extensive cemen-

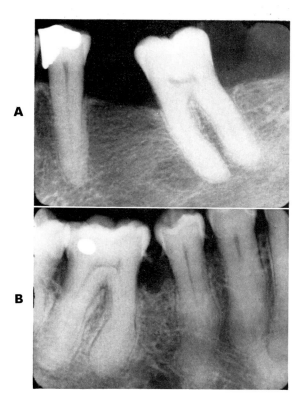

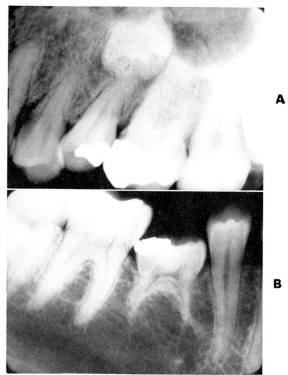

Fig. 8-18 Hypercementosis. Both the premolar and the molar in **A** exhibit mild enlargement of the apical one third of the roots. **B** demonstrates more dramatic, bulbous enlargement of all roots. In both examples, note that the radiopaque root enlargement is surrounded by normal periodontal ligament space and lamina dura.

Fig. 8-19 Ankylosis of teeth. **A** demonstrates an unusual instance of ankylosis of a deciduous tooth that eventually became surrounded by subsequent membranous bone growth. The succedaneous premolar has erupted ectopically. **B** exhibits the typical radiographic features of ankylosis of a deciduous tooth. This case is complicated by the mesial tipping of the first molar.

tum accumulation during passive eruption. Generalized hypercementosis is associated with acromegaly, Paget's disease of bone, and advanced attrition.

The radiographic appearance of hypercementosis is unique. Multiple examples should prompt diagnostic consideration of the conditions suggested above. No specific treatment of hypercementosis is required. However, extraction of affected teeth is complicated by retention of the bulbous apical portion of the root within the socket.

Ankylosis

Ankylosis is the fusion of two structures that are not normally joined. In reference to teeth, ankylosis is the fusion of the tooth root to the alveolar bone. This may affect teeth of the adult dentition in cases of localized inflammation, traumatic injury, or reimplantation of avulsed teeth. However, most examples affect retained deciduous teeth in the absence of a succedaneous tooth, although in some instances the replacement tooth has erupted ectopically (Fig. 8-19, *A*). The occlusal surface of the ankylosed tooth usually appears lower than the occlusal plane, as shown in Fig. 8-19, *B,* which explains the use of the phrase *submerged teeth* as a synonym for dental ankylosis. This results from continuing membranous bone growth of the cortical surface that essentially bypasses the tooth and its attachment to central bone. Percussion of ankylosed teeth produces a characteristic sharp sound in contrast to the duller resonance produced by healthy teeth suspended in a normal periodontal ligament. Focal obliteration of the periodontal ligament space may be radiographically apparent, but it is usually difficult to identify with the thin roots of deciduous teeth and if buccal or lingual surfaces are affected.

The combination of percussion results and tooth position apical to the occlusal plane is diagnostic of ankylosis affecting a deciduous tooth. Percussion results and evidence of inflammation or traumatic injury support a diagnosis of ankylosed permanent teeth. Removal and replacement with a prosthesis is often necessary to arrest supereruption of opposing teeth and tipping of adjacent teeth (Fig. 8-19, *B).* Extraction is complicated by the fusion of the tooth with bone. Nontender ankylosed teeth can be retained and restored to function in selected cases, but tenderness often develops because of the abnormal periodontal ligament function.

Internal Resorption

Internal resorption is the loss of dentin from within the pulp cavity. The dentinoclastic cellular activity is generally initiated by inflammation, and histopathologic examination typically demonstrates hyperplastic pulpitis. In some cases, however, a source of inflammation cannot be identified, and the process must be considered idiopathic. Initial identification of the condition is usually incidental during radiographic examination. The focal increase in pulpal size with associated thinning of the dentin as illustrated by Fig. 8-20 affects a single tooth in most instances. The tooth is usually

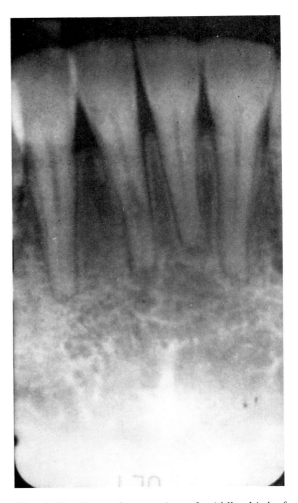

Fig. 8-20 Internal resorption of middle third of root of mandibular right central incisor.

nonpainful, although extensive resorption may produce pink coronal discoloration.

Internal resorption in the coronal portion of the tooth must be distinguished by clinical examination from more common superficial conditions that cause similar focal radiolucency such as dental caries and radiolucent restorations. Internal resorption within the root can appear similar radiographically to external resorption, except that radiolucency of

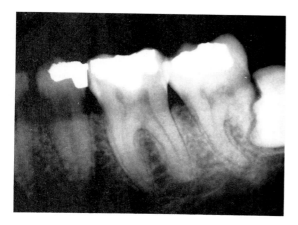

Fig. 8-21 External resorption of mandibular second molar associated with horizontally impacted mandibular third molar.

bone is usually present adjacent to the site of external resorption. Internal resorption is managed by endodontic treatment. Extraction of the tooth is usually necessary if the resorption has perforated the root.

External Resorption

External resorption is the cellular removal of tooth structure from nonpulpal surfaces. The mechanism is analogous to the osteoclastic resorption of bone, but what initiates the process is poorly understood. Most examples are identified radiographically as a root concavity of an erupted tooth adjacent to abnormalities such as chronic inflammatory lesions, cysts, and impacted teeth (Fig. 8-21). Idiopathic external resorption may affect impacted teeth without an associated lesion. External resorption is also a frequent complication discovered years after reimplantation of traumatically avulsed teeth. An occasional complication of orthodontic treatment is generalized external resorption of roots referred to as *root blunting.*

Determining the focus of tooth resorption as either internal or external is necessary to determine appropriate treatment. Radiographs exposed from several angulations usually demonstrate a parallax shift of the radiolucency relative to the radiolucency of the pulp cavity and the radiolucency of an adjacent bone lesion in cases of external resorption. Pulp testing may clarify if the cause is related to pulpal necrosis. Effective treatment of external resorption requires control of any initiating lesions by surgical removal or endodontic treatment. External resorption affecting reimplanted teeth is a poor prognostic sign. External resorption caused by orthodontic treatment typically ceases at the end of active tooth movement. If the remaining root support and mobility is minimal, poor prognosis is suggested. Periodic radiographic reevaluation is adequate management of idiopathic external resorption of impacted teeth, in most cases without an associated bone lesion.

Traumatic Injury and Fractures of Teeth

Numerous factors can contribute to the fracture of teeth. Examples include weakening of the tooth by carious lesions, cusps undermined by large restorations, loss of typical resilience following endodontic treatment, inadvertent mastication of solid objects, and traumatic injury. The patient is generally aware of the fracture as a consequence of the actual injury, sharp edges, sensitivity of exposed dentin, or discovery of tooth fragments. Assessment of dental fractures when tooth fragments have been displaced is uncomplicated. Cases of fracture without displacement of tooth structure can usually be clarified by gentle pressure at the fracture site or by percussion as described in Chapter 9. Radiographs are usually ineffective in demonstrating dental fractures unless the fragments are obviously displaced. Mobility, malposition, hemorrhage, and extreme tenderness following an episode of blunt trauma are the characteristic features associated with *subluxation,* which is displacement of a tooth. *Avulsion* refers to a tooth that has been physically forced completely out of the alveolus during an injury.

The evaluation of dental trauma requires identification of the fracture, pulpitis, mobility, and related findings. The treatment goals are to relieve symptoms and control pulpitis and to assess adjacent bone and soft tissue for signs of injury. Treatment options for coronal fractures include sedative temporary restoration if the pulpitis is considered reversible or endodontic treatment if the pulpitis is irreversible. Vertical fractures extending apically beyond the crest of the alveolar bone present a poor restorative prognosis, and extraction may be necessary. Repositioning and immobilization by splinting is optimal treatment for traumatically subluxated or avulsed teeth.

DENTAL CARIES

Carious lesions result from the gradual dissolution of tooth structure by metabolic acids produced by bacteria within the dental plaque matrix. The characteristic clinical features associated with carious lesions include softness of dentin and enamel to probing, discoloration of tooth tissues, and cavitation. Also, patients often describe symptoms such as sensitivity to sugar or extremes in temperature that are suggestive of pulpitis resulting from dentin exposure. Larger cavities can be demonstrated radiographically as focal radiolucency within enamel and dentin. Radiographic identification of dental decay is diagnostically less sensitive than direct clinical identification by probing, but radiographs are essential in discovering cavities affecting inaccessible proximal surfaces and in assessing decay extent. Differential diagnosis is generally uncomplicated, since (1) most other conditions that produce a loss of tooth structure such as abrasion and attrition are characteristic in pattern of occurrence, history, and location; and (2) the tooth structures near sites of abrasion, attrition, and erosion are solid to probing in contrast to decay. Diagnosis of carious lesions includes classification by the surface affected and by extent of the lesion. Both factors affect treatment decisions.

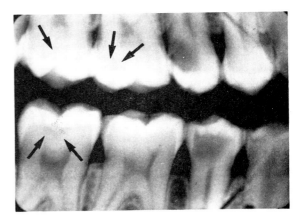

Fig. 8-22 Radiographic demonstration of pit and fissure decay of maxillary first and second molars and mandibular second molar as indicated by arrows. The extensive decay of the mandibular second premolar probably originated as an occlusal lesion because of the intact radiopacity of the peripheral enamel. The extensive decay of the maxillary second premolar represents advanced interproximal decay.

Classification of Carious Lesions by Location

Pit and fissure decay. Development pits and fissures of teeth are prone to decay because removal of plaque from these irregularities is difficult or impossible. Pit and fissure lesions are most accurately identified by systematically probing the defects in search of soft spots or "catches." Visual evidence of enamel discoloration can be helpful in locating suspected lesions, but probing is the definitive method of demonstrating decay. Staining and superficial discoloration of the pits and fissures without softness to probing should be considered enamel-limited decalcification, which generally does not justify restoration. Radiographs may reveal dentinal radiolucency adjacent to the dentinoenamel junction (DEJ) associated with extensive decay of developmental pits (Fig. 8-22). Visually obvious cavitation indicates extensive decay progression.

Interproximal decay. The occurrence of

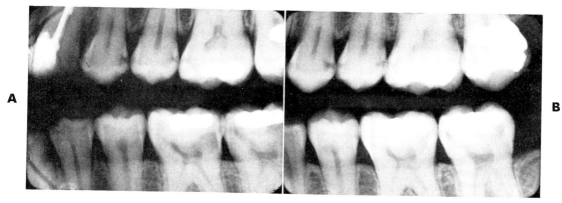

Fig. 8-23   Radiographic demonstration of interproximal decay. The effect of beam angulation on the radiographic demonstration of decay can be appreciated by comparing the appearances of the same lesion in the two radiographs. The radiolucencies in the center of the crowns of the mandibular molars are the result of extensive smooth-surface carious lesions.

interproximal lesions typically reflects one or more factors of dental caries susceptibility such as infrequent flossing, a diet rich in sucrose, or less than optimal fluoride availability during dentinogenesis. Advanced interproximal lesions can often be identified clinically by marginal ridge discoloration and probing, whereas radiographs are required to detect more superficial lesions. Most early lesions are triangularly shaped radiolucencies within the proximal enamel immediately apical to the contact point (Fig. 8-23). Deeper cavities and lesions that form in areas of unusual embrasure shape may appear semicircular or irregular in shape.

The open embrasure spaces of anterior teeth permit effective identification of early interproximal decay by probing, and the narrower facial-lingual thickness often allows visualization of decay by transillumination. Therefore radiographs are somewhat less important in the discovery of interproximal lesions affecting anterior teeth.

Smooth-surface decay.   Carious decalcification of smooth buccal and lingual enamel surfaces is usually associated with poor oral hygiene because these surfaces are much less plaque retentive than proximal surfaces or developmental irregularities. Most smooth-surface carious lesions affect the buccal surfaces of maxillary and mandibular molars near the gingival margin. The abnormal chalky, opaque white appearance of the enamel during early carious decalcification is a typical observation among patients with poor oral hygiene habits. Because the enamel and dentin overlying the pulp are thinner in this region than occlusal and proximal surfaces, smooth-surface lesions progress to pulpal involvement within a shorter time period. As with most types of decay, the discovery of one smooth-surface cavity increases the likelihood that additional lesions are present. Radiographs contribute less to the identification and progression assessment of early smooth-surface lesions than to interproximal lesions.

Cervical decay.   Vulnerability to decay of root surfaces increases dramatically with the increased root exposure caused by advanced periodontitis. Therefore this type of decay usually affects older adults. In addition, cervical decay is often associated with conditions that produce xerostomia. Early radicular lesions are identified as a mild tackiness to probing,

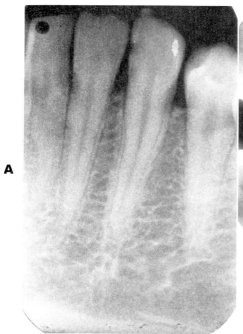

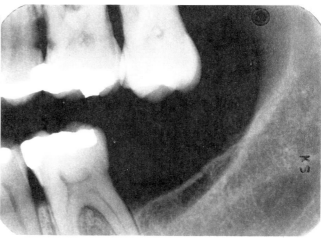

Fig. 8-24 **A,** The radiolucency of the distal root surface of the mandibular canine and mesial root surface of the lateral incisor is typical of cervical burnout. Interproximal decay of the mesial surface of the canine is present. **B,** Cervical decay of distal root surface of maxillary second premolar and mesial root surface of maxillary first molar. The radiographic features of cervical burnout and cervical decay are compared in Table 8-2.

whereas more advanced lesions are softer or leathery. Pulp exposures often complicate removal of cervical lesions because the cementum and dentin are relatively thin from the surface to the pulp. As with smooth-surface decay, radicular carious lesions are more directly related to obvious evidence of poor oral hygiene than occlusal and interproximal decay. Radiographs may aid in identifying cervical decay of proximal surfaces, but care must be taken to avoid misinterpreting a radiographic phenomenon referred to as *cervical burnout* as carious. Cervical burnout is a misleading radiolucent appearance of healthy root structures in the region apical to the cementoenamel junction and occlusal to the alveolar crest as shown in Fig. 8-24, *A.* Radiographic features of cervical burnout and cervical decay (Fig. 8-24, *B)* are compared in Table 8-2.

Recurrent decay. Recurrent carious le-

sions develop at the margins of an existing restoration. The most reliable method of demonstrating recurrent decay is probing the marginal regions with a dental explorer. Radiographs often demonstrate large recurrent lesions, but recurrent decay is easily obscured by the superimposed radiopacity of metallic restorative materials or may not be apparent if it is adjacent to radiolucent composite materials.

Evaluation of Dental Caries by the Pattern of Occurrence

To some degree in most patients, exposure of all teeth to the same diet, fluoride absorption during development, and quality of oral hygiene can be expected to yield a relatively consistent pattern of dental decay. Recognizing a patient's pattern of decay can contribute to lesion detection and treatment planning deci-

Table 8-2   Comparison of radiographic features of cervical burnout and cervical decay

Feature	Cervical burnout	Cervical decay
Shape of the radiolucency	Triangular, rectangular, angular	Semicircular
Occlusal border	Must be near CEJ*	Can be apical to the CEJ or extend occlusally and appear axial to the proximal enamel
Apical border	Must be near crestal bone height	Occlusal to crestal bone height
Axial border	Fades or follows an "anatomic" contour	Sharp delineation and ragged contour
Peripheral root contour	Peripheral outline appears intact	Peripheral outline appears cavitated
Multiple exposures (different x-ray beam angulation)	Radiolucency often disappears	May change, but radiolucency remains

CEJ, Cementoenamel junction.

sions. For example, decay affecting an interproximal surface suggests that a subtle lesion affects the adjacent tooth surface. Conversely, generalized resistance to interproximal decay formation should make the clinician skeptical that a vague radiolucency is actually carious. Superficial carious lesions exhibited by a patient prone to decay are more justifiably restored than precisely the same lesion in a decay-resistant individual.

Rampant caries refers to an extensive pattern of decay affecting numerous tooth surfaces. Clinical features include cavities affecting most of the teeth, numerous smooth surface lesions, rapid decay progression, poor oral hygiene, multiple lesions affecting individual teeth, and habitual ingestion of sucrose. *Radiation caries* is a special form of rampant decay observed following therapeutic head and neck irradiation. Direct exposure of the salivary glands during radiotherapy causes irreversible radiation-induced salivary gland atrophy and resulting xerostomia. This deprives the patient of the decay inhibition provided by saliva. Radiation caries is characterized by unrelenting progression of cervical and smooth-surface carious lesions of most teeth. Absence of facial hair overlying the major salivary glands indicates significant radiation exposure of the sali-

vary glands. A similar pattern of cervical and smooth-surface decay is also associated with xerostomia caused by medications and primary disease of the salivary glands. Decay progression associated with xerostomia can be slowed or arrested by daily application of nonacidic fluoride gels, exceptional oral hygiene effectiveness, and frequent dental prophylaxis.

Classification of Carious Lesions by Extent

The actual extent of a carious lesion is only revealed during decay removal. However, accurately predicting the extent is a necessary part of optimal treatment planning. Decay extent can be considered in the facial-lingual, axial, and crestal directions.

Facial-lingual carious extent. The size of the carious lesion in this dimension primarily determines the degree to which the functional strength of the tooth has been compromised by undermining and weakening of cusps or incisal edges. This effect is usually greater than initially suspected because the carious extent within dentin exceeds the visually apparent decalcification of enamel. Crowns or onlays are often required to restore the compromised strength or appearance of the tooth, whereas conservative restoration is adequate for smaller lesions. Clinical indications of advanced facial-lingual decay progression are extensive cavitation, enamel discoloration, and recurrent decay affecting large restorations.

Axial carious extent. The axial depth of decay influences the decision whether or not to restore superficial lesions and whether decay removal of deep cavities is likely to involve the pulp. Radiographs generally provide the best single indication of axial carious extent. However, the apparent extent of a carious lesion as demonstrated radiographically is always less than the actual extent demonstrated during removal for reasons described in this chapter under the heading "Factors Influencing Radiographic Demonstration of Carious Lesions."

Early carious decalcification limited to the enamel may not progress into dentin following alterations in cariogenic factors such as improved diet and oral hygiene. Whether or not the decay process has been *arrested* can only be confirmed by periodic radiographic reevaluation for axial progression. The expectation that the decay may not progress is the justification for delaying treatment of many enamel-limited or *incipient* carious lesions. The decay can be expected to progress, regardless of preventive measures, once the lesion has reached the dentin; in this case restoration is justified. Simply stated, evidence of axial decay progression to the DEJ indicates the need for restoration, whereas axial progression limited to enamel may not require immediate treatment.

Instances of deep axial carious extent challenge the dentist to predict during treatment planning whether or not pulp exposure will occur during decay removal. Pulp exposure generally requires endodontic treatment and restoration to maintain the tooth, whereas restoration alone is usually sufficient if the decay removal can be accomplished without causing pulpal necrosis.

Grading the radiographic extent of carious lesions can be an effective method of predicting the actual decay extent at the time of removal. Although developed for the assessment of interproximal lesions, many of the general implications of this grading scheme also apply to decay affecting other surfaces. Grade I carious lesions exhibit radiolucency extending less than one half of the enamel thickness without evidence of radiolucency within dentin and are expected to be limited to enamel. Grade II lesions are radiolucencies that extend more than one half of the enamel thickness without radiolucency of dentin; the corresponding lesion at the time of removal is expected to have actually progressed into dentin. Grade III lesions exhibit radiolucency of dentin extending less than one half of the dentin thickness from the DEJ to the pulp chamber. Decay removal of grade III lesions is likely to be extensive, but encroachment on the pulp is unlikely. Grade IV cavities exhibit radiolucency of dentin extending more than one half of the distance from the DEJ to the pulp, and encroachment on the pulp during decay removal is to be expected.

Crestal extent of carious lesions. The crestal extent of decay refers to how far the destruction of tooth structure has progressed apically relative to the gingiva and crest of the alveolar bone. Crestal decay extent can affect treatment planning decisions relative to cervical, smooth-surface, and large interproximal cavities. Minimal crestal extent implies an uncomplicated restorative procedure because the supportive tissues will not limit access during restoration. At the opposite extreme, apical extent approaching the alveolar bone crest indicates that restoration of the tooth will be complicated or unfeasible. Probing most accurately demonstrates crestal lesion extent in most cases, although radiographs often confirm it.

Factors Influencing Radiographic Demonstration of Carious Lesions

Radiographic demonstration of carious lesions is highly dependent on several exposure factors and their impact on image quality. For example, extremes in image density such as exceptionally dark or light radiographs limit the detection of carious lesions. Also, poor beam angulation can produce superimposition of structures that obscures lesions. Even when optimal image quality is achieved, several inherent limitations in the radiographic demonstration of carious decalcification produce images of decay that are always less extensive than the actual lesion.

Radiographic demonstration of carious lesions relies on the differential absorption of radiation by the normal enamel and dentin in contrast to that of decalcified lesions. Substantial decalcification of tooth structure must be present to yield a difference in x-ray absorption that is great enough to produce an image difference perceivable to the human eye. The macroscopic morphology of carious lesions consists of gradations in decalcification from maximal decalcification near the superficial surface to minimal decalcification at the most axial extent of the lesion. This means that the most axial extent of the decay process consists of significantly less than the minimal decalcification necessary for radiographic visualization.

Interproximal decay generally forms immediately apical to the contact point, and the initial facial-lingual extent of early lesions is somewhat greater than the width of the contact point (Fig. 8-25). For the optimal horizontal beam angulation to demonstrate the embrasure contours without superimposition of adjacent teeth, the radiation must pass through some amount of normal dentin and enamel located buccal and lingual to the carious lesion. This superimposes the radiopacity of these tissues on the radiolucency of the carious lesion and effectively masks the lesion to some degree, as illustrated in Fig. 8-25.

For optimal demonstration of interproximal carious lesions, the vertical angulation of the primary radiation beam is ideally directed parallel to the marginal ridge by passing through the greatest dimension of the lesion as demonstrated by Fig. 8-26. This also minimizes the superimposition of healthy buccal and lingual tooth structure over the image of the decay. Ideal vertical beam angulation cannot be consistently achieved, and conditions such as malalignment may yield unusual orientation of the lesion. In such cases the carious lesion may not be ideally demonstrated as suggested by Fig. 8-26. This effect explains the common clinical observation that bite-wing radiographs of a full mouth series reveal decay of a particular tooth, but the lesion is not apparent in the periapical radiographs. In general, given several radiographic representations of a particular tooth, bite-wing radiographs are most likely to provide optimal demonstration of interproximal carious lesions. However, carious lesions are occasionally more apparent in periapical projections because of an unusual embrasure form or other factors.

Factors such as tooth morphology, carious lesion shape, and radiographic beam angulation that influence the radiographic demonstration of interproximal decay similarly affect the appearance of decay affecting other tooth surfaces. The radiographic demonstration of molar occlusal lesions, for example, is minimized in axial extent by the superimposition of healthy, radiopaque enamel and dentin located buccal and lingual to the lesion. These factors must always be considered during the radiographic interpretation of decay.

PULPAL INFLAMMATION

The physiologic response to traumatic, thermal, microbial, and chemical stimulation of the pulp is inflammation. Pulpal inflammation produces clinical manifestations such as sensitivity and pain that are roughly proportional in severity to the inflammation. The edema that is an inherent component of the inflammatory process is particularly significant when the dental pulp is affected because the pulpal cavity cannot enlarge to accommodate the swelling. This confined edema during severe or chronic pulpal inflammation can produce com-

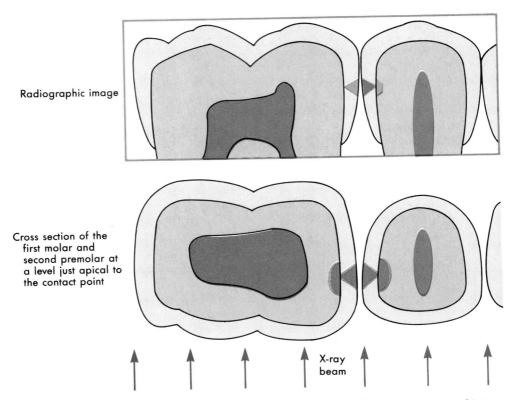

Radiographic image

Cross section of the first molar and second premolar at a level just apical to the contact point

X-ray beam

Fig. 8-25   Effect of buccal-lingual tooth thickness on radiographic demonstration of interproximal decay. The interproximal carious lesions of the distal surface of the mandibular second premolar and the mesial surface of the mandibular first molar are shown in the cross section of the teeth. The lesions are identical in size and axial extent and are approximately equal in size buccal-lingually to the size of the contact point. The radiographic image demonstrates the axial extent of both lesions as significantly less than the actual lesions because of the more narrow width of the decay at the most axial extent in comparison to the buccal-lingual thickness of the healthy tooth structure that obscures radiographic demonstration of the decay. Also, the premolar lesion appears more radiolucent and more extensive axially because less healthy enamel and dentin are present to "mask" the decay in comparison to the larger first molar.

pression of apical blood vessels, which produces ischemic pulp necrosis.

Pulpal inflammation is conceptually categorized as either *reversible* or *irreversible* on the basis of whether or not the inflammatory process can be controlled before pulpal necrosis occurs. Unfortunately, this clear conceptual difference does not mean that a clear clinical distinction is always possible. The cause of the pulpal inflammation, which is usually related to decay, is suggested in most instances by the patient history and clinical findings. However, the likelihood of pulpal necrosis cannot always be predicted on the basis of the source of inflammation. In most clinical situations the progression from mild pulpitis to obvious pulpal

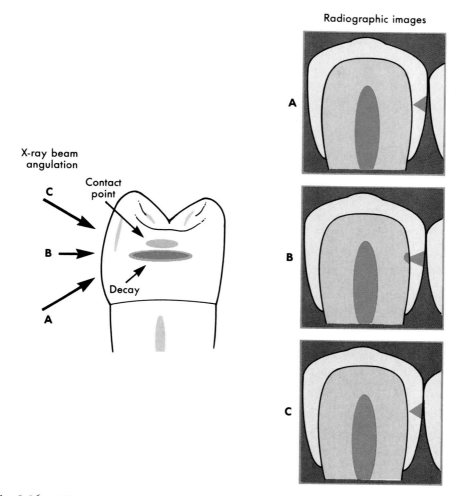

Fig. 8-26   Effect of vertical beam angulation on radiographic demonstration of interproximal decay. Beam angulation **(B)** is optimal to demonstrate the radiolucency of the carious lesion as shown by the corresponding radiographic image. This is because the beam at this level passes through the greatest amount of decay and is absorbed by relatively little healthy enamel and dentin. Both angulations **(A)** and **(C)** pass through a greater proportion of healthy tooth structure and a narrower zone of decay. This yields less radiolucency and less axial extent of the lesion in the radiographic image.

necrosis is gradual, and an overlapping of signs and symptoms frequently makes the diagnosis difficult. In addition, radiographs provide no evidence of the presence, absence, or severity of pulpal inflammation other than indicating possible causes. Pulp testing by stimulating the pulp with ice, heat, and electric shock and then evaluating the neural responsiveness is one effective method of distinguishing different forms of pulpal disease. Table 8-3 summa-

Table 8-3 Comparison of typical pulp testing responses for healthy teeth and various forms of pulpal disease

| Dental pulp status | Test stimulus* | | Electric shock |
	Ice	Heat	
Healthy pulp	Mild response Transient duration	Mild response Transient duration	Response
Reversible pulpitis	Hyper-response Short duration	Hyper-response Short duration	Response
Irreversible pulpitis	Painful response† Lingering duration	Painful response Lingering duration	Response
Pulpal necrosis	No response	No response	No response

Courtesy Dr. Gerald N. Glickman, Baylor College of Dentistry, Dallas, Tx.
*All test responses of suspect teeth must be interpreted in comparison with the response of adjacent or contralateral teeth that are clinically healthy.
†Cold may alleviate pain in end-stage irreversible pulpitis.

rizes the typical pulp testing results for the forms of pulpal disease described in the following paragraphs. However, pulp testing is subject to numerous variables. Therefore the results are not definitive but must be integrated and compared with other findings to achieve an accurate diagnosis.

Reversible Pulpitis

Reversible pulpitis can follow either a chronic or an acute clinical course. The most consistent features are that the severity of the sensitivity is mild and that the patient is usually free of discomfort. Patients frequently describe mild sensitivity of short duration following external stimulation of the tooth by exposure to cold, heat, direct pressure, and touching exposed dentin with a dental explorer. Spontaneous pain associated with reversible pulpitis is unusual. Intentional exposure of the suspected tooth to heat, cold, and electric shock during pulp vitality testing all produce a hypersensitive response of relatively short duration as compared to unaffected teeth. Sensitivity of teeth for several days following relatively superficial operative procedures is a typical example of reversible pulpitis. Treatment is by removal of decay or other possible causes

of inflammation, and symptoms generally improve within a few days.

Irreversible Pulpitis

Pulpal inflammation that will progress to pulpal necrosis is characterized by episodes of spontaneous pain, prolonged discomfort after external stimulation, and more severe discomfort in comparison to reversible pulpitis. Dramatic increase in pain intensity following an abrupt postural change is a typical complaint indicative of irreversible pulpitis. The clinical course of irreversible pulpitis is characterized by gradual progression in the severity of symptoms intermixed with periods of improvement, but some residual tenderness is usually present. Pulp testing by exposure of the tooth to heat, cold, and electric shock produces pain of lingering duration. In some cases of advanced irreversible pulpitis, cold may relieve pain. Treatment alternatives consist of extraction or endodontic treatment.

Hyperplastic Pulpitis

Hyperplastic pulpitis is an uncommon form of pulpal inflammation in which edematous enlargement of the pulp occurs. A *pulp polyp* is enlargement of the pulp into a large carious le-

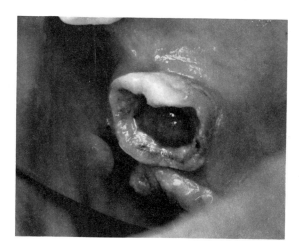

Fig. 8-27 Hyperplastic pulpitis or *pulp polyp* of maxillary second molar.

sion (Fig. 8-27), which generally affects a child or adolescent. The pulp polyp is erythematous, hemorrhagic, and mildly tender. Internal resorption is also a form of hyperplastic pulpitis. Endodontic treatment is required to maintain the tooth.

PERIAPICAL INFLAMMATORY LESIONS SECONDARY TO PULPAL NECROSIS

The confined edematous pressure of irreversible pulpitis destroys the vascular supply to the pulp, which causes pulpal necrosis and prevents the blood flow necessary for healing and repair. This leaves a source of necrotic, toxic material within the pulp chamber that eventually diffuses through the apical or accessory foramina and induces inflammation of adjacent tissues. The radicular or periapical inflammation persists as diffusion of necrotic pulp contents continues, which stimulates lysis and remodeling of periradicular bone. Periapical inflammation secondary to pulpal necrosis continues until the necrotic material is removed either by extraction of the tooth or endodontic treatment. Appearance of a radicular or periapical radiolucency in addition to findings suggesting a cause of pulpal inflammation is usually an adequate basis for a diagnosis of pulpal necrosis. Pulp testing yields minimal response to all forms of stimulation.

Periapical inflammatory lesions are generally considered on the basis of the degree of localization as either focal or diffuse. Focal lesions include the *periapical abscess, periapical granuloma,* and *periapical cyst.* Diffuse inflammation secondary to pulpal necrosis is referred to as *osteomyelitis* if the process is limited to the surrounding bone or *cellulitis* if the inflammation has extended into the adjacent soft tissues.

Periapical Abscess

An abscess by definition produces liquefaction degeneration of tissue and is clinically indicated by the presence of a purulent exudate and pain. This inflammatory response is most characteristic of bacterial infection associated with the pulpal necrosis. Patients complain of spontaneous throbbing pain that increases in severity with pressure. Percussion instantaneously produces severe pain by dramatically increasing the pressure on the acutely inflamed supportive tissues. In addition, digital pressure on the periapical region of the alveolar process demonstrates focal tenderness. More diffuse tenderness to palpation suggests osteomyelitis. Pulp testing of the tooth may produce a slight increase in pain with heat, some relief of pain with cold, and no response to electric stimulation. Radiographic examination reveals a periapical radiolucency characterized by widening of the periodontal ligament space and alteration in the contour and integrity of the lamina dura (Fig. 8-28).

Periapical Cysts and Periapical Granulomas

These lesions represent chronic, localized inflammation that result from diffusion of necrotic pulpal contents without superimposition of bacterial infection or abscess formation. Periapical cysts and granulomas can be considered an equilibrium between the continuous

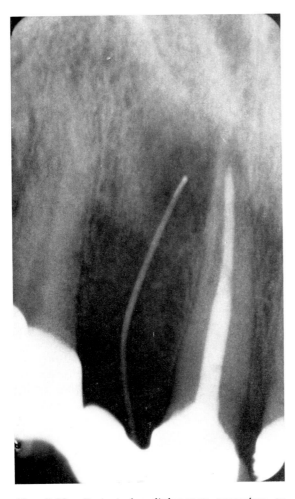

Fig. 8-28 Periapical radiolucency secondary to pulpal necrosis. This vague radiolucency near the apex of an endodontically treated central incisor was associated with a pathologic sinus. The radiograph was exposed with a gutta percha point inserted into the sinus tract to demonstrate the origin of the acute infection that prompted the patient to seek treatment. This lesion represents acute exacerbation of a chronic inflammatory lesion or a *phoenix abscess.*

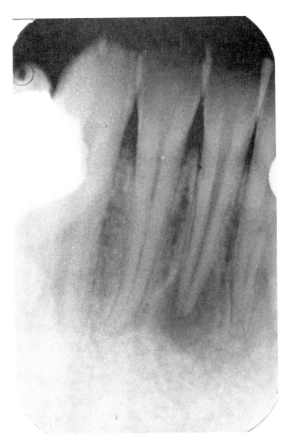

Fig. 8-29 Chronic periapical radiolucency secondary to pulpal necrosis. The patient is unaware of any problem with the tooth. Note the relatively large pulp chamber of the affected tooth in comparison with the adjacent incisor. This is the result of no secondary dentin formation from the time of pulpal necrosis.

periapical diffusion of necrotic pulpal contents and the physiologic mechanisms of containing and absorbing the noxious materials. These lesions are nonpainful; and percussion of the tooth, biting pressure, alveolar palpation, and pulp testing stimulation produce no response, or the patient may indicate that the "tooth feels different, but does not hurt." The lesion is often identified radiographically as a prominent periapical radiolucency (Fig. 8-29) with

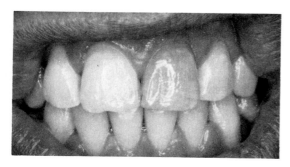

Fig. 8-30 Discoloration of the maxillary left central incisor. Isolated, uniform discoloration of a tooth is generally an indication of pulpal necrosis.

relatively well-delineated borders. The patient generally describes a chronic clinical course of intermittent discomfort interspersed with asymptomatic periods, or the patient may be unaware of any problem. Pulpal necrosis of long duration may produce discoloration of a single tooth (Fig. 8-30).

A *pathologic sinus* is a slender passage from a deep lesion or structure to the mucosal or skin surface. Pathologic sinuses often develop from periapical inflammatory lesions, and their formation allows release of exudate and inflammatory pressure. This drainage generally minimizes pain and tenderness. A soft, mildly tender, erythematous, edematous papule of the alveolar mucosa called a *parulis* represents the sinus opening and is located near the apex of the affected tooth. Gentle probing of the papule demonstrates extension of the tract into the alveolus and may produce exudate. Insertion of a radiopaque probe such as a gutta percha point into the sinus tract and exposure of a radiograph effectively localizes the affected tooth as illustrated in Fig. 8-28.

The dynamic equilibrium represented by chronic periapical inflammatory lesions may be disrupted by the sudden onset of a virulent bacterial infection or by deterioration of the host's general health and resistance to infection. This results in exacerbation of a chronic, asymptomatic lesion into an acute periapical abscess exhibiting the typical features of spontaneous pain and purulent exudate. This is referred to as a *recurrent* or *phoenix abscess.* Radiographic examination usually reveals a large periapical radiolucency with sharply delineated borders and other features indicative of a chronic bone lesion. This seemingly contradictory concurrence of acute clinical signs with chronic radiographic findings is explained by comparing the rate at which clinical and radiographic indications of inflammation become apparent. The inflammatory nature of a periapical lesion can change within hours or days, whereas bone resorption must progress for weeks or months before becoming radiographically apparent. Therefore radiographic manifestations of periapical lesions tend to lag behind the clinical status of the lesions, and diagnosis of periapical lesions on the basis of radiographs alone can be misleading. Clinical signs and symptoms more accurately reflect the current status of periapical inflammation.

Osteomyelitis. Osteomyelitis of the jaws usually represents diffuse progression of a focal inflammatory process into the surrounding marrow spaces. Clinical features indicating this process are diffuse and spontaneous pain, poorly localized tenderness to pressure, and fever. Additional features may include tenderness of regional lymph nodes and purulent drainage. Bacterial infection is the predominant cause of mandibular and maxillary osteomyelitis, although chronic, aseptic osteomyelitis can result from ischemia and other conditions. The distinctive forms of osteomyelitis that are recognized on the basis of the clinical course and radiographic features are discussed in Chapter 19.

Bacterial osteomyelitis can spread into the adjacent soft tissues and anatomic spaces. The terms *subperiosteal abscess* and *periostitis* refer to an enlarging abscess trapped between the cortex and the tough periosteum, whereas progression into connective tissue spaces is *cellulitis.* Swelling and increased prominence of systemic features such as fever and malaise indicate the potential gravity of these regional infections, which are described in Chapter 18.

The treatment of all focal periapical inflammatory lesions is removal of the causative necrotic pulp by endodontic treatment or removal of the tooth. Antibiotic treatment may be a beneficial adjunct if progression of the bacterial infection is suspected. Most periapical inflammatory lesions resolve following removal of the necrotic pulp as indicated by absence of symptoms and radiographic evidence of periapical healing within 6 to 12 months. Persistence of the periapical lesion following initial treatment may require endodontic retreatment or surgical curettage with retrograde obturation.

The sequential goals in treating disseminated infections are initial containment of the infection, then localization of the infection, and eventually resolution of the infection. Antibiotic treatment of suppurative, diffuse jaw infections should be instituted empirically with penicillin for nonallergic patients. A more specific antibiotic may be identified by microbial culture and antibiotic sensitivity testing, but the best results are attained if the microbial specimen is obtained before initiating empiric antibiotic therapy. Incision and drainage is an effective method of relieving pressure and promoting localization of cellulitis if an area of pooled pus or "pointing" can be identified as a site for the incision. Drainage can also be accomplished by opening the necrotic pulp chamber or removing the infected tooth. Both antibiotic treatment and drainage limit the spread and promote localization of the infection. Removal of the initial cause, if not previously accomplished, is the final step in achieving resolution.

INFLAMMATORY CONDITIONS OF THE DENTAL SUPPORTIVE TISSUES

Inflammation of the periodontium, *periodontitis,* with the resulting chronic degeneration of the supportive tissues, represents a complex diagnostic and therapeutic challenge to the dentist. Most adults exhibit some evidence of this disease, and the dentist's responsibility is to prevent the final consequence of periodontitis, which is loss of teeth. The causes of periodontitis can be generally categorized as either conditions that contribute to diminished host resistance to infection or those that promote the accumulation of bacterial plaque. Treatment goals are improved host resistance and elimination of the bacterial plaque by effective oral hygiene, removal of plaque retentive calculus, and surgical elimination of tissue defects.

Despite the complexity of etiologic and therapeutic considerations, the diagnostic features indicating the presence of periodontal inflammatory conditions are consistently demonstrated by clinical and radiographic examination. These diseases are categorized as either gingivitis or periodontitis.

Typical Forms of Gingivitis

Gingivitis is defined as inflammation of the gingiva, although in clinical usage the term generally implies that the inflammatory process is limited to the superficial soft tissue without involvement of underlying alveolar bone. The characteristic clinical signs of bacterial infection, including erythema, edema, exudate, and tenderness, can be identified visually and by palpation. Food and plaque present on tooth surfaces provide evidence of ineffective oral hygiene. Sulcular probing often causes hemorrhage and tenderness. Probing depths may be within the normal range of 1 to 3 mm or slightly increased, and cervical calculus may be present. Radiographs demonstrate normal crestal alveolar bone within 1 to 2 mm of the cementoenamel junction.

Specific forms of gingival inflammation are compared in Table 8-4 on pp. 154–155 by the modifying diagnostic terms used to distinguish variations in clinical features and the influence of causative factors. Regardless of the specific form of gingivitis, however, bacterial plaque is the primary causative agent. Typical forms of gingivitis are designated as marginal, hyper-

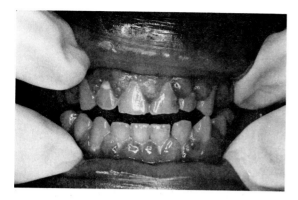

Fig. 8-31 Hyperplastic gingivitis characterized by generalized bulbous, edematous gingival enlargement. This patient did not practice any significant form of dental hygiene. No contributory conditions such as medications or pregnancy were identified.

plastic, and chronic gingivitis on the basis of the extent of the inflammatory response.

Marginal gingivitis. This mild form of gingivitis is insipient, superficial inflammation limited to the marginal gingiva and interdental papillae. Improved oral hygiene practices and thorough prophylaxis produce rapid resolution.

Hyperplastic gingivitis. Hyperplastic gingivitis may be either focal or generalized and is characterized by gingival enlargement. The interdental papillae are most conspicuously affected. Hyperplastic gingivitis produces increased pocket depths by greater coverage of the anatomic crowns as shown in Fig. 8-31 rather than by the apical migration of the gingival attachment that is characteristic of periodontitis. The phrase *pseudopocket formation,* although strictly a misnomer, is occasionally used to indicate that increased probing depths are related to soft tissue enlargement rather than bone destruction. Indications of inflammation such as erythema, edema, and prominent vascularity are also present and explain the common use of the term "boggy" to describe the clinical appearance. The condition

typically improves within weeks of dental prophylaxis and improved oral hygiene, although some enlargement usually persists.

Several forms of hyperplastic gingivitis are caused by cofactors in addition to local accumulation of bacterial plaque. *Hormonal, pregnancy,* and *puberty gingivitis* are clinical terms indicating the contribution of pronounced hormonal fluctuations in the progression of generalized gingival hyperplasia affecting some women. Prominent, generalized fibrotic gingival enlargement may indicate certain medications as a cofactor or the presence of a hereditary condition known as *fibromatosis gingivae* as discussed in Chapter 18.

Chronic gingivitis. Chronic gingival inflammation is characterized by a generalized pale, fibrotic appearance of the gingiva and inflammation of the sulcus surfaces and interdental papillae. Alteration of gingival contours such as loss of the gingival papillae often develops. This represents a chronic, cyclic reparative response to years of inflammatory gingival injury and is often associated with features of periodontitis.

Atypical Forms of Gingivitis

Unusual forms of gingivitis imply a significant contribution to the gingival inflammation by a variety of host factors and by the accumulation of bacterial plaque. The contribution of hormonal imbalance to hyperplastic gingivitis has been described. In general, the possible influence of systemic factors should be considered if the inflammation is inordinately severe relative to the bacterial plaque present or if dental prophylaxis and improved oral hygiene fail to yield improvement.

Desquamative gingivitis. This is a nonspecific clinical designation that refers to gingival inflammation with features of striking erythema, atrophic appearance, and sloughing of the superficial epithelium. Painful gingival ulcers result without purulence or other evidence of acute bacterial infection. Middle age—to-older females are most often affected. The

Table 8-4 Comparison of different forms of gingivitis

Form of gingivitis	Clinical features	Contributory factors	Significance
COMMON, LOCALIZED PROCESS			
Marginal gingivitis	Erythema, edema, tenderness limited to the marginal gingiva and interdental papillae; younger patients	None beyond poor oral hygiene and relatively short duration of the process	Superficial; resolves quickly with plaque elimination with no permanent defect
Hyperplastic gingivitis	Bulbous, edematous enlargement of the gingiva, may be focal or generalized; "boggy" and pocket depth is increased	Caused by poor oral hygiene over an extended time; hormonal or medication effect should be eliminated as contributing to the process	Deeper, hyperplastic response resolves with plaque removal, but mild enlargement may persist
Chronic gingivitis	Pale, fibrotic appearance of gingiva, loss of stippling; edema, exudate and hemorrhage from the sulcular surface on probing; increased pocket depth	Chronic inflammation produces a recurring cycle of active inflammation and reparative fibrosis	Usually associated with periodontitis; inflammation of the crevicular pockets can be controlled by plaque removal if pockets can be kept clean
UNUSUAL, LOCAL PROCESS PROMOTED BY SYSTEMIC CONDITIONS			
Desquamative gingivitis	Erythematous and atrophic appearance without enlargement; pain and sloughing of surface epithelium are characteristic	Autoimmune conditions such as lichen planus and cicatricial pemphigoid; similar features may be caused by contact hypersensitivity	Topical corticosteroid application during episodes of increased severity usually required to maintain symptomatic control

Condition	Clinical Features	Etiology/Association	Significance
Acute necrotizing ulcerative gingivitis	Severe pain, fetid odor, punched out papilla, pseudomembranous ulceration, exudate and erythema; usually most severe in anterior segments	Compromised host resistance to infection; unusual microbes, including spirochetes and fusiform bacilli, are usually involved	Rapid response to improved status of the host, antibiotic therapy, and superficial debridement of the tissues
Pregnancy, hormonal, or medication gingivitis	Indistinguishable from hyperplastic gingivitis, except that the erythematous enlargement is generalized and the patient history usually reveals the contributory factor	Pregnancy, puberty, and other conditions associated with hormonal fluctuation may be contributory; also, certain medications can produce similar changes (see Chapter 18)	Improved hygiene and oral prophylaxis usually yields significant improvement by minimizing the inflammatory component of the process; may persist to some degree
Hemorrhagic gingivitis	Edematous enlargement and erythema may be dramatic, but the consistent feature is dramatic hemorrhage after even slight pressure on the tissue	Associate with bleeding disorders, scurvy, leukemia, and hemopoietic suppression; may become severe	Diagnostic sign of the causative condition; improvement is usually dramatic following resolution of the systemic condition
Nephritic or uremic gingivitis	Painful, erythematous gingiva, as well as the odor of ammonia and excessive salivation	Associated with renal failure	Often persists to some degree despite local plaque control
Idiopathic gingivitis	Evidence of inflammation persists following elimination of plaque and calculus, as well as improved hygiene	Failure to respond to normally effective treatment usually suggests diminished host resistance or other contributory systemic disease that has not been diagnosed	Indicates the need for additional diagnostic evaluation to identify the underlying contributory condition

underlying condition is usually demonstrated to be either erosive lichen planus or cicatricial pemphigoid as described in Chapter 17.

Acute necrotizing ulcerative gingivitis. This gingival infection by fusiform bacilli and spirochetes is also known as *ANUG, Vincent's infection,* and *trench mouth.* It is usually an opportunistic infection caused by conditions of diminished host infection resistance such as malnutrition, systemic viral infection, emotional distress, and loss of immune system competence. ANUG produces severe pain, mild fever, fetid breath, pseudomembranous ulceration, exudate, and erythema. Necrosis of the interdental papillae produces a characteristic "punched out" appearance between teeth, which is usually most apparent in the anterior mandibular segment. Antibiotic therapy, superficial debridement of affected areas, and improved oral hygiene yield rapid improvement in most instances. Amelioration of symptoms allows more thorough dental prophylaxis within a few days. Identification of the underlying contributory condition becomes the primary diagnostic issue if local infection control measures are ineffective or if the condition recurs.

Hemorrhagic gingivitis. Hemorrhagic gingivitis is a nonspecific designation for the combination of gingival inflammation and dramatic hemorrhage following mild pressure or probing. Moderate enlargement and edema are also typically present. Vitamin C deficiency or *scurvy,* acute leukemia, and bleeding disorders should be considered as possible causes of hemorrhagic gingivitis.

Atypical gingivitis caused by other conditions. Other systemic conditions can exacerbate the effects of gingival inflammation. Uremic or nephritic gingivitis is excessive inflammation associated with pain, ammonia breath, and excessive salivation in patients suffering from renal failure. Diabetes mellitus, particularly when poorly controlled, produces more severe gingival inflammation than would be expected, based on the quantity of bacterial plaque. *Cyclic neutropenia* is an uncommon cause of recurring exacerbation of gingivitis corresponding to a periodic, idiopathic decrease in the number of circulating neutrophils approximately every 3 weeks.

Periodontitis

Periodontitis is chronic inflammatory deterioration of the supportive dental tissues resulting from the accumulation of bacterial plaque. The diagnosis of periodontitis requires evidence of apical migration of the gingival attachment to cementum, as well as crestal alveolar bone loss. The most dependable clinical indication of periodontitis is sulcular depths beyond 1 to 3 mm without gingival enlargement and radiographic evidence of crestal alveolar bone loss. Radiographic evidence of bone loss must be carefully evaluated, however, in the context of the clinical findings because technical factors such as the example illustrated in Fig. 8-32 can be misleading. Periodontitis may also produce mobility of teeth and gingival recession. Features of gingivitis such as edema, exudate, fibrosis, erythema, and bacterial plaque are associated with active periodontitis and reflect the inflammatory nature of the disease.

Several distinct forms of periodontitis are recognized on the basis of the clinical course and prognostic implications. The most easily identified distinguishing findings are the age of onset and rate of progression. Most forms other than the common adult type of periodontitis are believed to be caused by differences in the virulence of predominant microbes or conditions associated with diminished host resistance to the infection. In addition, the severity of the periodontal bone loss, regardless of the specific disease form, is often graded in an effort to anticipate probable methods of treatment and prognosis.

Adult periodontitis. Adult periodontitis is the most common form of inflammatory deterioration of the periodontal tissues. Apical migration of the periodontal attachment and alve-

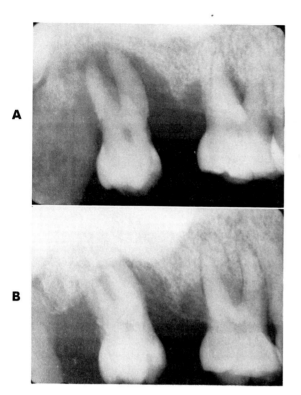

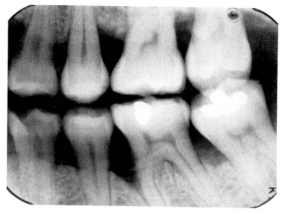

Fig. 8-33 Periodontal bone loss. This bite-wing radiograph reveals a generalized pattern of horizontal bone loss, as well as triangulation defects of vertical bone loss along the mesial root of the mandibular first molar and distal to the maxillary second premolar. Infrabony crater formation is suggested between the mandibular molars and between the maxillary molars. The focal radiolucency between the roots of the mandibular first molar is typical of an early furcation defect.

Fig. 8-32 Both periapical radiographs of these maxillary molars were exposed on the same day but with considerable difference in vertical angulation of the x-ray beam. Periapical **A** demonstrates destruction of nearly all supportive bone associated with the third molar, as well as infrabony cratering of the distal root of the first molar and a furcation defect. Periapical **B** reveals similar alveolar bone defects, but the extent of bone loss appears less severe because of steep vertical x-ray beam angulation.

olar bone loss are generally not identified until the third decade. Adult periodontitis typically progresses relatively slowly and is qualitatively proportional to the accumulation of calculus and bacterial plaque. The severity of alveolar bone loss is relatively uniform throughout the mouth, as indicated by radiographic demonstration of a horizontal pattern of alveolar bone loss (Fig. 8-33). Focally advanced periodontal lesions may be identified radiographically as vertical bone loss or infrabony defects (Fig. 8-33). These more rapidly destructive lesions are usually explained by unusual factors contributing to plaque retention such as overhanging restorations, prominent calculus formations, or malalignment. Effective elimination of bacterial plaque usually arrests disease progression in less advanced stages of the disease.

Juvenile periodontitis. This form of periodontitis has been referred to as *periodontosis* and is characterized by alveolar bone loss affecting healthy adolescents. Both a localized and a generalized pattern of juvenile periodontitis are recognized. Most of the teeth are involved in the generalized form, whereas the bone loss of the localized form is limited to the first molars and incisors as shown in Fig. 8-34. Females are affected more often than males, and a greater proportion of blacks are affected in comparison with other races. Deep sulcular pockets are identified clinically that

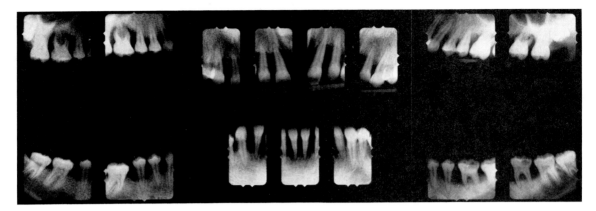

Fig. 8-34   Juvenile periodontitis affecting 18-year-old female. This full mouth series demonstrates severe bone loss associated with the incisors and first molars. The remaining teeth are less dramatically compromised.

correspond to angular or vertical bone defects demonstrated radiographically. The inflammatory bone loss appears disproportionally advanced compared to the amount of calculus and degree of inflammation. Demonstration of altered neutrophil function and identification of unusual bacterial species in juvenile periodontitis patients support the theory that the cause is related to a bacterial exotoxin. A similar clinical course affecting children before age 5 has been referred to as *prepubertal periodontitis,* which is a diagnostic feature of Papillion-Lefèvre syndrome as discussed in Chapter 20. Juvenile periodontitis may be arrested with combination therapy of antibiotics and antibacterial rinses such as chlorhexidine gluconate to control the virulent bacteria and strict plaque control and periodontal surgery to eliminate tissue defects.

Rapidly progressive periodontitis. Generalized vertical bone lesions affecting young adults are the characteristic feature of rapidly progressive periodontitis. Cyclic phases of active inflammation and rapid osseous destruction over several months followed by quiescence and recurrence is the typical course of the condition. Altered inflammatory cell chemotaxis may be demonstrated during the active phases, which suggests a bacterial exotoxin as a pathogenic mechanism. Rapidly progressive periodontitis typically responds to the same combination therapy described for juvenile periodontitis. The condition continues to progress rapidly without treatment until the teeth are lost or may spontaneously subside to the more gradual progression of adult periodontitis.

Necrotizing ulcerative periodontitis. This form of periodontitis is characterized clinically by generalized, painful interproximal craters of soft tissue (Fig. 8-35) and bone destruction with a predominance of vertical bone lesions. This form of periodontitis is most common among young adults but can occur at any age and is often associated with repeated episodes of acute necrotizing ulcerative gingivitis. Rapid, cyclic progression is the typical clinical course. Necrotizing ulcerative periodontitis is frequently associated with the compromised immune function of acquired immunodeficiency syndrome.

A variety of advanced systemic conditions can produce clinical features typical of rapidly progressive periodontitis by various defects in host resistance. Failure of periodontitis to resolve following conventional periodontal ther-

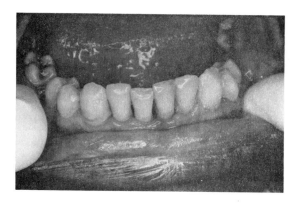

Fig. 8-35 Necrotizing ulcerative periodontitis following initial debridement and antibiotic therapy. The most acute features of the infection have resolved, but the destruction of the gingival papillae is still apparent. The condition causing compromised host resistance in this case was AIDS. Necrotizing ulcerative gingivitis is a common feature of the later stages of the syndrome.

apy of bacterial plaque control and surgical tissue defect elimination is generally referred to as *refractory periodontitis* and strongly suggests such underlying conditions.

Classification of Periodontitis Severity

A diagnosis of periodontitis is inadequate to determine specific treatment goals and prognosis without identifying the amount of alveolar bone destruction. Tissue characteristics, six-point sulcular probing depths, and radiographic variations in alveolar contour provide the detailed information needed to plan and evaluate the effectiveness of periodontal treatment. In addition, a categorization scheme is often useful to reflect the general profile of the patient's periodontal status and general treatment needs.

Case type I indicates gingivitis without evidence of significant bone loss. *Case type II* is early periodontitis characterized by gingivitis, mild increase in sulcular probing depths, and minimal evidence of alveolar bone loss. Both case types I and II are expected to resolve following elimination of bacterial plaque. The prognosis is excellent, assuming that plaque control is maintained.

Case type III is moderate periodontitis as demonstrated radiographically by significant alveolar bone loss that is limited to the coronal one third to one half of the root. Focal vertical lesions may be identified, but the general pattern of bone loss is horizontal. Sulcular probing depths are typically in the 5- to 7-mm range, and hemorrhage during probing is common. Gingival fibrosis and recession, calculus accumulations, and mild tooth mobility are additional clinical observations. Surgical elimination of tissue defects to facilitate plaque removal and other plaque control therapy are likely to be required to control the condition. The prognosis is good if effective plaque control can be achieved and maintained.

Case type IV or advanced periodontitis indicates generalized alveolar bone loss exceeding one half of the root length. Vertical bone loss, infrabony defects, and furcation involvement are frequent observations radiographically, in addition to the general horizontal pattern of bone loss. Sulcular probing depths may exceed 8 mm in areas with production of hemorrhage and purulent exudate. Tooth mobility (Fig. 8-36) and gingival recession are typical findings. Treatment can be expected to include surgical elimination of tissue defects and extraction of hopelessly compromised teeth. The prognosis is generally considered guarded or unfavorable, even with aggressive treatment.

All forms of early onset and rapidly progressive periodontitis are categorized as *case type V* or refractory periodontitis. This indicates the importance of recognizing the possible clinical influence of virulent bacterial species and underlying conditions of compromised host resistance to infection. Successful treatment must include antibiotic therapy, chlorhexidine gluconate rinses, plaque control, and efforts to improve underlying systemic conditions, if possible. The prognosis must be considered guarded.

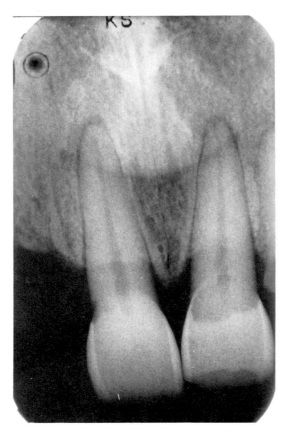

Fig. 8-36 Radiographic evidence of mobility. Both central incisors exhibit widening of the periodontal ligament space in the apical and crestal one third of the root and more narrow, normal width in the middle third of the root. The appearance reflects bone remodeling and periodontal ligament stretching caused by chronic mobility apical and crestal to the pivot point in the middle third of the root.

In addition to the features described in previous paragraphs, numerous clinical considerations influence the clinician's assessment of periodontitis severity. For example, comparing case type III periodontitis affecting a 40-year-old with the same findings in an eighty year-old implies different clinical considerations relative to progression and prognosis. Nevertheless, this case type categorization facilitates general comparisons.

SUMMARY

A definitive diagnosis of most abnormalities of the teeth and supportive structures can be made by a specific determination of the tissues affected, the clinical features, the results of specific diagnostic tests, and the response of abnormalities to empiric treatment. This provides the basis for additional treatment, prevention of future disease, and determination of prognosis.

BIBLIOGRAPHY

Barr JH, Stephens RG: Dental radiology: pertinent basic concepts and their applications in clinical practice, Philadelphia, 1980, Saunders.

Eversole LR: Clinical outline of oral pathology: diagnosis and treatment, ed 2, Philadelphia, 1984, Lea & Febiger.

Goaz PW, White SC: Oral radiology: principles and interpretation, ed 2, St Louis, 1987, Mosby–Year Book.

Langlais RP and others: Oral diagnosis, oral medicine and treatment planning, Philadelphia, 1984, Saunders.

Lynch MA, Brightman VJ, Greenberg MS, editors: Burket's oral medicine: diagnosis and treatment, ed 8, Philadelphia, 1984, Lippincott.

Regezi J and Sciubba J: Oral pathology. Clinical-pathologic correlations, Philadelphia, 1989, Saunders.

Shafer WG, Hine MK, Levy BM: A textbook of oral pathology, ed 4, Philadelphia, 1983, Saunders.

Wood NK, Goaz PW: Differential diagnosis of oral lesions, ed 4, St Louis, 1991, Mosby-Year Book.

Worth HM: Principles and practice of oral radiologic interpretation, Chicago, 1963, Mosby–Year Book.

CHAPTER *9*

Clinical Evaluation Of Pain

JOHN F. NELSON

Pain is a sensation of suffering resulting from a noxious stimulus, physical disorder, or mental derangement. Although this definition may not fully clarify all that is implied by the word, several points are apparent. First, pain originates from a variety of causes other than the direct stimulation of peripheral nerves by temperature extremes, pressure, sharp incision, and similar agents. Second, the sensation is perceived as negative, which prompts the sufferer to seek and expect relief. Also, the perception of pain as suffering is a subjective experience that is not easily evaluated objectively.

From a diagnostic perspective, the presence or absence of pain and its characteristics provides significant and reliable diagnostic information. For example, most inflammatory soft tissue enlargements are painful or tender, while neoplastic soft tissue enlargements seldom are. From a practical perspective, most patients gauge the competence of their dentist by how well the pain of dental procedures is controlled and by how effectively conditions that cause pain are treated. Therefore pain is a central diagnostic and therapeutic issue in the practice of dentistry.

GENERAL ASPECTS OF PAIN

Clinically significant aspects of pain include the origin, the assessment, the comparison, and the management of discomfort.

Classification of Pain by Origin

Classification of pain by origin (Bell, 1989) relies on the origin of oral and facial pain for categorization by the following designations:

1. *Somatic pain* is pain resulting from the noxious stimulation of normal neural structures that innervate body tissues.
2. *Neurogenous pain* is discomfort generated within the nervous system itself and is caused by an abnormality of the neural structures that innervate body tissues.
3. *Psychogenic pain* is pain resulting from

161

psychic causes and not from noxious stimulation or neural abnormality.

The clinical value of this categorization scheme is that the diagnostic features of pain often suggest its origin as illustrated in Fig. 9-1. Most dental patients complain of somatic pain. Examination generally reveals inflammation, tissue injury, or another condition that explains the discomfort. Neurogenous pain and psychogenic pain are not associated with an obvious lesion or are disproportionally severe in comparison to any abnormality that is present. These forms of pain are just as real as somatic pain to the patient and their diagnosis should be considered if no somatic source of pain is apparent.

Clinical Evaluation of Pain

An accurate diagnosis of pain and effective treatment requires an understanding of the patient's subjective perception of the discomfort. Most patients eagerly describe the following diagnostic features of their pain during the diagnostic interview. In instances of mentally compromised individuals, however, considerable prompting may be needed to obtain contributory information. A preliminary diagnosis should be delayed until the physical examination can be conducted to identify a source of somatic pain.

Onset of the Pain. How the pain started can reveal the cause, especially if traumatic injury is suspected. A brief duration from the onset of pain to the request for treatment can suggest inflammatory somatic pain and exclude typically chronic conditions. The duration of the pain in comparison with its severity may also indicate the patient's sensitivity to discomfort or attitude toward dental care.

Localization of the Pain. Somatic pain of the oral and perioral region nearly always emanates from the affected site, which is readily identified by the patient. The location of pain is the basis for organizing the discussion of specific painful somatic conditions within this chapter because location is a reliable indication of the origin of somatic pain.

Inability of the patient to localize pain may indicate somatic pain originating from deep tissues or that the pain is not somatic. The radiation of pain is the sensation of a spreading to adjacent areas from the primary source, which may suggest a neurogenic component to the problem. In rare instances pain is perceived at a site other than that of the somatic abnormality. This is *referred* or *projected pain* and can be distinguished from simple somatic pain by the failure to obtain relief by a local anesthetic injection at the painful site.

Characteristics of Pain. The patient's perception of pain is reflected by the choice of descriptive terms such as steady, bright, dull, pricking, itching, burning, aching, pulsating, stabbing, throbbing, vague, sharp, or pounding. The severity of pain can be graded as mild, moderate, or severe based on its disruption of routine activities such as sleeping, eating, or work.

Course of Pain. The course or pattern of discomfort often suggests possible causes. The temporal pattern of pain refers to the timing or spacing of the sensation. Episodic pain is classified as intermittent in contrast to continuous discomfort. Steady increase in the severity of pain is typical of the progressive, acute inflammation produced by a bacterial infection. Periods of relief followed by recurrences is a pattern of pain often caused by chronic periapical inflammatory lesions that episodically undergo acute exacerbation. Painful sequelae of nocturnal bruxism are more severe in the morning, while tension headaches are relatively constant in severity throughout the day.

Factors That Alter The Pain. Alteration of pain following exposure to certain agents and conditions can reveal its nature and possible causes. Application of ice, for example, soothes pain from most superficial inflammatory causes, and moist heat usually relieves the deeper discomfort of muscle spasms. Observa-

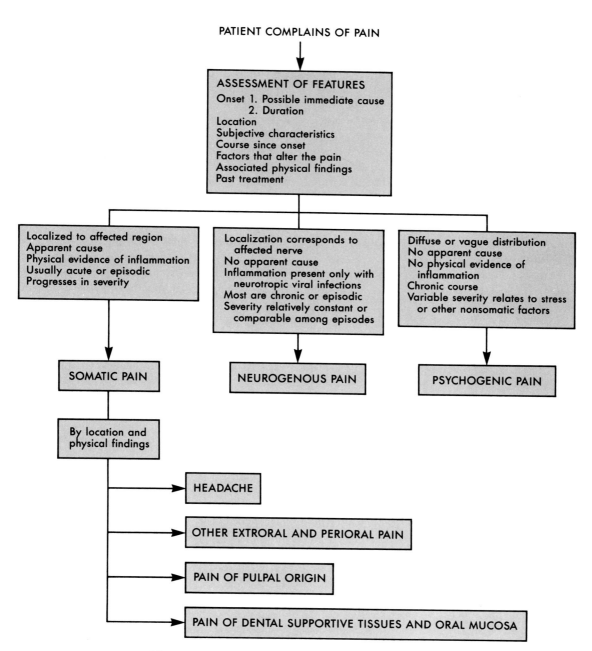

Fig. 9-1. Clinical assessment and categorization of pain.

tion of the patient's response when heat, cold, electric shock, and pressure are intentionally applied to a tooth is the basis of pulp vitality testing. External stimulation of an inflamed pulp produces a hypersensitive response whereas similar stimulation of a necrotic pulp does not bring about such a response. Spontaneous pain suggests that it may be neurogenous, psychogenic, or caused by severe inflammation. The effectiveness and nature of any prior treatment for the pain by another clinician should also be evaluated.

Associated Findings. Certain systemic conditions can cause or influence the nature of pain. Uremia, electrolyte imbalance, and a variety of medications can accentuate pain perception or produce neurogenous pain. Emotional stress may exacerbate somatic pain or suggest psychogenic complaints.

Treatment of Pain

Pain is the source of most chief complaints, which implies the expectation of expedient treatment and relief. Pain management can be approached in several different ways. *Curative* or *definitive treatment* provides relief by eliminating the cause. The goal of *palliative treatment* is to alleviate pain and other distressing symptoms without curing the condition. *Symptomatic treatment* attempts to eliminate symptoms as they develop without specific consideration of their origin.

Curative treatment is considered the optimal approach if a definitive diagnosis of the problem can be made and an effective treatment for the condition is available. Palliative treatment is the appropriate approach to provide relief when no curative treatment is available for the condition. Palliative treatment is also useful in conjunction with curative treatment to provide relief until curative treatment eliminates the pain. Symptomatic treatment is an unsuitable approach because control of pain may allow the progression of potentially harmful, undiagnosed diseases.

Several aspects of pain management influence the diagnostic process. Many patients suffering from pain initiate symptomatic treatment with analgesics or topical anesthetics before they consult the dentist. This must be considered during the diagnosis because it may interfere with attempts to localize or evaluate the problem. Also, the clinician is often tempted to provide symptomatic relief of pain while the definitive diagnosis remains uncertain. The decision to provide symptomatic relief for a distressed patient must be weighed against the value of an unaltered pain response in future attempts to reach a diagnosis. Finally, most complaints directed to the dentist are related to somatic pain of inflammatory origin, which is usually controlled by curative dental procedures. Ineffectiveness of normally curative treatment demands reconsideration of the diagnosis because this is often the initial indication that the original diagnosis is incorrect.

SOMATIC PAIN: HEADACHE

Headache or *cephalalgia* can be produced by numerous conditions and is an extremely common form of somatic pain. Vascular spasm is the causative mechanism of several characteristic types of cephalalgia including migraine and cluster headaches. Emotional and muscular stress contribute to many forms of cranial pain and are principal factors in the common tension headache. In addition, any source of increased intracranial pressure including edema following injury and enlarging neoplasms can produce cephalalgia.

The diagnosis and management of cephalalgia in general is beyond the scope of dental practice and a medical referral is indicated if dental conditions can be excluded as a possible cause. However, the features of several common and characteristic forms of cephalalgia provide a basis for comparison with the symptoms of dental and temporomandibular diseases. Pattern of occurrence and precipitating factors of cephalalgia are generally the most contributory diagnostic features.

Classic Migraine Headache

The classic migraine is caused by vascular spasm initiated by the release of endogenous vasoactive mediators such as serotonin and bradykinin. Pain results from vasoconstriction in or near the head followed by distant vasodilation. The patient often has a premonition of the attack followed by a *visual aura* described as flashing lights or blurred vision that is caused by ophthalmic artery spasm. This is immediately followed by numbness, tingling, nausea, vomiting, photophobia, and intolerance to loud noises. Severe unilateral pain then develops in the region of the eye, forehead, temple, jaw, or neck. The symptoms last from several hours to a day or two. Most patients are women between the ages of 10 and 30. Stress and menstruation appear to be precipitating factors, and most patients report familial occurrence.

Common Migraine Headache

The common migraine lacks the visual aura of the classic migraine and produces more diffuse pain but the duration of the attack is similar. The pain is accompanied by altered sensation, depression, sweating, nasal congestion, and lacrimation. Stress, specific foods, and certain medications, especially birth control pills, are often described as precipitating factors. A family occurrence of common migraine headache is also frequently reported.

Cluster Headache

Cluster headache or *paroxysmal nocturnal cephalalgia* is characterized by unilateral, intense, and steady orbital pain of 1 to 2 hours duration. Lacrimation, rhinorrhea, and facial edema also develop. The nightly attacks commence approximately 2 to 3 hours after falling asleep and usually occur during a 2 to 3 week period. The patient may then be free of symptoms for months or years, but the "cluster" of episodes generally recurs. Men are 4 times as likely to suffer cluster headaches as women. Individuals often relate onset of the attacks to stress, alcohol, specific foods, or drugs.

Tension Headache

The tension headache is the most common form of cephalalgia, and it is precipitated by demanding emotional situations leading to muscle strain. The mechanisms are probably more complex, but stress, overwork, and depression are definite initiating factors. The bilateral pain is described as fullness, pressure, or tightness with waves of superimposed aching. The typical throbbing sensation suggests a vascular component to the pain. Attacks may be acute with a duration of a few hours to a day or in some instances the pain can be relatively constant for days or weeks. The tension headache is one of the few types of cephalalgia that can be constant and continuous both day and night over an extended time period.

Other Causes of Headache

Headaches can also result from traumatic injury, severe hypertension, intracranial tumors, infection, systemic disease, and certain medications. The common feature of most of these conditions is an increase in intracranial pressure. Medical referral is indicated since diagnosis and management of unexplained cephalalgia is not an area of proficiency for most dentists. The dentist should, however, be prepared to rule out a dental origin of the pain. For example, headache associated with temporomandibular joint (TMJ) dysfunction is a common finding, but a history of episodic headaches alone seldom justifies diagnosis of "TMJ disease." Many patients have degenerative joint disease without headaches, many patients have headaches unrelated to joint dysfunction, and some patients have headaches that are caused by TMJ dysfunction. The diagnosis of jaw dysfunction as contributory to cephalalgia demands demonstration of additional evidence of the condition such as spasm of muscles of mastication.

SOMATIC PAIN: OTHER CAUSES OF EXTRAORAL AND PERIORAL PAIN

Other causes of extraoral and perioral pain that are of clinical importance to the dentist include conditions that affect the temporomandibular joint, the major salivary glands, the nasal sinuses, and the oropharynx. As with other forms of somatic pain, location of the pain and the pattern of occurrence are generally the most significant diagnostic features. The diagnosis of these painful conditions is often challenging because their features can be similar. Treatment is generally palliative except in cases of acute infection.

Myofascial Pain Dysfunction Syndrome

Myofascial pain dysfunction syndrome (MPDS) refers to the clinical condition characterized by pain, fatigue, and spasm of the muscles of mastication. Tenderness to palpation of one or more of these muscles is the most reliable diagnostic feature of MPDS. Muscle tenderness is generally most pronounced near the origin or insertion of an affected muscle, but the belly is often at least mildly tender. This tenderness is most easily demonstrated for the temporalis and masseter muscles by applying fingertip pressure during extreme opening and closing movements of the mandible. The symptom complex that defines the MPDS includes:

1. Spasm of one or more of the muscles of mastication
2. Tenderness to palpation of one or more muscles of mastication
3. Diffuse head pain that is similar to tension headache and is usually most severe in the morning
4. Pain on jaw opening
5. Limitation of opening measured to be less than 35 to 40 mm between incisal edges at the midline
6. Lateral deviation during jaw opening
7. Evidence of bruxism or clenching by history or presence of generalized wear facets
8. Malocclusion or evidence of occlusal disharmony
9. Unilateral or bilateral preauricular pain during palpation
10. Joint sounds such as clicking, popping, and crepitus during jaw opening

The patients are usually young to middle-aged females who experience constant or episodic emotional stress. The symptoms of MPDS tend to occur in cycles with asymptomatic periods interposed between acute bouts associated with demanding emotional situations. Occlusal disharmony may be a contributory factor.

The treatment approach that is most effective relies on elimination of contributory factors, if possible, and palliative treatment during acute periods of discomfort. Palliative treatment with analgesics and application of moist heat to the spastic muscles is generally adequate in mild cases. Elimination of occlusal disharmony by removal of isolated interferences and comprehensive orthodontic treatment of complex malocclusion may be appropriate. A bite splint to minimize the adverse effects of bruxism often relieves symptoms. Counseling to promote better adaptation by the patient to stress and dramatic emotional episodes may help some individuals. Any combination of these approaches may be necessary to achieve relief in a specific case.

Internal Derangements of the Temporomandibular Joint

Abnormal relationships of the soft tissue joint components relative to the osseous structures are collectively referred to as internal derangements of the joint. Inflammation, sclerosis, and distortion of the soft tissues gradually develop as a consequence of functional stress that is essentially magnified by these dysfunctional anatomic relationships. In most cases no direct cause is apparent other than conditions such as bruxism that appear to generate excessive "wear and tear" of the joint. However, other patients can relate symptoms to instances of a specific injury. The recurring muscle of mastication spasm of MPDS is believed to contribute to some cases of internal joint derangement. This is based on the observation that many patients with MPDS symptoms eventually develop internal derangements. Spasm of the internal pterygoid muscle has been speculated to actually pull the meniscus anteriorly and eventually cause elongation of the stabilizing posterior capsular ligament. However, many other patients do not progress from MPDS to internal derangement. This suggests that a cause and effect relationship of the two conditions is less than direct and that other factors contribute significantly.

Many patients with objective evidence of TMJ internal derangement may not be aware of the condition or may complain of mild pain in either or both joints. Not surprisingly, many of the previously listed features of MPDS are also associated with internal joint derangement, and the conditions are often concurrent to some degree. The distinguishing clinical features of internal derangement are "popping" or "clicking" during jaw opening or limited opening and tenderness to palpation of the joint. This is in contrast to the predominant tenderness affecting the the muscles of mastication with MPDS. The abnormal relationship of the articular disk or meniscus to the bony articulator surfaces of the condyle and the glenoid fossa can take four forms: anterior disk displacement with reduction, anterior disk displacement without reduction, disk perforation, or posterior disk displacement.

Anterior disk displacement with reduction. Distortion or stretching of the posterior ligament allows anterior displacement of the meniscus relative to the head of the condyle, which reduces to normal position during opening. This is collectively referred to as anterior disk displacement with reduction and is

the most common form of internal derangement affecting the TMJ.

A "pop" or "click" can be heard or felt during jaw opening as the condylar head shifts forward into the concavity of the meniscus. Auscultation of subtle joint sounds usually requires the aid of a stethoscope. Reduction usually occurs early in translation of the condyle on opening, although the pop may occur later in translation or during excursive movements. Deviation of the mandible toward the affected side on opening and closing is usually observed and suggests an unconscious adaption mechanism to minimize discomfort and facilitate "recapture" of the anteriorly displaced disk. The pattern of this deviation can become quite complex if both joints are affected. No evidence of limitation of opening is present unless caused by episodes of superimposed muscle spasm. Many patients with this condition do not complain of pain but are aware of the popping or clicking.

Anterior disk displacement without reduction. The same anterior disk displacement is present as described above, except that the meniscus does not reduce to normal position during opening. This implies greater degeneration of the soft tissues as compared with reducing anterior displacement, and it is more likely to be related to traumatic injury. Most patients can describe joint sounds when they were younger, which suggests that the trauma of recurring reduction has promoted soft tissue distortion and scarring until reduction is no longer possible. Limited opening is observed rather than a pop or click because the meniscus blocks complete translation. Deviation of the mandible toward the affected side is observed if the condition is unilateral. Bilateral involvement leads to limited opening with less dramatic deviation. This condition is more likely to result in episodic joint pain than anterior displacement with reduction, although some patients deny any discomfort.

Disk perforation. Chronic functional injury to the articular soft tissues related to anterior disk displacement can eventually cause perforation of the soft tissues. The phrase "disk perforation" is actually a misnomer in many cases because the perforation actually occurs in the posterior ligament rather than the disk, although the meniscus is also irreversibly damaged. The distinguishing clinical feature is the crepitus of bone grinding on bone during jaw movements, which requires a stethoscope to identify in most cases. Patients nearly always complain of joint pain and soreness, although the severity varies, and preauricular tenderness to palpation is a consistent feature. Radiographic evidence of osteoarthritis as described in Chapter 19 is generally present.

Posterior disk displacement. Posterior displacement of the meniscus with or without reduction is unusual clinically and is more likely to result from a traumatic injury than from chronic functional stress. Clinical observations are variable depending on the injury, but they may include an acquired Angle class III occlusal relationship, joint pain, popping on forced retrusion, crepitus from perforation of the anterior ligament, and muscle pain.

Osteoarthritis of the Temporomandibular Joint

Osteoarthritis is chronic degenerative alteration of the bone components of the joint secondary to minor injury and functional stress. This is usually a consequence of anterior meniscus displacement, although internal derangement is not the only cause. The essential diagnostic feature of osteoarthritis is radiographic evidence of altered bone morphology involving the head of the mandibular condyle and glenoid fossa. Typical features include flattening of the anterior aspect of the condylar head, osteophyte formation near the anterior aspect of the condylar head, and cortical abnormalities of the functional surfaces as described in Chapter 19. Panoramic radiographs may reveal pronounced osteoarthritic defects, but demonstration of more subtle features early in the disease course requires specialized techniques.

Many patients describe mild pain and tenderness to preauricular palpation, although others report no significant discomfort. This reflects the varying severity of pain produced by osteoarthritis, as well as its acceptance by many as "part of growing old," comparable to similar symptoms affecting other joints. These findings are unusual prior to the age of 30. Earlier onset suggests that the progress of osteoarthritis has been promoted by traumatic injury or that the condition is actually rheumatoid arthritis. Treatment relies on aspirin and nonsteroidal antiinflammatory drugs.

Rheumatoid Arthritis of the Temporomandibular Joint

Rheumatoid arthritis causes more severe bone degeneration and is observed at an earlier age than osteoarthritis. The pathogenesis of rheumatoid arthritis involves an abnormal immunologic response similar to other collagen or connective tissue diseases as discussed in Chapter 7. Multiple joints in a symmetric distribution are affected by pain, enlargement, and degenerative changes. Frequent concurrence of rheumatoid arthritis with other immune-mediated manifestations such as xerostomia is a significant diagnostic consideration. Degenerative joint disease and demonstration of serum immunoglobulins collectively known as *rheumatoid factor* provide the definitive diagnosis in most cases.

The clinical and radiographic features of rheumatoid deterioration of the TMJ among adults are essentially the same as osteoarthritis except that the severity is greater and the onset is earlier. Clinical findings that assist in differentiating osteoarthritis and rheumatoid arthritis among adults involve the hands as illustrated in Chapter 7. The aggressive juvenile form of rheumatoid arthritis known as *Still's disease* causes crippling joint degeneration of the extremities. Severe TMJ deterioration can result in limited opening, micrognathia, and ankylosis. Treatment in most cases consists of antiinflammatory medications, and medical referral is appropriate considering the diverse manifestations and implications of the disease.

Sialadenitis

Sialadenitis is a nonspecific term for salivary gland inflammation. Common causative conditions include mumps, sialolithiasis, and retrograde bacterial infections. All are associated with dull pain or tenderness to palpation that is localized within the substance of the affected major salivary glands.

Mumps. Mumps or *epidemic parotitis* is an infection caused by the paramyxovirus that usually affects children. Diagnostic features include acute onset of unilateral or bilateral parotid enlargement that is associated with malaise, fever, sore throat, and chills. The epidemic occurrence of the infection aids in the diagnosis. Parotid swelling progresses to maximum extent within 1 to 3 days and gradually resolves within approximately 1 week. Treatment is palliative in the absence of the rare complications such as pancreatitis and central nervous system involvement. Testicular inflammation (orchitis) affects approximately one third of infected postpubescent males.

Retrograde bacterial infection. Decreased saliva production increases the possibility of bacterial colonization and inflammation within the excretory duct, which is known as *sialodochitis*; and eventually a bacterial sialadenitis occurs. This is usually related to a dramatic decrease in salivary flow as occurs with radiotherapy, advanced Sjögren's disease, acute sialolithiasis, and some medications. Positive pressure in the oral cavity for extended periods can also force bacteria into Stensen's duct. This may develop following inhalation anesthesia and is referred to as *surgical mumps*.

The distinguishing clinical features of sialadenitis in addition to xerostomia are the acute onset or a recurring pattern of pain accompanied by purulent outflow while massaging the affected gland. Antibiotic treatment of the acute infection is generally effective. Salivary stimulants may decrease the probability of recurrence.

Sialolithiasis. Blockage of the excretory ducts by sialoliths or mucus plugs and the resulting intraglandular accumulation of saliva is a relatively common cause of episodic sialadenitis. The unilateral pressure, pain, and enlargement follows salivary stimulation and the submandibular gland is affected more often than the parotid. Suspected sialoliths can usually be demonstrated radiographically as discussed in Chapter 19. Demonstration of blockage by radiolucent mucus plugs requires *sialography,* which is the radiographic exposure of the gland and duct following injection of a contrast medium.

Asymptomatic sialoliths are occasionally identified during routine radiographic examinations. The absence of obstruction in these cases is explained by gradual dilation of the duct that allows passage of saliva as the sialolith enlarges. Obstruction may develop if the stone shifts and lodges in a narrower ductal segment. Bacterial infection secondary to saliva obstruction is indicated by purulent discharge during compression of the painful gland.

Definitive treatment usually requires surgical removal, which is complicated in some cases by scarring of the duct. Mild, episodic discomfort can be relieved by massage and analgesics in most instances, which is preferred by most patients as an alternative to surgery. Occasionally, dilation of the duct with successively larger lacrimal probes or injection of a lubricating, lipid-soluble contrast medium during sialography promotes passage of distal sialoliths.

Eagle's Syndrome

Ossification of the stylohyoid ligament is a common idiopathic process, which progresses gradually and is more pronounced among older patients. The ossification is usually revealed by panoramic radiographs of asymptomatic patients. Eagle's syndrome is the combination of radiographic evidence of stylohyoid ligament ossification and pain. The pain is caused by the resistance of the rigid, ossified ligament to the mobility of surrounding soft tissues. This is usually associated with a history of tonsillectomy, which has produced scarring and entrapment of the ligament. Symptoms develop years after the surgery as the ossification progressively increases the rigidity of the structure.

The complaints related to Eagle's syndrome include sharpness in the throat during swallowing or a chronic sore throat without erythema. The sensation may be described as that of a fish bone caught in the throat or as obstruction. Throat pain during extreme head movements or a burning sensation of the tongue secondary to rubbing of the lingual nerve are less common symptoms. In rare instances unilateral headaches or a burning sensation results from the rubbing of the ossified stylohyoid ligament on the sympathetic fibers of the carotid sheath. Definitive treatment is surgical removal.

Pharyngitis

Various forms of pharyngitis and their diagnoses are discussed in Chapter 16. All can produce the familiar discomfort that explains the colloquial term *sore throat.* Acute onset with variably severe fever and malaise is typical. Mucosal erythema in the tonsillar pillar region is adequate clinical evidence of the inflammatory nature of the condition in most cases. Medical referral for throat culture, definitive diagnosis, and treatment is appropriate.

Sinusitis

Inflammation of the nasal sinuses is a common source of pain. The symptoms of chronic sinusitis include bilateral tenderness, pressure, congestion, and nasal drainage. The typical cyclic pattern of symptomatic periods corresponding to seasonal pollen release or exposure to specific materials suggests allergic hypersensitivity in most cases. Despite the misnomer "sinus headache," the localization of pain corresponds to the nasal sinuses and the familiarity of the symptoms to the patient leaves little doubt about the diagnosis. Treatment includes nasal decongestants and suppression of the allergic response with medications such as corticosteroids.

Acute sinusitis is characterized by abrupt onset of unilateral pressure, pain, and focal tenderness near the affected sinus. Purulence indicates the bacterial nature of the infection and drainage usually provides relief. A common finding is that a postural change such as leaning forward increases or relieves the pain. Pharyngitis, otitis, and cervical lymphadenopathy are often associated features. Radiographic evidence of sinusitis and the possibility of dental infections as the origin of maxillary sinus inflammation are discussed in Chapter 19. Medical referral is indicated and treatment relies on nasal decongestants and antibiotic therapy.

Referred Pain of the Mandible

Diffuse, radiating pain of the lower jaw is occasionally caused by conditions such as angina pectoris, myocardial infarction, and thyroiditis. These conditions are usually suspected on the basis of additional clinical manifestations as described in Chapter 7. The dentist should be suspicious of diffuse mandibular pain without an apparent dental cause, particularly if additional features are associated with the discomfort. Medical referral is indicated.

SOMATIC PAIN: PAIN OF PULPAL ORIGIN

Toothache or *odontalgia* results in most instances from inflammatory stimulation of the neural fibers of either the dental pulp or the supportive alveolar tissues. Pulpitis exists to some degree in nearly all cases of pain originating within the tooth. The most reliable single feature to distinguish whether pain is of pulpal or alveolar origin is that with alveolar pain, percussion of the tooth increases severity, whereas with pulpal pain this is usually not the case. Although inflammation may affect both the pulp and alveolus, additional features such as radiographic findings generally suggest which is the primary source of inflammation.

Pulpitis

Pulpitis and its occasional progression to pulpal necrosis were discussed in Chapter 8. Blunt trauma, restorative trauma, dentin exposure, and thermal conduction by large metallic restorations are among the causes of pulpitis in addition to extensive carious lesions. Traumatic occlusion rarely causes significant pulpitis unless the tooth demonstrates conspicuous mobility. Traumatic occlusion can, however, aggravate or worsen the severity of pulpitis caused by other conditions. Pulpitis is classified as *reversible* if elimination of the source of inflammation is expected to promote resolution without pulpal necrosis. *Irreversible pulpitis* is pulpal inflammation that will progress to pulpal necrosis regardless of treatment. The distinction between reversible and irreversible pulpitis is often difficult but optimal treatment relies on this decision.

Reversible pulpitis is not spontaneously uncomfortable, but external stimulation of the tooth such as by temperature extremes evokes a mild "tingling" sensation that abruptly stops after removal of the stimulus. Pulpitis can be expected to progress in severity until the source of inflammation is eliminated. More severe discomfort indicates a greater probability of irreversible pulpitis and eventual pulpal necrosis. Spontaneous pulpal pain, sensitivity to percussion, and persistence of pain after the removal of external stimulation are reliable indications of irreversible pulpitis in most cases. Radiographs reveal normal periapical appearance, although findings suggesting the source of inflammation such as a deep cavity or advanced periodontal bone loss are usually present. The combination of symptoms and signs may not be adequate for a definitive diagnosis of whether the pulpitis is reversible or irreversible in some cases.

Reversible pulpitis is treated by removal of the source of inflammation with the hope that progression to necrosis can be averted. Placement of a sedative zinc oxide and eugenol temporary restoration after removal of axially extensive decay is a common example. Palliation with analgesics may be beneficial in cases of more severe discomfort. Irreversible pulpitis requires either endodontic treatment or extraction. If the diagnosis is in doubt, then the condition is managed conservatively as reversible pulpitis with reevaluation at a future date. Definitive evidence of pulpal necrosis following irreversible pulpitis may not become evident for years following conservative treatment.

Exposed Dentin

Attrition, abrasion, erosion, gingival recession, and tooth fractures can expose dentin to the oral environment. Sensitivity of the exposed surfaces results from direct stimulation of dentinal tubules and their cellular processes by chemical and physical insults such as bacterial plaque, abrasion by an explorer tip, and temperature extremes. The painful sensation stops immediately after removal of the stimulation. Gradually exposed dentin is usually not sensitive because concurrent dentinal tubule sclerosis provides pulpal insulation. Comparison of the minimal root sensitivity in cases of chronic gingival recession and the dramatic discomfort experienced by many patients following periodontal surgery illustrates this effect. Also, less secondary dentin formation and larger pulp size explains why younger patients with exposed dentin are more likely to experience discomfort than older individuals.

Significant pulpitis is unusual unless the insult is severe or abrupt as is the case with tooth fractures. Therefore pulp testing using percussion, heat, cold, and electricity on the enamel surfaces elicits essentially a normal response. The only radiographic finding is the loss of enamel or crestal bone height. Promotion of dentinal tubule sclerosis is the basis of treatment by root desensitization procedures and dentifrices.

Carious Lesions

Large carious lesions also cause tooth sensitivity and mild pulpitis by exposure of dentin. The irritation is increased, however, by the constant exposure of dentinal tubules to the acidic materials within the lesion. Pulpal stimulation and pain does not occur with decay limited to enamel, and it is minimal with most carious lesions limited to superficial dentin. Lesions that extend axially more than one half of the dentin thickness are likely to produce mild pulpitis as indicated by sensitivity to external stimulation. The pain abruptly ceases after the removal of the stimulation without spontaneous pain or sensitivity to percussion. A commonly reported symptom associated with deep decay and "leaky" restorations is abrupt, dull discomfort following exposure to high concentrations of sugar. Radiographs usually demonstrate the cavity or a deep restoration and no indication of periapical radiolucency.

Pulpitis Following Dental Treatment

Pulpitis after dental treatment is an understandable inflammatory response considering the physical trauma of many dental procedures. This is generally a reversible pulpitis as indicated by vague "soreness" and hypersensitivity responses to external stimulation such as thermal extremes. This can be pronounced if metallic restorations are involved. Analgesics and reassurance are usually adequate management until the reversible pulpitis resolves. The dentist's diagnostic responsibility in this situation is to identify irreversible pulpitis caused by the dental procedure, which can be challenging. Irreversible pulpitis should be suspected in cases of unusually severe, persistent, or spontaneous pain. Attention should also be directed to the possibility of contributing factors such as traumatic occlusion and soft tissue injury related to the procedure. Occlusal adjustment is often beneficial because normally tolerated interferences tend to amplify the pulpitis.

Vertical Tooth Fracture

Teeth that are weakened by large restorations or endodontic treatment become vulnerable to vertical fractures with or without displacement of the fragments. Nonrestored teeth also fracture but this is much less common. Often a crack can be identified in the enamel near an undermined cusp or crossing a marginal ridge. This should not be confused with commonly observed *crazing lines* in the enamel of asymptomatic teeth of older patients. Crazing lines are cracks limited to enamel that are nonpainful to external stimulation and are analogous to cracks in a car windshield that remain "sealed."

The vertical fracture may be limited to enamel and dentin or it may involve the pulp and extend apical to the crest of the alveolar bone. The patient reports sharp, stabbing pain of abrupt onset during chewing or "biting just right." Otherwise, additional symptoms of fractures limited to enamel and dentin may suggest mild pulpitis or exposure of dentin. Fractures that involve the pulp produce spontaneous or constant pain that increases dramatically with external stimulation of the tooth.

A reliable diagnostic sign of a subtle vertical fracture without displacement is sensitivity to percussion of a single cusp. Pressure on the other cusps of the tooth produces no pain. This procedure essentially stresses the crack and causes pain by movement of the smaller fragment. At times the same effect can be noted with wedging pressure of an explorer tine at the crack. Radiographs seldom demonstrate vertical fractures. Prognosis generally depends on the apical extent of the fracture because cracks that extend apical to the crestal bone can present restorative complications.

SOMATIC PAIN: PAIN ORIGINATING FROM THE DENTAL SUPPORTIVE TISSUES AND ORAL MUCOSA

Pain associated with inflammation of the dental supportive tissues is caused in most cases by acute exacerbation of chronic alveolar inflammation. This is usually related to periapical lesions secondary to pulpal necrosis or the manifestations of periodontitis. The diagnosis of alveolar inflammation may be complicated by the manifestations of an associated pulpitis. Sensitivity to percussion is a reliable indication that the source of the pain is around the tooth and not within the tooth. Additional conditions that cause alveolar and mucosal pain include eruption, tooth mobility, and oral mucosal ulcers.

Acute Bacterial Infections of the Alveolus

The pathogenesis, clinical course, and treatment of alveolar inflammation secondary to pulpal necrosis, periodontitis, and pericoronitis are described in Chapter 8. A definitive diagnosis of these typically chronic and nonpainful lesions can be based in most cases on clinical and radiographic findings. Pain related to these chronic conditions nearly always represents a superimposed acute bacterial infection, which is indicated by edematous swelling, erythema, and purulence. Localized discomfort progresses in extent and severity until spontaneous drainage or treatment leads to resolution.

Periapical inflammation secondary to pulpal necrosis. The pain of acute abscesses secondary to pulpal necrosis is spontaneous and continuous with tenderness to pressure and percussion of the tooth. Examination may reveal purulent drainage via a pathologic sinus tract. Single canal teeth are usually unresponsive to thermal or electrical stimulation, although in some cases cold may provide some relief or heat can dramatically increase pain. Teeth with multiple canals may demonstrate different stages of the pulpal degeneration in each canal, so a sensitivity response of one canal to pulp testing stimulation can falsely suggest vitality of the tooth. An asymptomatic or latent period of many years between the time

of pulpal necroses and the onset of pain related to periapical inflammation is common.

Periodontal abscess. The periodontal abscess generally develops from accumulation of exudate or impaction of food within a prominent periodontal defect. The pain is usually poorly localized and dull compared with the focal discomfort produced by periapical inflammation. Mobility, a pathologic sinus, and generalized evidence of periodontitis are often present and radiographs may reveal infrabony defects in the affected area.

Pericoronitis. Pericoronitis produces rapid onset of pain associated with a partially erupted tooth. A chronic course of recurring acute infections is typical. Pericoronitis associated with mandibular third molars often causes trismus by extension of the infection into the adjacent soft tissues.

Dissemination of acute alveolar infections. The dissemination of a localized alveolar infection is suggested by diffuse swelling and spontaneous pain, as well as by systemic manifestations such as fever, malaise, and regional lymphadenopathy. Spread of the infection within bone is osteomyelitis, as discussed in Chapter 19. Cellulitis is progression of the infections into adjacent soft tissue spaces, and it is described in Chapter 18.

Acute Necrotizing Ulcerative Gingivitis

Acute necrotizing ulcerative gingivitis *(ANUG)*, also known as *trench mouth*, is an acute, superficial infection of the gingiva by fusiform and spirochete bacteria. This is generally an opportunistic infection associated with diminished host resistance from malnutrition or immunosuppression. Pain is spontaneous, generalized, and of rapid onset. A "punched out" appearance of the interdental papillae and the fetid odor are the characteristic features related to the gingival necrosis caused by ANUG. Additional physical findings include dramatic gingival erythema, pseudomembranous ulceration, fever, malaise, and regional lymphadenopathy. Treatment includes antibiotics, improved hygiene, antibacterial rinses, gross scaling, and debridement of necrotic tissue.

Occlusal Trauma

Traumatic occlusal relationships are characterized by excessive nonaxial forces during functional and parafunctional contact of the teeth. Pain is related to abnormal stretching of the periodontal ligament, which is indicated by tooth mobility. Pulpitis may also develop with severe examples but the pulpal symptoms are generally mild in comparison with the periodontal discomfort. Traumatic occlusion alone rarely causes irreversible pulpitis. Other factors are nearly always the principle cause of the pulpal inflammation when irreversible pulpitis or pulpal necrosis is associated with occlusal trauma. This is illustrated by the common occurrence of pain after placement of a large restoration with occlusal interferences. The irreversible pulpitis that may develop in this situation results from the deep decay and the traumatic operative procedure, whereas occlusal trauma plays only a contributory role.

Radiographic indications of periodontal ligament space widening and lamina dura changes (Fig. 8-37) may be associated with mobility. Chronic occlusal trauma also produces wear facets on functional tooth surfaces. A reliable sign of occlusal trauma is the sensation of fremitus or vibration that can be sensed by placing a finger on the facial surface of the tooth and asking the patient to grind. The tenderness resulting from traumatic occlusion can alter mastication, which can initiate or aggravate symptoms of myofascial pain dysfunction syndrome.

Traumatic Injury of Teeth

The severity of blunt trauma determines the degree of the tissue injury and the associated pain. Most diagnostic issues in this context relate to radiographic evaluation for fractures, displacement of teeth, and clinical evaluation of soft tissue damage because the history clearly reveals the cause. Appropriate treatment includes palliative control of pain, stabilization of mobile teeth, closure of soft tissue injuries, and reduction and stabilization of fractures.

Tooth Eruption

"Teething" pain in infants usually generates more distress for the parents than the infant. The typical symptoms are excessive salivation, irritability, tenderness at the eruption sites, alteration of sleep patterns, and mild fever. Patience, reassurance, and acetaminophen are adequate management. Soreness of erupting teeth in older children is usually mild, localized, and of short duration. The principle diagnostic issue is the identification of pericoronitis as indicated by purulence and more severe discomfort.

Orthodontic Treatment

"Orthodontalgia" is the generalized soreness that follows the periodic alteration of the archwire during active orthodontic treatment. Tenderness and sensitivity of the teeth is most dramatic within 2 to 3 days of the appointment with gradual improvement until the next adjustment. Most patients adapt to this cycle during the course of the treatment. However, patients may contact the general dentist concerning unusual soreness following an error in archwire contour or placement. Exceptional tenderness to percussion of one or more teeth results from excessive stretching of the periodontal ligament. The orthodontist should be consulted if this develops.

Acute Maxillary Sinusitis

Acute maxillary sinusitis produces clinical signs and symptoms as previously described for acute sinusitis in general. The diagnostic challenge of acute maxillary sinusitis for the dentist is related to the close proximity of the maxillary posterior teeth. Acute maxillary sinusitis can cause odontalgia and tenderness to percussion of the posterior maxillary teeth. Periapical inflammatory lesions of these teeth can also be the proximal cause of acute maxillary sinusitis. Periapical radiographs provide the most reliable evidence of a primary dental infection by demonstrating the presence of radiolucent dental inflammatory lesions. Decongestant and antibiotic therapy is effective treatment of acute sinusitis. The dental treatment issue is whether or not endodontic treatment of one or more of the teeth in the region is necessary. Pulp vitality tests are often contributory if the radiographic findings are equivocal.

Pain of the Oral Mucosa

Pain of the oral mucosa typically results from cheek biting habits, functional injury, or irritation by materials such as spicy foods, hot beverages, caustic chemicals, tobacco, alcohol, and medications. Incidental injury during dental treatment, maladapted removable devices, and faulty restorations are forms of iatrogenic mucosal injury. In addition, numerous diseases that can cause painful oral ulceration are discussed in Chapter 17.

Mucosal pain is attributable in most cases to compromised integrity of the tissue by ulceration, epithelial thinning, or superficial infection. The discomfort is often described as burning soreness that is constant immediately after injury and improves within several days. Irritants can cause dramatic increase in severity. The relationship of local pain to a focal ulcer leaves little doubt about the diagnosis. If multiple ulcers are present or the discomfort does not improve rapidly, the conditions discussed in Chapter 17 should be considered. If chronic, burning mucosal pain is described but no definite lesions are present, neurogenous pain such as atypical neuralgia or burning mouth syndrome are possible explanations. Treatment is palliative during initial healing of focal mucosal abrasions. Topical anesthetic gels provide relief for exceptionally sensitive individuals.

NEUROGENOUS PAIN

Neurogenous pain is discomfort resulting from an abnormality of the peripheral nerve rather than the tissues innervated. *Neuropathy* is defined as any functional abnormality of nerves, and sensory neuropathy is generally either neuritis or neuralgia. *Neuritis* is inflammation of the nerve trunk that is perceived as a burning sensation in most instances. *Neuralgia* refers to paroxysmal pain along the distribution of a nerve that is caused by conditions such as vascular spasm and central nervous system disease.

Dentists manage somatic pain so routinely that a clinical bias develops that all oral and facial pain originates from inflammatory somatic lesions. The typically chronic and poorly localized nature of neurogenous pain often confuses the clinician's diagnosis because of the inconsistency with the typical acute onset and distinct localization of somatic pain. Also, patients with neurogenous pain seldom consult the dentist and such problems are not common, which limits the opportunities to develop experience with these conditions. Nevertheless, an appreciation of the features of neurogenous pain helps to avoid confusing it with pain of somatic origin. Management in most cases is palliative and requires consultation with a neurologist.

Burning Mouth Syndrome

The most common neurogenous oral pain is burning mouth syndrome, which has also been referred to as *burning tongue, glossodynia,* and *orolingual paresthesia.* This elusive neuropathy produces a diffuse burning sensation that usually involves the tongue or in some cases the lips or gingiva. The mucosal surfaces appear normal and intact in the areas of discomfort, although in some instances the mucosa may appear mildly atrophic. The pain tends to become more severe during the day and some patients report that eating or drinking provides some relief. This suggests that xerostomia may be a factor. Postmenopausal females are most often affected and psychogenic influences as well as hormonal fluctuations are believed to be contributory. Treatment is palliative and elimination of discomfort is unusual.

Trigeminal Neuralgia

The recurring pain of trigeminal neuralgia, which is also known as *tic douloureux, facial neuralgia,* and *Fothergill's neuralgia,* reaches maximum intensity abruptly after stimulation of a "trigger zone" in the region innervated by the affected nerve. The cause is related to compression of the gasserian ganglion resulting from enlargement or spasm of associated vascular structures. A single branch of the trigeminal nerve is usually involved and the site of pain is consistently the same, although pain may affect more than one branch and in some cases spontaneous pain occurs. The mandibular division is most frequently affected, while ophthalmic involvement is least common.

The unilateral pain is described as lacerating or like an electrical shock and the patient may be aware of an aura or premonition of the occurrence. Episodes may be separated by intervals of a few minutes or years. The patient is usually between 40 and 60 years of age and is aware of the diagnosis in most cases. Treatment by alcohol injections and sectioning of the nerve trunk seldom provides permanent relief because of the frustratingly persistent regeneration of the nerve fibers. More success has been observed with surgical gasserian decompression and administration of tricyclic antidepressants. The characteristic symptoms of trigeminal neuralgia allow a definitive diagnosis in nearly all instances.

Glossopharyngeal Neuralgia

This rare condition affects the distribution of the glossopharyngeal nerve with virtually the same manifestations as trigeminal neuralgia. The diagnosis is based on the triggering phenomenon and unilateral pain affecting the tonsillar fossa, base of the tongue, oropharynx, or middle ear.

Causalgia

Causalgia is the discomfort that occurs after traumatic damage to a peripheral nerve trunk; it is a common complication following limb amputation. Oral and facial occurrence is unusual. The onset of pain may be immediate or delayed for several weeks after surgery or traumatic injury. The diffuse pain is usually constant and is described as a burning or stinging sensation that is aggravated by stimulation. Palliative treatment may provide some relief.

Viral Neuralgia

Viral neuralgia is characterized by paroxysmal burning or aching following herpes zoster infection and recurrent herpes simplex outbreaks. This is understandable considering the neurotropic nature of the viruses that produce these lesions. The severity of viral neuralgia following the clearing of herpes zoster eruptions varies dramatically among patients but is generally most uncomfortable among elderly patients. The pain is described as a persistent burning sensation in the same region as the preceding viral eruptions. The oral cavity is an unusual site for herpes zoster lesions and viral neuralgia. Trigeminal involvement most commonly affects the ophthalmic branch. Herpes simplex neuralgia is much less common and less severe than neuralgia following herpes zoster. Viral neuralgia and atypical neuralgia are occasionally considered in the diagnosis of mucosal pain after more common somatic causes have been excluded as possibilities and treatment is palliative.

Atypical Neuralgia

Atypical or idiopathic neuralgia is distinguished clinically from more "typical" neuralgias by (1) the absence of trigger zone initiation of the pain and (2) the affected region varies from one episode to another. The pain manifestations are usually deeper, less "sharp," more gradual in onset, and less characteristic in comparison to typical neuralgias. The patient is usually younger than typical neuralgia sufferers. The cause is thought to be vascular spasm, and many clinicians believe emotional factors contribute significantly to atypical neuralgia. Palliative treatment with tricyclic antidepressants or ergotamine to stabilize vascular spasm may be effective.

PSYCHOGENIC PAIN

Psychological factors influence to some degree the subjective experience of all painful conditions. The normal patient's perception of somatic pain that is particularly severe or is of long duration tends to be clouded or exaggerated by the emotional distress it has caused. Important diagnostic features such as the time of onset or precise location become secondary issues to the patient in comparison to the urgent need for relief. Dentists frequently hear phrases such as "they all hurt" or "I want them all out," which contribute little to the diagnosis other than demonstrating the patient's distress.

The mouth serves as a central focus of personal appearance and pleasurable functions such as eating, speech, and sexual expression. Perceived or actual disturbances in these functions in the susceptible individual can result in psychological conversions that are perceived as painful. This does not imply that the patient isn't suffering. Although some of these patients are affected by psychiatric illness, dismissing their psychogenic pain by labeling them as emotionally unstable is counterproductive.

The diagnosis of psychogenic pain is generally by exclusion of somatic and neurogenous pain. Predominance of psychogenic discomfort is suggested by chronic duration, poor localization, and absence of a somatic cause. These manifestations are similar to those of neurogenous pain except that neural characteristics such as trigger zone initiation, preceding viral lesions, recent injury, and pain limited to the distribution of a peripheral nerve are not observed. In addition, the pattern of occurrence, location, severity, and effect of secondary stimuli are unpredictable and inconsistent. In some cases a somatic condition may be present but the pain described by the patient is disproportionate to the discomfort normally associated with the cause.

A history of emotional problems, current treatment with psychiatric drugs, and other indications of mental illness may be associated with psychogenic pain. However, such findings are certainly not essential to the diagnosis. Many patients with psychogenic pain appear well adjusted on the basis of conversation and social behavior. The vulnerability of a patient to atypical pain perception may be revealed by references to cultish health practices or exceptionally stressful situations such as divorce.

Treatment of psychogenic pain by either palliative or definitive procedures such as unwarranted endodontic treatment is generally ineffective. Occasionally, dental treatment may relieve psychogenic pain if the actual problem can be identified. For example, the patient's perceived pain may actually reflect dissatisfaction with the appearance of the teeth. The discomfort often resolves in such cases following treatment that improves the appearance of the painful teeth. Unfortunately, the basis of the psychogenic pain is not nearly this direct in most cases. Referral for diagnosis and management of psychogenic pain may be necessary after somatic and neurogenous forms of pain have been excluded.

SUMMARY

The diagnosis and management of pain is a central aspect of dental practice. Pain can be categorized by origin as somatic, neurogenous, or psychogenic. The clinical evaluation of pain relies on assessment of its onset, duration, location, descriptive characteristics, the pattern of painful episodes, and agents that alter the sensation. Treatment of pain can be approached by whether the therapeutic goal is curative, palliative, or symptomatic relief. Effective treatment of pain eliminates the patient's suffering and provides confirmation of the original diagnosis.

Most head and neck pain is somatic in origin. The location of somatic pain provides the most reliable indication of probable cause, which determines the diagnostic procedures necessary to identify the specific condition. Secondary features such as the pattern of occurrence and physical findings influence additional diagnostic decisions. Somatic pain related to the teeth is usually inflammatory and can be diagnosed on the basis of radiographic and clinical findings. Neurogenous pain is suggest by chronic duration, distribution corresponding to that of a peripheral nerve, a burning sensation, and the absence of a somatic cause. Occurrence following stimulation of a specific triggering zone, recent viral infection, traumatic nerve injury, or inflammatory lesions affecting the painful nerve are features that may indicate the specific neuropathy. Psychogenic pain should be suspected if no evidence of a somatic disease process can be identified and the pattern of pain is inconsistent with typical patterns of neurogenous pain. Psychogenic pain is often poorly localized, occurs in unpredictable patterns, has an inconsistent response to secondary stimulation, and is not relieved by normally effective treatment.

The treatment of most somatic oral pain, some extraoral somatic conditions, and some neurogenous oral problems can be accomplished by the dentist. The treatment approach should be curative if that is feasible. Palliative treatment is appropriate to provide relief early in the course of curative procedures and if the condition is incurable. Medical referral for definitive diagnosis and treatment is indicated for many somatic conditions such as cephalalgia, many forms of neurogenous pain, and most psychogenic discomfort. Somatic pain of dental origin should be excluded if possible before referral.

BIBLIOGRAPHY

Bell WB: Orofacial pains, ed 4, St Louis, 1989, Mosby−Year Book.

Langlais RP and others: Oral diagnosis, oral medicine and treatment planning, Philadelphia, 1984, Saunders.

Lynch MA, Brightman VJ, Greenberg MS, editors: Burket's oral medicine: diagnosis and treatment, ed 8, Philadelphia, 1984, Lippincott.

Shafer WG, Hine MK, Levy BM: A textbook of oral pathology, ed 4, Philadelphia, 1983, Saunders.

CHAPTER 10

Referrals and Consultations

GARY C. COLEMAN

Professional interactions with physicians, dental specialists, general dentists, and other professionals are an important part of daily dental practice. Severely compromised medical status, complex treatment regimens for a diagnosed condition, or the suspicion of an undiagnosed illness are among situations in which the dentist may seek the advice of the patient's physician. The general dentist also commonly requests the participation of other general dentists and dental specialists during the course of the patient's dental care.

Effective patient referrals and consultations are fostered by clear communication, professional courtesy, common sense, and a genuine concern for the patient's welfare. The patient and other practitioners form a favorable opinion of the dentist's clinical judgment when potential problems are solved by the coordinated participation of several professionals. However, failure to follow the "unspoken rules" that govern the conduct of referrals and consultations can adversely affect the process and leave a negative impression.

A *consultation* is the communication be-tween two professionals regarding the status of a patient and treatment options for any problems. This implies that the consultant does not take an active part in the actual treatment but serves in an advisory capacity to the primary care provider. A *referral* is contact between two professionals in which the primary care provider requests the active participation of another professional in some portion of the patient's treatment. These terms may be used interchangeably in cases in which the active treatment participation by the consultant depends on the opinion formulated during the initial consultation. Most contacts with physicians initiated by the general dentist represent consultations, while the general dentist refers patients to dental specialists for all or part of their dental care.

MECHANISMS OF PROFESSIONAL COMMUNICATION

Contacts with other professionals can be accomplished by referral letters, telephone conversations, communications using the patient record in an institution, and informal discussions. Each of these methods offers distinct advantages and entails certain disadvantages compared with the others. The common goal is the clear, concise exchange of information to promote the optimal health care of the patient.

Referral and Consultation Letters

The effectiveness of most consultations and referrals is enhanced when a letter from the referring dentist clarifies the specific details of the clinical situation. The referral letter and the consultant's written response provide a record of the communication, which can be included in the patient's chart as permanent documentation. The time required to exchange information is the primary disadvantage of written professional communications.

The essential information of the referral letter includes the patient identification, a summary of the referring clinician's evaluation, reference to any materials enclosed with the consult letter, the expectation of the consultation, and identification of the referring clinician. The example referral letter shown in the box on the opposite page illustrates the arrangement and concise discussion of this information.

Patient identification. Simply stating the patient's name is inadequate, especially if the referral is directed to an institution. Common names can cause confusion. Demographic data such as gender, age, and race not only provide more specific identification of the patient but also appropriately introduce the patient summary. Including the patient's social security number or address often avoids misidentification of patients with exceptionally common names or when contacting large institutions.

Patient summary. The patient's chief complaint, significant historical data, contributory observations of the physical examination, and the working diagnosis of the problem are briefly summarized. Clarification of other relevant information such as additional pending consultations may also be appropriate.

Reference to enclosed diagnostic materials. Any material such as radiographs, laboratory test results, or communications from another clinician that are enclosed are specifically referred to in the consult letter to avoid confusion. The consultant should be informed if the return of the enclosures is expected or if the materials are intended for the consultant's records.

Consult expectations. The referring clinician must explain what is expected from the consultant even if the problem and the appropriate course seem apparent. Misunderstandings are avoided when the referring dentist clearly states whether the consultant is expected to treat the condition or if only an opinion is expected. The consultant needs to know if the patient should make another appointment with the referring office following the consult or if the consultant's treatment of the problem is the only care required. Consults that request an opinion concerning the need for infective endocarditis prophylaxis, for example, should clarify whether the consultant is expected to write the antibiotic prescription or if that will be arranged by the referring clinician.

Identification of the referring clinician. The office stationery usually identifies the referring clinician, but this may not be evident when the referral is from a group practice or an institution. Also, clarification of referring clinician's practice as a general dentist or a dental specialist avoids confusion, particularly when consulting physicians.

Telephone Consultations and Referrals

Professional communications by telephone offer the advantages of immediacy in urgent situations and convenience in discussing uncomplicated problems. The disadvantage of using the telephone is that no written record of the consultation exists, which can cause essential information to be misunderstood or forgotten. Also, no documentation of consultation

October 1, 1991

Cedric Wilson, M.D.
Johnston Medical Center
1066 Herald Avenue, Suite 4D
Arlington, Texas 75555

RE: Anna Lawler (patient record #75463)

Dear Doctor Wilson:

This letter concerns your patient, Anna Lawler, age 44, who lives at 1915 Hawthorne Drive in Richardson. Ms. Lawler has come to Baylor College of Dentistry requesting routine dental care. She relates a history of heart damage and resulting murmur caused by rheumatic fever at age 6. She also indicates an allergy to penicillin manifested several years ago as a skin rash. She is taking birth control medication and specifically denies any other conditions affecting her health.

Our evaluation indicates that Ms. Lawler's dental needs include cleaning of the teeth, surgical removal of an impacted third molar, endodontic treatment of an anterior tooth, and a variety of routine dental restorations. These procedures will be accomplished with local anesthesia and are all expected to produce bleeding as well as a transient bacteremia. Please state your opinion of the risk of infective endocarditis during dental procedures for Ms. Lawler. Also, indicate to us if you recommend a variation in this case from the American Heart Association regimen for patients allergic to penicillin. In addition, please inform us if you would prefer to prescribe the prophylactic antibiotic coverage. She has been informed that the effectiveness of birth control medication may be adversely affected by antibiotic therapy.

Your written reply is required before any dental treatment can be provided. Your prompt response will expedite Ms. Lawler's dental treatment. Thank you for your time and help in this matter.

Sincerely,

Martin McKinney, Dental Student
Baylor College of Dentistry

exists if an issue of professional negligence later arises.

Essentially the same information is exchanged during telephone consultations as that listed for referral letters. The patient record that contains this information should be available when the call is initiated. It is appropriate to explain the purpose of the call to the consultant's staff and offer to either wait or have the consultant return the call. Few dental situations are so urgent that immediate access to the consultant is necessary. Also, this allows the consultant's staff to obtain the patient's chart if the patient has been seen previously. This promotes accurate information exchange without having to endure delays to locate records.

Documentation of the telephone consultation in the patient's record is necessary, particularly if significant clinical opinions have been expressed. Accurate notes made during the conversation minimize omissions. A confirmational letter should be sent to the consultant in most situations to verify the information discussed. The importance of this confirmational letter increases dramatically with more complex problems and if the advice provided is related to serious potential risks. Also, this confirmational letter should state that written documentation of the consultant's opinion is expected following a telephone conversation if that is the case.

Institutional Consultations

Institutional consultations rely on the patient's record as the mechanism for conveying information. This simplifies many aspects of the communication process because the relevant patient database and the identification of all participants is provided by the patient record. Consultations are accommodated in most institutional documentation schemes by a specific consultation form. Space is provided to record the basis for the consultation request as well as the consultant's response. The consultation request can be described with direct references to information such as prior treatment that is documented in other sections of the record without the need to specifically rewrite the information. The consult request should not be so brief, however, that the basis for the consult and what is expected of the consultant are unclear.

Informal Consultations

Clinicians commonly discuss both general and specific patient care issues in social situations. Although advice on general clinical topics and arrangements concerning a future consultation may be appropriately exchanged in this context, informal discussion of opinions related to a specific patient is unprofessional. Both the consultant and referring clinician must rely on memory, which can cause misunderstandings. Distractions may interrupt a significant qualifying remark related to a prior generalization, and an incorrect impression may be conveyed. Conversations concerning sensitive or confidential matters about a patient may be overheard. Almost without exception, conversations concerning the status of a specific patient should not be conducted informally in a social situation.

MEDICAL CONSULTATIONS AND REFERRALS

Medical referrals by the dentist are requests for the physician's opinion concerning conditions that are either likely to directly affect anticipated dental treatment or may be unrelated to dental care. In either case, the dentist's physical assessment of the patient should discern inconsequential medical problems from those that pose risks and require evaluation. The features from the patient history and clinical examination that suggest common systemic diseases and their relative severity with respect to the need for medical consultation are discussed in Chapter 7. In addition, medical complications that develop during actual dental procedures may warrant medical consultation.

Medical Conditions Without Direct Dental Treatment Implications

Most medical conditions that are unlikely to cause direct complications during dental treatment are chronic diseases or abnormalities that do not adversely affect cardiovascular, pulmonary, hepatic, or renal function. Borderline hypertension, many skin conditions, and most gastrointestinal complaints are typical examples. The limited risk of immediate problems is suggested by the long duration of the symptoms and the absence to date of any serious consequences. This implies that initiation of medical treatment to control symptoms or arrest progression of the conditions could eventually benefit the patient but that immediate complications are unlikely. For example, control of incipient hypertension is unlikely to produce any immediate improvement in the patient's health or make routine dental procedures any safer. However, the patient's health would be improved by elimination of chronic hypertension as a contributory factor in the progression of cardiovascular, cerebrovascular, and renal diseases.

Such referrals should be suggested to the patient on the basis of the signs and symptoms rather than as a presumptive diagnosis. In other words, a speculative diagnosis should not be suggested or discussed with the patient. Also, referral to the primary care physician rather than to a medical specialist is appropriate in most cases. These situations are usually managed most effectively by encouraging patients to seek their physician's advice rather than by arranging a formal referral.

Managing such situations diplomatically avoids forcing the dentist's health care values on the patient. The patient may have previously undergone several expensive and inconclusive diagnostic evaluations to identify an illness suspected on the basis of chronic symptoms described to the dentist. Insistence on repeating the process prior to dental treatment is unlikely to contribute to the health of the patient or the safety of dental care. Another patient may prefer to tolerate a minor medical problem rather than accept the cost and potential complications of treatment. Also, the patient who has not complied with prior medical treatment recommendations is unlikely to be any more receptive to the physician's advice than before. The dentist risks credibility and patient rapport by attempting to force health care decisions on the patient if the suspected condition is not directly related to dental care.

Medical Conditions With Direct Dental Treatment Implications

The conditions that may require modification of dental treatment methods generally involve cardiovascular, pulmonary, hemostatic, or metabolic dysfunction. The dentist's suspicion is that significant compromise of major organ system status may leave little functional reserve to accommodate additional physiologic demands during dental treatment. Complications such as arrest of organ system function may develop when this functional reserve is exceeded. The source of potential stress may be primarily emotional for an apprehensive patient, traumatic from an extensive oral surgical procedure, or related to the administration of drugs such as epinephrine.

The dentist's physical assessment of every patient must identify those who are at significant risk of adverse consequences during dental treatment and determine the most appropriate management to minimize these risks. Unfortunately, the dentist cannot be prepared by training or experience to fully evaluate every disease affecting every patient. Even if that were the case, the patient's primary care physician is more familiar with the disease course and unique variation of the disease that affects a specific patient. In addition, the dentist's assessment may be limited by the inability of the patient to describe current medical treatment methods. In other instances, the patient may be suffering from several systemic diseases, which inject additional complexities into the assessment beyond those recognized for each condition. Regardless of the specific issue from among these possibilities, medical consultations are most effective if the dentist clarifies several issues for the physician. Nonspecific medical consultation requests such as "please provide medical clearance prior to dental treatment" are often unproductive because they provide no guidance for the physician.

The consult request should summarize the dentist's interpretation of the patient's medical status in general terms. This informs the physician of the dentist's understanding of the patient's medical problems and should justify the consult request. In one sense this indicates to the physician that the dentist has tried to evaluate the potential problems and that the issues are beyond the dentist's assessment skills.

Next, the dentist must inform the physician about the nature of the anticipated dental treatment. The procedures should be described in general terms with emphasis on the physiologic implications of the dental treatment methods. This provides the physician a basis for judgments about the potential demands of the dental treatment relative to the patient's health status. The dental procedures are clearer if described in terms that the physician is likely to understand. For example, the phrase "two quadrants of periodontal therapy" is unlikely to convey any significant information. The explanation, "Superficial gingival surgery of the lower teeth will require approximately 1 hour, will be accomplished with local anesthesia, and is expected to cause a transient bacteremia." provides a better basis for the physician's assessment.

Finally, the consultant is more likely to provide the needed opinion if the specific complication of concern to the dentist is clarified. If the dentist's question is essentially whether or not the patient's heart murmur is associated with an increased risk of infective endocarditis and whether prophylactic antibiotic coverage during dental treatment is indicated, that should be specifically stated. The consultant

should not be expected to guess what the referring clinician wants to know.

Medical consultations that affect the conduct of routine dental procedures should be documented in most instances by a formal referral letter. The dentist must insist that the patient comply with the medical referral to determine the necessity of altering dental treatment methods. The patient should understand that potential medical risks during dental care have been identified and that safe dental treatment requires the physician's advice. Most individuals appreciate the referring dentist's concern and will comply. Others may resist. Dental treatment should be delayed until the required consultation is accomplished. The dentist accepts substantial responsibility for any complications that may develop during dental care for a patient who has refused the dentist's recommendation to consult their physician.

Medical Referrals Required By Complications During Dental Treatment

Despite efforts to prevent problems, both anticipated and unanticipated complications that require medical consultation occasionally arise during dental treatment. Examples include aspirating or swallowing of objects and acute episodes of chronic conditions such as epileptic seizures and angina attacks. Problems that require no immediate supportive care are best managed by contacting the patient's physician. More immediate problems may require initiating basic life support procedures, contacting emergency medical services, or transporting the patient to a hospital emergency room as dictated by the complication. The dentist should accompany the patient at all times in cases of acute distress until medical personnel can assume responsibility for supportive care. The availability of the dentist to provide a description of the episode is likely to be of diagnostic value. Also, the dentist's medical history can be invaluable in the initial evaluation and treatment of the patient. Regardless of the circumstances, the patient's primary care physician should be notified as soon as possible. The physician can then coordinate subsequent patient treatment.

CONSULTATIONS AND REFERRALS TO OTHER DENTISTS

Referrals and consultations between dentists are generally more comfortable for the general dentist than are medical consultations because all parties are familiar with the issues under consideration. However, complex treatment planning problems and differences in opinion among the dentists can make dental referrals and consultations more challenging in some respects than communications with physicians.

Referrals To Another Dentist

Referrals from a general dentist to another dentist are either to a dental specialist or to another general dentist. The distinction between these situations usually relates to the role that the dentist accepting the referral will play in the treatment of the patient. The specialty referral in most instances is to arrange the evaluation and treatment of conditions beyond the skill and training of the general dentist. The referral to another general dentist is an effort to achieve continuity of general dental care in most cases.

Dental specialist treatment. The referral from the general dentist to the specialist is for specialty-level care in the context of comprehensive dental care or for procedures that the general dentist chooses not to perform. The livelihood of the dental specialist relies on patient referrals from general dentists. Therefore the specialist invests considerable effort providing optimal treatment that complies with the wishes of the patient and the general dentist. Most problems that arise in the course of specialty referrals result from failure of the general dentist to adequately clarify the comprehensive treatment goals to the specialist.

Patient management problems can also develop if the patient fails to understand the role of the specialist.

Several specialty referral situations are seldom associated with misunderstandings. These situations include referrals to the oral surgeon for removal of third molars, to the orthodontist for correction of malocclusion, and to the pediatric dentist for comprehensive treatment of a child. The treatment and necessary arrangements are understood by both dentists because these referrals occur frequently and most general dentists establish professional relationships with a limited number of specialists. The referrals in these situations are well accepted by most patients because they are aware that these services are commonly performed by specialists.

Most problems that arise with these referrals relate to unusual circumstances. For example, the general dentist may delay restoration of several carious teeth pending an orthodontic referral with the thought that the restorations may be unnecessary if these teeth are selected by the orthodontist for serial extraction. However, orthodontists typically expect routine dental treatment to be completed prior to orthodontic referral and could interpret this as an oversight by the general dentist. These problems can generally be avoided by describing such circumstances in the referral letter to the specialist.

Other referral situations that are uncomplicated involve dental diagnostic problems. Radiographic exposures such as specialized TMJ, cephalometric, and panoramic projections require equipment that is often not available to the general dentist. Mucosal lesions, soft tissue enlargements, and bony abnormalities that are infrequently seen by the general dentist may be referred for evaluation by a more experienced clinician. Oral pathologists and oral medicine specialists may be available in larger cities or are associated with dental schools. In the absence of these specialists, the oral surgeon often serves in this role, particularly if the diagnosis is likely to rely on a biopsy procedure.

Referrals to periodontists, prosthodontists, and endodontists can be more complicated because the treatment provided by these specialists is often directly related to the care provided by other specialists and the general dentist. For example, treatment of a potential abutment tooth affected by a pulpal necrosis and advanced periodontal bone loss could depend on the opinions of these three specialists as well as that of the referring dentist. In general, referrals to these specialists require more attentive participation by the general dentist and more frequent communications between the clinicians involved to avoid problems.

Referrals to another general dentist. The referral of a patient to another general dentist typically seeks to maintain continuity of dental treatment. Examples of these referrals include patients moving to another community, requests for second opinions concerning treatment, and patients dissatisfied with past dental care.

Relocation of the patient. Dental patients who are planning to move to a new community often trust the advice of their dentist in finding a new dentist. The dentist may feel comfortable recommending a general dentist known personally or by reputation. Otherwise, the best recommendation of the dentist may be to encourage the patient to seek the advice of new neighbors or coworkers concerning competent practitioners. In either case, the conscientious dentist should make it clear that recent radiographs and a summary of treatment will be forwarded when requested by the new dentist. Giving such materials directly to the patient deprives the referring dentist of the opportunity to inform the new dentist of conditions that may require clinical reevaluation and other professional information.

Second opinions concerning planned treatment. Patients occasionally seek reassurance concerning the feasibility of a complex treatment plan by requesting a second opinion. This may reflect skepticism about investing in extensive dental care on the advice of one clinician rather than a confrontational patient attitude. In similar circumstances the dentist may request advice from a more experienced colleague, which is common in a group practice or an institutional setting.

Second opinion consultations should be approached by all participants as an opportunity to achieve optimal care for the patient rather than as a negative reflection on the original dentist. One method of achieving this is for the original dentist to suggest consultation for a second opinion when the patient appears hesitant to accept the treatment plan. Most patients respect and value the confidence of a dentist who encourages a second opinion on a complex treatment plan. One essential practical issue is that the consulting dentist should have access to the diagnostic information on which the original treatment plan was based.

Situations involving unsuccessful prior dental treatment. Clinical findings or patient complaints occasionally draw attention to the possibility that past treatment by another dentist has been deficient. Although substandard dental treatment certainly occurs, numerous factors other than the technical quality of the procedure, including patient compliance, also affect treatment success. For example, all dentists rely on the patient to indicate minor tissue adaptation deficiencies of a removable appliance during the period following insertion. The dentist cannot adjust these minor deficiencies if the patient becomes critical and refuses to return for adjustments. Also, it is not unusual to discover that critical patient complaints about a previous dentist actually relate to treatment performed by a different dentist. Some patient complaints may reflect the patient's unreasonable expectations more than deficiency of treatment.

Considering the nature of the financial, professional, and liability issues that can develop, the dentist confronted by this situation must maintain an attitude that is both positive and skeptical concerning substandard treatment. The patient should be referred to the previous dentist, if that is feasible, concerning the problem. Professional courtesy and most peer review procedures allow the original dentist the opportunity to evaluate and remedy any deficiencies. Professional courtesy also requires that the referring dentist contact the original dentist and objectively discuss the situation. This should be approached as a matter of solving the problem rather than assigning blame. Many misunderstandings become clear when the previous dentist describes the "other side of the story." If an actual deficiency does exist, most conscientious clinicians will make reasonable efforts to remedy deficiencies or satisfy the patient complaint. Negative opinions about prior care should not be stated to the patient unless absolutely no doubt exists, the previous dentist refuses to remedy the problem, and the referring dentist is prepared to justify the criticism in a peer review or legal proceeding.

Obligations of the Referring Dentist

Most of the implied responsibilities of the dentist who refers a patient to another clinician are a matter of common sense rather than rigid protocol. The patient's dental care is most effectively accomplished when the general dentist actively attends to the following issues.

Minimizing duplication of diagnostic procedures. Duplication of many diagnostic procedures can be avoided if the referring dentist provides the consultant with diagnostic materials prior to the consultation appointment. Radiographs are the most common example, but study models, laboratory findings, and opinions from other practitioners may also be contributory. Another example is documentation of a medical consultation for a patient with a complex dental treatment plan. The physician will appreciate one consultation request from the generalist who then informs the dental specialists of the results rather than several separate consultation requests related to the same problem.

Treatment coordination. The referring dentist assumes the role of coordinator among several specialists to minimize dental treatment inconsistencies. Treatment planning disagreements among specialists and the referring dentist can be awkward at times but several opinions from different perspectives can also achieve optimal care for the patient with complex treatment needs. Eventually, however, someone must decide what the final plan is going to be among the options and opinions. This is the responsibility of the general dentist and the patient.

It is the responsibility of the general dentist to avoid contradictory procedures such as the extraction of a critical abutment tooth or endodontic obturation of a tooth with a hopeless periodontal prognosis. This supervisory function is best accomplished by maintaining frequent contact with the involved specialists and the patient. For example, general dental care appointments can often be logically interspersed among specialty care appointments. Another method of minimizing the possibility of these problems is to arrange specialty consultations and the ensuing procedures in the general dental treatment sequence outlined in Chapter 12. Providing a copy of the patient's preliminary treatment plan to the specialists at their initial consultations and updated versions during active treatment minimizes such problems.

Support of the specialty treatment. The referring dentist should encourage the patient to accept the treatment recommendations of the specialist if they appear feasible and consistent with the comprehensive treatment plan. Patients often request what is essentially a second opinion from the general dentist concerning the specialist's plan because their relationship with the general dentist is more established. If the specialist's recommendations appear contrary to the opinion of the referring dentist, the referring dentist should contact the consultant to discuss the situation rather than revealing the inconsistency to the patient. In some cases the specialist may have identified clinical features overlooked during the generalist's examination.

Confirmation of the patient's compliance with the specialty treatment recommendations of the referring practitioner is another aspect of support for the specialist. This often involves recall or follow-up evaluation of the specialist's care during the later stages of comprehensive treatment. For example, the periodontist usually expects the generalist to monitor and encourage home care during the restorative phase of treatment.

Minor complications that result from the specialist's treatment can often be most efficiently managed by the referring dentist, particularly if the specialist's office is some distance away. The general dentist should not hesitate to provide this support as long as solving the problem is within the generalist's ability. The specialist should eventually be informed of the complication and the generalist's treatment in the event that the problem persists.

Arranging the referral. The patient should understand that the consultation requires an appointment to avoid leaving the impression that the consult can be accomplished on a "walk in" basis. Some patients prefer to have the referring dentist's staff arrange the consultation appointment, whereas those who prefer to schedule the appointment themselves need the consultant's telephone number and address and directions to the office. The patient should also understand that additional professional fees will be charged for the consultant's diagnostic opinion and treatment. The referring dentist should provide the patient with a general idea of the likely expense to avoid wasting everyone's time if the cost will be prohibitive for the patient.

Initiating productive referrals. Most dentists develop strong relationships with the dental specialists and physicians to whom they refer patients. These relationships can be invaluable when treatment complications arise and the immediate support of the specialist or physician is needed. Consultants, particularly physicians, can also be a source of patient referrals for general dental care if professional interactions leave an impression of competence. This relationship deteriorates rapidly, however, if the dentist's referrals consist primarily of inconsequential medical problems, problem patients, patients without financial resources, and requests to salvage deficient dental treatment. Physicians soon tire of providing unnecessary reassurance to the dentist about insignificant medical conditions. Habitual referral to the dental specialist of patients whose problems primarily reflect management difficulties or an unwillingness of the general dentist to accept patient care responsibilities soon becomes obvious.

Obligations of the Dental Consultant

The consultant or specialist provides evaluation and patient care to supplement or extend the dental care provided by the referring dentist. Many of the responsibilities of the consultant are direct extensions of the obligations described for the referring dentist. The priority and point of reference in all difficult situations is optimal patient care. This can best be achieved with good communication and respect for the situation of the general practitioner. Divergent opinions may occasionally emerge in complicated situations. However, most problems can be resolved with an effort to involve all parties, including the patient, in the decision process.

The consultant should provide the referring dentist with written documentation of the consultation that includes the specialist's opinion of the problem and the recommended solution or treatment. Information concerning planned procedures by the specialist is usually listed to allow the generalist to plan other aspects of treatment. The return of any radiographs or other materials supplied by the general dentist is expected unless they have been specifically designated by the referring dentist as copies for the specialist's records.

An additional priority for the consultant is to stress to the patient the importance of returning to the referring dentist for routine dental care. Patients occasionally assume that the specialist has accepted responsibility for all aspects of the dental care. This may be true for pediatric dental referrals and in some other circumstances. Otherwise, additional comprehensive dental care and routine recall examination remain the general dentist's responsibility after the specialty care has been provided.

CONSULTATIONS WITH OTHER PROFESSIONALS

Situations occasionally arise in which professionals other than physicians and dentists can contribute to the dental health and management of the patient. For example, the patient's pharmacist can certainly provide a listing of the patient's current medications, dosages, and the medication regimens. Of greater importance in many instances is the pharmacist's knowledge concerning drug interactions and other practical aspects of clinical pharmacology. The dentist is required to report cases of suspected child abuse to social services workers, who are better prepared to manage these complicated situations. The nursing staff of extended care facilities can be exceptionally helpful in advising the dentist of the patient's oral hygiene capabilities and supervising daily cleaning efforts to attain optimal results.

Interactions with such professionals are approached essentially in the same attitude as consultations and referrals with physicians and dentists. By the nature of these situations, the exchange of information is more likely to be by telephone conversation or personal contact than by formal consult letter. Nevertheless, the priorities of the interaction should still be to adequately describe the nature of the problem, provide a summary of the baseline information relevant to the problem, and explore possible solutions. Appropriate professional courtesy promotes the commitment of all involved professionals toward improving the patient's health care.

SUMMARY

Effective conduct of consultations and referrals with physicians, dentists, and other professionals is an important aspect of dental practice. The key elements of effective interprofessional contacts are clear communication, professional courtesy, common sense, and concern for the patient's welfare.

Consultations with physicians may be appropriate both for medical problems that are unrelated to dental care and those that could require modification of routine dental procedures. Suspected medical conditions that are unlikely to cause complications during dental care can be managed by encouraging the patient to contact their physician as health care advice rather than as a formal consultation. If the medical problem is associated with the risk of complications during dental treatment, then consultation should be required before dental treatment. Written documentation of the consult is sound practice in cases of potentially serious complications or complex medical conditions.

Referrals to dentists include those for continuity of routine dental care by other general dentists and for dental specialty evaluation and treatment. Continuity of general dental care referrals can result from patients moving to a new community, requests for a second opinion concerning planned treatment, and complaints concerning prior dental care. Referrals for specialty dental procedures require that the general dentist maintain responsibility for the comprehensive dental care of the patient while supporting the specialist's efforts. Both situations require the referring dentist to establish effective communication with other involved dentists while maintaining priority for the welfare of the patient.

BIBLIOGRAPHY

Brightman VJ: Rational procedures for diagnosis and medical risk assessment. In Lynch MA, Brightman VJ, Greenberg MS, editors: Burket's oral medicine: diagnosis and treatment, ed 8, Philadelphia, 1984, Lippincott.

Langlais RP and others: Oral diagnosis, oral medicine and treatment planning, Philadelphia, 1984, Saunders.

Little JW, Falace DA: Dental management of the medically compromised patient, ed 3, St Louis, 1988, Mosby–Year Book.

CHAPTER 11

Clinical Evaluation by Laboratory Methods

JOHN F. NELSON

Clinical pathology and *clinical laboratory medicine* refer to the discipline of medicine concerned with the analysis of fluids and other materials from the patient by microscopic, biochemical, microbiologic, and immunologic methods. *Surgical pathology* is the microscopic evaluation of intact tissues. These diagnostic methods expand the patient's diagnostic database beyond "macroscopic" signs and symptoms to include the "microscopic" realm of abnormal cellular morphology and biochemical dysfunction.

The clinician must consider several issues while interpreting clinical laboratory studies. Specimens from clinically healthy patients occasionally yield abnormal laboratory test results. This can represent a technical error, mislabeling of samples, poor specimen quality, or simply an individual at an extreme of the range of normal in the same sense as unusual height. Also, all quantitative laboratory tests are only accurate within a technical error range. For these reasons, the clinical opinion suggested by laboratory results must always be formulated in the context of the patient's condition. Contradictions between the implications based on laboratory results and those from clinical features justify repeating the tests.

Laboratory methods are considered as *screening tests* if their results provide evidence of disease but a specific diagnosis cannot be based on the information. *Definitive laboratory tests* support a specific diagnosis. Most of the laboratory studies discussed in this chapter are screening tests. Blood is an ideal testing material for many systemic conditions because the specimen can be obtained easily and many diseases produce detectable peripheral blood abnormalities. Blood tests are arranged by the component evaluated: erythrocyte studies, leukocyte counts, coagulation evaluation, serum chemistry, and serologic tests for common in-

Table 11-1 Classification of anemias

Types of anemia/general causes	Specific conditions
FACTOR DEFICIENCY ANEMIAS	
Malnutrition, malabsorption, and blood loss	Iron, folic acid, and vitamin B_{12} deficiency anemias
Intrinsic factor defect limits vitamin B_{12} absorption	Pernicious anemia
Isoniazid therapy alters B_6 absorption	Vitamin B_6 deficiency anemia
PRODUCTION DEFECT ANEMIAS	
Hypoplastic bone marrow	Myelofibrosis, cancer, cancer chemotherapy, drug-induced and idiopathic aplastic anemias
Chronic systemic disease	Chronic renal, hepatic, and autoimmune disorders, as well as chronic neoplastic disease and chronic infections
DEPLETION ANEMIAS	
Hemolytic	
Intracorpuscular defect	Genetic defects such as sickle cell anemia, thalassemia, and congenital spherocytosis
Extracorpuscular defect	Transfusion reactions, autoimmune diseases, disseminated intravascular coagulation, intoxications, malaria, hypersplenism
Hemorrhage	Acute and chronic blood loss such as gastrointestinal bleeding

Modified from Ravel R: Clinical laboratory medicine: clinical application of laboratory data, ed 5, St Louis, 1989, Mosby—Year Book.

fectious diseases. In addition, urinalysis and microbiologic methods are briefly described.

Surgical pathology provides essential information to the diagnosis of many oral lesions. The accuracy of this diagnostic approach depends on the method of tissue acquisition, the information submitted with the specimen, and the clinician's interpretation of the pathologist's opinion.

ERYTHROCYTE STUDIES

Erythrocyte studies primarily reflect the capacity of the blood to transport oxygen and carbon dioxide. *Anemia* refers to a compromise of this function by an inadequate number of erythrocytes, deficient hemoglobin within the erythrocytes, or a combination of both. Specific causes of anemia are categorized in Table 11-1. Clinical features such as pallor, weakness, fatigue after minimal exertion, and atrophic glossitis may suggest severe anemia. However, anemia screening tests are necessary to detect more mild examples of erythrocyte deficiency. An additional laboratory test involving red blood cells that indicates illness unrelated to anemia is the erythrocyte sedimentation rate.

Screening Tests for Anemia

The hematocrit, red blood cell count, and hemoglobin concentration are the screening tests relied on to identify anemia. These tests are summarized in Fig. 11-1. The *hematocrit* (Hct) is the percentage of total blood volume that is composed of cells. The determination is made by centrifuging a capillary tube that contains the blood sample and then measuring the total length of the sample compared with the

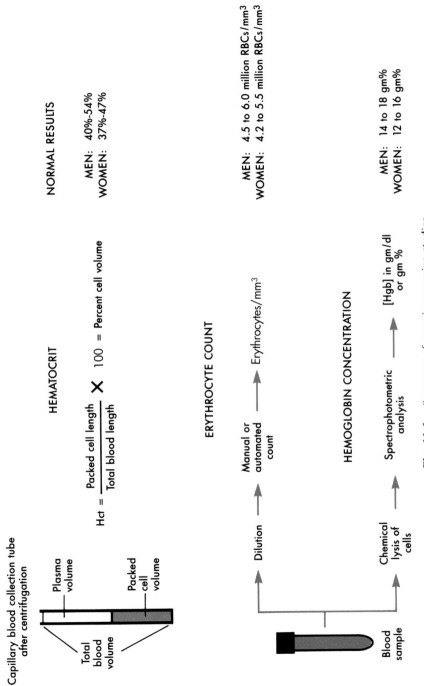

Fig. 11-1 Summary of anemia screening studies.

length of packed cells. The *red blood cell count* (RBC) can be performed manually with a microscope and a volumetric glass slide, but automated counting devices are less tedious and yield comparable or superior accuracy. The *hemoglobin concentration,* [Hgb], is a relatively accurate indication of the oxygen carrying capacity of the blood because the test reflects the hemoglobin content of the erythrocytes as well as the number of erythrocytes. The density of hemoglobin pigment is measured spectrophotometrically after chemical lysis of the erythrocytes and compared with reference standards.

Low values from these tests indicate anemia but without specification of the cause. An abnormally high erythrocyte count is defined as *polycythemia,* which can be caused by dehydration, excessive production of erythrocytes (polycythemia vera), or pathophysiologic compensation for conditions of diminished oxygen transport such as cardiopulmonary insufficiency.

Peripheral Blood Smear

Microscopic examination of a peripheral blood smear reveals erythrocyte morphology and may provide an indication of the type of anemia. The following terms refer to the morphologic features of a significant proportion of the erythrocytes:

Normocytic refers to normal erythrocyte size.

Microcytic refers to abnormally small red blood cells.

Macrocytic indicates a significant number of abnormally large red blood cells.

Normochromic indicates normal pigmentation as a reflection of hemoglobin content.

Hypochromic reflects pale pigmentation and low hemoglobin concentration.

Hyperchromic refers to dark color indicative of excessive hemoglobin content.

Reticulocytosis and *normocytosis* refer to the presence of erythrocyte precursors in the peripheral circulation.

Anisocytosis is used when variation in erythrocyte size is apparent.

Poikilocytosis applies to variation in red blood cell shape, including sickle-shaped features indicative of sickle cell anemia.

Spherocytosis describes the loss of typical biconcave erythocyte shape as identified by absence of the central pale area of the cells.

A significant proportion of erythrocytes that exhibit abnormal cell size or color, or both, suggests certain types of anemia. The most frequent cause of microcytic-hypochromic anemia, for example, is iron deficiency. The erythrocytes are morphologically normal in acute hemorrhagic anemia. The correlations of erythrocyte size and hemoglobin concentration to different forms of anemia are summarized in Table 11-2. The presence of immature erythrocytes such as normoblasts and reticulocytes in the peripheral blood indicates severe anemia or advanced systemic disease.

Wintrobe Indices

Estimates of erythrocyte size and hemoglobin content referred to as the *Wintrobe indices* can be calculated from the results of the hematocrit, RBC, and hemoglobin concentration determination. These calculated values can provide initial direction in the differential diagnosis of anemia. Microscopic examination of a peripheral blood smear is still necessary in many cases to detect other morphologic abnormalities. The advantage of the Wintrobe indices, however, is that they are readily derived from the results of screening anemia studies performed by automated methods.

The Wintrobe indices consist of the mean corpuscular volume, mean corpuscular hemoglobin, and mean corpuscular hemoglobin concentration. The *mean corpuscular volume* (MCV) is an estimation of average red blood cell size in cubic microns. The *mean corpuscular hemoglobin* (MCH) provides an estimate of the average hemoglobin content of the erythrocytes expressed in picograms (pg). The *mean corpuscular hemoglobin concentration*

Table 11-2   Correlation of erythrocyte morphology with various forms of anemia

| | Hemoglobin content* | |
Cell size	Normochromic	Hypochromic
Microcytic	Uncommon, possible in some cases of infection and chronic systemic diseases	Iron deficiency anemia Thalassemia major and minor Anemias of chronic systemic diseases
Normocytic	Hemolysis Hemorrhagic anemia Aplastic anemia Anemia of renal failure Hypersplenism	Anemias of systemic diseases in some cases Lead poisoning
Macrocytic	Pernicious anemia Folic acid deficiency Malabsorption conditions Reticulocytosis (release of precursors) Chronic hepatic disease Some cases of aplastic anemia Alcoholism	Macrocytic anemias with superimposed iron deficiency

Modified from Ravel R: Clinical laboratory medicine: clinical application of laboratory data, ed 5, St Louis, 1989, Mosby—Year Book.
*The category for hyperchromic hemoglobin content is excluded because this form of anemia is rare.

(MCHC) also quantifies hemoglobin content as the average percentage of hemoglobin in the average erythrocyte. The MCHC is generally a more reliable indication of hemoglobin concentration than is the MCH. The range of normal values and the diagnostic implications of the Wintrobe indices are summarized in Table 11-3.

Erythrocyte Sedimentation Rate

Immunoglobulins increase erythrocyte surface adherence and cause agglutination or clumping in an undisturbed blood sample that contains an anticoagulant. The erythrocyte sedimentation rate (ESR or "sed rate") quantifies this phenomenon by determining the rate at which visible erythrocyte clumps settle in a glass column. Normal values are less than 15 mm/hour for males and 20 mm/hour for females.

Accelerated erythrocyte agglutination is a feature of many inflammatory diseases that stimulate the production of immunoglobulins or alter the cell membrane properties of erythrocytes. Therefore elevated ESR indicates generalized inflammatory disease but is not specific for any condition. The test is typically applied as a "barometer" to monitor the course of a chronic disease process such as rheumatoid arthritis after a definitive diagnosis has been made by other methods. Comparison of a series of ESR results during a period of weeks or months provides evidence of improvement or deterioration in the patient's status.

LEUKOCYTE STUDIES

Many systemic diseases produce changes in the number of circulating leukocytes, as well as changes in the proportions of the different white blood cell types. Abnormalities may reflect a pathophysiologic response to infection, leukocytic neoplasm such as leukemia, or sup-

Table 11-3 Calculation of the Wintrobe indices from the anemia screening tests provides an estimate of the erythrocyte size and hemoglobin concentration

Index	Calculation*	Normal range	Clinical significance
MCV	$\dfrac{\text{Hct} \times 10}{\text{RBC count}}$	82-100 μ^3	↑ Macrocytic anemia → Normocytic anemia ↓ Microcytic anemia
MCH	$\dfrac{[\text{Hgb}] \times 10}{\text{RBC count}}$	26 to 34 pg	↑ Hyperchromic anemia (rare) → Normochromic anemia ↓ Hypochromic anemia
MCHC	$\dfrac{[\text{Hgb}] \times 100}{\text{Hct}}$	31% to 37%	↑ Hyperchromic anemia (rare) → Normochromic anemia ↓ Hypochromic anemia

*Calculations by these formulas rely on the numerical value of the Hct and Hgb without designation of units. The RBC count for calculation is in number of millions, that is 5.0 is used in these formulas for an RBC count of 5,000,000 per cubic millimeter.

pression of leukocyte production by drugs or severe illnesses. Peripheral leukocyte changes develop rapidly or early in the course of many diseases, which can provide valuable diagnostic information in the assessment of an acute illness. The two principal peripheral leukocyte studies are the total white blood cell count and the differential white cell count. These two determinations are usually requested together because each is of limited value without the other.

White Blood Cell Count

The white blood cell count (WBC) is the total number of all leukocytes per cubic millimeter in the peripheral blood. The determination can be made microscopically with a volumetric slide, although automated methods have virtually replaced the manual technique. In many instances the WBC is combined with a count of the peripheral erythrocytes and platelets, which is referred to as a *complete blood count* or CBC. Many physiologic conditions, other than disease states, such as age, sex, physiologic status, physical stress, and pregnancy can affect the WBC. A low count is referred to as *leukopenia* and can result from

severe debilitation, cancer chemotherapy, blood dyscrasias, and overwhelming infection. A high WBC or *leukocytosis* may be stimulated by infections and tissue destruction or represent neoplasia of leukocytic origin.

Differential White Blood Cell Count

The differential leukocyte count (or "diff") is performed by microscopic examination of a peripheral blood smear or by automated methods to quantify the different white blood cell types present in the circulating blood. The results are reported for each leukocyte type both as percentages and as absolute counts per cubic millimeter. Absolute counts are calculated by multiplying the total leukocyte count by the percentage determined for each leukocyte type. The normal ranges for adults are relatively broad as illustrated by Table 11-4.

The differential white blood cell count is invaluable in many clinical situations because the pathophysiologic response to many diseases is represented by numeric changes in specific leukocyte groups. Table 11-4 summarizes the diseases frequently associated with numeric changes of specific leukocyte types. Certain diseases such as infectious mononucle-

Table 11-4 Differential white blood cell count: normal adult values and clinical significance of abnormal results

Leukocyte type	Normal %	Normal Absolute count per mm³	Low absolute count	High absolute count
Total neutrophils	50-70	3000-6000	Neutropenia: specific infections including typhoid, hepatitis, infectious mononucleosis, and malaria; hypersplenism related to hepatic or rare metabolic diseases; autoimmune diseases such as systemic lupus erythematosus and severe nutritional deficiencies; idiopathic conditions such as cyclic neutropenia and agranulocytosis	Neutrophilic leukocytosis: bacterial infections, especially "coccal" diseases such as pneumonia, otitis media, osteomyelitis, appendicitis, and strep throat; tissue necrosis following stroke and myocardial infarct; cancer of any kind including myelogenous leukemia; physiologic causes such as exercise, stress, temperature extremes, and childbirth
Segmented (polys)	50-70	3000-6000		
Immature forms				
Band (stab)	3-5	<500	Neutropenia with many immature forms ("shift to the left") suggests progressive, overwhelming infection; myelocytes suggest myelogenous leukemia	Neutrophilic leukocytosis with many immature forms indicates progressive, acute infection; myelocytes suggest myelogenous leukemia
Metamyelocytes	<1	Few		
Myelocytes	None	None		
Lymphocytes	20-40	1500-3000	Lymphocytopenia: immunodeficiency such as rare genetic conditions, AIDS, corticosteroid medication, and other immunosuppression	Lymphocytosis: viral infections, some "noncoccal" bacterial infections, autoimmune conditions, other immunologic responses, and lymphocytic leukemia
Monocytes	0-7	300-500	Low monocyte, eosinophil, or basophil counts reflect technical or sampling error or leukopenia if all are low	Monocytosis: malaria, tuberculosis, typhus, hepatitis, syphilis, granulomatous diseases, autoimmune diseases, and many cancers, including monocytic leukemia
Eosinophils	0-5	50-250		Eosinophilia: parasitic infestations, scarlatina, psoriasis, pemphigus, asthma, erythema multiforme, pernicious anemia, leukemias, and lymphomas
Basophils	0-1	<50		True basophilia is very rare
Total leukocytes	100	5000-10,000	Leukopenia: overwhelming infection, severe systemic disease, drug-induced aplastic anemia, chemotherapy, poisoning, and advanced malignancy	Leukocytosis: identify increase of specific leukocyte type(s)

Modified from Platt WR: Color atlas and textbook of hematology. Philadelphia, 1979, Lippincott.

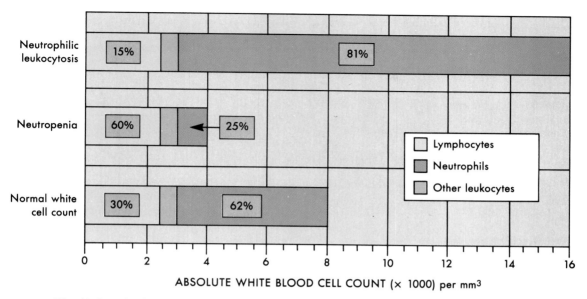

Fig. 11-2   Absolute versus relative changes in white blood cell populations. This chart represents the white cell counts of three patients who all have a normal absolute lymphocyte count. The bottom bar represents a healthy individual with typical absolute numbers and percentages of lymphocytes and neutrophils. The neutropenic patient represented by the middle bar has a normal number of peripheral lymphocytes, but the decreased total leukocyte count yields an increased lymphocyte percentage that falsely suggests lymphocytosis. The top bar represents neutrophilic leukocytosis that is a typical response to a bacterial infection, but the decreased percentage of lymphocytes falsely suggests lymphopenia. Clinical opinions should always be based on absolute leukocyte counts rather than on relative changes in the percentages of leukocytes.

osis and the leukemias produce morphologically characteristic peripheral white cells that can be identified microscopically. In addition, comparison of the results from a series of differential leukocyte counts during the course of an illness can demonstrate improvement or deterioration in the patient's condition.

The white cell differential results can be misinterpreted if the opinion is based strictly on the relative proportions of specific leukocyte types without considering the total leukocyte count. For example, a disease that destroys circulating neutrophils produces a decreased total leukocyte count as well as a decreased percentage and absolute number of neutrophils in the differential white blood cell count. This is referred to as an *absolute* neutropenia and accurately represents the patient's status. The unaffected lymphocyte population is reflected by a normal absolute lymphocyte count in the differential, but the percentage of lymphocytes is greater because the total leukocyte count is decreased. This falsely suggests a lymphocytosis in response to the disease and is referred to as a *relative* lymphocytosis. This relative change in the percentage of a leukocyte group is a misrepresentation when it results from an absolute change of another leukocyte group (Fig. 11-2). The clinical interpretation of the differential leukocyte

Table 11-5 Summary and categorization of bleeding disorders

Category/condition	Mechanism(s)	Associated features
CAPILLARY FRAGILITY		
Osteogenesis imperfecta	Genetic collagen defect	Bone fractures, blue sclera
Ehlers-Danlos syndrome	Genetic collagen defect	Hyperelasticity of skin
Hereditary hemorrhagic te-langiectasia	Genetic vessel malformation	Multiple bluish skin lesions
Scurvy, malnutrition, malab-sorption	Acquired, limited collagen synthesis and repair	Weight loss, anorexia, gas-trointestinal symptoms
PLATELET DEFICIENCIES		
Thrombocytopenia (limited platelet availability)	Hemopoietic disease or sup-ply exhausted	Pancytopenia, malnutrition, chemotherapy, or hemor-rhage
Thrombocytopathia (deficient platelet function)	Genetic platelet deficiencies, von Willebrand's disease, analgesic inhibition, uremia, immune disorders	History
COAGULATION DEFICIENCIES		
Hemophilia, Christmas disease	Genetic factor deficiency	Congenital, family history
von Willebrand's disease	Genetic factor deficiency	Congenital, family history
Severe hepatic disease	Deficient factor production	Jaundice, other liver disease signs
Anticoagulant therapy	Heparin or coumarin	Recent history of stroke, myo-cardial infarction, throm-bophlebitis

Modified from Widmann FK: Clinical interpretation of laboratory tests, ed 9, Philadelphia, 1979, Davis.

count results must always be based on abso-lute changes rather than relative or percentage changes.

HEMOSTASIS

Abnormal hemostasis represents potentially serious complications for the patient following minor injuries as well as surgical procedures. A hemorrhagic tendency or *bleeding diathesis* can result from abnormal capillary fragility, in-adequate platelet function in "plugging" vessel injuries, and deficiencies in the coagulation process that stabilize the platelet plug. Com-mon and well-recognized bleeding disorders are categorized in Table 11-5.

The clinical suspicion of a bleeding ten-dency is based in most cases on the indication by the patient of bleeding episodes following minor wounds or medical conditions that are known to affect hemostasis. Screening hemo-stasis tests are designed to identify whether capillary fragility, platelet function, coagula-tion, or a combination of hemostatic elements is adversely affected. These screening tests in-clude the tourniquet test, platelet count, bleeding time, partial thromboplastin time, and prothrombin time. More specific tests are often required to determine the specific hemostatic deficiency after the affected element has been identified by these screening tests.

CONDITIONS THAT CAN CAUSE PANCYTOPENIA

General illnesses

Overwhelming infection
Hemorrhage
Severe systemic disease
   Renal failure
   Hepatic failure
Severe malnutrition

Hemopoietic failure

Antimetabolic agents such as radiation,
   chemotherapy, and poisoning
Bone marrow replacement
   Advanced malignancy
   Myelofibrosis
Idiopathic aplastic anemia
Drug-induced aplastic anemia

Screening for Capillary Fragility

The *tourniquet* or *Rumpel-Leede test* evaluates capillary fragility by blocking venous blood return, which increases intraluminal pressure stress. Visible evidence of vessel rupture indicates capillary fragility. The test is performed by placing a sphygmomanometer cuff over the upper arm and inflating the cuff between the systolic and diastolic pressures. After 15 minutes the pressure is released, then 5 minutes later the small petechial hemorrhages of the skin are counted in a 2 x 2 cm square proximal to the antecubital crease. Fewer than 10 petechiae is normal and more than 20 indicates capillary fragility. Tourniquet test results are generally considered to be of limited clinical value because the test is heavily reliant on technique and subjective interpretation. Most instances of capillary fragility can be adequately identified by patient history and diagnosis of the underlying condition by the features suggested in Table 11-5.

Screening Tests for Platelet Deficiency

Platelet count. The complete blood count includes the number of platelets per cubic millimeter in the peripheral blood. Normal counts in the range of 2 to 5 million/mm^3 indicate adequate platelet availability. Platelet deficiency or *thrombocytopenia* is usually associated with *pancytopenia,* which is a deficiency of all cellular elements of the blood caused by cancer chemotherapy, advanced malignancy, radiation exposure, hemorrhage, or other conditions listed in the box above. Platelet counts less than 100,000/mm^3 indicate the possibility of difficulty establishing hemostasis with small wounds. Spontaneous hemorrhage is likely for patients with platelet counts less than 50,000/mm^3 and below 25,000/per mm^3 spontaneous hemorrhage can be expected.

Bleeding time. Bleeding time provides information about both platelet availability and platelet function in arresting blood flow from a small, precise incision made on a finger or earlobe with a template device. The wound is blotted every 30 seconds and the result is the time at which a drop no longer forms. The normal value varies with different approaches. The Duke and Ivy methods are examples of bleeding time tests that differ by the site, depth, and length of the incision. Elevated bleeding time for a patient with a normal platelet count suggests abnormal platelet function, which can be evaluated by additional tests. A common cause of deficient platelet function is high dosages of analgesics such as aspirin or nonsteroidal antiinflammatory agents.

Screening Tests of Coagulation Deficiency

Stabilization of the temporary platelet plug into a permanent clot requires the conversion

Fig. 11-3 Summary of coagulation.

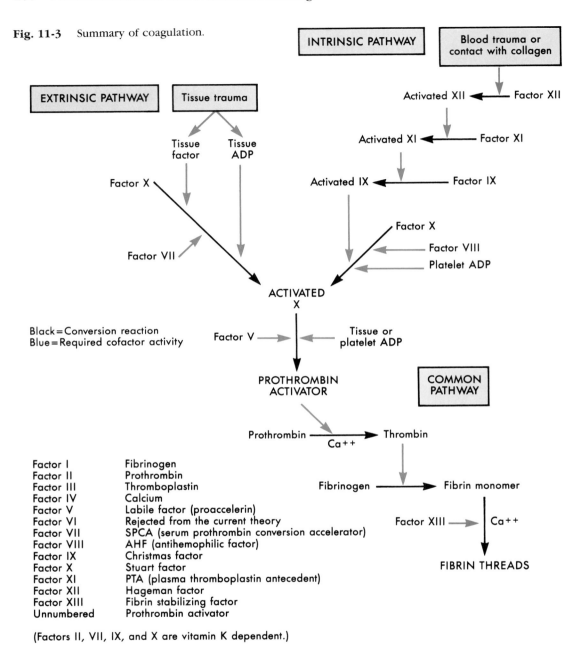

Black = Conversion reaction
Blue = Required cofactor activity

Factor I	Fibrinogen
Factor II	Prothrombin
Factor III	Thromboplastin
Factor IV	Calcium
Factor V	Labile factor (proaccelerin)
Factor VI	Rejected from the current theory
Factor VII	SPCA (serum prothrombin conversion accelerator)
Factor VIII	AHF (antihemophilic factor)
Factor IX	Christmas factor
Factor X	Stuart factor
Factor XI	PTA (plasma thromboplastin antecedent)
Factor XII	Hageman factor
Factor XIII	Fibrin stabilizing factor
Unnumbered	Prothrombin activator

(Factors II, VII, IX, and X are vitamin K dependent.)

of prothrombin to thrombin, which promotes coagulation by the formation of fibrin. This process may be initiated by either the intrinsic or extrinsic pathways as illustrated in Fig. 11-3. The partial thromboplastin time (PTT) evalu- ates the intrinsic pathway, and the extrinsic pathway is tested by the determination of the prothrombin time (PT). Abnormal results of both tests suggest a defect of the common pathway.

Partial thromboplastin time. Normal clot formation is observed within 35 to 50 seconds after mixing the commercial PTT test kit reagents with the patient's plasma. Greater PTT clotting time indicates genetic defects of intrinsic factors including classic hemophilia (factor VIII) and Christmas disease (factor IX) as well as factors XI and XII to a lesser degree. The PTT is also an effective quantitative monitor of the results of heparin anticoagulant therapy.

Prothrombin time. The test of the extrinsic pathway is the prothrombin time (PT). The patient's citrated plasma is added to the commercial kit reagents to activate factor X directly without activation of the intrinsic factors. The normal clot forms in 11 to 13 seconds. The PT evaluates the extrinsic and common coagulation pathways both qualitatively and quantitatively. A normal result requires adequate fibrinogen, factor X, factor VII, factor V, and prothrombin. Because these are primarily vitamin K-dependent factors synthesized by the liver, the PT detects acquired coagulation disorders caused by liver disease and dietary deficiency. The prothrombin time is also used to monitor outpatient anticoagulant therapy with coumarin because this drug inhibits hepatic synthesis of these factors.

BLOOD CHEMISTRY

Blood chemistry evaluation contributes to the diagnosis of common hepatic, renal, and metabolic diseases. The automation of blood chemistry analysis allows numerous individual serum chemistry tests to be performed on a single blood sample, and because of this automation the tests are relatively inexpensive, accurate, and rapidly available. Identification of blood chemistry abnormalities generally indicates the affected organ system, which provides direction in ordering and interpreting more specific diagnostic procedures. Blood chemistry tests can be categorized by the substance evaluated as serum electrolytes, metabolic molecules, serum proteins, intracellular enzymes, and serologic tests.

Electrolytes and Blood pH

Maintenance of physiologic electrolyte and fluid concentrations is accomplished by balanced intake and excretion of water and salts. Severe renal disease, dramatic fluid loss, and respiratory abnormalities can overcome physiologic mechanisms to produce electrolyte imbalance and abnormal blood pH. In general, electrolyte imbalance and acid-base abnormalities are so closely related that separate consideration can be misleading.

Blood pH and the blood concentrations of sodium (Na^+), potassium (K^+), chloride (Cl^-), and bicarbonate ion (HCO_3^-) are qualitatively and quantitatively the most significant indicators of acid-base and electrolyte balance. The anion gap is also listed in most reports as reflecting the unmeasured difference in charge between measured cations (Na^+ and K^+) and anions (Cl^- and HCO_3^-). This represents the anionic effect of serum proteins and metabolic molecules.

Acid-base imbalance is categorized as either acidosis or alkalosis as indicated by the blood pH and as either metabolic or respiratory to reflect the cause. Respiratory acidosis and alkalosis result from abnormal pulmonary CO_2 exchange, which affects the bicarbonate blood buffering capacity by altering $[HCO_3^-]$. All other causes of acid-base abnormality are considered metabolic including dehydration, renal disease, diabetic ketoacidosis, and shock. Table 11-6 summarizes the common causes of acid-base abnormalities with associated clinical and laboratory features.

The normal cationic balance of primarily extracellular sodium and intracellular potassium can be adversely affected by conditions such as fluid loss, renal failure, decreased renal profusion from congestive heart failure, excessive dietary intake, and dietary deficiency. In addition, iatrogenic forms of cationic imbalance include excessive dosages of some diuretics and intravenous administration of large volumes of saline fluids without regard to cationic balance. In general, the fluctuations in one cation are compensated for by an intracellular-ex-

Table 11-6 Summary of simple acid-base imbalances of the blood

Physiologic status	Blood pH	[HCO_3^-]	Causes	Clinical features
Normal values	7.37-7.43	19-25 mEq/liter	—	—
Metabolic acidosis	<7.37	<15	Ethanol toxicity, diabetic ketoacidosis, renal failure, gastrointestinal fluid loss, shock	Shock, coma, hypokalemia
Metabolic alkalosis	>7.43	>27	Persistent vomiting, decreased blood volume, hyperaldosteronism, excessive diuretic dosage	Paresthesias, tetany, weakness, hypokalemia
Respiratory acidosis	<7.35	>27	Acute or chronic respiratory failure	Oxygen starvation, hypoventilation, cyanosis
Respiratory alkalosis	>7.45	<20	Hyperventilation	Light-headedness

Modified from Nairas RG, Gardner LB: Simple acid-base disturbances, Med Clin North Am 65:321-346, 1981.

Table 11-7 Summary of conditions that can cause cation imbalance

Serum cation status

ABNORMAL [NA^+]	DECREASED ECF*	NORMAL ECF*	INCREASED ECF*
Hyponatremia (decreased [Na^+])	Gastrointestinal fluid loss Burns, ascites	Increased ADH* Glucocorticoid deficiency Severe hypokalemia	Acute renal failure Congestive heart failure Cirrhosis, nephrotic syndrome
Hypernatremia (increased serum [Na^+])	Fever, gastroenteritis Thyrotoxicosis Diabetes insipidus Profuse sweating	None	Excessive salt ingestion Inappropriate intravenous therapy
ABNORMAL [K^+]	**ABNORMAL METABOLISM**	**ABNORMAL EXCRETION**	**ABNORMAL POTASSIUM INTAKE**
Hyperkalemia (increased [K^+])	Insulin deficiency Acidemia Hypoaldosteronism Cell necrosis	Acute renal failure Chronic nephritis Hypoaldosteronism	Excessive use of salt substitutes High doses of potassium salt medications
Hypokalemia (decreased [K^+])	Alkalemia Rapid cell turnover (e.g., malignancy)	Vomiting/diarrhea Diuretic overdose Hyperaldosteronism Renal tubular acidosis	Anorexia Diet deficient in meats or vegetables

Modified from Widmann FK: Clinical interpretation of laboratory tests, ed 9, Philadelphia, 1979, Davis.
*ECF, extracellular fluid; ADH, antidiuretic hormone.

tracellular shift in concentration of the other cation, and anionic balance is maintained by passive diffusion of chloride anion. If cationic balance is severely affected, then basic physiologic functions governed by sodium-potassium flux across cellular membranes are affected. This is usually first apparent clinically as tetany and cardiac conduction defects. Abnormalities of cationic balance are summarized in Table 11-7.

Metabolic Molecules

Numerous small molecules are present in the circulating blood either as supply elements for basic metabolic processes or as by-products of these reactions. Identification of abnormal metabolic molecule concentrations in the circulating blood indicates the effects of metabolic dysfunction, such as diabetes mellitus, or diseases affecting centers of metabolic activity, such as the liver. In addition, monitoring the concentrations of certain metabolic molecules over a period of time is often essential to the determination of the current status of a previously diagnosed metabolic disease. Table 11-8 summarizes the clinical significance of abnormal findings for metabolic molecules.

Calcium and phosphorus. Calcium and

Table 11-8 Summary of frequently tested metabolic molecules and the possible causes of abnormal blood concentrations

Metabolic molecule and condition	Possible causes of abnormal blood concentration
Calcium	
Hypercalcemia	Malignancy, hyperparathyroidism, thiazide diuretics
Hypocalcemia	Hypoparathyroidism, malabsorption, renal failure, sepsis, vitamin D deficiency, alkalosis, pancreatitis
Phosphate	
Hyperphosphatemia	Renal failure, severe muscle injury, hypoparathyroidism
Hypophosphatemia	Parenteral hyperalimentation, diabetic acidosis, alcohol withdrawal, severe alkalosis
Glucose	
Hyperglycemia	Diabetes mellitus, hyperthyroidism, obesity, shock
Hypoglycemia	Insulin overdose, fasting, insulin-producing adenomas, other endocrine conditions, alcoholism
Cholesterol	
Hypercholesterolemia	Tendency for atherosclerosis and coronary artery disease
Blood urea nitrogen (BUN)	
Azotemia	Renal disease, decreased renal blood flow, urinary obstruction, infection, electrolyte loss, shock
Creatinine, elevated	Renal disease
Nonprotein nitrogen, total (NPN), elevated	Renal disease
Uric acid, hyperuricemia	Gout, cancer treatment, polycythemia, renal failure, ketoacidosis, certain drugs
Bilirubin, hyperbilibubinemia	
Unconjugated	Hemolysis, cholecystitis, cardiac disease, generalized infection, inflammatory gastrointestinal disease, cancer
Conjugated	Biliary obstruction
Both elevated	Hepatic disease, biliary obstruction

Modified from Ravel R: Clinical laboratory medicine: clinical application of laboratory data, ed 5, St Louis, 1989, Mosby—Year Book.

inorganic phosphorus are necessary for bone mineralization, and calcium is an essential factor in blood coagulation, neuromuscular function, and other physiologic processes. Serum calcium concentration is primarily regulated by parathyroid hormone, and it is influenced by dietary availability and vitamin D promotion of absorption. Elevated serum calcium concentration can result from hyperparathyroidism, certain malignant tumors, severe hyperthyroidism, and primary bone diseases. Clinical features of hypercalcemia include nonspecific neurologic symptoms, muscle weakness, peptic ulcers, and constipation. Hypocalcemia is produced by hypoparathyroidism, uremia, vitamin D deficiency, and acute pancreatitis, and it is indicated clinically by neuromuscular hyperexcitability, altered myocardial function, and tetany.

Serum phosphate concentration is controlled primarily by the amount of renal excretion. Therefore elevated phosphate concentration is a feature of renal failure. Hypophosphatemia is most commonly associated with diabetic ketoacidosis.

Glucose and cholesterol. Glucose is the basic substrate for cellular energy production, and its blood concentration is affected by insulin release from the pancreas, as well as by dietary intake. Elevated blood glucose usually indicates diabetes mellitus, although other conditions can be associated with persistent hyperglycemia. The reliability of the test in the diagnosis of diabetes depends on the timing of blood sampling relative to ingestion and absorption of food with a significant carbohydrate content. Therefore the definitive diagnosis of diabetes usually requires a fasting blood glucose test and a glucose tolerance test, which is a monitoring of the blood glucose level following a loading dose of glucose under strictly defined conditions. The most common cause of hypoglycemia is insulin overdosage.

Cholesterol is a component in the synthesis of cell membranes, adrenal cortical steroids, estrogens, and androgens. Dietary intake and synthesis by the liver provide adequate cholesterol concentration for these purposes. The primary issue in routine serum testing is to indicate hypercholesterolemia as a risk factor for atherosclerosis, ischemic heart disease, and stroke.

Metabolic by-products. Excessive blood concentration of metabolic by-products indicates disease affecting the primary metabolic organ, a defect in the metabolic process, or defective excretion. *Azotemia* is the condition of elevated blood urea nitrogen (BUN), nonprotein nitrogen (NPN), and creatinine concentrations; the presence of azotemia indicates the failure of the kidneys to clear these metabolic wastes from the blood. *Uremia* is the term to describe the clinical condition resulting from a toxic accumulation of these materials in the blood. High uric acid concentrations indicate either excessive purine metabolism or limited renal excretion that is clinically termed *gout.*

Bilirubin is produced by the metabolism of hemoglobin generated by hemolysis of erythrocytes in the spleen. Normally the bilirubin is then conjugated into a soluble form in the liver and excreted as bile. Elevated unconjugated bilirubin concentration suggests excessive hemolysis, hepatic dysfunction, or cardiac disease; elevated conjugated bilirubin implies biliary obstruction; and elevation of both may result from severe hepatic disease. The clinical manifestation of hyperbilirubinemia is *jaundice.*

Serum Proteins

Serum proteins function in coagulation, transport of insoluble metabolites, immunologic defense, maintenance of osmotic pressure, and similar physiologic processes. Total serum protein and the A/G ratio are the two screening tests routinely performed as a part of automated blood studies. Highly specific tests to determine the serum concentration of many hormones, binding proteins for certain metabolites, and other specific blood proteins are also available.

Table 11-9 Intracellular enzymes of diagnostic importance when significant serum concentrations are present

Enzyme	Primary diagnostic implications
Alkaline phosphatase	Active bone metabolism: normal growth in children, rickets, healing fractures, hyperparathyroidism, osteosarcoma, and Paget's disease of bone Hepatic disease and biliary obstruction
Acid phosphatase	Prostatic carcinoma
Amylase	Pancreatitis, sialadenitis
Alanine aminotransferase (ALT) (formerly referred to as GPT)	Hepatic disease excluding cirrhosis
Aspartate aminotransferase (AST) (formerly referred to as GOT)	Hepatic disease (hepatitis, cirrhosis), infectious mononucleosis, myocardial infarct (peak at 24-48 hours postinfarct), pancreatitis
Lactic dehydrogenase (LDH)	Hepatic disease (obstructive jaundice, cirrhosis, metastatic carcinoma); myocardial infarct (peaks 48-72 hours postinfarct); also, renal disease, skeletal muscle disease, and hemolytic anemia
Creatinine phosphokinase (CPK)	Myocardial infarct (peaks within 48 hours), skeletal muscle injury

Total serum protein. Albumins and globulins are quantitatively the most important serum proteins reflected in the determination of total serum protein concentration. Total serum protein concentration below the normal level of 6 to 8 gm% usually indicates hypoalbuminemia resulting from urinary loss caused by nephrosis, decreased synthesis caused by hepatic disease, extensive burns, or other debilitating conditions.

A/G Ratio. The A/G ratio is the proportion of albumin to globulins, and it is normally between 1.5 and 3. Comparison of an abnormal A/G ratio to the total protein concentration indicates whether the albumin or globulin component of total serum protein is affected. A high A/G ratio and low total serum protein suggests humoral immunodeficiency. A low A/G ratio and low total serum protein suggests hypoalbuminemia. A low A/G ratio and elevated total serum protein indicates increased globulins as observed with certain infections, autoimmune diseases, and multiple myeloma.

Intracellular Enzymes

A significant serum concentration of what is normally an intracellular enzyme indicates either excessive enzyme production or necrosis of the producing cells. The diagnostic value of this is that certain enzymes are only produced in significant quantities by the cells of certain organs. Therefore high serum concentration of a particular enzyme indicates disease or hyperactivity limited to one or a few specific sites. Table 11-9 lists the diagnostic significance of detecting several of the most commonly tested intracellular enzymes in serum.

Serologic Tests

Serologic tests rely on immunologic mechanisms to demonstrate the presence of either antibodies or antigens associated with specific infections and autoimmune diseases. Most serologic tests are designed either to identify a current infection or to demonstrate antibodies stimulated by past exposure to an organism and the current immunity to the disease.

Different infections and autoimmune diseases stimulate different immunologic response patterns. This determines the testing strategy that most effectively demonstrates a specific disease. For example, antibodies to the core antigen of the hepatitis B virus appear early in the infection, while antibodies to the hepatitis B viral surface antigen develop later in the infection. Therefore such factors must be considered when ordering and interpreting serologic tests. In contrast, tuberculosis stimulates primarily a cellular rather than a humoral response, which means that serologic testing is ineffective. The tuberculin test for tuberculosis relies on subcutaneous injection of inactivated tuberculin material to elicit the delayed hypersensitivity reaction mediated by the cellular immune system.

Screening serologic tests usually rely on indirect reactivity by immunologic mechanisms and are designed to be inexpensive, simple, and quick. Most screening tests are more likely to produce false-positive results that occasionally indicate healthy individuals are infected in comparison with definitive serologic tests. This demands that a definitive diagnosis should not be based on the results of a screening test. Definitive serologic tests rely on direct interaction of specific antigens with corresponding antibodies. These tests are highly specific and sensitive but they are also expensive and require sophisticated quality control measures. Therefore these tests are usually reserved for the definitive diagnosis of individuals identified by screening tests or clinical findings as likely to have the disease.

Serologic tests are usually quantitated by serial dilutions of the patient serum called *titers*. The weaker the dilution that still reacts, the stronger the antibody or antigen concentration was prior to dilution. The titer reflects the effectiveness of the patient's immune response to a current infection, the severity of the infection, the stage of the disease when compared with prior results, or the patient's humoral immunity against a specific organism.

Syphilis. The diagnosis of syphilis by serologic methods is particularly valuable because microbiologic demonstration of the organisms is notoriously difficult. Two commonly used syphilis screening tests rely on detection of a nonspecific antibacterial antibody called *reagin*. The *rapid plasma reagin (RPR) card test* is simple to perform and inexpensive. False-positive results are common, particularly with individuals suffering from autoimmune diseases or infectious mononucleosis. The *Venereal Disease Research Laboratory (VDRL) test* is based on similar mechanisms and is associated with the same limitations. The *Treponema pallidum hemagglutination test (TPHA)* and the *fluorescent treponemal antibody with absorbed serum (FTA-ABS) test* are the definitive serologic studies for syphilis and are highly specific and sensitive.

Infectious mononucleosis. Infectious mononucleosis is the infection that results from initial contact with the Epstein-Barr virus. The serologic hallmark is the formation of a *heterophil* or *Paul-Bunnell antibody* that causes sheep red blood cells to agglutinate. The antibody appears shortly after the initial symptoms develop and disappears approximately 6 months after the symptoms resolve. Definitive diagnosis is usually based on clinical findings in combination with a positive screening test.

Acquired immunodeficiency syndrome. Detection of human immunodeficiency virus (HIV) relies on the presence of either the antigenic viral components or antibodies formed by the patient in response to the HIV virus. The most common antibody test is the *Western blot test*. Test HIV antigens are separated by electrophoresis, then the patient's serum is exposed to the test strips. The antigen-antibody complexes are then demonstrated by an ELISA (enzyme-linked immunosorbent assay) sensitive to the complex. The test is complicated and expensive, but it is highly sensitive and specific. The antigen test relies on similar mechanisms, but the known component is the HIV antibody and the patient's serum serves as the test source for antigen. Both HIV antigen and antibody reactivity may not appear for 6 months or more following infection.

Viral hepatitis. *Hepatitis* refers to inflammation of the liver parenchyma. Nonviral forms of hepatitis include bacterial infections, biliary obstruction, and various intoxications. Clinical evidence of jaundice and fever or elevated serum enzyme studies (see Table 11-9) support only a nonspecific diagnosis of hepatitis.

Many disseminated viral infections, such as Epstein-Barr virus and cytomegalovirus, can cause liver inflammation as well as the more characteristic features of these infections. However, five distinct viruses infect the liver primarily and are designated hepatitis virus A, B, C, delta, and E. The features of these infections are summarized in Table 7-5. The diagnosis depends on clinical features of the infection and serologic demonstration of the infective virus. The serologic diagnostic strategy involves demonstration of both the viral antigen and the humoral antibody response of the patient by ELISA or similar immunologic techniques.

Hepatitis A and E. Hepatitis A is transmitted by oral-fecal contamination and is generally a mild infection of short duration. The most clinically significant aspect of identifying hepatitis A antigen or antibody is that this excludes the possibility of hepatitis B, C, or E infection. Hepatitis E is similar in most clinical respects to hepatitis A.

Hepatitis B. Hepatitis B is transmitted by blood-to-blood or intimate contact and is among the most communicable blood-borne human infections. The condition can linger for months, is usually more severe than hepatitis A, and occasionally produces serious complications. One such complication of hepatitis B is that certain patients fail to generate an effective immune response to the virus, which results in progression of the disease known as *chronic active hepatitis*. Also, a *carrier state* can develop in which a recovered, asymptomatic individual carries the virus and is infectious. An additional diagnostic problem with hepatitis B is that many cases are subclinical and nonicteric, which yields no historical indication of the past infection. Detection of the hep-

atitis B virus is a priority concern to avoid spreading the virus by blood donation and in health care settings.

A positive serologic test for hepatitis B surface antigen (HBsAg) can generally be obtained prior to the onset of jaundice and during the icteric phase of the infection. HBsAg typically disappears from the serum of the recovering patient within 1 to 2 months of the onset of jaundice. A positive HBsAg test indicates hepatitis B virus (HBV) as the infectious agent and that the blood is currently infectious. This test is the usual method of testing donated blood for HBV. Unfortunately, approximately 10% to 25% of jaundiced patients do not test positive for HBsAg and the diagnosis must be based on demonstration of an antibody response to HBV.

A positive serologic test for hepatitis Be antigen (HBeAg) is only seen in conjunction with a positive result from HBsAg. This indicates that the serum contains the intact virus and that the patient is highly infectious. A positive HBeAg test may occur prior to the appearance of antibodies to the disease or as an indication of inadequate immunologic response. It can also suggest the development of chronic active hepatitis and is typical of the carrier state if no evidence of antibodies to HBV is present.

A positive serologic test for hepatitis B core antibody (anti-HBc) is the earliest immunologic response of the patient to the virus. This implies that HBV is the infectious agent and that the patient is responding immunologically to the virus. Serologic demonstration of hepatitis B surface antibody (anti-HBs) involves roughly the same diagnostic implication as demonstration of anti-HBc. The surface antibody appears later in the course of the disease, represents the long-term immunity against hepatitis B, and is the usual method of testing acquired immunity following either infection or vaccination. A positive test for anti-HBs excludes the possibility of the carrier state. Testing for hepatitis Be antibody (anti-HBe) is usu-

Table 11-10   Summary of hepatitis B virus (HBV) serology and clinical implications of results

Serologic test	Abbreviation	Clinical significance
Hepatitis B surface antigen	HBsAg	Proves HBV is present and patient is infectious, but 10% to 25% of test results are false-negative
Hepatitis B core antigen	HBcAg	Seldom used since it provides no more information than the HBsAg test
Hepatitis Be antigen	HBeAg	Intact virus is present, patient is highly infectious; test reveals carrier state if antibody response is absent
Hepatitis B surface antibody	Anti-HBs	Indicates immune response, appears late in recovery and is used for testing long-term immunity
Hepatitis B core antibody	Anti-HBc	Indicates immunologic response, appears within weeks of onset of jaundice
Hepatitis Be antibody	Anti-HBe	Positive test excludes carrier state
Hepatitis A antigen/antibody	HAAg/anti-HA	Either may exclude HBV from differential diagnosis of hepatitis

ally undertaken to exclude the possibility of a carrier state, although demonstration of anti-HBs or anti-HBc typically supports the same conclusion. Hepatitis B serology is summarized in Table 11-10.

Delta hepatitis can only develop simultaneously with hepatitis B infection because replication of the delta virus relies on the HBV genetic codes. The primary significance of the combination of HBV and delta hepatitis infections is that this combination is associated with a greater probability of complications, such as the progression to chronic forms of viral hepatitis.

Hepatitis C. Hepatitis C was referred to as non-A, non-B hepatitis until recently because specific serologic demonstration of the disease had not been developed. The virus has now been identified, and the clinical features as well as serologic testing are similar in most respects to hepatitis B.

Serology of Autoimmune Diseases

Autoimmune diseases, such as rheumatoid arthritis, systemic lupus erythematosus, and systemic sclerosis, are usually suspected on the basis of clinical abnormalities, an elevated erythrocyte sedimentation rate, or decreased A/G ratio. However, specific serologic findings are particularly helpful in the diagnosis of relatively frequent instances of patients who exhibit autoimmune manifestations that do not clearly match the typical features of a specific autoimmune disease. Also, the reactive serologic titer at the time of diagnosis is often a significant prognostic indicator, as well as a baseline value for comparison during the course of the disease.

Rheumatoid factor. Rheumatoid factor (RF) actually refers to a heterogeneous group of immunoglubulins that react with the IgG immunoglobulin molecule. Complement activation by this antigen-antibody complex and the resulting inflammatory response contribute to the damage to synovial membranes that characterizes rheumatoid arthritis. The most commonly used test to detect RF is called the *latex agglutination test,* although other methods are available. Approximately 80% of rheumatoid arthritis patients are RF positive and high titers at the time of diagnosis are generally a poor prognostic indicator. RF is also an occasional observation in other autoimmune diseases.

Antinuclear antibodies. Antinuclear antibody (ANA) formation to various nuclear components is a diagnostic feature of several autoimmune diseases. An indirect immunofluorescence approach called the *fluorescent antinuclear antibody test (FANA)* is used to react patient serum with nonhuman nuclear components. Fluorescence is present in nearly all patients with lupus erythematosus. A positive FANA test is also noted in approximately two thirds of patients with Sjögren syndrome, over one third of systemic sclerosis patients, and in some cases of rheumatoid arthritis. Titers generally correspond to progression and prognosis of the disease.

Organ specific antibodies. Immunologic testing is also available for a variety of organ specific antibodies. Positive results contribute to the diagnosis of certain thyroid conditions, some renal diseases, myasthenia gravis, and several forms of hemolytic anemia.

BACTERIAL CULTURE AND SENSITIVITY TESTING

Culture and sensitivity tests identify causative microorganisms of a specific infection and the antibiotics that will be effective in controlling that infection. A representative, uncontaminated specimen of the infection is required, and this can be difficult to obtain in the oral cavity.

Direct Preparation

Certain organisms are adequately characteristic morphologically to allow identification by direct preparation and microscopic examination. Lesion contents are aspirated or smeared on a glass slide, fixed, and stained. This is useful for superficial "coccal" infections and actinomycosis. The advantage of direct preparation is that the results are immediately available.

Microbial Culture

Isolation of a specimen by aspiration or a sterile swab and introduction of the material into an appropriate culture medium are more commonly used techniques than is direct preparation for several reasons. Growth of the culture allows testing with antibiotic disks to demonstrate specific antibiotic sensitivity as well as identification of the organism, if necessary. The major disadvantage of bacterial culture is that the process requires several days. Also, the normal flora often grow better in culture than the pathogens, which may yield misleading results. An empiric course of antibiotics prior to securing the specimen can also adversely affect culture and sensitivity studies. Special techniques are required if infection by an anaerobic organism is suspected.

URINALYSIS

The examination of the urine is a routine screening procedure that is useful for detecting renal disease and common metabolic disorders, such as diabetes. Most of the tests are relatively simple and inexpensive. Screening urinalysis is summarized in Table 11-11.

General Features

Normal urine appears clear and amber in color. Blood, bile, some foods, and certain drugs can alter the color. Cloudiness usually indicates the presence of pus, bacteria, or protein. Normal urine is slightly acidic with a pH range from 4.7 to 8.0. A lower or higher pH suggests acidosis or alkalosis. Normal specific gravity of urine ranges from 1.010 to 1.025 and low values suggest minimal renal concentration resulting from medullary or tubular damage. High specific gravity suggests the presence of glucose or protein. Urine volume is usually measured following collection for 24 hours, and the normal range is adjusted relative to the patient's size and fluid intake. Excessive volume can indicate diabetes, while decreased volume usually results from renal failure.

Microscopic Features

The microscopic examination of the urine is made on the solid sediment following cen-

Table 11-11   Summary of urinalysis and clinical implications of abnormal results

Evaluation method	Normal	Clinical implications of abnormal results
Appearance	Clear, amber	Cloudiness: Pus, bacteria, protein
		Discoloration: Blood, bile, metabolic disease, certain foods, medications
pH	4.7-8.0	Metabolic acidosis suggested below 4.7, alkalosis indicated above 8.0
Specific gravity	1.010-1.025	Lower results suggest tubular or medullary damage
		Higher results suggest the presence of protein or glucose
Volume	Varies	Polyuria or anuria, judged in relation to patient size and fluid intake
Microscopic	Few cells or casts	Bleeding, infection; erythrocyte or bacterial casts indicate kidney disease, and separate cells or bacterial colonies suggest lower urinary tract origin; numerous hyalin casts suggest proteinuria and/or stasis
Chemical tests		
Protein	Negligible	Usually albumin indicative of glomerular damage (nephrotic syndrome)
Glucose	Negligible	Diabetes mellitus
Acetone	Negligible	Fat metabolism, either diabetes mellitus or calorie deficient diet
Bilirubin	Negligible	Biliary obstruction or hepatitis
Others	Negligible	Specific tests can identify materials in urine suggestive of pregnancy, multiple myeloma, illicit drug use, and other conditions

trifugation. The most common findings that are considered abnormal include blood cells, bacterial colonies, and urinary casts.

Urinary casts are tubular-shaped bodies composed of gelled protein (hyaline) and tubular epithelial cells. A few casts are normally present in urine, particularly with older patients. Numerous casts indicate tubular or glomerular disease. Red cell or white cell casts suggest bleeding or infection within the kidney. Scattered erythrocytes or white cells indicate that the bleeding or infection involves the lower urinary tract. The association of bacterial colonies with casts reflects renal infection, while free colonies suggest the infection affects the urethra, bladder, or ureter.

Tests for Specific Substances

Urine normally does not contain significant concentrations of metabolic molecules or pro-

tein. Screening tests to identify specific abnormal substances in the urine are available as convenient and inexpensive "dip" sticks that are impregnated with the necessary reagents. Positive findings demand referral for more comprehensive analysis.

Protein in the urine, particularly albumin, implies glomerular loss of blood protein, referred to as the *nephrotic syndrome.* Certain specific proteins are indicative of pregnancy, multiple myeloma, and other diseases. Glucose in the urine without protein reflects the hyperglycemia of either undiagnosed or uncontrolled diabetes mellitus. Acetone in urine indicates ketoacidosis resulting from incomplete lipid metabolism, which is characteristic of diabetes, starvation, or cachexia. Bile in the urine suggests biliary obstruction or hepatitis. Several other definitive tests are available for comprehensive analysis of urine contents.

SURGICAL PATHOLOGY

Microscopic or *histopathologic* examination of tissues that have been surgically removed from the patient is referred to as *surgical pathology*. Surgical pathology is the only definitive diagnostic method for many superficial mucosal lesions and soft tissue enlargements. Unfortunately, the diagnostic value of surgical pathology can leave the clinician with the impression that histopathologic examination is the only source of definitive diagnostic information for *all* diseases. This incorrect assumption may promote less complete clinical evaluation of the patient's condition. Effective application of surgical pathology requires correlation of histopathologic findings with all available diagnostic information.

Methods of Tissue Acquisition

A *biopsy* is the controlled and deliberate removal of tissue from a living organism for the purpose of microscopic examination. This is warranted if the clinical assessment of a lesion does not support a definitive diagnosis. This is particularly important if findings suggest even a remote possibility of malignant neoplasia. A biopsy is also justified if the clinical course of a lesion diagnosed on the basis of clinical features is inconsistent with the initial diagnosis. A biopsy is not justified if a definitive clinical diagnosis of an inconsequential abnormality can be achieved. The technique selected for acquiring a tissue specimen is determined by the nature of the lesion and the possible conditions considered in the differential diagnosis.

Excisional biopsy. The goals of excisional biopsy are to obtain the entire abnormality for histopathologic examination and to provide definitive treatment by the total removal of the lesion. Excisional biopsy is the optimal approach for relatively small, isolated oral lesions.

Adequate deep and lateral margins of normal appearing tissue must be excised to ensure that no remnants of the lesion remain as a po-

tential source of recurrence as suggested in Fig. 11-4. The width of peripheral normal tissue to be included in the excision depends on the diseases considered in the differential diagnosis. A relatively narrow periphery of normal tissue is excised if the differential diagnosis is limited to lesions that seldom recur. Consideration of lesions that often recur justifies excision of wider margins. Inclusion of adjacent normal tissue also indicates the tissue orientation during the histopathologic examination. The cellular features in the area of transition from normal to abnormal tissue of many lesions is an essential element of the pathologist's assessment.

The recommendations of the Joint Commission on Accreditation of Hospitals specify that microscopic examination by a qualified pathologist is required in all instances of tissue excision. The rationale is that if removal of a lesion is justified, then histopathologic examination is also justified. This recommendation has been accepted as a general guideline in the handling of tissue in all health care settings. Therefore tissue excised primarily as a therapeutic procedure should be submitted for examination to confirm the diagnosis even though this may not be the clinician's clinical priority.

Incisional biopsy. The goal of incisional biopsy is to obtain an intact tissue specimen for histopathologic examination without attempting to treat the abnormality by removal. This is indicated for conditions such as multiple ulcers that cannot be eliminated by surgical excision and for large lesions that require a definitive diagnosis in order to plan optimal treatment.

The specimen must contain representative tissue of the lesion and at least one periphery of normal tissue for specimen orientation and demonstration of the interface between normal and abnormal tissues. The wedge incisional approaches shown in Fig. 11-5, *A* and *B*, generally produce tissue representative of the central, deep, and peripheral portions of the lesion.

CROSS-SECTIONAL VIEWS

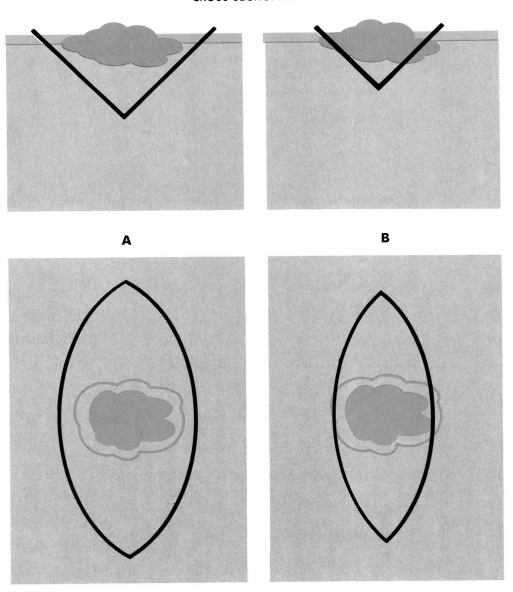

SURFACE VIEWS

Fig. 11-4   The goal of the excisional biopsy is to completely remove the lesion. This is accomplished with the surgical design illustrated in **A,** which includes an adequate border of normal appearing tissue at the lateral and deep margins of the lesion. Close approximation of the excision to the visually obvious abnormal tissue margins as shown in **B** risks leaving abnormal tissue and dramatically increases the probability that the lesion will still be present after healing.

CROSS-SECTIONAL VIEWS

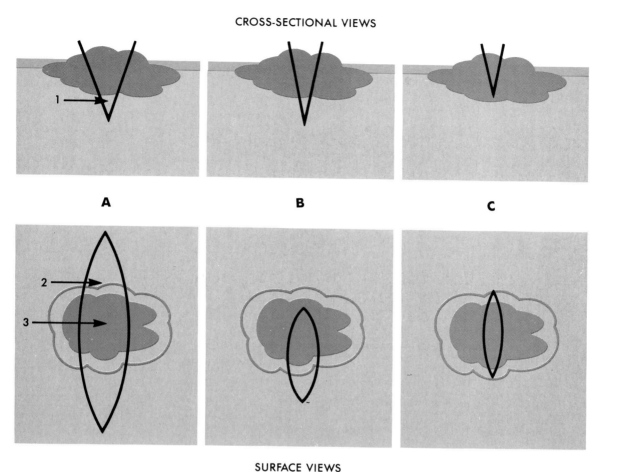

SURFACE VIEWS

Fig. 11-5 The goal of the incisional biopsy is to obtain a diagnostically representative specimen including a periphery of normal tissue at the deep margin (1), normal tissue at the lateral margin (2), and abnormal tissue from the center of the lesion (3). The incision designs illustrated in both **A** and **B** accomplish all three of these goals. The conservative incision approach illustrated in **C** will fail to include the diagnostically critical transition from abnormal to normal tissue at the deep and lateral borders.

Exfoliative cytology. This procedure is the collection and examination of cells scraped with a blunt instrument or tongue blade from the surface of a suspected lesion. The scrapings are immediately spread on a glass slide and sprayed with an aerosol fixative. Commercial hair spray may also be used if fixative is unavailable. Exfoliative cytology or a "Pap smear" is a common and effective method of screening women for malignant and premalignant cervical lesions. Screening of oral lesions for evidence of malignancy by exfoliative cytology is considered somewhat unreliable and difficult to justify in view of the accessibility of oral surface lesions for biopsy procedures. Exfoliative cytology is, however, an effective method for demonstrating mucosal candidiasis and some viral lesions.

Specimen Handling During Biopsy Procedures

Irrespective of the specific biopsy approach, careful manipulation of the tissue provides the pathologist with an optimal specimen.

Surgical technique. Sharp dissection is preferable to blunt dissection during biopsy procedures since this minimizes tissue stretching and tearing. Anesthetic solution and surgical markers such as India ink produce artifacts and should be introduced away from the planned tissue specimen. Grasping the specimen with forceps should be minimized to avoid crushing the specimen.

Tissue fixation. The fixative for routine pathologic examination is a 10% formalin solution in a volume at least 10 times the volume of the specimen to ensure complete fixation. The tissue should be immersed immediately after removal to minimize desiccation. Thin tissue specimens are spread on a piece of glazed paper prior to fixation to avoid tissue shrinkage and curling. Fixation for special diagnostic techniques such as immunofluorescence and electron microscopy requires special fixation techniques that should be arranged prior to the biopsy. These special procedures are severely compromised or impossible after formalin fixation.

Submitting The Specimen

Many clinically diverse conditions exhibit similar histopathologic features. The pathologist can offer the most accurate diagnosis by drawing on both the histopathologic findings and significant clinical information. Also, inconsistency of the clinical and microscopic features alerts the pathologist to the possibility that the tissue specimen may not fully represent the lesion of concern to the clinician. The information provided by the clinician should include identification of the specimen, the case history, a description of the lesion represented by the specimen, and the specific biopsy technique. Surgical pathology services provide forms to organize this information.

Identification of the specimen and case history. The identification of the specimen includes the patient's name and demographic data that may influence the diagnosis such as gender, age, and race. The clinician's name, address, and the date of the biopsy are also included. The patient's insurance carrier and other facts may be requested for administrative purposes.

The history of the abnormality is concisely summarized. This includes the lesion duration, symptoms described by the patient, and the clinical course. The presence of any other similar lesions in the mouth, history of a prior lesion at the same site, or possible contributing factors such as a tobacco habit are described. Significant findings of the clinical examination, such as fever or palpable regional lymph nodes, and data from the patient's medical history that conceivably could be related to the lesion are also included.

Lesion description. The description of the lesion includes the location stated in anatomic terms, the size as measured in metric units, and the color compared with normal mucosa. The shape of the lesion is usually described in geometric terms as oval, rectangular, or irregular, and the consistency of the lesion to palpation is communicated by words such as firm, indurated, or fluctuant. Sessile, pedunculated, exophytic, or cavitated are expressions of the lesion's relationship to adjacent tissue contours. Abnormal enlargements are often described as fixed or movable to convey whether or not the lesion is attached to surrounding normal tissues. Erythema, ulceration, and other features of the lesion should be stated along with any suspicion that these findings might be caused by incidental trauma or similar secondary influences. Submission of contributory clinical photographs or radiographs with the tissue specimen often aids the pathologist and simplifies the lesion description.

Clinical impression and biopsy method. The practitioner provides the pathologist with insight into the character of the abnormality by relating the clinical impression and listing other abnormalities considered in the differential diagnosis. The clinician's priority may be to exclude a serious disease such as squamous cell carcinoma from diagnostic consideration. This is conveyed by stating the clinical impression followed by the phrase "rule out" and the serious condition as, "Clinical impression: physiologic hyperkeratosis, rule out squamous cell carcinoma." The clinician can communicate that two conditions are considered equally probable by the use of the word "versus" in the clinical impression statement: ". . . physiologic hyperkeratosis versus squamous cell carcinoma." Specifying whether the tissue acquisition procedure was excisional or incisional informs the pathologist if complete removal of the lesion was the clinician's goal.

Interpreting The Surgical Pathology Report

The surgical pathology or biopsy report communicates the pathologist's opinions concerning the tissue specimen to the practitioner. The most significant element of the surgical pathology report is the diagnosis. However, the clinician must often consider other information contained in the report to fully appreciate the pathologist's diagnosis. The format includes the patient summary, gross description of the specimen, microscopic description of the tissues, the diagnosis, and any additional comments by the pathologist.

Patient summary. The patient summary restates the patient information provided by the clinician. The clinician should review this information to identify any inaccuracies that may affect the diagnosis. The only new information in this section is the reference number or *accession number* assigned to the specimen by the pathologist. Any future communications with the pathologist about the case should include this accession number.

Gross and histopathologic descriptions. The macroscopic features of the tissue specimen including color, general shape, and metric dimensions are detailed in the gross description section. Macroscopic features can provide confirmational diagnostic information in some cases.

The microscopic features of the specimen include the composition of normal tissues and any abnormal findings. The use of special stains other than hematoxylin and eosin to demonstrate specific tissue components or microorganisms is reported in this section. The histopathologic description can supplement the clinician's understanding of the pathologist's diagnosis and may reveal the severity of some lesions. In addition, the microscopic description should indicate if the lesion extends to the specimen margins, which in cases of excisional biopsy may suggest the possibility of recurrence.

Diagnosis. This is the pathologist's opinion of the patient's condition based on the tissue specimen and the clinical information provided. The anatomic location of the lesion is usually specified after the diagnosis. *Comments* are occasionally added to the biopsy report by the pathologist to clarify an unusual or nonspecific diagnosis, suggest additional diagnostic procedures, or recommend treatment methods.

Any photographs or radiographs submitted with the specimen are returned to the clinician with the biopsy report unless such materials were identified as intended for the pathologist's files. Many surgical pathology services also send a prepared microscopic section of the specimen with the biopsy report.

The Pathologist's Approach To Diagnostic Limitations

The pathologist's goal is to provide the most specific diagnosis justified by the clinical information and the histopathologic characteristics of the tissue specimen. Unfortunately, the combined clinical and histopathologic findings of individual cases may not fulfill the criteria for a specific diagnosis or contradictory features may be present. The pathologist can communicate the diagnostic limitation of such cases to the clinician in three ways: (1) A relatively nonspecific diagnosis can be made. (2) A specific diagnosis can be made that includes a qualifying term to indicate a degree of diagnostic reservation. (3) A descriptive diagnosis can be provided. In all three situations, the pathologist usually explains the diagnostic limitation with a comment.

Nonspecific histopathologic diagnosis. A nonspecific diagnosis defines the lesion as specifically as possible within a disease category. This can be illustrated by the example of a patient with a cystic lesion associated with an unerupted third molar. If the histopathologic features of a dentigerous cyst are present and the clinical description or a radiograph indicates that the molar is impacted, then a specific diagnosis of dentigerous cyst can be made. The pathologist may be forced to make a less specific diagnosis of follicular cyst if the eruption status of the molar is not described, because this diagnosis includes the possibility of either a dentigerous cyst or an eruption cyst. The pathologist may be limited to a diagnosis of odontogenic cyst for the same tissue specimen if the association of the lesion with a tooth is not clarified. In each case the diagnosis of a cyst is clearly demonstrated by the specimen, but diagnostic specification among cystic lesions cannot be made without additional information.

Diagnostic qualifying terms. Several phrases can be combined with the most probable diagnosis to reflect the pathologist's reservations. Using the cyst example, the pathologist could assign the diagnosis "suggestive of dentigerous cyst" if uncertain about the eruption status of the third molar. This conveys that the lesion is probably a dentigerous cyst, but an eruption cyst is also possible. The diagnosis of "consistent with dentigerous cyst" for the same specimen if the location of the lesion were not specified conveys that this could be a dentigerous cyst if clinical findings can confirm the diagnosis. The designation "compatible with dentigerous cyst" is reserved for situations in which unusual histopathologic features are present but clinical information strongly supports the diagnosis. This translates to mean that the lesion might be a dentigerous cyst, but the histopathologic features are inconsistent enough that additional clinical information could support a different diagnosis.

Descriptive diagnosis. A descriptive histopathologic diagnosis states the principal histopathologic features of the specimen as the diagnosis. An example could involve tissue fragments surgically removed from the region of a partially erupted third molar, and the tissue exhibits microscopic features of acute inflammation. Pericoronitis, periodontal abscess, inflammation of a dentigerous cyst, or a periapical abscess are all possible diagnoses depending on the relationship of the lesion to the teeth and other features. The pathologist may offer the diagnosis "epithelial lined connective tissue with acute inflammation" as the best indication of the disease process without speculating on the specific cause of the inflammation.

The pathologist's choice of how to communicate diagnostic limitations in a specific situation depends on several factors including the clinical information provided by the clinician, the histopathologic features of the specimen, and the training of the pathologist. The priority for the clinician is to appreciate that the pathologist's diagnosis is made with reservation and that a definitive diagnosis requires additional evaluation of clinical information by the dentist.

Diagnostic Responsibilities of the Pathologist and the Clinician

Both the pathologist and the clinician contribute to the diagnosis of a lesion examined microscopically, but the diagnostic responsibilities for the pathologist and the clinician are distinctly different. The pathologist accepts responsibility for the diagnosis of a tissue specimen with the additional input of clinical information. The clinician assumes responsibility for the diagnosis of the patient's condition as supported by the histopathologic opinion of the pathologist. Stated simply, the pathologist makes a diagnosis of a tissue specimen, while the clinician makes the diagnosis of the patient's condition. The clinician must, therefore, assess the consistency of the pathologist's diagnosis with the clinical manifestations of the abnormality in making the definitive clinical diagnosis as suggested by the case illustrated in Fig. 11-6.

Indication of diagnostic limitation, such as a nonspecific diagnosis, by the pathologist forces the clinician to reassess the clinical findings with the added insight of the histopathologic findings. Prior information must be reevaluated for accuracy or supplemented with new information to overcome, if possible, the diagnostic problem. A comment by the pathologist in the surgical pathology report often suggests methods of reaching a definitive diagnosis.

SUMMARY

Clinical laboratory methods provide an effective, efficient, and relatively inexpensive approach to obtaining diagnostic information from blood, urine, and other patient specimens. Both screening and definitive laboratory test results can provide a comprehensive profile of the patient's health status when considered in the context of clinical findings. Laboratory tests are categorized as red cell studies, white cell counts, evaluation of hemostasis, blood chemistry tests, microbial techniques, and urinalysis.

Red cell studies primarily identify anemia, which can affect the patient's ability to resist infection and surgical stress and which can also indicate an underlying illness. White cell studies can demonstrate the integrity of the patient's cellular defense against infection and

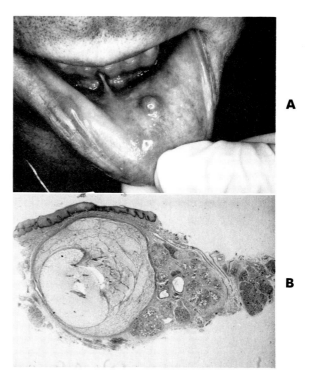

A

B

Fig. 11-6 The lesion shown by **A** was a compressible, slightly pale, nontender, dome-shaped enlargement of the lower lip that fluctuated in size over its 4 week duration. These features are characteristic of a mucous retention phenomenon as described in Chapter 18. Following excision and preparation of the specimen, the pathologist observed a region of pooled saliva with the connective tissue adjacent to minor salivary gland tissue (**B**). This justified a tissue diagnosis of mucous retention phenomenon. The clinician can comfortably make the clinical diagnosis when the original clinical features of the abnormality are consistent with the histopathologic findings and the pathologist's tissue diagnosis. The patient history, clinical findings, and the surgical pathology report must all be reconsidered before making a definitive diagnosis if inconsistencies become apparent.

provide evidence of the type of organism causing an active infection. Tests of hemostasis can reveal deficiencies of platelets or coagulation factors in instances of a suspected bleeding tendency. Blood chemistry tests reflect the status of basic metabolic functions, the health of internal organs, and the possibility of certain infections. Microbial preparations can reveal the organism causing a specific infection and the most effective treatment by antibiotic sensitivity testing. Urinalysis provides evidence of renal function, as well as evidence of certain other metabolic diseases, such as diabetes mellitus.

Many conditions affecting the oral cavity require histopathologic examination to achieve a definitive diagnosis. Methods of obtaining tissue include excisional biopsy, incisional biopsy, and exfoliative cytology. Excisional biopsy attempts to remove the entire lesion as definitive treatment in addition to obtaining the tissue. Incisional biopsy removes a portion of a lesion to obtain the histopathologic diagnosis needed to plan definitive management of conditions not treatable initially by excision. Exfoliative cytology is microscopic evaluation of superficial scraping from oral surface lesions, and it is most effective in confirming a working diagnosis of oral candidiasis and some viral lesions. Interpretation of opinions of the pathologist as stated in the surgical pathology report requires an understanding of the pathologist's diagnostic perspective, particularly in situations associated with diagnostic limitations. Effective communications between the pathologist and the clinician is essential in achieving the most accurate diagnosis and optimal management of the patient's condition.

BIBLIOGRAPHY

Brightman VJ: Diagnostic laboratory procedures. In Lynch MA, Brightman VJ, Greenberg MS, editors: Burket's oral medicine: diagnosis and treatment, ed 8, Philadelphia, 1984, Lippincott.

Greenspan D and others: AIDS and the mouth: diagnosis and management of oral lesions, Copenhagen, 1990, Munksgaard.

Langlais RP and others: Oral diagnosis, oral medicine and treatment planning, Philadelphia, 1984, Saunders.

Nairas RG, Gardner LB: Simple acid-base disturbances, Med Clin North Am 65:321-346, 1981.

Platt WR: Color atlas and textbook of hematology, Philadelphia, 1979, Lippincott.

Ravel R: Clinical laboratory medicine: clinical application of laboratory data, ed 5, St Louis, 1989, Mosby—Year Book.

Sabes WR: The dentist and clinical laboratory procedures, St Louis, 1979, Mosby—Year Book.

Shira RB: Biopsy in oral diagnosis and treatment planning, Dent Clin North Am 7:41-54, (March) 1963.

Widmann FK: Clinical interpretation of laboratory tests, ed 9, Philadelphia, 1979, Davis.

CHAPTER 12

Dental Treatment Planning

GARY C. COLEMAN

Dental treatment planning is the formulation of a strategy to solve as many of the patient's dental problems as possible. This is the final aspect of the diagnostic process for common dental conditions before active treatment. The problem-oriented patient record provides an effective organizational format for the complex information that must be correlated during dental treatment planning. The diagnostic database identifies abnormalities and problems that require treatment in the general order of urgency. The nature of these dental problems and opinions expressed by the patient direct the clinician in determining treatment goals. Specific treatment goals then direct the selection from among the treatment options for each of the patient's problems, as well as suggesting the optimal treatment sequence. Finally, the *case presentation* allows the dentist to describe the diagnostic findings in the patient's case, the preliminary treatment plan for the patient, and available treatment options to the patient.

LISTING OF PROBLEMS

The patient's complaints, conditions, lesions, and other problems are listed in the general order in which they have been identified during the patient interview and clinical examination. The results of specialized diagnostic tests and consultations may still be unavailable, but the best current assessment of each problem is listed. Patient problems are categorized as related to the chief complaint, potential medical complications, and oral conditions. Each entry in the listing of problems concisely indicates the clinician's current understanding of the problem without extraneous detail. One indication of the items to be listed is that any clinical procedure in the treatment plan must be justified by a corresponding problem. Accurately listing the patient's problems allows the treatment plan to be directly derived.

Chief Complaint

Many chief complaints such as pain, acute infection, bleeding, and traumatic injury require immediate attention. The chief complaint may also be a request for less urgent care, as in the case of patients requesting a "cleaning." The listing of the chief complaint should be the working diagnosis of the condition rather than the chief complaint as stated by the patient. For example, the entry "#8-subluxation caused by blunt trauma" is more meaningful in the treatment planning process than the patient's indication that the "front tooth is sore and loose since the car accident." Patients may report several complaints, which are listed in the order of priority as stated by the patient.

Potential Medical Complications

The patient's medical conditions that could present complications during routine dental treatment are listed as problems. This does not imply that the dentist will treat these conditions, but that recognition and prevention of potential complications by modification of dental procedures is an active problem solving process. These potential problems are categorized as diagnosed medical conditions, current medications, known hypersensitivity to medications, and undiagnosed medical conditions.

Diagnosed medical conditions. Conditions of compromised cardiovascular function are most likely to increase the risk of serious complications during routine dental procedures. Examples of other conditions that can cause complications during dental treatment include asthma, epilepsy, bleeding disorders, pregnancy, and diabetes. Patients' understanding of the effectiveness of current medical treatment, physical limitations, and potential complications of their own diseases can be dependable. This may be an adequate basis for the dentist to decide the necessary modifications of dental procedures. The need for a medical consultation is often indicated by poor patient understanding of the condition, failure to comply with medical treatment, long duration since the condition was evaluated, or features suggesting ineffective treatment. The expected physiologic and emotional demands during the patient's dental treatment are additional factors in determining whether or not a medical condition represents a potential complication. The minimal stress of routine operative procedures may be well tolerated by a medically compromised patient who would be at risk for complications during the extraction of numerous teeth.

Current medications. Certain medications may pose the threat of altered response of the patient during dental treatment or potentiation of the effects caused by drugs that are routinely used during dental procedures. Anticoagulant therapy and the resulting alteration of hemostatic function is an obvious consideration in the planning of surgical procedures. Other commonly encountered examples are described in Chapter 13. The problem listing contains any alteration of routine dental treatment that the dentist decides is necessary to accommodate the patient's medications. Sometimes, the appropriate solution to the problem is to list the need for consultation, particularly if alteration of the drug regimen prescribed by another clinician is necessary.

Hypersensitivity. Allergic and idiosyncratic responses to medications or materials that may come into contact with the patient during dental treatment should be listed as potential problems. This listing will help to avoid inadvertent exposure to drugs and other sources of allergic complications such as latex gloves. All drug hypersensitivities are listed regardless of whether or not the drug is commonly prescribed by the dentist. The indication of an idiosyncratic reaction to a rarely used drug in dentistry such as morphine may suggest the possibility of hypersensitivity to codeine, which is often prescribed by the dentist.

Undiagnosed medical conditions. Any undiagnosed diseases that are suspected by the dentist should be listed as problems. This confirms the importance in the problem-solving process of informing the patient of the suspicion and suggesting medical consultation.

Oral Diseases and Conditions

The patient's dental problems other than the chief complaint are categorized as periodontitis, degenerative dental lesions, complications of eruption, missing teeth, and other less common conditions. This sequence of listing dental problems reflects higher treatment priority for infectious conditions, while less rapidly progressive problems are given a lower priority.

Periodontitis. A summary of the patient's periodontal condition is the initial item listed among dental problems. Exceptional conditions such as rapidly progressive periodontitis or acute necrotizing ulcerative gingivitis should be specified. Poor prognostic indicators such as mobility, furcation involvements, and infracrestal cratering should be identified as specific problems after the general periodontal assessment.

Degenerative dental lesions. This category of dental problems includes periapical inflammatory lesions secondary to pulpal necrosis, pulpitis, and carious lesions in that order of importance. Periapical lesions with purulent drainage or other evidence of active infection are given priority over asymptomatic lesions identified radiographically. Examples of pulpitis that are likely to be listed at this stage of the priority sequence rather than as a chief complaint involve episodic or mild symptoms indicative of reversible pulpitis. Carious lesions are usually listed in the order of greatest axial extent, although esthetic considerations and other factors may alter priorities. Multiple lesions of one tooth are listed separately if the typical restorative approach involves separate restorations.

Complications of eruption. The dental conditions resulting from abnormal eruption assume priority after degenerative dental diseases in the listing of problems. This includes chronic pericoronitis, ectopic eruption, impaction, and malalignment of teeth. With the exception of the acute pericoronitis, treatment of these problems is generally less urgent than are periodontitis and active, degenerative dental lesions. Many problems such as an impacted, asymptomatic tooth or minor malalignment of teeth may not justify any treatment. In other cases, correction of malalignment or ectopic eruption may be essential to the effective control of periodontitis or other problems.

Consequences of missing teeth. This category includes edentulous spaces, supereruption, unfavorable esthetics, and compromised masticatory function. These problems are less urgent than the treatment of active carious, periodontal, and periapical lesions. Therefore their treatment is usually in the final stage of active dental treatment. This is also the appropriate category in which to list current dental prostheses that are unsatisfactory.

Nondental oral conditions. This group of nondental problems consists of mucosal lesions, soft tissue enlargements, bone lesions, and findings that suggest a clinical syndrome. These lesions generally represent diagnostic challenges beyond routine dental conditions and require specialized management. Subsequent chapters are devoted to the discussion of their differential diagnosis and treatment. Treatment priority for such problems may be justified at any stage of the treatment sequence depending on the condition.

LISTING POSSIBLE SOLUTIONS FOR PATIENT PROBLEMS

Many of the patient's problems can only be solved by a specific procedure, and for some problems several alternative solutions are available. General treatment options for dental conditions are described in Chapter 8. The following sections correlate categories of patient problems with typical options to solve the problems. In the process of formulating the treatment plan, the possible solutions for each problem are written adjacent to the corresponding condition in the listing of patient problems. This provides a reminder of the treatment options during the formulation of the comprehensive treatment plan for a specific patient. Table 12-1 summarizes the general treatment planning options available for common patient problems.

Problem-Solving Options for Chief Complaints

The immediate solutions available for chief complaints may be considered either *palliative* or *curative treatment*. Palliative care attempts to control the symptoms of a diagnosed problem and definitive treatment is directed to eliminating the problem. Palliative treatment in the cases of a painful periapical abscess might include prescription of a pain medication and an antibiotic. Curative treatment would entail either extraction of the tooth or initiation of endodontic treatment. Whenever possible, curative treatment is the optimal goal. Palliative care may be necessary until curative treatment can be arranged, such as in cases of severe infection, potential medical complications requiring consultation, and the need for specialty care.

Less urgent chief complaints may involve lost restorations, coronal tooth fractures, mild symptoms of pulpitis, and carious lesions. Sedative restorations using zinc oxide and eugenol cements are an effective approach to relief of symptoms and allow reevaluation of pulpitis before restoration. Permanent restoration can often be accomplished if irreversible pulpitis is considered unlikely. Prefabricated temporary crowns can provide interim restoration of large carious lesions until a more comprehensive treatment can be accomplished. Less urgent complaints can typically be deferred until a definitive treatment plan can be formulated later in the treatment sequence.

Problem-Solving Options for Potential Medical Complications

The dentist's principle alternatives in solving the problems posed by potential medical complications are either to make the decisions concerning necessary modification of dental procedures or to obtain definitive medical assessment by consultation. The treatment planning goal is always prevention of complications.

Chapter 13 discusses recommended modifications of dental treatment to minimize the risks associated with various common medical conditions. The treatment modification is listed as the appropriate solution for the problem in the treatment planning process. A common example is the requirement for prophylactic antibiotic coverage against infective endocarditis during dental treatment for the patient with a history of mitral valve prolapse with regurgitation. The confidence to make these decisions depends on the reliability of the patient's medical history, the dentist's understanding of the condition, the control achieved by current medical treatment, and how recently the physician has reevaluated the patient. Significant doubts about the patient history, the status of the condition, or appropriate clinical management suggests the need for consultation.

Alterations of dental procedures necessary to avoid complications related to current medications should be specifically listed in the problem-solving section of the treatment plan. The contraindication to the use of epinephrine-containing anesthetics for patients taking MAO inhibitors or tricyclic antidepressants is a frequently encountered example. Drugs for which the patient has a documented hypersensitivity are also listed in the problem-solving section of the treatment plan.

Specific Solutions for Dental Problems

The dentist's determination of the best solutions for the patient's dental problems de-

Table 12-1   General treatment planning options for common patient problems

Patient problems	Potential solutions
CHIEF COMPLAINT(S)	
1. Conditions involving pain, injury, infection, or bleeding	A. Expeditious care to control acute conditions usually involves extraction, endodontic therapy, infection control procedures, or repair of injury
GENERAL HEALTH PROBLEMS	
1. Diagnosed medical conditions	A. Modify dental treatment procedures as necessary (Chapter 13) B. Medical consultation for complex medical problems not clarified by the patient history and physical assessment
2. Medications	A. Investigate actions, drug interactions, contraindications, and side effects B. Modify dental treatment procedures as necessary (Chapter 13)
3. Allergic/idiosyncratic drug reaction	A. Avoid use of the drug B. Avoid use of cross-reactive drugs
4. Undiagnosed conditions suspected	A. Advise medical consultation for problems without direct dental treatment implications B. Require medical consultation for problems with potential implications relative to dental treatment
DENTAL HEALTH PROBLEMS*	
1. Nondental lesions of the oral cavity	A. Clinical reevaluation if features are predominantly suggestive of benign or reactive conditions; excisional biopsy if reevaluation is inconclusive B. Incisional or excisional biopsy if malignancy is a possibility
2. Gingivitis/periodontitis	A. Initial therapy of preventive instruction, scaling, removal of plaque retentive conditions, and similar procedures B. Maintenance therapy consisting of repetition of initial therapy procedures C. Surgical elimination of tissue defects D. Combination antimicrobial therapy in addition to A and C E. Extraction
3. Reversible pulpitis	A. Eliminate noxious pulpal stimulation by decay removal B. Eliminate noxious pulpal stimulation by sedative restoration C. Eliminate noxious pulpal stimulation by occlusal adjustment D. Eliminate noxious pulpal stimulation by root desensitization treatment
4. Irreversible pulpitis and pulpal necrosis	A. Endodontic therapy B. Extraction
5. Carious lesions	A. No treatment of enamel-limited lesions B. Decay removal and restoration (see Fig. 12-1) C. Extraction
6. Malalignment/malocclusion	A. Orthodontic treatment B. No treatment, particularly if condition is relatively mild
7. Ectopic eruption and impaction of teeth	A. Extraction B. No treatment, periodic radiographic reevaluation
8. Missing teeth	A. Fixed prosthesis B. Removable prosthesis C. Dental implant D. No treatment

*Referral or consultation with an appropriate dental specialist is a problem-solving option for most dental conditions.

mands simultaneous consideration of numerous interrelated factors. The treatment options for each problem must be considered on the basis of feasibility, effectiveness in solving the problem, and anticipated prognosis. The list of solutions for all problems then must be reviewed to eliminate contradictory procedures such as planning periodontal treatment of a tooth that must be extracted because of an irreparable carious lesion. The advantages and disadvantages of various prosthetic appliances must be considered as possible solutions for missing teeth, while at the same time the treatment benefits are weighed against the expense. This entire process can be challenging but it can be simplified somewhat by listing all treatment options for each problem independently. Contradictory, unsatisfactory, and unfeasible solutions can then be eliminated until the dental treatment planning decisions are clarified. The experienced clinician learns to accomplish this selection and elimination process mentally. Inexperienced clinicians can learn and develop this skill by actually writing out the treatment alternatives for each dental problem.

Treatment options for periodontitis. The treatment options for periodontitis include plaque control by improved oral hygiene, removal of plaque retentive conditions such as calculus, surgical elimination of tissue defects, combination antimicrobial therapy, and extraction of teeth for which the prognosis is hopeless. The appropriate treatment corresponds to the severity of the disease as graded by the periodontal case typing scheme as described in Chapter 8. Improved oral hygiene and removal of local irritants by scaling and root planing are required for nearly all patients with inflammation of the supportive tissues. This generally solves the problem for periodontal case types I and II, while serving as initial therapy for more advanced disease.

Case type III severity dictates that focal lesions are likely to require surgical procedures to eliminate tissue defects and control inflam-

mation. The need for periodontal surgery is indicated by the continued presence of tissue defects that the patient cannot adequately clean after initial therapy. The advanced destruction of type IV periodontitis implies that extensive periodontal surgery will be required to control the disease and that removal of severely affected teeth may be necessary. Type V or rapidly progressive forms of periodontitis involve the same treatment implications as advanced adult periodontitis with the additional need to control atypical bacteria by antibiotic therapy and antimicrobial rinses. The response to treatment of both type IV and type V periodontitis varies dramatically among patients. Therefore reevaluation of the response to initial therapy is essential before planning definitive periodontal treatment.

The severity of the periodontitis, its prognosis, and the effectiveness of initial therapy may influence problem-solving decisions for other dental problems. The prognosis of case types I and II is good to excellent and alteration of other dental treatment for periodontal reasons is unusual. The fair prognosis of type III periodontitis suggests that plans to solve most other dental treatment can be made if the response to initial plaque control efforts is favorable. However, isolated teeth may not tolerate functional stress as an abutment for a fixed or removable prosthesis. Also, extraction of compromised teeth may be an economic treatment option in some cases. The guarded prognosis associated with the advanced, progressive destruction of periodontal case types IV and V demands that all other dental treatment will be affected by the response to periodontal therapy. Teeth with poor prognosis as indicated by advanced mobility, furcation involvement, concurrent periapical inflammatory lesions, and extensive restorative needs will probably require extraction. Plans for other dental treatment must be reevaluated after the effectiveness of periodontal treatment can be assessed. Table 12-2 summarizes the treatment options in solving periodontal problems.

Table 12-2 Summary of treatment options for inflammatory disease of the dental supportive tissues

	Severity of inflammatory disease and tissue destruction				
	Type I	Type II	Type III	Type IV	Type V
Clinical features	Gingivitis, no evidence of bone loss, minimal increase in pocket depth	Evidence of minimal bone loss, moderately increased pocket depth	Evidence of moderately advanced bone loss, substantial increase in pocket depth	Severe bone loss, severe increase in pocket depth	Significant bone loss, significant increase in pocket depth, rapid progression, younger patient
Treatment options					
Improved oral hygiene prophylaxsis, scaling, elimination of plaque retentive conditions	Indicated for all patients who exhibit inflammatory disease of supportive tissues				
Surgical elimination of tissue defects	Not indicated in most situations	Not indicated in most situations	Usually limited to specific sites of advanced tissue destruction	Generalized surgical treatment usually necessary	Generalized surgical treatment usually necessary
Combination antimicrobial therapy (antibiotics, antimicrobial rinses, etc.)	Not indicated in most situations	Not indicated in most situations	Possible use as adjunctive treatment	Possible use as adjunctive treatment	Essential for control
Extraction of teeth	Not indicated	Not indicated	May be a treatment option or necessity for severely affected teeth	Depends on response to initial therapy; extraction may be necessary for teeth with severe vertical lesions, concurrent periapical lesions, mobility, furcation involvement, and complex restorative needs	
Prognosis	Excellent	Good	Fair, may be guarded for isolated teeth	Guarded	Poor
Impact on other aspects of dental treatment planning	Insignificant with control	Unlikely except with chronic progression	Minimal; compromised abutment teeth may alter prosthetic approach	All other aspects of dental treatment affected by response to periodontal therapy	

Treatment options for pulpal necrosis. Evidence of a periapical inflammatory lesion, irreversible pulpitis, or pulpal necrosis indicates the need to remove the pulp either by extraction of the tooth or by endodontic therapy. Endodontic treatment must generally be considered optimal care since this allows retention of the tooth. However, several associated conditions affect the treatment decision. Poor prognostic indicators for the success of endodontic treatment include advanced periodontitis, mobility, root fractures, internal resorption, and external resorption. In addition, endodontic treatment can only be justified if restoration of the tooth is feasible. Endodontically treated teeth develop significant compromise of the coronal strength and often require restoration by placement of a post and core build-up and a crown. Patients frequently select extraction of a tooth with pulpal necrosis rather than endodontic treatment because of the considerable expense associated with both the endodontic and restorative treatment required.

Periapical inflammatory lesions occasionally persist and progress after endodontic treatment. Endodontic retreatment or periapical surgery with retrograde obturation are the two alternatives for such situations. Endodontic retreatment may be justified if there is evidence of deficiency of the original treatment and access for retreatment is possible. Periapical surgery is a more traumatic procedure, but removal of the periapical lesion more consistently leads to resolution of inflammation. Also, periapical surgery may be the only alternative if posts or other materials prevent conservative retreatment.

Treatment options for pulpitis. Treatment for pulpitis depends on whether the condition is reversible or irreversible. Irreversible pulpitis must be considered as early pulpal necrosis and treated by endodontic therapy or extraction. The practical problem is that a definitive distinction on the basis of clinical findings between reversible and irreversible pulpitis is not always possible. In such cases the condition should be managed as reversible with periodic reevaluation after treatment.

Reversible pulpitis is treated by elimination or limitation of the inflammatory stimulus to control the inflammation and discomfort. Such treatment usually requires removal of deep decay, placement of obtundent zinc oxide-eugenol temporary restorations, or desensitization of exposed radicular dentin. Minimizing both axial and nonaxial forces on the affected tooth by selective grinding, referred to as *occlusal adjustment,* often yields improvement of symptoms. Pulpitis associated with mobility caused by traumatic injury or periodontitis can be controlled in some cases by splinting the mobile tooth to adjacent teeth. Resolution of tenderness and other symptoms within a 7 to 10 day period suggests successful control of pulpitis. Persistence or increase in the severity of symptoms usually indicates progression to irreversible pulpitis.

Treatment options for carious teeth. Treatment options for carious lesions include no treatment, restoration, and extraction of teeth when restoration is not justified. The decision among these options is generally determined by the axial and cervical extent of the carious lesion. Once the decision has been made to restore a carious tooth, the commitment to one among various possible restorative procedures is determined by facial-lingual extent of decay, the number of carious surfaces, existing restorations, and the esthetic expectations of the patient. The inability to precisely predict the extent of carious lesions and existing restorations before actual removal is frequently the source of uncertainty during treatment planning. The possibility that alteration of the treatment plan will become necessary at the time of treatment must be accepted as part of the treatment planning process. Fig. 12-1 illustrates the most significant factors in the decision sequence for the treatment of carious lesions.

Carious decalcification limited to enamel,

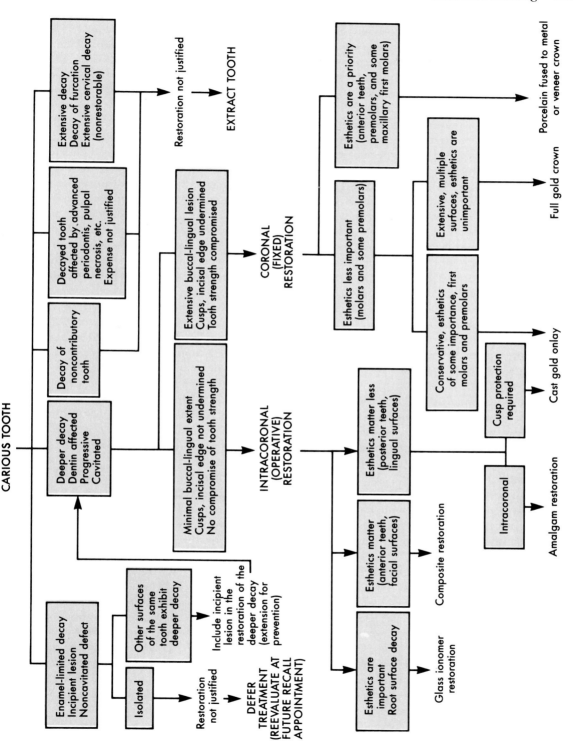

Fig. 12-1 Treatment options for carious teeth

also referred to as *incipient decay,* may not require removal and restoration. The assumption is that improved oral hygiene, a less cariogenic diet, and topical fluoride application may arrest the carious process before actual cavitation or decalcification of dentin occurs. If reevaluation at a 6 month or 1 year recall interval reveals decay progression into dentin, then removal can be accomplished before the decalcification extends beyond the need for a conservative operative restoration. One justification for removal of incipient carious lesions arises when other surfaces of the tooth contain decay requiring treatment and the surface with the incipient lesion would typically be included in the required restoration. This is an application of the operative dental concept of extension for prevention since the incipient lesion must be considered vulnerable to decay. The most common application of this approach occurs when an occlusal cavity is present and the radiographs reveal an enamel-limited lesion of an interproximal surface. Both surfaces are then included in the final restoration.

Several situations justify extraction rather than restoration of a carious tooth. Cervical decay may extend apically beyond the crest of the alveolar bone or into furcation areas to a degree that restoration is not feasible. Conditions in addition to decay such as pulpal necrosis and advanced periodontal bone loss may require complex treatment for which the prognosis is relatively poor or the patient is unwilling to make the financial commitment to save the tooth. Partially erupted or malopposed third molars that are carious represent a situation in which restoration may be technically feasible, but the procedure is not justifiable because the tooth is nonfunctional. Extraction is often a more rational solution than restoration in such situations.

The restoration extent and restorative material must be determined in planning treatment for those carious teeth for which restoration is considered necessary, feasible, and preferable to extraction. The factors determining

the extent of restorative treatment are the surfaces affected by decay and whether the decay has compromised the strength of the tooth.

Conservative operative restorations are optimal treatment for carious lesions that have not significantly compromised the strength of the tooth. This usually involves three or fewer affected tooth surfaces with limited facial-lingual decay extent. Composite is the material of choice for anterior teeth where esthetics must be considered, whereas amalgam is the restorative material of choice for most posterior teeth. Glass ionomer compounds offer advantages in the restoration of cervical lesions. Designation of the tooth to be restored, the surfaces involved, and the restorative material is adequate specification during treatment planning.

Extensive carious destruction of enamel and dentin compromises the inherent strength of the tooth, particularly when the lesions approach functional surfaces. Restoration with amalgam or composite adds no strength to such teeth and results in vulnerability to fracture, as well as compromised esthetics, in many situations. A coronal restoration that includes the function surfaces of the tooth supports and protects the tooth against fracture. Endodontically treated teeth also require coronal restoration in many cases because of large carious lesions that originally caused the pulpal necrosis and the tendency of endodontically treated teeth to become somewhat brittle.

The composition and design of the crown is determined by the esthetic demands of the situation. Cast gold crowns and onlays are preferred if esthetics are of minimal concern because gold is less abrasive to the opposing teeth. Porcelain-fused-to-metal crowns offer the best esthetic alternative for the coronal restoration of anterior and premolar teeth but are somewhat more abrasive. The treatment plan should also specifically list the preliminary operative procedure required to "build up" an extensively decayed tooth with amalgam or composite in addition to the coronal restoration.

The decision between an operative or a coronal restoration for teeth with intermediate decay extent can be difficult. There are no absolute rules that can be expected to apply to all instances, but some guidelines may be helpful in borderline situations. Operative restorations of posterior teeth expected to exceed more than one half of the coronal volume of the tooth with a restorative material should be reconsidered for a crown. Posterior teeth for which a three-surface restoration would exceed one half of the intercuspal distance may require a crown. Loss of a cusp or an incisal edge suggests that a crown is necessary. Restorative involvement of more than three tooth surfaces, excluding conservative developmental pit restorations, often indicates that a crown should be considered. Crowns can be justified on an esthetic basis in selected cases where an operative restoration might suffice in terms of strength.

Treatment options for complications of eruption. The optimal solution for most complications of eruption is either orthodontic treatment or extraction of teeth. Interceptive orthodontic treatment can be beneficial in minimizing the sequelae of ectopic eruption during the mixed-dentition stage of development. Orthodontic treatment should be advocated in cases of dysfunctional relationships, poor esthetics, and malalignment in the late mixed dentition period and later in life. This may be *elective treatment,* treatment at the patient's discretion, if the existing malalignment is functional and the primary treatment goal is esthetic. Clinical examination and cephalometric analysis may indicate the need to correct skeletal abnormalities by orthognathic surgery in conjunction with orthodontic treatment. Orthodontic treatment requires preparatory dental treatment to eliminate dental disease. This minimizes the destructive progression of decay, periodontitis, and other dental lesions during active orthodontic treatment.

Partially erupted, impacted, and severely malaligned teeth often must be extracted to minimize adverse effects on adjacent teeth. Other complications of impaction and ectopic eruption are generally less urgent but also require treatment. These complications include external resorption of adjacent teeth, cystic enlargement of the dental follicle, and formation of an interproximal relationship that is difficult to clean. The trauma and potential complications of the surgical procedure must always be justified by the benefits to the patient of removing the teeth. For example, many asymptomatic, impacted third molars with no radiographic evidence of adverse effects can be reevaluated radiographically at yearly intervals as an alternative to surgical removal. Conversely, surgical removal of a painless impaction may be justified during the surgical removal of several uncomfortable third molars since the additional surgical trauma and related discomfort to the patient would be negligible. Unique clinical situations often require consideration of other factors in the treatment planning relative to the removal of teeth. The acute manifestations of pericoronitis are common examples of eruption complications that must be managed by infection control measures in the context of a chief complaint before eventual removal of the tooth.

Treatment options for missing teeth. The treatment options for missing teeth include fixed prostheses, removable prostheses, and dental implants. The treatment goals are restoration of function and esthetics and prevention of deterioration of the health of remaining teeth by minimizing supereruption or drifting into edentulous spaces. In some situations prosthetic replacement is not justified because the treatment will not achieve these goals.

Prosthodontic treatment planning is challenging because the numerous biologic and technical factors that influence treatment success are relatively unpredictable. Four distinct difficulties apply to most cases of missing teeth:

First, the success of prosthetic treatment depends on the health and stability of the abutment teeth because these teeth must eventually bear additional mechanical forces. Unfortunately, the reasons that teeth are usually missing such as periodontitis and intermittent past dental care also affect the potential abutments. How well compromised abutment teeth will withstand the functional demands after placement of the prosthesis is difficult to anticipate.

Second, the patient's biologic and functional condition must change considerably from the time of initial treatment planning to the actual fabrication of the prosthesis. Active dental disease must be eliminated, abutments must be restored, and periodontitis must be eliminated. This means that the conditions originally confronted by the dentist during treatment planning will be quite different by the time the final aspects of the dental treatment are provided.

Third, many initial prosthetic decisions depend on the success of preparatory treatments, which can be difficult to predict. The dentist frequently contends with situations involving a treatment plan for a removable or fixed partial denture that relies on an abutment tooth that is found during decay removal to be nonrestorable.

Fourth, and finally, the success of prosthetic treatment depends on factors over which the dentist may have little or no direct control. The skill of the laboratory technician, the handling of impressions by office assistants, and the compliance of the patient with instructions are only a few of the unpredictable elements that can adversely affect prosthetic results.

Table 12-3 lists various factors influencing the replacement of missing teeth by fixed and removable prostheses. The optimal application of a fixed prosthesis is the replacement of a single missing tooth by a three unit bridge abutted to adjacent teeth. This generally provides physiologic distribution of masticatory forces and the most esthetically pleasing prosthesis. *Ante's rule* attempts to predict the requirement for abutments by prescribing that the periodontal support of the abutment teeth should equal or exceed that of the tooth or teeth to be replaced. This quantitative assessment is difficult to determine practically and is hardly absolute, but it does provide a qualitative indication that bridges involving periodontally compromised abutments or a long-span bridge replacing several teeth may not withstand functional demands.

An additional factor affecting the feasibility of some long-span fixed partial dentures is the leverage effect of force applied to pontics not aligned with the abutments, as shown in Fig. 12-2. This may produce nonaxial forces beyond the support of the abutment teeth. A "double abutment" design to include two adjacent teeth at one end of a bridge to compensate for a compromised abutment tooth or for a long-span bridge must be considered against the added difficulties in cleaning, technical complexity, and additional expense. Other designs such as the cantilever and the acid-etched or "Maryland" bridges may be applicable in certain clinical situations.

Removable prostheses are the primary treatment option for the problem of missing teeth in situations in which abutments are unavailable. Removable prostheses can be considered as complete, immediate, partial, and transitional dentures.

Complete dentures are the only available treatment for edentulous patients unless dental implants can be accomplished to provide abutments. The major treatment planning consideration for edentulous patients is whether preprosthetic surgery is necessary to successfully adapt complete dentures. Surgery may be indicated to eliminate obstructive alveolar prominences, hyperplastic alveolar soft tissue, retained root fragments, inflammatory lesions, and unerupted teeth or to augment atrophic alveolar ridges. The decision must be based on the feasibility of providing a complete denture with the existing alveolar conditions as com-

Table 12-3   Comparison of favorable and unfavorable clinical factors for fixed and removable partial dentures

	Favorable factors	Unfavorable factors
Fixed partial dentures	Minimal pontic span Linear alignment of abutments and pontic (see Fig. 12-2) Abutment teeth uncompromised by periodontitis or other conditions Good oral hygiene practices	Long pontic span Nonlinear relationships of abutments and pontic Abutment teeth compromised by periodontitis or other condition Poor home care Mesial tipping of abutment Supereruption of opposing tooth (teeth) Short clinical crowns of abutments
Removable partial dentures	"Balance" of abutments (see Fig. 12-3) Abutment teeth uncompromised by periodontitis or other conditions Both canine teeth present Posterior abutment present (tooth borne) Uncomplicated path of insertion Good oral hygiene practices	Lack of abutment "balance" Abutment teeth compromised by periodontitis or other condition One or both canine teeth missing No posterior abutment (distal extension) Complex path of insertion Poor home care Mesial tipping of abutment(s) Patient intolerance of framework Isolated abutment teeth (Fig. 12-3) Narrow edentulous gaps Short clinical crowns of abutments Prominent tori

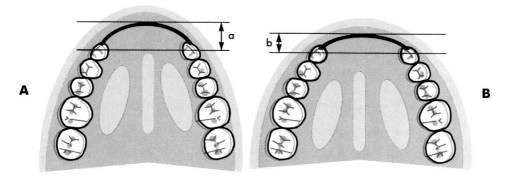

Fig. 12-2   The effect of abutment and pontic alignment on leverage forces. In **A,** the arch contour demands that the pontics of the bridge extend a greater distance (*a*) beyond the alignment of the abutment teeth than in example **B.** The situation in **A** will produce greater leverage forces on the abutment teeth and is associated with a poorer extended prognosis than is the situation illustrated in **B.**

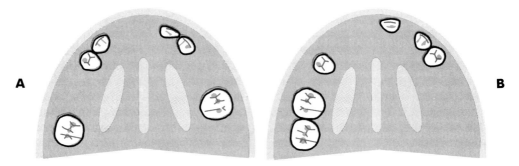

Fig. 12-3   Comparison of favorable and unfavorable arch "balance" for a removable partial denture. Although both examples **A** and **B** exhibit the same number of abutment teeth, the prognosis in example **A** is more favorable. Both canine teeth are present in **A,** abutments are positioned throughout the arch, and posterior abutments are available, which allows a tooth borne design. Example **B** requires a distal extension design; one canine is missing, isolated teeth complicate the design, and the distribution of abutment support is "unbalanced."

pared with the trauma and possible complications of the surgical procedure. A successful complete denture can often be fabricated without removal of small tori and deeply impacted teeth. Impacted teeth and root fragments near the alveolar crest and residual inflammatory lesions generally must be removed or the functional pressure of the denture may eventually induce symptoms or expose impacted teeth.

The immediate complete denture involves placement of the denture at the same appointment at which the teeth are removed. This provides the esthetic and functional advantage of having the prosthesis in place during healing. The disadvantage is that the denture generally must be relined within a year because the alveolar ridge atrophies during the healing and repair process.

Replacing missing teeth with a removable partial denture should be considered in situations of two or more edentulous gaps in the dental arch. Removable partial dentures must be considered if no maintainable posterior abutment for a fixed prosthesis is present in the arch unless a dental implant is feasible. Table 12-3 lists favorable factors including stable

abutment teeth, relatively large edentulous gaps, minimal supereruption of opposing teeth, and "balance" in the arrangements of abutments as shown in Fig. 12-3. Mobility and unfavorable crown-to-root relationships of abutments, isolated teeth, and nonretentive clasp areas are among the unfavorable factors. The dentist must frequently decide between fixed bridges and a removable partial denture to replace multiple missing teeth in an arch. Table 12-4 summarizes several of the general clinical factors the dentist must compare in making this decision.

Fabrication of a transitional removable partial denture provides replacement of one or more missing teeth with minimal expense for a short duration until more permanent treatment can be accomplished. The cold cured acrylic "flipper" to replace an anterior maxillary tooth is a typical example, although more complicated designs that rely on wrought wire clasps are possible. Reliance on a temporary partial denture for a relatively short duration is often a necessary aspect of dental care. The difficulty from a treatment planning perspective is that temporary partials are often ac-

Table 12-4   General treatment planning considerations compared for fixed and removable prostheses

Clinical factor	Fixed prosthesis	Removable prosthesis
PATIENT'S PERSPECTIVE		
Expense	Greater	Less, particularly if numerous teeth are missing in an arch
Soft tissue coverage	Minimal, more natural sensation	Greater, sensation like "hardware"
Esthetics	Usually more favorable	Clasps unsightly, but can be more favorable for severely atrophic maxillary anterior ridge
DENTIST'S PERSPECTIVE		
Mastication's forces	Favorable, more axially directed	Harmful lateral forces and "rocking" often develop with time
Edentulous span	Smaller spans are more easily replaced by fixed bridge	Larger edentulous gaps are more easily replaced by removable appliance
Posterior abutment	Required	Improves prognosis, but not necessary
Abutment tooth reduction	Must be fully reduced	Minimal unless abutments require coronal restoration for strength
Hygiene	Cleaning under pontic can be difficult, tedious	Can be removed for cleaning
Recurrent decay	Greater vulnerability, extensive margins	Less vulnerability, only clasps, rests, and guide planes covered.
Compromised abutment teeth	Abutments bear entire functional force, but forces are more axial	Soft tissues bear some force, but lateral forces are more likely
Modification after insertion	Little modification possible	Can be adjusted or relined and, in some cases, teeth can be added
Technique sensitivity	Greater vulnerability to failure because of technical errors	Less vulnerable to failure because of technical errors

cepted by patients as inexpensive permanent treatment. Since no occlusal rests or other mechanical features of rigid removable partial denture design are possible, the temporary partial rests entirely on soft tissue. Over time this adversely affects periodontal health, which explains why many dentists refer to temporary partial dentures as "gum strippers."

Dental implants are an emerging option in the replacement of missing teeth. Although technical aspects and the prognosis of various techniques are somewhat controversial, dental implants have been shown to be successful in selected clinical situations. General requirements include adequate alveolar bone for implant placement and effective oral hygiene by the patient. In addition, the expense and surgical trauma must be justified by the additional benefit to the patient of the implant as compared with traditional prosthetic treatment methods. Such a situation might involve implants to replace the mandibular first and second molars rather than a unilateral removable partial denture. In general, treatment planning consideration of dental implants should be made in consultation with clinicians skilled in providing such care.

In many clinical situations *not* replacing missing teeth is optimal management of the problem. Replacement of missing second and third molars is seldom justified if no other teeth are missing from the dental arch. The resulting "first molar occlusion" and in some cases "premolar occlusion" can provide adequate function and stability. Often the teeth adjacent to the gap left by a missing tooth gone for a long duration will have drifted to close the gap, which yields a stable, functional, and esthetically pleasing relationship. Initial treatment of advanced periodontitis or other conditions affecting potential abutment teeth may be ineffective or yield a poor prognosis for either fixed or removable prosthetic care. The additional forces generated by the prostheses in such cases may be more detrimental to the abutment teeth than the benefit provided by prosthetic replacement can justify and must, therefore, be deferred.

Treatment options for nondental oral problems. Treatment options for nondental oral conditions vary considerably depending on the nature of the specific conditions, as discussed in Chapters 15 through 20. Incorporation of treatment into the dental treatment plan is generally uncomplicated once a definitive diagnosis of these problems is achieved.

Implications and Consequences of Specific Treatment Options

Most treatment options create additional treatment needs or entail definite consequences in the treatment planning process. In

the situation of pulpal necrosis of a lower first molar, for example, the potential solutions for the problem are extraction or endodontic treatment of the tooth. If the tooth is extracted, then the missing tooth should be replaced if feasible by a three-unit bridge. Drifting and supereruption of teeth in the area is a consequence of extracting the tooth and not fabricating the replacement bridge. Endodontic treatment usually requires restoration with a post and core and a crown.

These additional treatment implications are listed adjacent to each treatment option. This prevents oversights and can be helpful in considering the ramifications of various treatment decisions. Table 12-5 illustrates this process for a hypothetical patient by listing the patient problems, possible solutions for each problem, and treatment implications for each potential solution. This process can be helpful in formulating complicated dental treatment plans and developing conceptual understanding of the treatment planning process by less experienced clinicians. Experienced dentists compare and consider the numerous problems, treatment options, and the implications of each option mentally, but the process is essentially the same.

DETERMINATION OF DENTAL TREATMENT GOALS

The premise that an ideal treatment plan exists for a specific patient's oral condition is false and misleading. A complex treatment plan with priority for conservation of compromised teeth and restoration of missing teeth may be technically sound and consistent with the highest standards of dental care. Unfortunately, this technically superior treatment plan fails because the patient will refuse the treatment if the expense is excessive and the procedures ignore the patient's preferences. An alternative plan formulated with primary considerations for cost limitation and patient concerns may be the "ideal" treatment for this patient even though conservation of teeth and other techni-

Table 12-5   Problem list for a hypothetical patient with possible solutions for the problems and the treatment planning implications of each solution

Problem list	Solutions	Treatment planning implications
1. Pericoronitis, tooth #17* (chief complaint)	A. Lavage, antibiotic therapy	Advise patient of altered birth control pill (BCP) effectiveness, must confirm resolution of infection, and extraction will eventually be necessary
	B. Immediate extraction	Risks extension of infection
2. Nonspecific history of heart murmur	A. Medical consultation	May delay treatment of chief complaint
	B. Proceed without coverage	Risk of infective endocarditis
	C. Proceed with coverage	Possible unnecessary antibiotic therapy
3. History of migraine headaches	A. Dental treatment as usual	May precipitate migraine episode
	B. Dental procedures with stress reduction	May decrease efficiency of dental treatment
4. BCP	A. Avoid use of antibiotics	Avoids altered BCP effectiveness, but may not be possible (#1 and #2)
	B. Use of antibiotics	Advise patient of altered BCP effectiveness
5. Allergy to penicillin	A. Use alternate antibiotics	Attention for possible cross-sensitivity
6. Periodontitis, type II	A. Initial therapy	Must evaluate disease control
7. Reversible pulpitis, deep occlusal decay of tooth #30	A. Amalgam restoration	Risks causing irreversible pulpitis
	B. Decay removal, sedative temporary restoration	Less risk of pulpal necrosis, but a second procedure for final restoration is needed
8. Pulpal necrosis, tooth #8	A. Endodontic therapy	Requires a crown after post and core buildup
	B. Extraction	Requires a three-unit bridge
9. Superficial decay of several teeth	A. Restoration	Specify teeth, surfaces, and restorative materials
	B. No treatment	Progression of decay, more complex problems
10. Other third molars (#1, #16, #32) are impacted, no current complications	A. Surgical removal	Can be accomplished when #17 is removed
	B. Periodic radiographic reevaluation	An additional surgical procedure may become necessary if complications develop later
11. Tooth #19 is missing (extracted)	A. Three-unit bridge, #18 through #20	Requires uprighting of #18 and crown for #14 to level the occlusal plane
	B. No treatment	Mesial drift of #18 and supereruption of #14 will progress

*All numerical abbreviations for teeth are by the Universal Numbering System.

cal considerations are given a lower priority.

The practical issue is that many potential treatment plans can be justified for the unique problems posed by a patient. The differences among the possibilities are related primarily to the specific factors that are given priority consideration during the treatment planning process. The priority considerations that are most appropriate for a patient are collectively referred to as the *dental treatment goals.* The dentist and the patient determine these goals during the case presentation. However, the dentist effectively guides this decision process by understanding the influence of both the patient's perspective and the dentist's perspective of what the treatment priorities should be. Several general treatment planning approaches are available to guide the treatment decisions from among the available treatment options for each specific patient problem after dental treatment goals are determined.

The Patient's Perspective

Assessment of the patient's attitudes about dental treatment relies on information beyond what the patient actually verbalizes. For example, when asked what they expect from their dental care, many patients say what they think the dentist wants to hear rather than what they truly believe. Nonverbal clues, the nature of past dental care, and questions asked by the patient all provide clues to attitudes and priorities.

Chief complaint. The problem that brought the patient to the dentist is obviously a treatment priority, and successful practitioners soon learn that the patient's chief complaint should become the dentist's chief treatment priority. Essential diagnostic procedures, such as radiographs, should not be circumvented and more urgent problems should not be ignored in treating the chief complaint, but the treatment plan must include prompt attention to the problem that brought the patient to the dental office. Otherwise, the patient will seek treatment elsewhere.

The patient's dental expectations. The patient's dental expectations include the general aspects of patient's dental treatment interests beyond care for the chief complaint. Patient expectations range from care limited to treatment of painful teeth at one extreme to the patient who wants to retain teeth regardless of treatment complexity. Past dental care as suggested by history or clinical findings is a reliable indicator of the patient's real attitude if the dentist suspects what the patient claims. The dentist should assume that the patient who expects comprehensive restorative treatment also expects a result with a favorable extended prognosis. The dentist must be suspicious of unreasonable patient expectations when highly detailed specifications for esthetics or denture retention results are stated. Unreasonable expectations are also suggested by harsh criticism of past dental care.

Financial limitations. Few patients can afford to accept a comprehensive dental treatment plan without asking the cost and patients generally prefer to keep dental expenses to a minimum. However, many will pay for the care needed to solve their dental problems if they believe that the problems exist. The challenge for the dentist in many cases is to convince the patient that painless dental diseases with adverse long-term effects are actually a problem.

Financial limitations may reflect inadequate income, adequate income but a preference to spend for other things, or policies dictated by third parties such as insurance companies. Unfortunately, many people on limited incomes must consider comprehensive dental treatment as an expensive luxury rather than essential health care. In addition, most dental care is considered by many patients as less urgent than other forms of health care. The dentist's initial responsibility during the case presentation is patient education relative to the needed treatment, the treatment options, the consequences of refusing treatment, and the related expense. This allows the patient to make an informed decision about dental treatment goals.

If the motivation exists, dollars can be stretched. Examples include payment plans, delaying the most expensive restorative procedures, omitting truly elective procedures, and giving priority to disease-control procedures. Unfortunately, there are times when even minimal care is beyond the patient's means.

The patient's dental attitudes. The patient's attitudes about dentistry reflect a unique mixture of accurate knowledge, misinformation, impressions from past experiences, and opinions. This is occasionally referred to collectively as the patient's *dental IQ.* Ignorance about dentistry is alleviated by the dentist's efforts to educate the patient, but the patient's dental attitudes extend beyond knowledge to include opinions and values.

Negative attitudes about dentistry cannot be effectively addressed by patient education alone since the dentist is frequently perceived by the patient as biased or self-serving. For example, if the patient believes that root canals always fail, then informing the patient of the high success rate of endodontic treatment will not change the belief. Patients often nod in agreement to avoid additional "education" but then fail to arrive for the endodontic appointment. To change this bias the dentist must win the patient's confidence, so that a positive opinion of the dentist's knowledge and ability overrides the prior negative attitude. Development of such confidence requires time and positive experiences. Direct challenge of strongly-held patient opinions in the early stages of the dentist-patient relationship becomes confrontational and counterproductive. This situation may require delaying treatment planning commitments until a stronger dentist-patient relationship emerges.

Alterations in treatment plans to accommodate fear of pain, gagging, and other emotional responses to the dental treatment environment are necessary and important aspects of patient management. Few patients will tolerate unnecessary pain, but tolerance for the unpleasant sensations of dental treatment varies remarkably. Nitrous oxide analgesia and pretreatment sedation are just two of the possible approaches to such problems. Discreet questions about unpleasant aspects of past dental care reveal the types of dental discomfort that may exceed the patient's tolerance threshold. In addition, many patients regard convenient appointment times and minimizing the number of appointments as important factors in planning treatment.

In summary, patient treatment priorities generally include attention to the chief complaint, solving the patient's perceived problems within financial resources, and obtaining a reasonable prognosis while minimizing inconvenience, pain, and complications. The dentist's challenge is to accomplish these goals while solving the patient's dental problems as considered from the dentist's perspective.

The Dentist's Perspective

The effective clinician must appreciate that the dentist's attitudes and biases may seem unreasonable to the patient. Significant aspects of the dentist's treatment planning perspective include the patient's dental condition, the anticipated prognosis, possible complications, the optimal treatment, and the possible need for specialist care.

The patient's dental condition. The most direct factor influencing treatment planning are the patient's dental problems, since the treatment plan is essentially a listing of solutions to these problems. The dentist's perspective gives high priority to problems associated with active disease, while the patient is more concerned with problems that produce pain or unfavorable esthetics. The dentist's obligation is to confirm the accuracy of the diagnostic findings and to plan treatment that will solve the problems. Any diagnostic uncertainty should be resolved before the treatment options are selected and the treatment plan is formulated. The patient is more favorably impressed if corrections in the final treatment plan are unnecessary during the case presentation.

Prognosis. The expectation for success of various procedures or *prognosis* often affects selections from among treatment options. Both dentists and patients seek long-lasting dental treatment. Most dentists tend to recommend treatment options with the best prognosis because successful treatment reflects most positively on the practitioner. Considered another way, the dentist often hesitates to recommend treatment with a guarded or poor prognosis because patients who experience unsuccessful results tend to blame the dentist.

However, some extreme cases may justify treatment options with a poorer prognosis. A patient with a terminal illness, for example, would benefit from procedures to control infections and improve function, but complex procedures to promote an extended dental prognosis would be unjustified. A hopeless periodontal outlook may still warrant restorative care designed as transitional until the teeth must be removed.

Potential complications of dental treatment. Complications are a risk of almost all dental procedures. Treatment planning options are occasionally selected specifically to avoid the possibility of certain treatment complications. The dentist should carefully reconsider a preliminary treatment plan for a removable partial denture if the patient relates inability to wear a previously made partial because of a gagging sensation or intolerance to the "hardware" sensation. Vulnerability to infective endocarditis may require an increase in the treatment provided per appointment to avoid repeated administration of antibiotics.

Referral for specialty treatment. The need for specialty treatment may affect the dentist's treatment plan. Ideally, such considerations should not influence the general dentist's decisions about the best care for a patient, but from a practical standpoint this is often not the case. A comfortable working relationship between the general practitioner and a periodontist may encourage consideration of such treatment even if the prognosis is relatively poor. Inability to expeditiously arrange a difficult endodontic procedure may force the general practitioner to consider extracting the tooth. The general practitioner located in a remote community can find this to be a particularly difficult problem.

Financial considerations. The dentist must consider the cost of specific dental procedures in formulating the treatment plan, particularly if third parties such as a dental insurance company are involved. The patient often cannot understand why certain procedures are covered and others are not. Many programs allow only certain procedures in specific situations, which may not be optimal care. Some procedures, although they may be technically superior to others, are not sufficiently superior in quality and prognosis to warrant their increased cost. The dentist's goal is to weigh such issues and provide the patient with a treatment plan that realistically provides treatment quality proportional to cost.

Specific Dental Treatment Goals

Formulating the optimal approach to solving the patient's dental problems can be simplified somewhat by defining several general approaches to dental treatment planning based on the dental treatment goals agreed to by the dentist and patient. The treatment goals are usually not discussed in detail and agreed to until the case presentation, but most clinicians form an impression of the patient's expectations early in the diagnostic process. General dental treatment goals and their corresponding treatment plans are referred to as emergency, limited, disease control, tentative, and comprehensive dental treatment.

Emergency dental treatment. Emergency treatment plans provide solutions for chief complaints that involve some degree of urgency, such as pain and acute infection. These problems are usually solved by extraction, palliative pulpotomy, periodontal infection control, or similar treatment. The commitment for emergency treatment is relatively simple because the patient clarifies during the patient interview that solving the chief complaint is the patient's *only* treatment goal. The dentist should plan to expeditiously solve the uncomfortable problem and defer discussion of other dental problems until the emergency is controlled. Chief complaints related to less urgent dental problems, such as an ill-fitting removable partial denture or a request for a "check up," can be more appropriately accommodated by one of the other treatment planning approaches.

Limited dental plan. A limited dental treatment goal specifies a treatment solution for a specific problem that is not urgent. Dental specialists provide care for patients referred from a general dentist on the basis of a limited treatment plan. The periodontist, for example, focuses on the periodontal treatment needs of the referred patient while relying on the general dentist to evaluate and treat all other dental problems. The general dentist also uses limited treatment plans in certain circumstances. For example, a patient might request that an anterior tooth be restored before a special event such as a family gathering. The goal becomes expeditious treatment for a specific problem at the patient's request without specific attention to general dental problems. Such treatment must be evaluated to confirm that it is consistent with sound dental treatment principles.

Planning on the basis of limited treatment goals should represent the exceptional situation rather than a routine method of dental practice. The danger associated with frequent reliance on limited treatment plans by the general dentist is that treatment becomes tooth-by-tooth problem solving at the patient's request rather than a comprehensive health care service. The dentist who adopts a limited treatment approach should strongly encourage the patient to arrange for comprehensive dental diagnosis and treatment in the future.

Dental disease control treatment. This treatment goal reflects agreement between the dentist and the patient that all identified problems cannot be solved because of limitations such as money or available time. The treatment goal becomes elimination of progressive lesions and stabilization of the patient's dental condition. The assumption is that comprehensive restorative care such as replacement of missing teeth will eventually be accomplished when circumstances allow. Additional deterioration of the patient's dental condition is prevented during the interim by controlling active diseases. Therefore the prognosis of necessary restorative treatment will not be additionally compromised by the delay. Treatment of periodontitis, pulpal necrosis, and carious lesions, as well as preventive procedures, are typical features of the disease control treatment plan. Similar procedures may represent either definitive treatment in the case of an operative procedure to restore a small carious lesion or transitional treatment such as a large amalgam restoration intended to eventually serve as the build-up for a crown.

Tentative dental plan. The goal of the tentative treatment plan is to specifiy initial disease control procedures for cases in which the initial treatment outcome cannot be confidently predicted. The specification of additional treatment decisions is deferred or listed in general terms until the effectiveness of initial treatment can be assessed. Tentative treatment plans are useful in cases of advanced periodontitis and in cases of extensive carious lesions and missing teeth. For example, often the clinician cannot predict the ability of potential abutment teeth to function under various prosthetic appliances without knowing the results of periodontal treatment. In such cases the preventive, periodontal, pulpitis, and decay removal procedures are listed. The patient is then reevaluated before the formulation of a definitive treatment plan for advanced restorative procedures and replacement of missing teeth.

Comprehensive dental plan. The goal of comprehensive dental treatment is the decision by the patient and dentist to plan the procedures necessary to solve all of the patient's dental problems. Comprehensive dental treatment is the preferred approach to patient management because all aspects of care can be integrated and coordinated by the dentist for optimal results. Referral for specialty care and the delaying of certain elective procedures are consistent with comprehensive treatment planning as long as the plan clearly provides for the elimination of all problems. As indicated above, the tentative treatment approach is required if a comprehensive treatment cannot be confidently planned because of the advanced nature of the dental problems.

The dentist should always recommend either a comprehensive dental treatment plan or a tentative treatment plan. However, the dentist who agrees to proceed toward a limited or disease control treatment goal has the opportunity to convince the patient by the success of initial procedures to reconsider comprehensive treatment. For example, a patient indicating limited financial resources, an interest in achieving better dental health, and rather complicated dental problems would be a good candidate for a disease control treatment plan. The same patient with adequate financial resources would be appropriately managed by comprehensive dental treatment, while a patient with little motivation for better dental health beyond pain control will usually be treated on an emergency basis. In addition, identifying the patient's treatment goals provides guidance in selecting the best procedures for solving specific problems from among treatment options. This is illustrated by the patient with pain related to irreversible pulpitis and attitudes suggesting a dental treatment goal is limited to elimination of pain. The most logical treatment would be extraction of the tooth rather than initiating endodontic treatment.

SETTING PRIORITIES: THE OPTIMAL TREATMENT SEQUENCE

The final step in formulating the dental treatment plan is to rearrange all the treatment procedures necessary to solve the patient's problems in the most logical treatment sequence. The order in which dental procedures are completed is determined by consideration of the priorities from the perspectives of both the patient and the practitioner. Unfortunately, esthetic problems of high priority to the patient may seem rather secondary to the dentist compared with extensive decay affecting several molars. Despite this divergence of opinion, planning the sequence of procedures should allow high-priority problems to be solved early in treatment and prevent treatment complications resulting from delaying treatment or poor sequencing. For example, fabrication of a porcelain-fused-to-metal crown to improve esthetics before completing periodontal therapy risks the possibility that the newly crowned tooth will eventually be extracted if delayed periodontal therapy is unsuccessful. Also, preparatory procedures must be planned prior to the final procedures involving the same teeth, as in the case of placing crowns on abutment teeth to improve strength and retention before making an impression for a removable partial denture. The sequencing of dental treatment procedures is usually grouped in phases based on treatment priority and treatment goals satisfied by various procedures. Table 12-6 summarizes the optimal dental treatment sequence and indicates the commitment to various phases of dental care that is associated with the different dental treatment goals.

Pretreatment Phase

The pretreatment phase allows the dentist to resolve any unclear diagnostic issues that may affect how dental procedures are performed. Additional diagnostic procedures, such as specialized radiographs or study models, may be needed to complete all aspects of the diagnostic process. Medical and dental consultations may be necessary before active treatment procedures can be safely and confidently performed. This information is obtained during the pretreatment phase. The clinician can omit the pretreatment phase in cases uncomplicated by unresolved diagnostic issues.

Table 12-6 Optimal dental treatment sequence and commitment to treatment depending on different treatment goals

Treatment category	Dental treatment goals				
	Emergency	Limited	Disease control	Tentative	Comprehensive
Pretreatment phase					
Diagnostic procedures	X	X	X	X	X
Phase I					
Treatment of chief complaint	X	X	X	X	X
Excision of oral lesions suggestive of malignancy	X	X	X	X	X
Phase II					
Complaint(s) not treated in phase I		X	X	X	X
Preventive evaluation and instruction			X	X	X
Initial management of gingivitis/periodontitis			X	X	X
Removal of extensive decay			X	X	X
Extraction of teeth with poor prognosis			X	X	X
Endodontic treatment of nonacute pulpal necrosis			X	X	X
Definitive periodontal therapy			X	X	X
Phase III					
Restoration of superficial carious lesions			X	*	X
Orthodontic treatment				*	X
Fixed prosthodontic treatment				*	X
Removable prosthodontic treatment				*	X
Phase IV					
Reevaluation of treatment			X	X	X
Phase V					
Recall			X	X	X

*Reassessment of additional treatment and treatment goals following the evaluation of initial treatment results.

Phase I: Treatment of Acute Problems

The initial phase of treatment consists of procedures to control pain and acute infection, which are usually the patient's chief complaint. Phase I treatment may include extraction of painful teeth, incision and drainage of abscesses, and management of traumatic injuries. Pulpectomy, excavation of deep carious lesions, sedative temporary restoration, and pulp capping procedures are other examples of phase I treatment. An additional element of phase I treatment is biopsy of any lesions believed on the basis of clinical findings to be malignant. The implications of oral malignancy justify treatment priority on the same order as symptomatic dental conditions. The completion of phase I treatment generally represents all of the dental care necessary for the patient whose treatment goal is control of symptoms.

Phase II: Treatment to Control Active Disease

Phase II dental treatment procedures generally attempt to arrest active disease processes by controlling causative factors and eliminating lesions. Phase II treatment is also referred to occasionally as the *preparatory treatment phase* in the sense of preparing the patient for restorative treatment.

The initial obligation of phase II treatment is attention to any patient complaints that have not been previously managed. In many instances patients will relate several complaints at the beginning of the patient interview, some of which require phase I attention, and other less pressing problems that can be managed at the beginning of phase II. The limited treatment approach is typically completed when these complaints have been treated. The dentist must occasionally encourage the patient to wait for treatment of minor complaints until other conditions have been treated. A common example involves the complaint of poor appearance of an anterior tooth requiring a crown. The patient should understand that superior esthetics at the gingival margin will result if the crown is completed after gingivitis and periodontitis have been effectively treated.

Procedures to solve the problems associated with inflammatory disease of the dental supportive tissues are the first major priority of phase II treatment after management of complaints. For most adult patients this will include elimination of local irritants by oral hygiene instruction, scaling, and root planing. Limited surgical periodontal treatment may be accomplished after plaque control therapy, concurrent with other elements of phase II treatment, or at the end of phase II. The clinician determines the timing of periodontal surgery within phase II based on the patient's oral hygiene effectiveness, the tissue improvement following initial therapy, the complexity of the periodontal surgery planned, and the complexity of other phase II treatment. Regardless of the precise sequence, all surgical periodontal therapy will be completed by the end of phase II.

Decay removal of extensive carious lesions and any necessary pulp capping procedures are the next priority of phase II treatment. Decay removal to be accomplished in phase II includes teeth that are likely to involve pulpal exposure, teeth planned for crowns, and cavities affecting abutment teeth. Extensive decay and related complications that could alter the treatment plan are treated early in phase II so that the need to change the treatment plan will be appreciated early in the treatment sequence. The restorations may be temporary in the case of sedative cement restorations, transitional in the case of build-ups for crowns, or final restorations. Restoration of superficial carious lesions is generally delayed until the beginning of phase III treatment because the slow progression of these lesions makes their treatment primarily a restorative procedure rather than a pressing issue of disease elimination.

The next stage of phase II treatment is extraction of irreparable teeth not previously removed in phase I. Delaying extraction of compromised, painless teeth until after initial periodontal treatment and the removal of extensive carious lesions allows the clinician a better opportunity to determine which "borderline" teeth can be saved. The extractions are accomplished early enough in the treatment sequence, however, so that the probability of irreparable teeth adversely affecting adjacent teeth or becoming acutely inflamed is minimized. Surgical removal of impacted teeth should also be accomplished at this stage if the situation involves the possibility of surgical trauma adversely affecting adjacent teeth. Any subsequent treatment necessary to maintain surgically traumatized teeth will generally be simpler if accomplished prior to restorative treatment of the injured tooth. The surgical removal of impacted third molars as part of simple treatment plans for young adults can be delayed in most cases until operative dental treatment is completed.

Indicated endodontic procedures not completed during phase I are accomplished after the necessary extractions. The chronic, slowly progressive, or static nature of asymptomatic periapical lesions caused by pulpal necrosis does not justify a high treatment priority compared with the more progressive lesions treated earlier in phase II. In many instances, pulp exposures during the removal of deep carious lesions earlier in phase II treatment require completion of endodontic therapy prior to oral surgical procedures. Also, fabrication of a post and core build-up following endodontic treatment of badly decayed teeth is often required at this stage to provide an effective foundation for the fabrication of a stable temporary restoration.

Any surgical periodontal therapy not completed earlier in the phase II sequence should be accomplished as the final aspect of phase II treatment. The variability of periodontal lesions and patient response to initial treatment often requires an extended reevaluation period prior to extensive periodontal surgery. Combining the treatment time required for other aspects of phase II care with this periodontal reevaluation period increases treatment efficiency and allows frequent reinforcement of oral hygiene instructions.

All surgical periodontal therapy and the elimination of all active oral disease will be accomplished at the completion of phase II treatment with the exception of superficial carious lesions. As the preceding discussion suggests, considerable variation in the sequence of phase II treatment may be appropriate in individual cases to accommodate unique circumstances. The clinician must consider, however, the possible consequences of altering the phase II treatment sequence. Also, good communication between the general dentist and any dental specialist providing a portion of phase II care is essential to avoid contradictory treatment. The completion of phase II treatment is the stage during tentative treatment plans at which the patient's dental condition and response to prior treatment are reevaluated before phase III treatment is specifically planned.

Phase III: Restoration of Esthetics and Function

The goal of phase III treatment is the restoration of esthetics and function. The success of phase III treatment relies on the effectiveness of phase II treatment in providing a healthy environment for the final elements of active dental treatment.

The initial stage of phase III treatment consists of operative dental restoration of superficial carious lesions. Only relatively superficial carious lesions should be delayed until this portion of the treatment sequence. This is based on the expectation that superficial decay is unlikely to progress significantly within the time needed to complete higher priority procedures. Also, the outcome of less extensive operative procedures is sufficiently predictable that other aspects of treatment can be planned without the likelihood of unexpected results. The operative treatment at this stage should also include fabrication of post and cores and large coronal build-ups if this has not previously been accomplished. Final restoration of teeth managed by pulp capping procedures and temporary cement restorations during phase II care should be accomplished at this stage if possible.

All active disease should have been treated, and all decayed teeth should have at least transitional coronal build-ups or temporary crowns in place at this stage of treatment. This represents the completion of a disease control treatment plan. Assuming all preceding dental care has been successful, the patient who has completed this stage of the treatment sequence has reached a stable dental status. More expensive and time-consuming prosthetic treatment can be delayed for a time until the patient's finances allow such care without the risk of significant additional deterioration.

Adult orthodontic treatment is undertaken after the completion of all operative procedures. Carious lesions and active periodontitis must be eliminated before orthodontic treatment. Prosthetic procedures are typically less complex after a stable occlusal relationship has been achieved by orthodontic treatment. In addition, the orthodontic treatment is often preparatory for optimal prosthetic treatment as in cases of molar uprighting and the elimination of malalignment. Orthognathic surgery in conjunction with orthodontic treatment is also undertaken at this stage of comprehensive treatment.

Fixed prosthodontic treatment follows operative and orthodontic treatment during phase III. The final treatment element of phase III is completion of any necessary removable prosthetic procedures. Many fixed procedures such as crowning abutment teeth are preparatory for removable appliance fabrication and must be completed first. In cases of fixed bridges to oppose planned removable prostheses, the best results are usually obtained by completing the fixed procedures first. Placement of implants is usually accomplished early in the prosthetic treatment phase. The provision of the prosthetic care completes the phase III and the active treatment portion of the comprehensive dental treatment plan. All disease has been eliminated and esthetics and function have been restored.

Phase IV: Reevaluation of Treatment

Clinicians are obligated to reevaluate all treatment after phase III treatment is completed. The goal of reevaluation is to confirm that all treatment has been adequate, that inadvertent omissions have not occurred, that no new lesions have developed, and that the patient has adapted to any appliances. Deficiencies in home care can be identified and improved oral hygiene encouraged. This reevaluation of treatment is approached with the assumption that the patient will not be examined again by the dentist for an extended time period. Conditions that could lead to deterioration of the patient's dental status over this interval should be corrected. Correction of problems during treatment reevaluation can prevent understandable patient dissatisfaction with new dental problems shortly after completing comprehensive dental treatment. From another perspective, the phase IV reevaluation can be considered as a quality control procedure by the dentist to identify treatment deficiencies, such as restoration overhangs, and to improve the long-term prognosis.

Simple dental treatment regimens can usually be reevaluated at the final treatment visit. More complicated treatment can be reevaluated as an ongoing process throughout the course of treatment, as well as after active treatment is complete. New radiographs may be appropriate after an extended treatment duration or if the patient is unusually vulnerable to decay or periodontitis. Reevaluation of endodontic and pulp capping procedures by radiographs or pulp testing procedures is often appropriate during the reevaluation phase. Complex prosthetic treatment should be evaluated after a period of weeks or months to ensure that the long-term adaptation is optimal by evaluating for mobility and hygiene difficulties involving abutments. These problems may only become apparent following an interval of weeks or months.

Phase V: Recall

The goal of the recall phase of patient care is the early identification by periodic reexamination of new lesions and oral conditions. The assumption is that treatment of any oral condition is simplified if identified early in the progression of the lesion. Also, the recall phase offers additional opportunities to reevaluate past dental treatment.

The time interval between the completion of dental treatment and the next recall examination must be determined by the patient's past dental disease experience. A 3 month recall interval may be justified for the patient who has completed complex restorative and periodontal care, while the decay-resistant patient without evidence of periodontitis could be reexamined in 12 to 24 months with negligible dental health risk. The clinician's decision on the appropriate recall interval and radiographs to supplement the recall examination must be based on individualized consideration of the patient. The outdated approach recommending dental recall appointments at 6 or 12 months intervals for all patients without respect to individual needs and disease patterns cannot be justified.

CASE PRESENTATION

The process of explaining the diagnostic findings, the necessary dental treatment, and the possible complications of dental treatment to the patient and obtaining the patient's consent to begin treatment is referred to as the case presentation. As conceptually challenging as the treatment planning process can be, a greater challenge in interpersonal communications is often confronted by the dentist in gaining the patient's confidence during the case presentation. This is essentially an instructional discussion in which the clinician informs the patient of the problems present and the best solutions for these problems. It should not become a lecture because most patients have questions, input about past treatment, or disagreements with the dentist's opinions that cannot be ignored without losing the patient's confidence. In addition, a positive attitude and a certain measure of salesmanship help in obtaining the patient's consent for needed health care. Appealing to a person's esthetic concerns, for example, may be a realistic approach to gaining acceptance of fixed prosthetic treatment that is also functionally optimal.

The clinician initially describes the diagnostic findings to help the patient understand the nature of the existing problems before describing the possible solutions or treatment options. The patient must be informed of the consequences of treatment and be allowed the opportunity for questions and clarification to make an informed decision about the dental treatment plan. The last stage of the case presentation, the reassessment of treatment goals, allows the dentist and patient to agree on the best approach to solving the patient's dental problems.

Presentation of Diagnostic Findings

The presentation of the dentist's diagnostic findings should begin with an orienting statement, which informs the patient that this discussion will describe the dentist's opinions about the problems and the possible solutions. The patient should understand that questions are welcomed and that every effort will be made to promote the patient's understanding.

The diagnostic findings are described in the order in which the information was collected. The dentist's opinion concerning the chief complaint should be described initially. This is followed by opinions about any medical conditions that will alter routine dental procedures or require medical consultation before treatment. Next, the implications of the dental history such as past dental treatment, negligence in seeking regular care, excessive dietary sugar, or other general factors related to the patient's dental condition should be described. The dental findings should then be described without bias toward specific treatment. The use of radiographs, study models, and educational materials improves the clarity of the discussion. The amount of detail provided concerning dental problems depends on the extent of the findings and the patient's dental knowledge. The use of clearly understandable terms is essential. All diagnostic findings should then be briefly summarized.

Presentation of Planned Treatment

Presentation of the planned treatment is simply a description of the best solutions to the identified patient problems. The treatment plan considered most consistent with the patient's dental treatment goals is referred to as the *preliminary treatment plan*, and other possible approaches are considered *alternative treatment plans.*

Refusing dental treatment is, unfortunately, the dental care option that many people select and the patient should be informed of the ramifications associated with that decision. Describing the consequences of refusing treatment immediately after the summary of diagnostic findings allows the patient to understand the predictable progression of carious, periodontal, and other dental lesions. This also underscores how the current situation developed and supports many treatment recommendations as preferable to the consequences of rejecting treatment. The future progression of current lesions should be related as much as possible to the patient's past dental experiences and painful complaints. Consequences to emphasize for most patients include small carious lesions progressing to pulpal involvement, progression of periodontitis resulting in mobility, and malalignment of teeth caused by shifting into edentulous spaces. The rate of progression for most routine dental lesions should clearly be described as involving years rather than weeks or months, but the patient must understand that treatment of all routine dental diseases becomes more complicated as they progress.

Preliminary treatment plan. The preliminary treatment plan is described after the consequences of refusing treatment have been explained. The preliminary treatment plan typically recommended by the dentist is based on the goal of comprehensive treatment. For a patient concerned about financial limitations, the best preliminary treatment plan may be disease control treatment without the expense of phase III prosthetic procedures. If the same patient were to state interest in only symptomatic treatment of the chief complaint, then the preliminary treatment plan should be based on the emergency treatment planning approach. The tentative or limited treatment planning approaches would provide the best basis for pre-

paring the preliminary treatment plan in other situations. Simply stated, the dentist's goal is to present a preliminary treatment plan consistent with sound dental practice and with the patient's preferences and resources. The probability of the patient accepting the treatment recommendations increases when the preliminary treatment plan is designed as the best compromise between the dentist's and the patient's perspectives.

Alternative treatment plans. Alternative treatment plans should be described to the patient after the preliminary treatment plan has been discussed. Treatment options usually represent plans to complete fewer or more of the dental treatment phases as compared with the recommendation in the preliminary treatment plan. Alternative treatment plans can be easily described for the patient by comparing them with the approach presented as the preliminary treatment plan. For example, if a disease control treatment plan was initially presented, then the patient can be encouraged to consider the addition of phase III prosthetic procedures as an alternative plan. A patient hesitant to accept the comprehensive treatment approach as the preliminary treatment plan may agree to the disease control treatment approach in the interest of arresting additional dental deterioration.

Many patients will agree to phase I and phase II treatment as an opportunity to evaluate treatment results before agreeing to more complex and costly phase III procedures. The goal is to encourage acceptance of as much of the comprehensive treatment plan as possible while remaining flexible in offering less than total care as an alternative. Irrespective of the amount of treatment planned, the patient should be encouraged to accept follow-up care of phase IV and phase V procedures.

Specific treatment alternatives. Possible treatment procedure alternatives within the treatment plan should also be presented as options to the patient. Different procedures are frequently available to solve the problems of complicated treatment plans, while simpler treatment plans generally offer fewer options. Fabrication of a single removable partial denture rather than several fixed prostheses as replacement for multiple missing teeth within an arch is a common example of such an option. The comparative advantages and disadvantages of these alternative procedures should be explained to the patient. This provides the information the patient needs to assist in the decision process. The specific treatment options presented to the patient should be limited to those treatment options that are feasible and consistent with sound dental practice.

Consequences of Treatment

The patient has the right to know the consequences of planned treatment before agreeing to proceed. Most patients are eager to know the more predictable consequences such as the cost, number of treatment visits, and likelihood of pain associated with the planned treatment. The prognosis or expectation for success and longevity of the procedures should also be discussed in general terms. The patient's obligation to maintain effective oral hygiene as a prognostic factor should also be emphasized. The patient is then informed of the risk of complications and the sequelae associated with the planned treatment. Even if such complications are rare, the patient must be informed before agreeing to accept such risks as a prerequisite of dental treatment. Failure to obtain this *informed consent* can cause the dentist to be held liable for damages if complications develop.

The most efficient approach to providing this information to the patient in complex cases involving numerous treatment options is to describe treatment consequences for the preliminary treatment plan first. The cost, prognosis, risks and other consequences of alternative treatment plans can then be related or compared with those of the preliminary treatment plan. Providing this information to the patient in written form helps to avoid confusion and misunderstandings.

Questions and Clarification

The patient should be encouraged to ask questions and request clarification concerning the preliminary treatment plan, the possible treatment alternatives, and the consequences of treatment. Regardless of previous questions asked by the patient, the dentist should specifically request additional questions and provide the answers after the discussion of treatment consequences. If the patient asks no questions, then the dentist should confirm that the patient understands key aspects of the case presentation such as the general nature of the dental problems, treatment planned, and expected cost.

Reassessment of Treatment Goals

The only purpose of the case presentation discussion between the dentist and patient is to reach an agreement on how to proceed in solving the patient's dental problems. The dentist has presented a preliminary treatment plan based on comprehensive treatment or an approach believed to be most consistent with the patient's wishes and welfare. However, the cost, prognosis, or other treatment consequences may be unacceptable to the patient. The patient may have expected a few simple procedures to solve symptomatic problems and may be surprised by the nature or extent of the dental problems and the treatment needed to solve them. The dentist and patient must reassess treatment goals together in an effort to identify a compromise treatment approach that will solve the most important problems within available resources. Reaching the compromise usually relies on additional clarification of the dental problems and the treatment options.

The final treatment agreement, referred to simply as the *treatment plan,* should be documented by both the patient's and the dentist's signatures. As with all agreements, this treatment commitment must be made with a responsible adult. All aspects of the treatment plan and informed consent issues for a minor or adult of diminished capacity must be discussed with a parent or guardian. The patient should understand that certain aspects of the treatment may change as a result of unexpected and unpredictable conditions.

Several case presentation practices commonly lead to rejection of treatment. Patients become skeptical of unrealistic claims and assurances, such as promised results that cannot be predictably achieved. Also, procedures that are likely to be uncomfortable should be described as such. Patients often need to consider extensive treatment plans for a few days and prefer not to be pressured into a rushed decision. Whatever portion of comprehensive treatment the patient agrees to accept initially, the dentist should clarify that the decision can always be made later to proceed to more advanced treatment.

SUMMARY

Effective dental treatment planning is one of the most challenging aspects of dentistry. The dentist must simultaneously consider diagnostic findings indicative of dental problems, possible solutions to these problems, and the preferences of the patient while designing the best possible treatment approach. Dental treatment planning can be simplified by approaching the procedure in stages:

1. Listing the identified problems starting with the chief complaint, then those involving the medical status, and finally the oral conditions

2. Listing possible solutions and treatment planning implications for each of the identified problems

3. Selecting the best possible solution for each problem while considering the patient's concerns, the technical considerations, and implications of the patient's other dental treatment needs

4. Arranging the solutions for the patient's problems in a priority sequence starting with symptomatic care, followed by treatment for disease control, and completing active treatment with restorative procedures

5. Selecting the appropriate treatment planning approach for the patient's dental treatment goals from among emergency, disease control, comprehensive, limited, or tentative treatment schemes

Finally, the case presentation is the opportunity for the dentist to inform the patient of the diagnostic findings, the treatment options, and the consequences of the various options. The patient and dentist can use this information to reassess treatment goals and agree on the optimal treatment plan.

BIBLIOGRAPHY

Barsh LS: Dental treatment planning for the adult patient, Philadelphia, 1981, Saunders.

Langlais RP and others: Oral diagnosis, oral medicine and treatment planning, Philadelphia, 1984, Saunders.

Little JW, Falace DA: Therapeutic considerations in special patients, Dent Clin North Am 28:455-469, 1984.

Wood NK, editor: Treatment planning: a pragmatic approach, St Louis, 1978, Mosby–Year Book.

CHAPTER 13

Modification of Dental Treatment for Patients with Compromised Health

BYRON W. BENSON

Advanced medical treatment methods and greater access to sophisticated medical care have produced an active and ambulatory population of patients who suffer from serious systemic conditions and who need dental care. The diagnosis and treatment of these diseases are beyond the scope of dental practice, but the dentist must recognize evidence of compromised health to avoid potential complications during dental treatment. Modifying dental procedure methods or delaying dental care temporarily are often necessary to minimize the risk of problems. The dictum *primum non-nocere,* "first do no harm," concisely states the management obligation for patients with compromised health.

This chapter discusses the more common systemic conditions associated with potential dental treatment complications and general management recommendations. Unfortunately, a general discussion cannot address management decisions for all clinical situations and every rare disease. The intent is to illustrate frequently encountered potential problems associated with compromised health rather than to provide comprehensive coverage of the subject. The conscientious practitioner will frequently need to consult medical references, the patient's physician, dental specialists, and other resources for information and guidance in unique and complex clinical situations.

POTENTIALLY INFECTIOUS PATIENTS

Risks. Patients suffering from infectious diseases may represent a potential source of infection to dental office personnel and to other patients by contact with blood or saliva. Examples of such infections include hepatitis B, hepatitis C, HIV infection, and tuberculosis. Unfortunately, consistent identification of the potentially infectious patient in the dental office by history and examination is ineffective.

Management. The term *universal precautions* refers to the management of all patients as if they are infectious. The current standards for surface disinfection, use of barriers, sterilization of instruments, and disposal of contaminated material are regularly updated in professional journals.

CARDIOVASCULAR CONDITIONS
Hypertension

Risks. The physiologic demands, emotional stress, and vasopressors associated with dental treatment often cause temporary elevation of blood pressure. The normal patient tolerates this without consequence. However, stressful episodes entail increased risk of cerebrovascular accident or myocardial infarction for the severely hypertensive patient. Increasing difficulty in achieving hemostasis is proportional to elevated blood pressure. Antihypertensive medications may cause vertigo following abrupt postural changes, which is referred to as *orthostatic hypotension*. Calcium channel blockers have been reported to precipitate gingival hyperplasia.

Management. Medical consultation is appropriate for patients with blood pressure readings consistently above 150/90 mm Hg. Surgery and other stressful procedures are relatively contraindicated if the blood pressure is above 160/100 mm Hg. Hypertensive patients should not be allowed to stand immediately after being raised from a reclined position.

Increased Vulnerability to Infective Endocarditis

Risks. Infective endocarditis, formerly known as *subacute bacterial endocarditis,* is an infection of deformed heart valves or other endocardial surfaces by blood-borne pathogens. The infection can cause additional valvular damage, septic emboli, septicemia, and death.

Transient bacteremia is believed to occur during any dental procedure involving significant tissue manipulation or bleeding. This implies that most dental procedures could be the proximate cause of infective endocarditis for a vulnerable individual. Table 13-1 lists common cardiac conditions as categorized by the associated risk of infective endocarditis. Heart valve deformity or abnormal valvular function as suggested by a history of heart murmur and a history of a prosthesis in contact with the blood flow are the two characteristics that are most often associated with increased endocarditis risk. Medical consultation is often necessary to clarify the patient's cardiac condition. It must be stated to the physician that the specific consultation issue relates to the patient's vulnerability to infective endocarditis from transient bacteremia caused by dental procedures.

Management. The initial goal in minimizing the risk of infective endocarditis from oral microbes is to decrease the oral microbial reservoir by prevention and control of chronic oral infections. Therefore optimal oral hygiene, fluoride rinses, chlorhexidine gluconate rinses, and routine dental care should be a priority for patients vulnerable to infective endocarditis.

The dentist is also obligated to minimize as much as possible the duration, frequency, and severity of the bacteremia resulting from dental treatment. Topical use antimicrobials such as chlorhexidine gluconate by rinsing or direct application prior to extractions and other procedures limits the number of viable bacteria available to enter the blood at the site. Administration of antibiotics before dental procedures decreases the duration and the number of organisms of the bacteremia.

The American Heart Association (AHA) recommends antibiotic prophylaxis before any dental procedure that might cause bleeding, including periodontal probing and prophylaxis, for patients at risk for infective endocarditis. Dental procedures that are unlikely to induce gingival bleeding such as conventional anes-

Table 13-1   Relative risk of infective endocarditis associated with common cardiac conditions and recommended clinical management during dental procedures that are likely to cause bleeding

	Risk not significantly increased	Significant risk	High risk
Conditions	Physiologic (functional, innocent) murmurs Isolated atrial septal defects Nonvalvular surgical repair of the heart without residua (over 6 months postoperatively) Coronary artery bypass/vascular surgery (over 6 months postoperatively) Mitral valve prolapse without regurgitation History of rheumatic fever without valvular dysfunction Kawasaki's disease without valvular dysfunction Cardiac pacemakers Implanted defibrillators	Most congenital cardiac malformations Rheumatic valvular defects (including those surgically repaired) Other acquired valvular dysfunction (including those surgically repaired) Hypertrophic cardiomyopathy Mitral valve prolapse with regurgitation Heart surgery of any type within 6 months	Prior occurrence of infective endocarditis Prosthetic heart valve(s) Other intravascular prosthetic devices (e.g., shunts and conduits)
Management Regimen	Endocarditis prophylaxis not recommended None	Endocarditis prophylaxis recommended Standard oral antibiotic regimen in most cases Appropriate alternate regimen for patients unable to take oral medications or who are allergic to the standard antibiotics	Endocarditis prophylaxis recommended Standard oral antibiotic regimen in most cases Appropriate alternate regimen for patients who are allergic to the standard antibiotics or who are unable to take oral medications Some practitioners may prefer to use alternate parenteral prophylaxis for high-risk patients even though the standard oral regimen is considered adequate

Table 13-2   Summary of infective endocarditis prophylaxis regimens for patients with no history or other indication of allergic hypersensitivity to ampicillin, amoxicillin, or penicillin

| | Standard regimen (Oral) | Alternate regimens (Parenteral) | |
		For patients unable to take oral medications	For patients considered high risk
For adults and children over 60 pounds (27 kg)	Rx: Amoxicillin 500 mg Disp: 9 tablets Sig: Take 6 tablets 1 hour prior to dental treatment, then 3 tablets 6 hours after initial dose ***or*** Rx: Penicillin V 500 mg Disp: 6 tablets Sig: Take 4 tablets 1 hour prior to dental treatment, then 2 tablets 6 hours after initial dose	Rx: Ampicillin Disp: 2 gm Sig: 2 gm IM/IV 30 minutes prior to dental treatment ***then*** Ampicillin, 1 gm IM/IV 6 hours after initial dose, **or** amoxicillin 1.5 gm PO (if oral medication can be tolerated postoperatively) 6 hours after initial dose	Rx: Ampicillin Disp: 2 gm Sig: 2 gm IM/IV given 30 minutes prior to dental treatment ***and*** Rx: Gentamicin Disp: Per patient's mass Sig: 1.5 mg/kg IM/IV given 30 minutes prior to dental treatment, not to exceed 80 mg ***then*** Amoxicillin (500 mg tablets) 1.5 gm PO 6 hours after initial dose, **or** repeat parenteral regimen 8 hours after initial dose
For children under 60 pounds (27 kg)	Initial dose amoxicillin (250 mg tablets) 50 mg/kg or penicillin V (250 mg tablets) 1 gm; follow-up should be one half of the initial dose, not to exceed the total adult dosage Weight ranges may be used for initial pediatric dose of amoxicillin as follows: <15 kg, 750 mg; 15 to 30 kg, 1500 mg; and >30 kg, 3000 mg (full adult dose)	Initial dose ampicillin 50 mg/kg IM/IV; follow-up should be one half of the initial dose, not to exceed the total adult dosage	Initial doses: ampicillin 50 mg/kg IM/IV, gentamicin 2.0 mg/kg; follow-up amoxicillin (250 mg tablets) 25 mg/kg; doses are not to exceed the total adult dosage

thetic injections, supragingival restorations, and adjustment of orthodontic appliances do not require antibiotic prophylaxis. The AHA guidelines specify three antibiotic regimens. The *standard oral regimen* is appropriate for all dental procedures and for all conditions of increased infective endocarditis risk. The *alternate parenteral regimen for patients unable to take oral medications* is for just that circum-

stance. Some practitioners may prefer to use the *alternate parenteral regimen for patients considered high risk,* although the standard regimen has been shown to be adequate for dental procedures. The high-risk regimen is designed to provide additional antibiotic protection for conditions such as prosthetic valves or a history of infective endocarditis. The recommended antibiotic regimens for infective en-

Table 13-3   Summary of infective endocarditis prophylaxis regimens for patients who are hypersensitive to the routinely recommended antibiotic (ampicillin, amoxicillin, or penicillin)

	Alternate standard regimen for patients hypersensitive to amoxicillin/penicillin (Oral)	Alternate regimens for patients hypersensitive to ampicillin/amoxicillin/penicillin (Parenteral)	
		For patients unable to take oral medications	For patients considered high risk
For adults and children over 60 pounds (27 kg)	Rx: Erythromycin ethyl-succinate (ESS) 400 mg Disp: 3 tablets Sig: Take 2 tablets 1 hour prior to dental treatment, then 1 tablet 6 hours after initial dose *or* Rx: Erythromycin stearate 500 mg Disp: 3 tablets Sig: Take 2 tablets 1 hour prior to dental treatment, then 1 tablet 6 hours after initial dose *or* Rx: Clindamycin 150 mg Disp: 3 tablets Sig: Take 2 tablets 1 hour prior to dental treatment, then 1 tablet 6 hours after initial dose	Rx: Clindamycin Disp: 300 mg Sig: 300 mg IV 30 min prior to dental treatment: then 150 mg IV or PO 6 hrs after initial dose.	Rx: Vancomycin Disp: 1 gm Sig: 1.0 gm IV given slowly over 1 hour, starting 1 hour prior to dental treatment; no repeat dose is necessary
For children under 60 pounds (27 kg)	Initial doses erythromycin ethylsuccinate (200 mg tablets) or erythromycin stearate (250 mg tablets) 20 mg/kg 1 hour prior to dental treatment; clindamycin (150 mg tablets) 10 mg/kg; follow-up should be one half of the initial dose, not to exceed the total adult dosage	Initial dose clindamycin 10 mg/kg IM/IV; follow-up should be one half of the initial dose, not to exceed the total adult dosage	Vancomycin IV 20 mg/kg, not to exceed total adult dosage; no follow-up necessary

docarditis prophylaxis for patients who are not hypersensitive to the drugs are summarized in Table 13-2. Antibiotic recommendations for individuals who are hypersensitive to standard antibiotics are shown in Table 13-3.

Several treatment procedures should be combined, if possible, at each appointment to limit the number of antibiotic administrations required. Also, a 1-week interval between appointments is recommended to decrease the potential for the emergence of resistant bacterial strains.

Angina Pectoris

Risks. A history of angina pectoris indicates compromised coronary circulation and the possibility that the stress of dental treatment may cause an ischemic attack or myocardial infarction. This is a remote possibility for patients with stable angina, while the probability of an ischemic episode with unstable angina increases proportionally with the emotional and physiologic demands of the dental procedure. The clinical features of stable and unstable angina are described in Chapter 7.

Management. Routine dental treatment of stable angina patients rarely precipitates cardiac ischemia, although their nitroglycerin tablets should be readily available during dental treatment. Patients with unstable angina require medical consultation before even routine dental treatment. Eventual management in concert with the patient's physician may include prophylactic administration of long-acting nitrates or dental treatment in a hospital setting.

Myocardial Infarction

Risks. Individuals who have suffered one myocardial infarction (MI) are likely to have another. The demands of dental treatment can precipitate ischemic episodes as described for angina pectoris. Congestive heart failure and cardiac arrhythmia also predispose the patient to MI during stressful situations.

Management. The condition of a patient who has had a heart attack within 1 year demands medical consultation prior to dental treatment. Elective dental treatment should be temporarily deferred for patients who have had an MI in the previous 6 months. Minor dental treatment may be rendered if the MI occurred between 6 and 12 months previously but major dental treatment should be delayed. Methods of minimizing stress such as short appointments, morning appointments, and attainment of profound anesthesia before starting procedures are mandatory.

Relatively routine dental treatment methods may be relied on more than 1 year after an MI if ischemic symptoms such as angina appear well controlled. Attention to minimizing treatment stress is appropriate. Persistence of angina, hypertension, continuation of adverse personal habits, and other significant risk indicators suggest the need for a medical consultation. Dental treatment in a hospital setting may be appropriate for many patients with ischemic heart disease contingent on the physician's opinion.

Congestive Heart Failure

Risks. The immediate adverse consequence of congestive heart failure is that stressful dental treatment will exceed the compromised ability of the heart to pump blood and thereby precipitate cardiac ischemia.

Management. The use of epinephrine should be minimized to avoid the increased peripheral circulatory resistance of an inadvertent generalized vasopressor effect. Congestive heart failure patients usually take several medications including diuretics, digitalis preparations, and vasodilators. This requires careful consideration before administering additional drugs. Patients in a fully reclined position during dental treatment may experience labored breathing, and this position should be avoided. Medical consultation and hospitalization for stressful treatment may be appropriate in severe cases.

Cardiac Arrhythmia

Risks. Patients with therapeutically controlled cardiac arrhythmias risk an arrhythmic episode during dental treatment when stress or epinephrine absorption exceeds the physiologic limit of current treatment. Patients with atrial arrhythmias and unifocal premature ventricular contractions are considered low risk, especially if chronic medical treatment has not been necessary. Asymptomatic atrial arrhythmias with chronic medication represents a moderate risk. Asymptomatic ventricular arrhythmias with chronic medication present a significant risk, while symptomatic patients with a pulse rate greater than 100 or less than 60 and an irregular pulse rhythm are high risk. In addition, older pacemakers may be vulnerable to electromagnetic interference from devices such as ultrasonic scalers and microwave sterilizers.

Management. Minimization of stress including accomplishing profound anesthesia by the cautious use of epinephrine is appropriate dental management for low and moderate risk cardiac arrhythmias. Medical consultation and hospitalization for dental care should be considered for high risk patients. Electrosurgery is contraindicated in all patients with a history of arrhythmia and the susceptibility of a pacemaker to electric interference should be determined before the use of electric devices.

PULMONARY CONDITIONS
Asthma

Risks. The reversible airway constriction and labored breathing of asthma may be precipitated in the dental setting, but the patient is generally well prepared to control the acute episode. Most of the management problems posed by patients with asthma are related to the chronic side effects of the medications, such as corticosteroids and theophylline taken to control symptoms.

Management. Patients experiencing rare attacks and not on continuous medication may be managed in a routine manner. More frequent attacks and more complex drug regimens needed for control suggest the need for consultation and therapeutic coordination with the patient's physician. Stress and exposure to any known stimulus common to the dental environment should be avoided during dental treatment, and the asthmatic should have a bronchodilator inhaler readily available during dental treatment.

Use of aspirin and antihistamines are contraindicated for asthmatics. Acetaminophen is recommended for relief of minor pain. Administration of clindamycin and erythromycin

with theophylline is contraindicated. Use of epinephrine should be minimized. Supplemental steroids and antibiotic prophylaxis may be appropriate for the patient whose asthma is controlled by corticosteroids, as described in the section on adrenal suppression.

Chronic Obstructive Pulmonary Disease

Risks. The most common forms of chronic obstructive pulmonary disease (COPD) are chronic bronchitis and emphysema. The respiratory compromise during stress differs from asthma in that it is not reversible and it may progress to cor pulmonale (right side heart failure). In addition to the medications commonly prescribed for asthma, patients with COPD may be receiving chronic oxygen therapy, antibiotics, digitalis, and diuretics.

Management. Therapeutic contraindications are generally the same as for asthmatics. Well controlled individuals may be treated routinely. Poor control of the condition and frequent exacerbations contraindicate nonemergency dental care. All medications given to patients with advanced COPD should be discussed and coordinated with their physician. When surgical dental procedures are necessary, hospitalization may be appropriate for individuals whose conditions are poorly controlled.

BLEEDING DISORDERS

Risks. Difficulty achieving hemostasis following dental procedures is unusual in the absence of historical or clinical findings suggestive of an underlying bleeding disorder. Relatively common inherited disorders such as von Willebrand's disease and hemophilia will be promptly reported by the patient in most cases prior to any dental treatment. Identification of an acquired bleeding diathesis may be more difficult. Liver cirrhosis, severe hepatitis, peptic ulcers, other gastrointestinal bleeding, and malnutrition are among the conditions that can cause ineffective coagulation. Drug-induced hemostatic defects caused by aspirin, nonsteroidal antiinflammatories, chemotherapeutic agents, coumarin, and heparin are the typical examples confronted clinically.

Management. Virtually all bleeding disorders are detectable with laboratory tests including platelet count, bleeding time, prothrombin time, and partial thromboplastin time as described in Chapter 11. A congenital history or recent onset of bleeding abnormalities necessitates consultation with the patient's physician before dental treatment.

GASTROINTESTINAL CONDITIONS
Peptic Ulcer Disease

Risks. Dental treatment of the patient with peptic ulcers entails few direct risks. However, in severe cases the patient may develop a bleeding tendency attributable to the continuous consumption of platelets and coagulation factors.

Management. Substances that aggravate peptic ulcers such as aspirin, corticosteroids, and nonsteroidal antiinflammatories should not be administered. Tetracycline is contraindicated if the patient is taking antacid preparations containing aluminum. Preoperative evaluation of coagulation functions may be indicated if clinical findings suggest the possibility of a bleeding tendency.

Intestinal Disease

Risks. Dental treatment of patients with intestinal conditions presents few direct complications. Severe malabsorption conditions may produce oral ulcers, diminished host resistance to infection, a bleeding tendency, anemia, and other conditions related to poor general health. Treatment of inflammatory bowel diseases such as ulcerative colitis and regional enteritis commonly relies on chronic corticosteroid therapy, which may cause adrenal suppression.

Management. Medical consultation and treatment of severe malabsorption conditions improve the patient's response to dental treatment. Management of adrenal suppression is described in the discussion on adrenal cortical disorders.

Hepatitis and Liver Cirrhosis

Risks. The primary clinical consequence of hepatitis and cirrhosis for the dentist is the resulting decreased functional reserve, which implies the possibility of inefficient metabolism of drugs and decreased production of coagulation proteins. Also, the patient suffering from viral forms of hepatitis represents a source of infection. This risk to office personnel and other patients is minimized by infection control procedures, but inadvertent contamination may still occur.

Management. Elective dental care should be deferred during the acute phase of hepatitis until liver function tests have returned to normal. The dosage and administration of any medication primarily metabolized by the liver or with known hepatotoxic effects should be carefully considered in patients with compromised liver function. These drugs include the following:

lidocaine	mepivacaine
procaine	acetaminophen
codeine	meperidine
diazapam	barbiturates
ampicillin	tetracyclines

Patients with chronic active hepatitis may be on long-term steroid therapy, which may cause adrenal suppression. The routine infection control procedures for all patients should be designed to be adequate for the patient with viral hepatitis, whether identified or not.

ENDOCRINE CONDITIONS
Diabetes Mellitus

Risks. The most serious risk to the diabetic during dental treatment is that a combination of stress, inadequate insulin administration, and lack of available carbohydrates will adversely affect the balance of insulin and blood sugar. This imbalance can develop into either diabetic coma (hyperglycemia) or insulin shock (hypoglycemia). This is most likely if initial control is poor and for those who are difficult to control, the "brittle diabetics." Also, diabetes is associated with delayed healing and is among the conditions known to cause diminished host resistance to infection.

Management. Undiagnosed patients with signs and symptoms suggestive of diabetes and diagnosed patients with poor control of their disease should be referred to their physician before dental treatment. The patient with well-controlled diabetes may undergo dental care with attention to several factors. Patients taking oral hypoglycemic agents should take them as usual before the appointment. Diabetic patients should be instructed to eat a normal meal before treatment. Those using insulin may need to divide their normal morning dosage if the dental care alters their meal schedule. The second half of the insulin may be administered when a normal meal cycle is resumed. Medical consultation is appropriate whenever a medication routine must be altered.

Antibiotic prophylaxis might be considered for periodontal, endodontic, or oral surgical procedures. The AHA standard regimen for infective endocarditis prophylaxis is appropriate. Hospitalization may be required to adequately manage potential complications if extensive surgical procedures are planned.

Thyroid Disorders

Risks. Most patients with thyroid disorders have well-controlled conditions, and dental treatment presents little direct threat. However, the thyrotoxic patient is at risk for a thyrotoxic crisis precipitated by the physiologic stress of trauma, surgery, or severe infection.

Management. Individuals with diagnosed thyroid disease may be treated routinely if they are asymptomatic and recent thyroid function tests are normal. Stress and the use of epinephrine and central nervous system depressants should be minimized. Dental treat-

ment should only be rendered subsequent to medical consultation if the patient exhibits signs and symptoms of thyrotoxicosis (Chapter 7).

Adrenal Cortex Disorders

Risks. Corticosteroids offer effective treatment for numerous inflammatory conditions such as arthritis, autoimmune diseases, asthma, dermatologic disorders, and inflammatory bowel conditions. Unfortunately, chronic corticosteroid therapy often produces adrenal suppression, which leaves the patient without an adrenal reserve during episodes of stress and increases the risk of an adrenal crisis. Some degree of adrenal suppression must be presumed for patients who have received the equivalent of 20 mg of prednisone per day for more than 1 week during the preceding year. Use of topical steroids, maintenance regimens of less than 20 mg per day, and alternate day maintenance regimens are less likely to produce significant adrenal suppression.

Management. The patient's physician should be consulted if adrenal suppression is suspected to determine the need for corticosteroid supplementation. The physician needs to be informed of the anticipated degree of emotional and physiologic stress anticipated with the dental procedures in order to make this judgment.

Corticosteroid supplementation will generally not be necessary for the adrenally suppressed patient during routine dental treatment involving minimal stress. The corticosteroid dosage should be augmented by 20 to 40 mg of prednisone equivalency on the day of the procedure and half that dose the following day for moderately demanding procedures. For moderate to severe stress, the dosage of prednisone should be increased to a total equivalent to 60 mg of prednisone on the day of the procedure followed by gradual dose reduction to the maintenance dose or zero within 3 days. Prophylactic antibiotic coverage for 3 days starting on the day of treatment may be indicated to compensate for the patient's compromised resistance to infection.

GENITOURINARY CONDITIONS
Pregnancy

Risks. The most significant complications from dental treatment during pregnancy include developmental injury to the fetus and miscarriage. Ionizing radiation, stress, infection, and the use of drugs related to dental care may all pose the risk of harm. The fetus is most vulnerable during the first trimester of pregnancy, but confirmation of the pregnancy may be difficult until after a large portion of the first trimester has passed. Women of childbearing age should be assumed to be pregnant before the administration of drugs or the exposure of radiographs until the condition is specifically denied.

Several aspects of pregnancy can make dental treatment awkward and uncomfortable. The nausea of "morning sickness" can be aggravated by dental treatment during the first trimester. The reclined position of dental treatment becomes uncomfortable and many women develop a tendency for syncope, dyspnea, and hypotension during the third trimester.

Management. Elective dental care should be deferred until after pregnancy. Dental care that cannot be deferred is most comfortable for the patient and involves the least risk to the fetus during the second trimester. Development of pregnancy gingivitis resulting from hormonal fluctuations may require prophylaxis and oral hygiene instruction. Management of pregnant patients during dental treatment should include monitoring blood pressure and pulse. Alteration of the usual dental chair position will usually be necessary, especially during the third trimester.

The ADA Recommendation of Radiographic Practices suggests that pregnancy is not an indication to alter dental radiographic examinations. This implies the use of lead aprons, fast speed film, and other radiation dose limitation techniques that should be routine procedure for all patients. However, limitation of radiographic procedures that can be delayed until after delivery may be prudent management for patients who are particularly concerned.

The patient's obstetrician should be consulted before the administration of *any* drug to a pregnant or lactating woman. The use of penicillin, erythromycin, acetaminophen, or lidocaine is usually approved. Vasopressors, respiratory depressants, and aspirin should be avoided. Sedatives, tetracycline, and nitrous oxide are completely contraindicated in the context of dental care.

Renal Disease

Risks. The most significant complications from dental treatment for the patient with diminished renal function are related to the use of medications. Dosage or dose frequency of drugs primarily excreted by the kidneys may require alteration for the renal patient. Other drugs that can cause nephrotoxicity may not be tolerated at standard doses by the patient with compromised renal reserve.

Medical treatment of chronic renal failure requires hemodialysis several times a week for life or until renal transplantation can be arranged. The hemodialysis procedure includes use of heparin to prevent coagulation, which produces a residual bleeding tendency for approximately 12 hours following the procedure. In addition, hemodialysis tends to destroy platelets and many patients with chronic renal failure also develop abnormal platelet function. Peritoneal dialysis is an alternative to hemodialysis that does not require the use of heparin, therefore, bleeding following the procedure is a less likely source of complications. Patients who are undergoing renal dialysis will have semipermanent vascular shunts or catheter sites that are susceptible to infection.

Management. Few complications are associated with routine dental treatment of the patient with chronic renal disease if the need for the modifications described below is recognized. However, the patient's physician should be consulted, particularly if a bleeding diathesis is suspected. Dental appointments should not be scheduled for the day of hemodialysis. The day after hemodialysis is best because the residual heparin effects and the predictable azotemia prior to the next dialysis session are avoided. A course of prophylactic antibiotics may be recommended subsequent to medical consultation. The AHA standard regimen for infective endocarditis prophylaxis (Table 13-2) is appropriate for this purpose in most instances. Hospitalization may be necessary for extensive surgical procedures.

Some nephrotoxic drugs, such as tetracycline and acetaminophen, are contraindicated in chronic renal failure. Other drugs including aspirin, penicillin, cephalexin, and ampicillin may be used but their dosages must be decreased.

CONDITIONS AFFECTING THE NERVOUS SYSTEM
Cerebrovascular Disease

Risks. A patient with a recent history of cerebrovascular accident (CVA or "stroke") or transient ischemic attack (TIA) must be considered at risk for a CVA during stressful dental treatment. The probability of a CVA is substantially increased if the patient is hypertensive. Prevention of cerebrovascular accidents in patients with a history of CVA or TIA relies on anticoagulant and antiplatelet aggregation drugs such as coumarin and aspirin, which may make hemostasis difficult.

Management. Elective dental care is contraindicated for most patients in the 6 to 12 months after a CVA. Emergency dental care may be rendered following a medical consultation with proper attention to bleeding problems. Medical consultation is still recommended if more than 6 to 12 months have passed subsequent to the TIA or CVA. Routine dental care may be provided with proper attention to bleeding problems. The physician will often alter the anticoagulant regimen to accommodate necessary dental treatment. However, most physicians prefer to avoid repeated alterations of the anticoagulation regimen. Therefore each appointment should be planned to accomplish as much dental care as possible. Surgical procedures may require hospitalization.

Seizure Disorders

Risks. The principal complication for patients with seizure disorders during dental treatment is that a seizure may occur in the dental operatory. Although this rarely causes any permanent injury, it should still be avoided. Also, certain medications used to control seizures may require alteration of the use of medications for dental treatment.

Management. Routine dental treatment should pose no complications for the patient whose disorder is well controlled. Poor control—as indicated by a seizure more frequently than once per month—requires delaying elective dental treatment pending medical consultation.

The dosage of a narcotic analgesic should be reduced for seizure patients taking central nervous system depressant drugs. Phenytoin therapy has been associated with gingival hyperplasia, which should be managed aggressively. Tetracycline is contraindicated when the patient is taking phenytoin, primidone, or phenobarbital.

Should a seizure occur during dental treatment, place the patient in a supine position, protect him or her from injury, and monitor vital signs. Most seizures will end within 5 minutes, after which the patient may be confused for up to 1 hour. The patient may be discharged to the custody of another responsible individual when coherent. Should the seizure persist, intravenous diazepam may be administered if adequate respiratory and cardiovascular support equipment and training are available. If they are not available, transportation to a hospital emergency room is indicated.

COMPROMISED FUNCTION OF THE IMMUNE SYSTEM

Risks. Compromised function of the immune system is a feature of several rare congenital diseases and acquired conditions. These patients are exceptionally vulnerable to numerous common infections, as well as unusual infections caused by opportunistic organisms. HIV infection leading to AIDS, organ transplantation patients taking immunosuppressive drugs on an indefinite basis, and patients taking doses of corticosteroids are common examples of acquired immunodeficiency.

Management. Prevention of infection, control of common chronic infections such as periodontitis, and aggressive treatment of acute infections are priorities for the patient with compromised function of the immune system. Important methods of limiting the extent of oral infections are to establish good oral hygiene and to maintain routine dental care. A prophylactic antibiotic regimen may be beneficial in preventing incidental bacterial infections after routine dental treatment. The AHA standard regimen has been suggested for these patients.

Oral candidiasis is a common opportunistic infection among immunocompromised individuals. Nystatin oral suspension and clotrimazole troches are effective topical preparations for most oral infections:

Topical

Rx: Nystatin (Mycostatin) oral suspension 100,000 units/ml
Disp: One 60 ml bottle
Sig: Rinse with 2 to 5 ml of suspension for 2 minutes, then swallow
(Medicated "popsicles" can be made by adding 2 ml of the solution to each cube in an ice tray.)
* or *
Rx: Clotrimazole troches 10 mg
Disp: 70 troches
Sig: Melt one troche in mouth five times daily
* and *
Rx: Chlorhexidine gluconate 0.12%
Disp: 480 ml bottle

Sig: Rinse mouth with 15 ml of undiluted solution twice daily after brushing and flossing; expectorate after rinsing

Systemic

Rx: Ketoconazole 200 mg
Disp: 20 tablets
Sig: Take one tablet each day with a meal
* or *
Rx: Fluconazole 200 mg
Disp: 29 tablets
Sig: Take two tablets on the first day and one tablet each subsequent day

Fluconazole may be necessary to control candidiasis that is extensive or is unresponsive to topical antifungal agents. Antiviral agents such as acyclovir may be beneficial in treating herpes simplex, herpes zoster, and other viral infections:

Oral

Rx: Acyclovir capsules 200 mg
Disp: 50 capsules
Sig: Take one capsule five times daily

Topical

Rx: Acyclovir topical ointment 5%
Disp: 15 gm tube
Sig: Apply to area q2h

PROSTHETIC JOINTS

Risks. Prosthetic joints may be prone to hematogenous infection caused by bacteremias from dental procedures. Hip prostheses are considered most vulnerable, and the infection is often caused by penicillin-resistant staphylococcal organisms.

Management. There is no accepted prophylactic regimen to protect patients with joint prostheses during dental treatment. Therefore consultation with an orthopedic surgeon is appropriate before any dental procedure known to cause a bacteremia. Several regimens that are frequently recommended are the following:

Rx: Cephalexin (Keflex) 500 mg
Disp: 6 tablets
Sig: Take 4 tablets 1 hour before dental treatment, then 2 tablets 6 hours later
* **or** *
Rx: Erythromycin 500 mg
Disp: 3 tablets
Sig: Take 2 tablets 1 hour prior to dental treatment then 1 tablet 6 hours later
* **or** *
Rx: Cloxacillin 500 mg
Disp: 3 tablets
Sig: Take 2 tablets 1 hour before dental treatment, then 1 tablet 6 hours later

The orthopedic surgeon may also recommend that antibiotic coverage is not indicated during dental treatment.

RADIOTHERAPY AND CHEMOTHERAPY
Radiotherapy

Risks. Individuals treated with radiotherapy for tumors of the head and neck may experience a variety of oral complications including mucositis, candidiasis, xerostomia, loss of taste, and rampant caries. The patient may also be at increased risk for osteoradionecrosis of the mandible if the radiation dose was greater than 50 grays (5000 rads).

Management. Prevention is the optimal management approach for severe complications, such as osteoradionecrosis, following radiotherapy. Therefore it is imperative that the dentist be consulted before radiotherapy of the head and neck. Dental infections should be eliminated at that time by the extraction of nonrestorable teeth, control of periodontitis, and treatment of periapical infections. Tooth removal after radiotherapy should be avoided if possible. However, should it become necessary to remove teeth, it is preferable to wait until 1 year after radiotherapy and a broad spectrum antibiotic should be administered in conjunction with the procedure.

Acute mucositis during radiotherapy can be treated symptomatically with topical anesthetic agents or a coating suspension of Kaopectate and diphenhydramine:

Rx: Lidocaine HCl viscous 2%
Disp: 450 ml bottle
Sig: Swish 1 tsp before meals and then spit out
* **or** *
Rx: Diphenhydramine elixir HCl 12.5 mg/5 ml
Disp: 4 oz bottle
Sig: Rinse with 1 tsp for 2 minutes before meals, then spit out
* **or** *
Rx: Diphenhydramine HCl elixir 12.5 mg/5 ml to 120 ml mixed with anhydrous Kaopectate, 50% mixture by volume
Disp: 8 oz
Sig: Rinse with 1 tsp before meals and as needed for pain

Potential sources of irritation such as rough tooth surfaces should be removed. Sugar-free lemon drops, artificial saliva, and a bland tooth powder may lessen the symptoms of xerostomia. The antimicrobial effect of chlorhexidine rinses helps control superficial infections and nystatin or clotrimazole rinses may be necessary to control candidiasis.

Carious lesions should be restored and a neutral pH sodium fluoride gel prescribed to increase resistance to the development of radiation caries. Effective oral hygiene and frequent dental recall appointments are essential in maintaining oral health for xerostomic patients following radiotherapy.

Chemotherapy

Risks. Many of the oral complications described for radiotherapy also apply to chemotherapy. Each chemotherapeutic agent produces different side effects affecting the oral cavity. Two general implications of significance while providing dental care to a patient undergoing chemotherapy is that the patient will be immunocompromised and prone to bleeding because of hematopoietic suppression.

Management. Mucositis, xerostomia, and candidiasis may be present and managed as described for the radiotherapy patient. Agents that cause neurotoxicity can produce odontogenic pain that requires palliative treatment. Management of increased vulnerability to infection and a bleeding tendency are as previously described.

CLINICAL CONSIDERATIONS RELATED TO MEDICATIONS

Certain medications taken by the patient may necessitate modifications of dental procedures. Also, many of the drugs that dentists routinely prescribe and administer necessitate consideration of current medications and the patient's compromised health. Several points should be underscored:

1. A detailed listing of the patient's current medications is essential. Any changes should be determined before administering or prescribing any therapeutic preparation.
2. References should be consulted for information about unfamiliar drugs. The prescribing physician or pharmacist should be consulted if uncertainty still exists.
3. Medications of certain drug groups, such as monamine oxidase (MAO) inhibitors, are likely to interact with other drugs. The possibility of drug interaction should be investigated before a new medication is used.

The following examples listed by therapeutic groups illustrate the need for concern.

Analgesics

Both aspirin (ASA) and nonsteroidal antiinflammatories (NSAI) cause thrombocytopathy and gastric irritation and should be avoided by patients with bleeding disorders and peptic ulcers. Aspirin is contraindicated for asthmatics, its use by pregnant women is discouraged, and it may decrease the effectiveness of gout medication. To minimize the risk of Reye's syndrome, aspirin should not be given to children suffering from chickenpox or influenza. Acetaminophen should be used with caution by patients with abnormal liver function.

Antibiotics

Broad spectrum antibiotics such as tetracycline, penicillin, and cephalosporins decrease the effectiveness of contraceptive pills and can cause candidiasis by suppression of the normal oral and vaginal flora. Some antibiotics may cause an acquired thrombocytopathy. Ampicillin and tetracycline may adversely affect patients with abnormal liver function. Tetracycline is also contraindicated for pregnant women, children with developing teeth, and renal failure patients. It may also cause complications for patients with seizure disorders and individuals taking antacids that contain aluminum salts. Erythromycin potentiates theophylline toxicity. Both erythromycin and clindamycin are relatively contraindicated when methylxanthine preparations are taken for pulmonary dysfunction. Cephalosporins may enhance nephrotoxicity in patients with congestive heart disease who are taking furosemide and ethacrynic acid.

Corticosteroids

Corticosteroids may cause adrenal suppression, xerostomia, and diminished host resistance leading to candidiasis and exacerbation of chronic, asymptomatic dental infections. The action of the steroid medication is altered when it is administered concurrently with antidiabetic agents. Corticosteroids should not be prescribed for patients with peptic ulcers or a history of tuberculosis.

Gold Salts

Gold salts used to treat rheumatoid arthritis may precipitate drug-induced stomatitis.

Immunosuppressants

Immunosuppressants decrease host resistance to infection, which can cause opportunistic infections and exacerbate chronic dental infections. Cyclosporine may precipitate gingival hyperplasia.

Local Anesthetics

Amide-linked local anesthetics such as lidocaine and mepivacaine may be ineffectively metabolized by patients with compromised liver function.

Psychotropic Medications

MAO inhibitors contraindicate the use of vasopressors or central nervous system depressants. Tricyclic antidepressants and phenothiazines are relative contraindications for the use of vasopressors or CNS depressants. Many psychotropic medications cause xerostomia.

Vasodilators

Vasodilators may cause orthostatic hypotension.

Vasopressors

Vasopressors are contraindicated when patients are taking MAO inhibitors or tricyclic antidepressants. They are relatively contraindicated in pregnant women and should be minimized in patients with hyperthyroidism.

SUMMARY

Safe and effective dental treatment for the medically compromised patient relies on the identification of the patient's medical conditions and determination of potential complications related to those conditions. The need to modify dental procedures or delay dental treatment is determined by the relative probability and severity of potential complications. Medical consultation is often necessary to clarify the status of the patient and for management recommendations. Hesitance to contact the physician should never be a barrier to appropriate dental management of the medically compromised patient.

BIBLIOGRAPHY

Cioffi GA, Terezhalmy GT, Taybos GM: Total joint replacement: a consideration for antimicrobial prophylaxis, Oral Surg Oral Med Oral Path 66:124-129, 1988.

Council on Dental Materials, Instruments, and Equipment: Recommendations in radiographic practices: an update, 1988, J Am Dent Assoc 118:115-117, 1989.

Council on Dental Therapeutics: Management of dental patients with prosthetic joints, J Am Dent Assoc 121:537-538, 1990.

Council on Dental Therapeutics, American Heart Association: Preventing bacterial endocarditis: a statement for the dental profession, J Am Dent Assoc 122:87-92, 1991.

Dajani AS and others: Prevention of bacterial endocarditis recommendations by the American Heart Association, JAMA 264:2919-2922, 1990.

Fiese R, Herzog S: Issues in dental and surgical management of the pregnant patient, Oral Surg Oral Med Oral Path 65:292-297, 1988.

Langlais RP and others: Oral diagnosis, oral medicine and treatment planning, Philadelphia, 1984, Saunders.

Little JW, Falace DA: Therapeutic considerations in special patients, Dent Clin North Am 28:455-469, 1984.

Munroe CO: The dental patient and diabetes mellitus, Dent Clin North Am 27:329-340, 1983.

Sonis ST, Fazio RC, Fang L: Principles and practice of oral medicine, Philadelphia, 1984, Saunders.

PART III

Differential Diagnosis

CHAPTER 14

Concepts of Differential Diagnosis

GARY C. COLEMAN

The specific diagnosis of the disease process that has produced dental cavities, periodontal bone loss, or other common dental lesions is seldom as challenging as the diagnosis of nondental oral lesions. The clinical manifestations of routine dental diseases such as dental caries and periodontitis can be recognized by their characteristic appearance because virtually no other diseases produce these lesions. This diagnostic approach has been described as the *appearance recognition method.* The challenge in the evaluation of dental lesions in most cases is the appreciation of their extent and determination of optimal treatment rather than what disease caused them. With this experience in the diagnosis of dental diseases, dentists often develop the unrealistic expectation that mucosal and other lesions of the oral cavity should be as easily diagnosed by the same appearance recognition approach. Unfortunately, this is not the case. Most oral ulcers, for example, have more appearance features in common than distinguishing characteristics despite the diversity of the possible causes.

The diagnostic approach for nondental conditions must accommodate the possibility that the lesion could be caused by any of several diseases and that a diagnosis on the basis of appearance alone is likely to be incorrect. This method should allow comparison of several diseases known to produce the primary manifestation of the patient's abnormality in the expectation that some of the possible causes can be eliminated on the basis of contradictory features. This approach is referred to as *differential diagnosis.* The following discussion introduces the differential diagnosis method that will be applied for nondental oral lesions in Chapters 15 through 20.

DIFFERENTIAL DIAGNOSIS

Differential diagnosis is the determination of which of two or more diseases with similar signs and symptoms is the one from which the patient is suffering. This requires a comparison of the patient's signs, symptoms, and other information against known features of all diseases that can produce the observed primary

Table 14-1 Conceptual stages of the differential diagnostic process

Stage	Questions to be resolved
Stage 1: Classification of the abnormality	A. Could the suspected abnormality be an unusual presentation of healthy tissues? B. What is the primary manifestation of the suspected abnormality?
Stage 2: Listing secondary features	A. What secondary features of the abnormality provide additional evidence of the nature of the disease process? (See Table 14-2) B. What secondary features are of differential diagnostic importance among the diseases known to cause the primary manifestation?
Stage 3: List conditions capable of causing the primary manifestation	A. What conditions are known to cause the primary manifestation?
Stage 4: Eliminate improbable causes	A. Are any of the secondary features of the patient's condition inconsistent with the features of any of the conditions that are known to cause the primary manifestation?
Stage 5: Rank possible causes by probability	A. How well does each of the remaining possible causes compare with the secondary features of the patient's condition? B. How common or rare is each of the possible causes?
Stage 6: Determination of a working diagnosis	A. What is the most likely cause of the patient's condition? B. What procedure, test, or additional diagnostic information will most effectively differentiate the correct diagnosis from among the remaining possible causes? C. If no distinguishing test is available or if immediate treatment is necessary, then is it appropriate to treat the patient's condition on the assumption that the working diagnosis is correct?

manifestation. Differential diagnosis is considered conceptually and procedurally in several distinct stages as summarized in Table 14-1. These stages are the categorization of the abnormality by primary manifestation, the listing of additional clinical features, the listing of conditions that can cause the primary manifestation, elimination of unlikely causes, and ranking of possible causes by probability.

Categorization of the Abnormality by Primary Manifestation

Nearly all intraoral abnormalities are characterized by a prominent feature that demonstrates the general nature of the lesion as different from normal tissues. These *primary manifestations* of intraoral lesions serve as a basis for categorization before differential diagnosis. Nearly all intraoral abnormalities can be considered as predominantly an alteration of mucosal color, a loss of mucosal integrity, a soft tissue enlargement, an osseous lesion with radiographic manifestations, or a combination of dissimilar abnormalities suggestive of a clinical syndrome. Additional characteristics of the abnormality are considered *secondary features*.

Listing of Secondary Clinical Features

The appreciation of a suspected abnormality based on primary manifestations should be followed by an objective determination of the secondary features of the lesion. The inexperienced clinician is frequently tempted to make a diagnosis on the basis of one or two obvious characteristics without thoroughly examining the lesion. If a specific diagnosis is initially considered, then the tendency is to misinterpret the secondary features because of diagnostic bias. Skilled diagnosticians reserve judgment about the diagnosis until as much objective information about the lesion as possible can be determined.

Several features that should be identified for all nondental abnormalities are listed in Table 14-2. Careful visual examination after removal of saliva and food debris allows observation of the lesion size, shape, and location. The patient should be reexamined to ascertain if the lesion is isolated or if other similar abnormalities are present indicating a multifocal process. The lesion margins should be examined to determine the degree of delineation and contour. The appearance pattern of the abnormality should be identified as either homogeneous or heterogeneous. Palpation may illicit tenderness associated with the lesion and indicates whether or not alteration of underlying tissue consistency exists. Probing and other applicable examination techniques may reveal exudate or other significant diagnostic features for certain lesions. These secondary features of the lesion along with contributory information about the patient such as age, gender, race, and medical history provide the basis for differential diagnostic decisions.

Listing of Conditions Known to Cause the Primary Manifestation

As previously indicated, an accurate differential diagnosis of most nondental abnormalities usually requires consideration of many possible causes. The challenge for inexperienced clinicians is often simply to remember the conditions that can produce a specific type of lesion. The tendency is to consider a few common conditions and interpret the clinical findings to "fit" one of these diseases. This can

be an efficient method of misdiagnosis. The chapters covering each lesion category provide a more complete listing of possible causes for each type of lesion. The differential diagnosis is more likely to yield a correct diagnosis if the typical features of many possible conditions are compared with those of the patient's abnormality.

Elimination of Unlikely Causes

After the diagnostic features of the lesion and the possible causes of the primary manifestation have been listed, secondary findings and additional clinical information can be compared to eliminate unlikely causes. This relies on the identification of contradictions between the features of the patient's lesion and the known characteristics of the diagnostic possibilities. The most efficient differential diagnostic strategy in most cases relies on several easily interpreted diagnostic characteristics that can be consistently relied on to eliminate certain conditions. The lesion category determines which secondary features are most reliable. The specific differential diagnostic strategy within each lesion category represents much of the discussion in the following chapters. The goal is to eliminate as many causes from consideration as possible, which simplifies the consideration of more likely causes. Also, elimination of particularly serious conditions such as malignant neoplasia as a possible cause is often more important than achieving a definitive diagnosis.

Ranking of Possible Causes by Probability

After elimination of impossible conditions as potential diagnoses, the next stage of differential diagnosis is to rank the diseases that could explain the abnormality by probability. The ranking of possible diagnoses is based on the number of secondary features exhibited by the patient's condition that correspond with the typical features of each possible diagnosis. This is relatively subjective in many situations. Different diagnosticians assign different values

Table 14-2 Summary of the features that should be specifically determined for a suspected abnormality

Feature category	Features
Primary disease manifestation	The abnormality should be characterized as predominantly 1. A white mucosal discoloration without loss of mucosal integrity or enlargement 2. A dark discoloration without loss of mucosal integrity or enlargement 3. Loss of mucosal integrity or ulceration without enlargement 4. Enlargement of soft tissues 5. Radiographic manifestations of a lesion originating in bone 6. Concurrence of several dissimilar abnormalities suggestive of a syndrome
Secondary clinical features	Visual 1. Specific location 2. Lesion shape and tissue contours 3. Lesion size 4. Occurrence as isolated, multifocal, or diffuse 5. Delineation of the borders of the abnormality from adjacent tissues 6. Consistency of appearance as homogeneous or heterogeneous 7. Surface color and texture 8. Alteration of adjacent structures such as displacement of teeth Palpation 1. Degree of compressibility 2. Tenderness during compression 3. Alteration in color during compression Probing 1. Tissue defects 2. Exudate Patient Awareness 1. Pain, discomfort, or altered function 2. Duration 3. Course as constant, healing with recurrence, or steady progression 4. Response to factors such as stress and certain foods
Contributory factors	Demographic 1. Age 2. Gender 3. Race Habits 1. Alcohol 2. Tobacco 3. Oral habits Recent history 1. Injury 2. Infection 3. Surgery Medical conditions 1. Chronic diseases 2. Recent acute illnesses Current medical treatment 1. Medications 2. Other treatment

to various clinical features during differential diagnostic comparisons. This tendency and the unpredictable biologic behavior of a disease process affecting an individual at a particular stage in the disease course explains in part why few absolute "rules" apply to all situations. Simply stated, virtually every differential diagnostic generalization that is discussed in the remaining chapters will have exceptions. Nevertheless, comparing the features of a patient's lesion with the typical features of a possible diagnosis usually yields an impression that the diagnosis is likely, possible but not as probable, or unlikely but possible.

The condition considered the most likely cause of the lesion is referred to as the *working, tentative,* or *preliminary diagnosis* or the *clinical impression.* The working diagnosis and the less likely diagnostic possibilities provide the basis for additional diagnostic procedures, such as a biopsy or clinical laboratory tests, and for the initial clinical management of the condition. If all but one disease are eliminated from the differential diagnosis, then that is the *definitive* or *final diagnosis.* Definitive treatment can be instituted once a definitive diagnosis has been made assuming that a definitive treatment is available for that condition and that the problem has not resolved.

The final aspects of differential diagnosis are reevaluation and recall. The course of the condition over a period of time with or without specific treatment is one source of confirmational diagnostic information. If the definitive diagnosis is incorrect, then an unexpected clinical course of the abnormality often reveals the diagnostic error. In other situations, certain correctly diagnosed lesions are likely to recur and require additional treatment. For both reasons, reevaluation and recall are essential elements of the differential diagnosis process.

INITIAL CATEGORIZATION OF SUSPECTED ABNORMALITIES

Two decisions must be made early in the differential diagnosis of a suspected nondental abnormality of the oral cavity: (1) Could the suspected abnormality be a variation of normal tissues or is it actually evidence of disease? (2) If the abnormality is evidence of disease, which lesion category would provide the most appropriate differential diagnosis of the condition? Both decisions can be difficult, particularly for the inexperienced clinician. An error in either decision ensures that the differential diagnosis will proceed on the wrong track and usually means an incorrect assessment of the abnormality. These initial decisions are summarized in Fig. 14-1. The following observations provide a basis for making correct decisions on these two issues.

Features of Normal Tissue Variations Compared with Evidence of Abnormality

Several clinical features are typical of normal variations of anatomic structures and tissues. Exceptions to all of the following observations are common, which makes reliance on a single feature a probable source of error. However, concurrence of several of the features described below for a suspected abnormality is strong evidence that it is a variation of normal tissues.

Bilateral symmetry. Most variations of normal structures exhibit bilateral symmetry. Symmetry both in the location and the degree or extent of the unusual appearance is typical. Certain diseases can produce lesions affecting symmetric locations, but the degree or the extent of the abnormal features caused by disease are usually different from one side to the other.

Predictable locations. Many variations of normal structures occur in predictable locations. Radiographic misinterpretation of a prominent mental foramen as a periapical inflammatory lesion of mandibular premolars is a commonly encountered example. Misinterpretation of a prominent parotid papilla as a soft tissue enlargement is another frequent error.

Asymptomatic. Normal tissues that appear unusual are asymptomatic. When tenderness

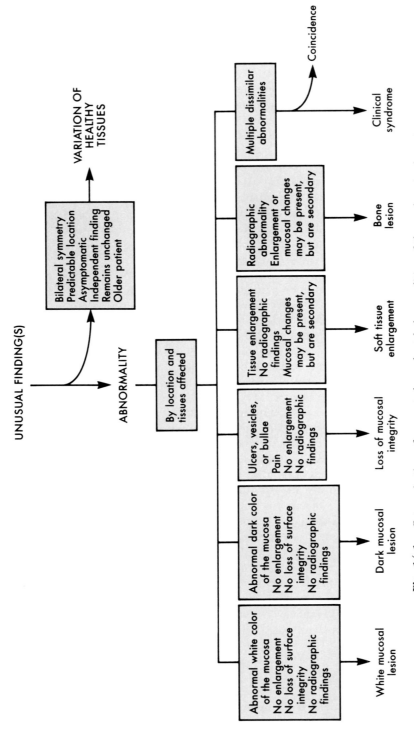

Fig. 14-1   Categorization of suspected nondental abnormalities of the oral cavity by primary manifestation.

drainage, or other symptoms have definitely been produced by a suspected abnormality, then a disease process is the likely explanation.

Independent finding. Most variations of normal are identified as an independent finding. Intraoral lesions often present secondary changes such as erythema or altered tissue consistency along with the primary manifestation.

Static. Normal anatomic variations remain unchanged. Diseases produce manifestations that either resolve or progress during a reevaluation period.

Increased prominence with age. Variations of healthy tissues become more common or more prominent with increased age of the patient. This may be because the atypical appearance is actually more common among older patients or the primary manifestations become more dramatic or noticeable after years of exposure to the oral environment. In either case, unusual appearing oral tissues of a child warrant greater suspicion of disease.

Remain unchanged following empiric treatment. Normal tissues that appear unusual remain unchanged following empiric treatment. Most lesions either improve or worsen under the influence of treatment.

As previously stated, one or two of these features is weak evidence that variation of normal structures is the explanation of an unusual clinical observation. However, several provide convincing evidence and can essentially end the differential diagnosis. In addition, clinical reevaluation within a few weeks or months of the initial observation of the suspected abnormality demonstrates whether the lesion remains unchanged. If a strong case cannot be made that the suspected abnormality is a variation of normal, then the clinician should proceed with the differential diagnosis as if the atypical appearance represents disease and categorize the lesion. Clinical situations commonly arise in which the decision between a normal anatomic variation or disease cannot be made with certainty. Therefore several common variations of normal anatomic structures are included in the discussion of the differential diagnosis for various lesion categories.

Categorization of Abnormalities by Tissues Affected and Primary Manifestation

Categorization of abnormalities on the basis of the tissues affected and by the primary manifestation simplifies the differential diagnosis by allowing the clinician to focus on conditions capable of producing the abnormality. From a different perspective, many diseases that cause different primary manifestations can be excluded from consideration early in the differential diagnosis. The initial oral lesion categorization is based on the tissues affected as either the surface mucosa, deeper soft tissues, or bone. In addition, some conditions are characterized by multiple abnormalities affecting several different tissues or anatomic sites.

For an abnormality to be considered in the mucosal lesion category the primary manifestation of the abnormality is altered appearance of the superficial oral mucosa. Evidence of enlargement, an associated lesion of bone, or additional lesions affecting other tissues suggests that the mucosal changes may be secondary to another disease process as shown in Fig. 14-2. Therefore these additional findings imply that the condition should be considered within another differential diagnosis category. Oral mucosal lesions without enlargement are divided on the basis of appearance as white lesions, dark lesions, and loss of surface integrity.

White mucosal lesions. Several secondary clinical features of white mucosal lesions are essential to their differential diagnosis. The surface appearance and texture of white lesions as smooth or rough provides an indication of the nature of the lesion. Some white lesions rub off with lateral pressure using a cotton gauze, which indicates that the white appearance is caused by superficial material. Any mixture of white mucosal changes with areas of ulceration should be categorized under oral

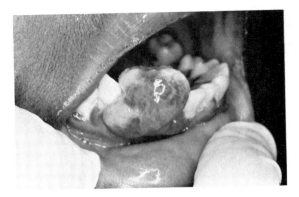

Fig. 14-2 This 32-year-old black female complained that this lesion had been present for 6 months and interfered with her ability to eat. The abnormality exhibits white and dark discoloration of the mucosa as well as focal ulceration and tissue enlargement. In this case, the primary clinical manifestation is the enlargement. Approaching the differential diagnosis in that disease category is much more likely to yield an accurate assessment than to categorize the lesion on the basis of secondary mucosal features.

ulcerations. Whether the condition is characterized by a single focal lesion, a diffuse area of abnormal white appearance, or multiple focal lesions is also contributory to the initial differential diagnosis. Habitual use of substances such as alcohol and tobacco is often related to the development of certain white lesions and should be clarified by the patient history.

Dark mucosal lesions. Dark lesions of the oral mucosa in most cases represent abnormal visibility of blood, accumulation of blood pigments, excessive melanin concentration, or dark foreign materials. The nature of the pigmentation is often suggested by whether the specific color of the dark lesion is red, brown, or black. The number and distribution of dark lesions is essential to the differential diagnosis. All dark lesions of the oral mucosa should prompt an examination to determine if any similar lesions are present on the skin as an indication whether the process is localized to the oral cavity or is a generalized condition. All red lesions should be palpated to determine if they blanch. This is a reliable secondary feature in their differential diagnosis.

Loss of mucosal integrity. This group of lesions includes ulcers and lesions that typically precede ulceration. Certain conditions that cause ulcers can be distinguished by whether the onset of lesions is acute or gradual. Lesion distribution as isolated or multifocal is another contributory diagnostic feature. The patient should be asked if ulcers affect other skin or mucosal surfaces, because several conditions that produce intraoral ulcers also affect the skin, genital mucosa, or conjunctiva. Because ulcers are painful, the patient can usually provide a dependable description of the severity of pain, duration, precipitating factors, and other helpful clinical information in their differential diagnosis.

Soft tissue enlargements. The palpation characteristics of soft tissue enlargements provide an indication of the composition of the abnormality, as well as eliciting whether or not the enlargement is tender to pressure. Most intraoral enlargements are solitary, but careful examination should determine if additional enlargements are present. Alteration of the surface mucosa should be noted because this may indicate the composition or possible cause of the enlargement. The precise location of the enlargement should be determined because this can suggest the origin of the lesion.

Radiographic lesions. Most osseous abnormalities are initially identified radiographically. The relative degree of radiation absorption by the abnormality compared with normal, adjacent structures is the basis for further classification. The typical designations are radiolucent, radiopaque, or mixed radiolucent-radiopaque lesions. As with all abnormalities, the size, shape, precise location, and the character of the margins of the abnormality contribute to the differential diagnosis. The patient should be clinically reexamined to identify any associated clinical findings that might be related to the radiographic lesion. These features include bone expansion, tenderness of overlying structures, abnormalities of the teeth in the region, and associated mucosal changes.

Clinical syndromes. The presence of multiple manifestations implies the possibility that the abnormalities may be related by a common developmental or metabolic condition. If that is the case, the condition represents a clinical syndrome. Several factors complicate the identification and evaluation of clinical syndromes. First, a disease that produces multiple lesions of similar character should be categorized by the primary manifestation as multifocal rather than as multiple abnormalities of a clinical syndrome. Second, multiple manifestations of one underlying process can be difficult to distinguish at times from the primary manifestations of several different conditions that affect the patient by coincidence. Many patients, particularly with advancing age, may exhibit abnormalities caused by dozens of different diseases that are totally unrelated except that they all affect the same patient. Finally, the clinician is challenged by the rare occurrence and large number of different syndromes that can affect the oral and perioral structures. Often the only way to identify the syndrome is to recognize the combination of clinical features that characterize the syndrome. The diagnostic problems related to clinical syndromes are considered in more detail in Chapter 20. The important diagnostic issue to appreciate is that the possibility of a clinical syndrome must be considered when a patient exhibits several apparently dissimilar abnormalities. The possibility can then be evaluated by comparing the patient's abnormalities with the known features of syndromes affecting the head and neck.

TERMINOLOGY USED TO DESCRIBE MUCOSAL ABNORMALITIES

The descriptive terms applied to oral lesions can quickly facilitate appreciation of primary and secondary features. This is particularly important during the differential diagnosis when making comparisons with the terminology of written lesion descriptions in reference materials. Most of the terms discussed below have become standardized by dermatologists in the differential diagnosis of skin lesions and can be directly applied to mucosal lesions with equal diagnostic effectiveness. The descriptions of specific white lesions, dark lesions, ulcerative conditions, and soft tissue enlargements in Chapters 15 through 18 rely heavily on this terminology. The terms used in radiographic interpretation are discussed in Chapter 19.

Descriptive Terms Applicable to Lesions of Mucosal Discoloration

The degree of thickening and surface texture of white mucosal lesions are the two features that are related to specific terms. A *plaque* is a mild elevation with a flat surface of more than 1 cm in diameter. Plaques typically exhibit a "stuck on" or patchy appearance. Surface texture that is pebbly or papillary in appearance is described as *verrucous* in contrast to lesions with a smooth or wrinkled texture.

A *scar* is an area of abnormal appearance that represents repair of an injury or large ulcer with dense fibrous connective tissue. The relative avascularity of scars located on nonkeratinized mucosal surfaces often yields a pale appearance. An example of scarring that exhibits enlargement is the hyperplastic reparative response known as *keloid formation,* which commonly affect black patients.

Dark mucosal lesions are usually flat, sharply-delineated areas of altered pigmentation known as a *macules.* The term *macule* can also apply to abnormal focal loss of melanin pigmentation. *Erythema* indicates inflammatory redness. Erythematous skin rashes are described as macular and if multiple small "bumps" are also present, then *maculopapular* is an appropriate descriptive term.

Several additional terms are used to describe macules that appear to contain blood or blood pigments. *Telangiectasia* is discoloration of an area caused by abnormally dilated blood vessels. *Petechiae* are reddish subepithelial hemorrhagic discolorations that are less than 2 to 3 mm in diameter. *Ecchymosis* or a bruise is identical hemorrhagic discoloration except that the size is larger. *Purpura* is a term often incorrectly used to refer to ecchymosis or petechiae, but which actually means a *condition* that causes a tendency to form such hemorrhagic lesions.

Descriptive Terms Applicable to Loss of Mucosal Integrity

Lesions characterized by a loss of surface integrity and that are the initial presentation of a disease are referred to as *primary lesions.* Primary lesions of the oral cavity and perioral skin include erosions, atrophy, vesicles, pustules, and bullae. These lesions are too fragile to exist for more than a few hours or days in the harsh environment of the oral cavity. They predictably degenerate to a *secondary lesion,* which is the stage of the process generally observed by the dentist. This is usually an ulcer in the oral cavity and a crust on the skin. In addition, chronic infections can produce specific defects of surface integrity known as fissures and sinuses.

An *erosion* is focal loss of epithelium superficial to the basal layer that can be caused by abrasion, superficial chemical burns, and several autoimmune diseases. The more generalized thinned, smooth, and fragile appearance of *mucosal atrophy* is usually a manifestation of malnutrition, hormonal abnormality, or advanced systemic disease. A *vesicle* is a focal, fluid-filled elevation less than 1 cm in diameter. These lesions are most often caused by viral infections that produce a cluster of vesicles referred to as a *zosteriform pattern.* A *pustule* is a vesicle that contains pus, which indicates a bacterial rather than a viral infection. A *bulla* is a fluid-filled elevation or "blister" greater than one cm in diameter. These lesions often form when intraepithelial or epithelial-connective tissue attachments

are compromised by recurring traumatic injury, genetic deficiency, or autoimmune degeneration. *Nikolsky's sign* is bulla formation following mild lateral pressure to an apparently normal tissue surface. This consequence of epithelial attachment deficiency is a reliable clinical sign of these conditions.

An *ulcer* is loss of epithelial integrity that extends deep to the basal layer of the epithelium. This can be a primary lesion caused by traumatic tissue injury or it can be a secondary degeneration of one of the primary lesions affecting surface integrity described above. In contrast to oral ulcers, loss of epithelial integrity affecting the skin usually appears as a *crust* or "scab" that is a dried concretion of blood cells and plasma proteins.

The primary and secondary lesions described above in most cases represent an acute process. Loss of surface integrity for an extended time period can produce lesions with somewhat different clinical features. A *fissure* is a linear defect that extends to the dermis. The characteristic and common example of a fissure is caused by the fungal infection known as "athlete's foot." The dentist occasionally observes fissures near the corner of the mouth that also represent a mycotic infection and are known as angular cheilitis. A *sinus* in this context is a narrow epithelium-lined tract connecting one epithelium-lined space to another. A *fistula* refers to a similar tract that connects an epithelial-lined space with the skin surface. These formations often develop secondary to the pressure of a chronic inflammatory lesion or an abscess. Sinuses can also represent developmental abnormalities or be associated with cysts.

Descriptive Terms Applicable to Mucosal Enlargements

The terms *polyp* and *exophytic* nonspecifically indicate any tissue enlargement that projects beyond the normal tissue surface contour. More specific terms refer to the shape and the size of the enlargement.

Enlargements with an attachment or base that is smaller than the exophytic portion are described as *pedunculated,* and *sessile* is the descriptive term for lesions with a broader base or dome-shaped contour. Enlargements that are identified by palpation and do not project beyond the surface are referred to simply as *submucosal enlargement. Fusiform* is the term applied for diffuse, "spindle-shaped" distention of tissue contours.

A *papule* is a solid, focal enlargement less than 1 cm in diameter. A *wheal* is an erythematous papule, which is the typical appearance of allergic reactions and insect bites. A *nodule* is a solid enlargement between 1 and 5 cm in diameter. A *tumor* is a solid enlargement of greater than 5 cm in diameter. "Tumor" in this context does not specifically mean a neoplasm, although that may be the case with such large size, and small neoplasms can present as nodules. A *cyst* is an encapsulated, epithelial-lined, fluid-filled body located deep to the superficial epithelium. This is indicated by compressibility during palpation as compared with the solid nature of papules, nodules, and tumors.

SUMMARY

The clinical evaluation of nondental oral lesions requires a different diagnostic approach than routine dental conditions do, because nondental lesions may appear similar even though several diseases could be the underlying cause. Differential diagnosis provides the diagnostic approach needed to compare the diagnostic findings exhibited by the patient with those of several diseases capable of producing the clinical findings. The differential diagnostic sequence consists of:

1. Categorization of the abnormality by primary manifestations
2. Listing the secondary clinical manifestations and findings
3. Listing the conditions that are known to cause the primary manifestation
4. Elimination of unlikely causes
5. Ranking of possible causes by probability
6. Determination of a working diagnosis and a plan to arrive at a definitive diagnosis

Classification of lesions is based on the tissue affected and the primary manifestation of the abnormality. Lesion categories are white mucosal lesions, dark mucosal discolorations, loss of mucosal integrity, soft tissue enlargements, osseous lesions, and the multiple manifestations of clinical syndromes. Various secondary clinical features are particularly helpful in the differential diagnosis of each lesion category, and these features should be listed before possible diagnoses are considered. Once secondary features of the abnormality have been evaluated, they allow elimination of many conditions as possible diagnoses on the basis of inconsistencies with the patient's condition. A relatively standardized terminology has emerged to facilitate differential diagnostic comparisons of mucosal lesions. The following chapters discuss the differential diagnosis within each category of nondental abnormality.

BIBLIOGRAPHY

Bengel W and others: Differential diagnosis of diseases of the oral mucosa, Chicago, 1989, Quintessence.

DeGowin RL: DeGowin and DeGowin's bedside diagnostic examination, ed 5, New York, 1987, MacMillan.

Harvey AM, Bordley J: Differential diagnosis: the interpretation of clinical evidence, ed 3, Philadelphia, 1979, Saunders.

Seidel HM and others: Mosby's guide to physical examination, St Louis, 1987, Mosby—Year Book.

Wood NK, Goaz PW: Differential diagnosis of oral lesions, ed 4, St Louis, 1991, Mosby-Year Book.

CHAPTER 15

Differential Diagnosis of White Mucosal Lesions

GARY C. COLEMAN

White lesions of the oral mucosa are among the most commonly encountered diagnostic challenges for the dentist. Fortunately, most are benign and justify little clinical concern once a definitive diagnosis of the lesion is made. However, a small proportion of these lesions represent dysplastic or early malignant neoplastic lesions of the surface epithelium. The most effective management of these squamous cell carcinomas relies on early identification and total excision of the lesion. Therefore the primary diagnostic issue for white lesions of the oral mucosa is the identification by differential diagnosis of those white lesions that are most likely to be dysplastic or malignant. The diagnostic goal is usually to exclude the possibility of early squamous cell carcinoma by assembling clinical evidence that the white lesion is a benign condition. If the possibility of epithelial dysplasia or early squamous cell carcinoma remains in differential diagnostic consideration, then excision and histopathologic diagnosis are mandatory.

The phrase *white lesions* in the context of oral abnormalities refers to any alteration of the mucosa characterized by an opaque, pale, or white appearance without evidence of significant enlargement, erythema, or ulceration. The term *leukoplakia* has been used in the past as a clinical reference to any white lesion without implying a specific diagnosis. In recent years leukoplakia has come to mean specifically those white lesions of the oral mucosa that are not explained clinically by a specific cause or clinically recognized condition. *Idiopathic leukoplakia*, therefore, has come to imply the possibility that the white lesion is dysplastic or early neoplastic disease. The phrase *white lesion* is most appropriately used as a nonspecific clinical reference to any oral lesion of this group without diagnostic implications. *Idiopathic leukoplakia* is reserved for white lesions suspected of cancerous or precancerous character when no direct cause or specific benign condition explains the abnormal appearance.

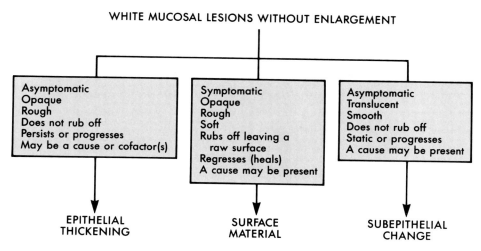

WHITE MUCOSAL LESIONS WITHOUT ENLARGEMENT

Asymptomatic
Opaque
Rough
Does not rub off
Persists or progresses
May be a cause or cofactor(s)

Symptomatic
Opaque
Rough
Soft
Rubs off leaving a
   raw surface
Regresses (heals)
A cause may be present

Asymptomatic
Translucent
Smooth
Does not rub off
Static or progresses
A cause may be present

EPITHELIAL
THICKENING

SURFACE
MATERIAL

SUBEPITHELIAL
CHANGE

Fig. 15-1   Initial differential diagnosis of white mucosal lesions.

DIAGNOSTIC FEATURES AND CLASSIFICATION OF WHITE MUCOSAL LESIONS

White mucosal lesions appear white because some tissue alteration obscures visualization of the normal pink appearance that results from the underlying connective tissue vascularity. This may be caused by epithelial thickening, the presence of a superficial material, or a submucosal alteration producing a decrease in blood vessel density. These features will serve as a basis for the differential diagnostic classification of oral white lesions because these three mechanisms consistently produce differences in clinical features that are easily identifiable. The initial differential diagnosis of oral white lesions is illustrated in Fig. 15-1.

Clinical Features of Lesions Caused by Epithelial Thickening

Thickening of the superficial epithelium produces a distinct combination of clinical features in addition to the white appearance. Thickened epithelium consists primarily of excessive keratin that exhibits a rough or grainy surface texture when dried with air or a cotton gauze. The additional keratin produces an opaque appearance rather than the translucence of some other white lesions. The attached keratin is difficult to dislodge so the lesion appears unchanged after it has been wiped with gauze or scraped with a dull instrument. Since the epithelium is intact there is no sensation of pain, burning, or tenderness when the area is abraded. This combination of clinical findings is strong evidence that a white lesion is characterized by surface thickening.

Most common conditions that produce epithelial thickening are further characterized by whether the patient exhibits an isolated white lesion or a multifocal distribution is present. Further differential diagnosis of white lesions within the surface thickening group is based on location, history, and other physical findings.

Clinical Features of White Lesions Caused by Superficial Material

White lesions of the mouth characterized by superficial material also appear opaque and rough or grainy when dried. In contrast to lesions of surface thickening, however, the white material often appears soft or friable and rubbing the white lesion removes a significant proportion of the white appearance. In many cases an ulcer or erythematous appearance of the mucosa is revealed after removal of the superficial debris. This explains the frequent complaint of burning discomfort associated with these lesions. If the superficial material is simply food remnants, a dense accumulation of *materia alba*, or plaque, then the site is painless and the underlying mucosal surface appears normal.

The differential diagnosis of white lesions composed of superficial material is relatively simple once the removal of the white appearance has been demonstrated because only a few conditions produce these findings. Most of these are actually ulcerative mucosal conditions that are revealed by the removal of a white surface coagulum. Therefore the differential diagnosis shifts to the ulcerative lesion category.

Clinical Features of White Lesions Caused by Submucosal Change

White or pale lesions characterized by diminished underlying vascularity are covered by normal epithelium, which appears smooth and translucent as compared with the rough, opaque appearance of other white lesions. No pain or burning sensation is present because the epithelium is intact and attempts to rub or scrape off the abnormality produce no change in appearance. The specific diagnosis among white lesions of submucosal change is usually clarified by the patient history or the distribution of the lesions.

WHITE LESIONS OF EPITHELIAL THICKENING

The distribution of the abnormal appearance as either focal or multifocal is the most helpful single feature in further evaluating white lesions of epithelial thickening. Additional helpful features of the differential diagnosis are summarized in Fig. 15-2. Although a number of other conditions can produce white oral lesions, they are either characterized by a more significant primary manifestation such as

enlargement or are so rare as to be considered diagnostically improbable in routine clinical practice.

Physiologic Hyperkeratosis

Definition. Physiologic hyperkeratosis consists of thickening of the mucosal epithelium in response to recurring friction. This is analogous to callus formation of the skin at sites subjected to a period of rubbing or physical irritation. *Focal keratosis, focal hyperkeratosis, frictional hyperkeratosis,* and other diagnostic terms have all been used to convey the cause and effect relationship of these lesions. This is by far the most common oral white lesion of epithelial thickening. *Linea alba* is such a common form of physiologic hyperkeratosis as to have been considered as a variation of normal anatomic appearance. Chronic chewing and sucking of the cheeks produces a thin white band of the buccal mucosa located bilaterally at the level of the occlusal plane. Other common causes of physiologic hyperkeratosis include sharp tooth surfaces, appliances, and masticatory function of edentulous ridges in the absence of a prosthesis. Galvanic irritation by the weak electric current generated by dissimilar restorative metals has also been reported to cause physiologic hyperkeratosis.

Clinical features. The opaque white appearance is homogeneous with sharply delineated borders as shown by the lesion in Fig. 15-3. The process is usually focal and its location can be directly related to a source of recurring friction. The patient is asymptomatic and unaware of the presence of any abnormality unless additional tissue injury has inadvertently occurred. Physiologic hyperkeratosis remains unchanged with time unless the source of irritation is removed. In these cases resolution is usually observed within a few weeks. Multiple or diffuse hyperkeratosis may develop if multiple or large sites are affected by friction as is the case with orthodontic brackets and the edentulous patient functioning without dentures.

Differential diagnosis. Demonstrating the

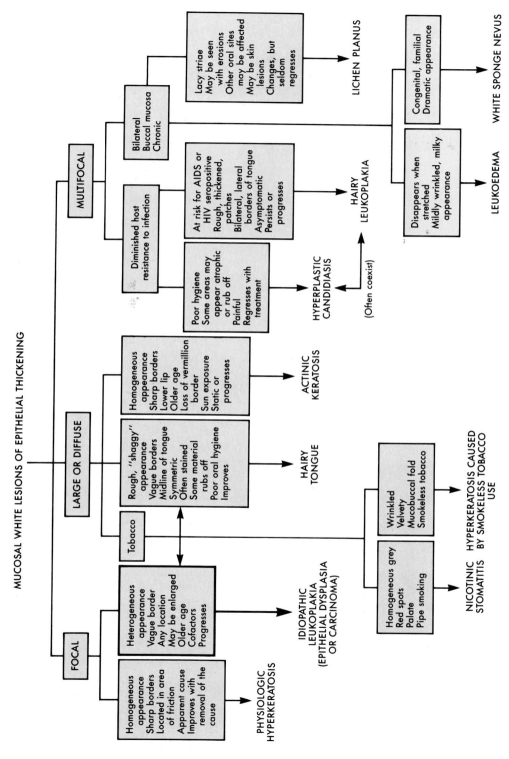

Fig. 15-2 Differential diagnosis of white lesions of epithelial thickening.

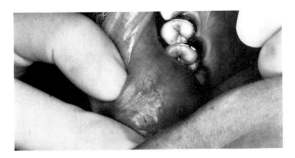

Fig. 15-3 Physiologic hyperkeratosis. This rough white lesion near the labial commissure is located immediately adjacent to a prominent orthodontic bracket when the tissues are in a resting position.

proximity of a source of friction to the location of the white lesion and resolution following removal of the cause are the essential elements of the diagnosis. Vague borders, focal ulceration, variation of thickening, or heterogeneous color of the white area are more suggestive of epithelial dysplasia and early squamous cell carcinoma. Location on the soft palate, floor of the mouth, and at the depth of the facial vestibule are unusual for physiologic hyperkeratosis unless an overextended prosthesis is present.

Management decisions. Removal of the source of irritation and reevaluation of the lesion in 1 to 2 weeks is appropriate management for a working diagnosis of physiologic hyperkeratosis. In cases in which removal of the cause is impractical, as with cheek biting, periodic reexamination to confirm the static nature of the abnormality may be justified. The frequency and duration of reexamination depends on the clinician's confidence that the lesion represents a physiologic response. Failure of the lesion to resolve after removal of the cause necessitates biopsy and histopathologic examination.

Epithelial Dysplasia and Early Squamous Cell Carcinoma

Definition. Epithelial dysplasia is nonmalignant alteration in the differentiation, development, and maturation of lining epithelial cells. Squamous cell carcinoma is malignant neoplastic proliferation of lining epithelial cells. Both conditions can produce identical lesions of focal epithelial thickening consistent with the clinical term *leukoplakia*. Also, squamous cell carcinoma is the most common malignant disease of the oral cavity and one of the few potentially fatal conditions the dentist is likely to initially identify. Unfortunately, these definitions and the histopathologic findings that form the basis of their diagnosis cannot be directly and consistently correlated with the clinical features of white lesions at the time of discovery. The implication is that a proportion of these lesions will eventually produce tissue destruction characteristic of malignant neoplasia. Therefore early diagnosis and removal of these lesions is the clinical priority in the differential diagnosis of white mucosal lesions in general.

The most common causes implicated in the development of oral epithelial dysplasia and squamous cell carcinoma are habitual exposure to tobacco and alcohol. The development of dysplastic lesions apparently requires several decades of exposure because leukoplakia is unusual among patients before age 40 and is more typical after age 50. Increased vulnerability to the development of premalignant and malignant epithelial lesions of the oral cavity is also associated with several conditions that affect other systems such as Fanconi's anemia, Plummer-Vinson syndrome, and erosive lichen planus.

Clinical features. Epithelial dysplasia and early squamous cell carcinoma can both produce focal white patches of the oral mucosa that superficially appear similar to physiologic hyperkeratosis. Closer examination after drying the mucosal surface usually reveals that the surface texture of dysplastic lesions is rougher or more wrinkled. Variation in color is typical and there may be an admixture of different shades of white, speckled foci of red, and ulceration, all of which reflect variable epithelial thickness. The borders are often vague or ir-

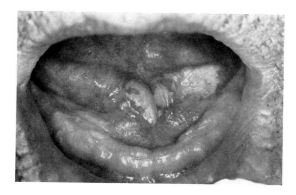

Fig. 15-4 Squamous cell carcinoma. These rough, wrinkled, plaquelike white patches are located in the floor of the mouth of an older male patient with a long history of cigarette smoking and alcoholism. Although most lesional margins appear sharply delineated, the subtle white appearance near the borders of the patches suggests the process is actually poorly delineated.

regular in contour (Fig. 15-4) in some areas, or several separate lesions may be grouped in the same general region. The patient is likely to be past 50 years of age with a history of alcohol and tobacco use.

Differential diagnosis. Identification of a specific source of recurring irritation or friction is the most useful feature in distinguishing between physiologic hyperkeratosis and dysplasia or early neoplasia. Absence of a specific cause or failure of the lesion to resolve after removal of a suspected cause are strong indications that a focal white lesion may be premalignant or malignant. This is particularly true when the lesion is located on the soft palate, the floor of the mouth, and the facial vestibule where frictional irritation is unusual. Additional observations such as heterogeneous appearance, vague borders, advanced patient age, or chronic use of carcinogens require the clinician to assume that the lesion is dysplastic or malignant until proven otherwise.

Diffuse and multifocal white lesions of epithelial thickening that are benign can usually be distinguished from dysplastic white lesions by their location, distribution of multiple lesions, homogeneous surface appearance, and the patient history. Some of these conditions such as actinic keratosis, lichen planus, and lesions associated with tobacco use are associated with an increased incidence of squamous cell carcinoma. The development of dysplasia or malignant neoplasia within these benign lesions is suggested by the presence of focal areas of heterogeneous appearance, ulceration, or nodular thickening.

Management decisions. The suspicion of dysplasia or malignant neoplasia warrants excision and histopathologic diagnosis of the lesion because of the serious threat of morbidity and mortality posed by these lesions. The suspicion may arise at the initial examination, after a period of observation reveals progression of the lesion, or when a white lesion fails to resolve after removal of a suspected source of irritation. Incisional biopsy may be preferable in cases of large lesions to obtain a definitive diagnosis of dysplasia or squamous cell carcinoma as justification for an extensive surgical procedure to remove the entire lesion. The incisional site should be carefully selected to represent the full spectrum of clinical features observed. Cytologic examination of surface scrapings from oral lesions suspected of dysplastic or neoplastic changes is generally unproductive and delays a definitive histopathologic diagnosis.

The biopsy report should receive particular attention for indications of the cellular features of the lesion, extension of the cellular abnormalities to the margins, and any treatment recommendations made by the pathologist. The pathologist should be contacted if any uncertainty remains concerning the histopathologic diagnosis.

Nicotinic Stomatitis

Definition. Nicotinic stomatitis is the response of the palatal tissues to the recurring irritation from tobacco smoke usually from a pipe or cigar habit. The heat of the smoke seems to be a significant contributory factor to

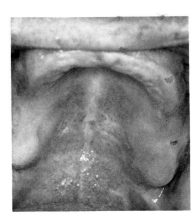

Fig. 15-5 Nicotinic stomatitis. This 56-year-old man smokes a pipe and wears his maxillary denture only while eating. The palate exhibits a uniform white appearance with a mild wrinkled surface texture and a uniform distribution of erythematous foci.

the lesion since the hotter smoke of cigars and pipes appears to produce more prominent lesions than does a cigarette habit.

Clinical features. The hard palate exhibits a diffuse, dull grayish-white, opaque discoloration that gradually fades to a normal pink color on the soft palate. More dramatic examples of nicotinic stomatitis exhibit a wrinkled or fissured surface texture with a suggestion of mild thickening. The discoloration is relatively homogeneous with the exception of numerous erythematous spots (Fig. 15-5) uniformly distributed on the surface of the lesion in the posterior portion of the hard palate. This relatively characteristic appearance is produced by inflammation of the ductal orifices of the underlying minor salivary glands. In addition, the tonsillar pillars are usually erythematous. Tobacco stains of the teeth and the odor of tobacco in addition to the patient history confirms the cause of the lesion.

Differential diagnosis. The combination of a pipe or cigar habit and the characteristic appearance of the palate provides a definitive diagnosis in most situations. The differential di-

agnostic issue in some cases is the suspicion that epithelial dysplasia or neoplasia may be developing from nicotinic stomatitis of long duration. This occurrence is unusual with this lesion, but the possibility is suggested by non-healing ulceration, focal heterogeneous appearance, and focal thickening.

Management decisions. A definitive clinical diagnosis of nicotinic stomatitis can be made in most cases, which makes biopsy and histopathologic examination for confirmation difficult to justify. The patient should be informed of the abnormality and encouraged to discontinue the tobacco habit. In the unlikely event that the patient should comply, gradual resolution of the lesion over several months may be expected. Biopsy is appropriate if unusual clinical features suggest the possibility of epithelial dysplasia or neoplasia.

Hyperkeratosis Caused by Smokeless Tobacco

Definition. The plaquelike epithelial thickening produced by smokeless tobacco use has been referred to clinically by a variety of terms such as "snuff dipper's pouch." The cause and effect relationship of the tobacco use is demonstrated by the location of the abnormality precisely where the tobacco is habitually placed. Awareness of the established carcinogenic effects of tobacco often promotes the suspicion that carcinoma may be developing within these lesions. With the tobacco products used in the United States, the progression to carcinoma is unusual and typically results from decades of exposure. The most likely forms of oral cancer caused by smokeless tobacco use are low grade squamous cell carcinoma and verrucous carcinoma. Smokeless tobacco use as practiced in many Asian countries is associated with a greater probability of carcinoma as a consequence of other carcinogenic materials added to the tobacco.

Clinical features. The hyperkeratotic white lesions produced by smokeless tobacco use exhibit a uniform, plaquelike thickening

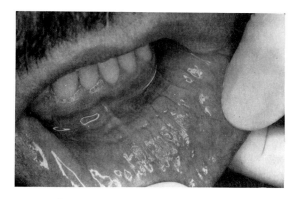

Fig. 15-6 Hyperkeratosis caused by smokeless tobacco use. This patient described an 8-year habit of placing snuff inside the lower lip.

with homogeneous white, grayish-white, or dark color. The surface texture exhibits a grainy roughness with a uniform reticular pattern of wrinkles and folds as illustrated by the lesion in Fig. 15-6. The lesions affect the labial, buccal, and facial alveolar mucosa in locations where the patient habitually places the tobacco. This can produce large focal lesions, multiple sites of involvement, or relatively diffuse mucosal alteration depending on the patient's habit. Focal lesions generally exhibit relatively well delineated margins. Tobacco stains of the teeth and residual specks of tobacco reveal the habit.

Differential diagnosis. The combination of the mucosal appearance and history of the habit are pathognomonic of the lesion. As with nicotinic stomatitis, the differential diagnostic question with hyperkeratotic lesions caused by smokeless tobacco is the carcinogenic effect of recurring tobacco exposure. The features indicating a transition from a reactive to a neoplastic lesion are heterogeneous appearance, non-healing ulceration, and excessive verrucous thickening in one or more areas of the lesion. This is most likely for patients with a habit of several decades duration or a habit of chewing a combination of materials, as practiced in Asia.

Management decisions. The patient should be informed of the consequences of the habit and encouraged to discontinue smokeless tobacco use. Hyperkeratotic lesions will improve to some degree within a few weeks or months if the patient complies. Lesions that persist more than a few months after the habit has been discontinued should be excised and submitted for histopathologic examination. Excision is also indicated for lesions that exhibit clinical findings suggestive of malignant neoplasia.

The clinical approach to these lesions when there is no physical evidence of malignancy and the patient refuses to discontinue the smokeless tobacco habit is less clear. Surgical excision is not justified because of the large wound size and the tendency of many patients to simply use a different site. Incisional biopsy is unnecessary to confirm the diagnosis, and early identification of dysplastic or early neoplastic lesions is unlikely because an incisional specimen cannot be fully representative of the entire lesion. Some clinicians advise that the tobacco be placed in several sites to disperse the carcinogenic effect, although no direct evidence supports this recommendation. Periodic clinical reevaluation for signs of dysplastic or neoplastic disease is usually the most reasonable approach in these cases.

Hairy Tongue

Definition. Hairy tongue is a diffuse elongation of the filiform papillae of the dorsum of the tongue. *Candida* organisms are commonly associated with hairy tongue as demonstrated by exfoliative cytology. This suggests that superficial candidiasis stimulates epithelial hyperplasia to produce the thickened matte. The condition is most often observed in smokers and patients with poor oral hygiene, which suggests that these are contributory factors. Secondary staining of the thickened surface by coffee, tea, or tobacco explains the common use of phrases like "black hairy tongue" to describe the condition.

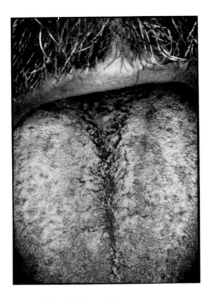

Fig. 15-7 Hairy tongue.

Clinical features. A symmetrical, "shaggy" matte is present on the dorsal surface of the tongue. The extent of the appearance varies, but the lateral borders and tip of the tongue that are exposed to continuous friction are rarely involved. The color of these lesions varies from grayish-white to black depending on the patient's habits. Firm scraping with a blunt instrument will remove some of the superficial material and reveal the unstained white appearance. The lesion is usually thickest near the midline and becomes gradually less prominent near the tip and lateral borders (Fig. 15-7).

Differential diagnosis. The location, symmetry, and filamentous appearance of the tongue should leave little doubt about the diagnosis. Generalized candidiasis may have a similar appearance, but additional lesions are usually present, the superficial material can be more easily rubbed off, and a history suggesting diminished host resistance to infection can usually be identified. Hairy leukoplakia also exhibits a similar surface texture, but these lesions are typically located on the lateral borders of the tongue rather than the central dorsal area. Hairy leukoplakia is also distinguished by sharper margins, the white surface will not rub off, and the patient generally exhibits other clinical features of AIDS.

Management decisions. No treatment is warranted beyond improvement of the patient's oral hygiene. When the patient is instructed to brush the tongue or routinely scrape the tongue surface with a spoon, rapid improvement occurs in most cases.

Actinic Cheilitis

Definition. Actinic cheilitis is a common alteration of the lower lip caused by chronic exposure to sunlight. The ultraviolet (UV) portion of the spectrum produces cellular damage to both the epithelium and the underlying connective tissue. Other designations for the condition are *solar cheilitis* and *solar keratosis*. *Actinic keratosis* is the term used to describe similar chronic sun damage to the skin. Fair-skinned individuals are much more vulnerable to actinic skin and lip damage than are black and Hispanic patients. The injury is a chronic process requiring decades of excessive sun exposure. Therefore affected patients are usually over 60 years of age and report an outdoor vocation or hobby. Actinic cheilitis is considered a premalignant lesion and biopsy usually reveals dysplastic cellular features. Progression to carcinoma of the lip is often associated with cofactors such as smoking.

Clinical features. The patient affected by actinic cheilitis is generally over 60 years of age and fair skinned with a history of excessive sun exposure. The sun-exposed surface of the lower lip appears thinned and atrophic in most areas with indistinct delineation of the vermilion border. Fig. 15-8, *A*, demonstrates the focal, homogeneous, milky-white patches of the atrophic lip surface that are typical of the condition. These areas appear smooth and mildly thickened with sharply-delineated peripheral borders of irregular or jagged contour. These white patches persist for years and remain un-

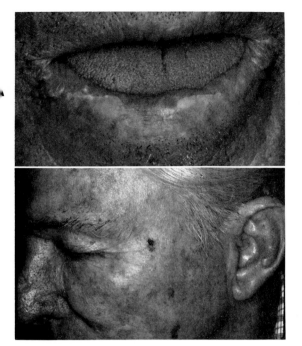

Fig. 15-8 **A,** Actinic cheilitis. This 73-year-old man has farmed for most of his life and enjoys outdoor sports including hunting and boating. The sun-exposed lip surface exhibits several sharply-delineated, milky-white patches. Note the atrophic, thinned appearance of the mucosa in other exposed areas and poor delineation of the junction of the skin and mucosa. **B,** Actinic keratosis. This patient's facial skin exhibits variation in pigmentation, patchy thinning with mild erythema, and an ulcer of several weeks duration lateral to the outer canthus. The pale area inferior to the eye healed with scarring following removal several years previously of a "skin cancer."

changed over an observation period of several months. Evidence of sun damage to the facial skin is invariably associated with actinic cheilitis. This may consist of splotchy variation in skin pigmentation, scaly atrophic patches (Fig. 15-8, *B*), or thick, dark plaques called *seborrheic keratosis.* The patient may report the removal of one or more "skin cancers" also caused by the actinic damage.

Differential diagnosis. Actinic cheilitis can be distinguished from acute injury caused by sunburn, drying or "chapping," or secondary herpetic lesions by healing of these lesions within a few days or weeks. Physiologic hyperkeratosis affecting the lip may appear similar, but a habit or appliance is usually the obvious cause and the patient will not exhibit actinic skin lesions. The occasional transition of actinic cheilitis from a premalignant, reactive condition into carcinoma of the lip occurs gradually over a period of years or decades. Altered appearance of the white patches including heterogeneous color, rough thickening, poor delineation of the borders, and nonhealing ulcers are early signs of carcinoma.

Management decisions. Protection from sun exposure by the use of wide-brimmed hats and a sunscreen lip balm is sound clinical advice for fair-skinned patients of any age. The causes of actinic lip injury and the possibility of lower lip cancer should be explained to the patient with actinic cheilitis to encourage limitation of sun exposure and discontinuation of contributory habits such as smoking. In addition, the visible location of the lesion allows the patient to watch for changes suggestive of carcinoma. Periodic reexamination for altered appearance or progression of the lesion at dental recalls is adequate management in most instances. Any indication of progression or features suggestive of early carcinoma warrant excisional biopsy. This is generally accomplished by a "lip stripping" procedure that removes all of the sun-exposed lip surface. In contrast to intraoral squamous cell carcinoma, the prognosis for cancer of the lower lip and for most UV-induced skin cancers is good to excellent.

Leukoedema

Definition. The cause of leukoedema is unknown, but the frequent occurrence among certain patient groups, such as blacks, indicates a hereditary influence. The predictable location and nonprogressive course of the condition justifies approaching leukoedema as a variation of normal tissue appearance among frequently affected patient groups.

Clinical features. A diffuse, homogeneous, mildly wrinkled, "milky" white appearance of the buccal mucosa is present in a symmetric distribution. The areas do not appear thickened, are not palpable, and do not rub off. A pathognomonic feature of leukoedema is that the whiteness disappears or decreases significantly when the buccal mucosa is stretched.

Differential diagnosis. The location of the white appearance and the dissipation when stretched provide a definitive diagnosis. The symmetric distribution of white lesions caused by white sponge nevus and lichen planus is similar to leukoedema. White sponge nevus, however, appears more dramatically thickened. Reticular or hyperplastic lichen planus produces a more distinct lacy pattern of white lines and patches rather than homogeneous whiteness and these lesions do not fade with stretching.

Management decisions. No treatment is indicated.

White Sponge Nevus

Definition. White sponge nevus is a genetic condition that produces white, rough epithelial thickening of the oral mucosa in a symmetric distribution. The familial occurrence pattern demonstrates autosomal dominant transmission. The condition usually becomes apparent during childhood and other mucosal surfaces may also be affected.

Clinical features. The lesions of white sponge nevus exhibit a thickened, white appearance and rough, fissured surface texture as shown in Fig. 15-9. Diffuse or patchy involvement of both buccal mucosal surfaces and symmetrical lesions limited to other oral and nonoral mucosal surfaces is typical. The lesions are asymptomatic, do not rub off, and do not progress.

Differential diagnosis. Appreciation of the thickened white lesions, the familial occurrence, the onset during childhood, and the

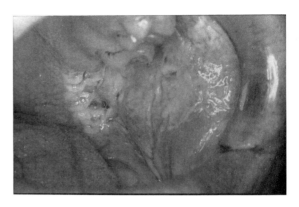

Fig. 15-9 White sponge nevus. The dramatic rough surface texture and white, wrinkled appearance was located bilaterally of the buccal mucosa and soft palate. Several of the patient's family members were also affected. (Courtesy of Dr William H Binnie, Baylor College of Dentistry, Dallas, Texas.)

symmetric distribution of lesions justifies exclusion of most other lesions of epithelial thickening. The oral lesions of white sponge nevus are similar to those of several rare genetic conditions such as *hereditary benign intraepithelial dyskeratosis,* but the effects of these other conditions are also demonstrated by abnormalities of the conjunctiva, skin, or nails.

Management decisions. No treatment or period of clinical reevaluation is necessary because the condition is asymptomatic and benign in all regards. It is appropriate to reassure the patient and the patient's family of the benign nature of the lesions. Incisional biopsy to confirm the diagnosis is unwarranted except in sporadic cases in which family members are unaffected or if other genetic epithelial conditions are suggested by lesions of nonmucosal surfaces.

Lichen Planus

Definition. Lichen planus is a common condition characterized by the chronic occurrence of multiple lesions affecting the skin, mucous membranes, or both. The disease is caused by an immune-mediated degeneration at the interface of the surface epithelium and connective tissue. Oral lesions can exhibit a variety of clinical appearances, which are the basis for classification into five distinct types. The *reticular* and *papular* forms of lichen planus produce oral white lesions of surface thickening and are appropriately discussed here. The *atrophic, erosive,* and *bullous* types of lichen planus are most commonly confronted by the clinician as ulcers and are discussed in Chapter 17.

Lichen planus is a condition of middle age without predominance by gender. A diagnosis of lichen planus before age 30 is unusual. The typical clinical course of the disease is one of chronic persistence of the lesions in affected sites with alternating periods of improvement and progression. A variety of factors have been related to lesion severity including emotional stress, local irritation, and certain drugs. Spontaneous resolution of the lesions, however, is unusual. Approximately one third of the patients with oral evidence of lichen planus exhibit characteristic skin lesions.

A variety of drugs, the most commonly prescribed examples being the thiazides, can produce lesions identical to those of lichen planus as a side effect. This is referred to as a *lichenoid reaction.* Discontinuation of the medication eventually yields resolution of the lesions.

A controversial issue is whether or not an increased probability of oral squamous cell carcinoma exists among patients affected by lichen planus. Some evidence suggests that much of the increased incidence of oral cancer actually represents the original misdiagnosis of dysplastic lesions as lichen planus. The best interpretation is that there may be some increased incidence of oral cancer among lichen planus patients, but the increase is low. Also, the increased cancer incidence is more often associated with the erosive form of lichen planus rather than the more common reticular form.

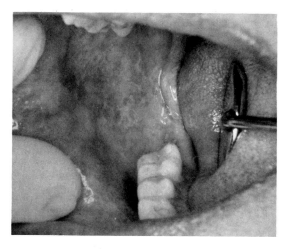

Fig. 15-10 Lichen planus. Clinical examination revealed the illustrated delicate, reticular pattern of thin white lines and mild erythema in additional locations including the contralateral buccal mucosa, tongue, and gingiva.

Clinical features. The oral lesions of the reticular lichen planus exhibit a lacy network of white lines (Fig. 15-10) often referred to as *Wickham's striae.* The peripheral borders may be sharply delineated or may fade gradually to a normal appearance. The lesions are asymptomatic and do not rub off. Multiple lesions are usually found in a symmetric distribution and the buccal mucosa is most commonly affected. Lesions of the tongue, floor of the mouth, labial mucosa, and palate are less common. The lesions of papular lichen planus appear focal and slightly raised with a flat surface and a smooth to slightly rough surface. Careful examination usually reveals subtle peripheral striations in some areas. When skin lesions are present, they are nonscarring papules that occur in aggregates and may coalesce. These lesions are pruritic and, therefore, the surface may be crusted from scratching. In other cases erythema and wrinkled striae as shown in Fig. 15-11 are predominant. Typical sites are flexor surfaces of the limbs, although any skin surface may be affected.

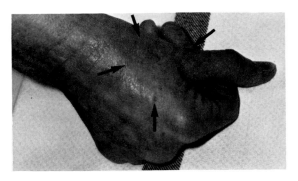

Fig. 15-11 Lichen planus. These skin lesions developed within the last few years and have varied in severity. The skin near the elbow and the genital region were similarly affected. The lesion in the region indicated by the arrows is erythematous and mildly elevated with a fine reticular pattern of white, linear thickening described as Wickham's striae. Oral examination revealed lesions similar to those shown in Fig. 15-10.

Differential diagnosis. Recognition of the lacy, reticular appearance and the symmetric distribution in addition to the characteristic skin lesions is strong evidence of lichen planus. The bilateral white lesions of the buccal mucosa are similar in distribution to white sponge nevus and leukoedema. White sponge nevus can usually be distinguished by the more dramatic appearance, the early age of onset, and the familial occurrence. The white lesions of leukoedema disappear when stretched, while lesions of lichen planus do not. The papular oral lesions may appear similar to leukoplakic lesions and cause concern about the possibility of epithelial dysplasia or early squamous cell carcinoma. Papular lichen planus usually produces multiple lesions while dysplastic lesions are generally isolated. The differentiation of lichen planus from a lichenoid drug reaction for a patient taking a medication known to cause the reaction can be made by discontinuation of the drug in consultation with the prescribing physician. The lichenoid reaction will resolve and lichen planus will not, although the im-

provement may not become apparent for several months. In many instances, discontinuation of the drug may not be possible.

Management decisions. Incisional biopsy may be necessary to confirm the working diagnosis of lichen planus, particularly if no skin lesions are present. The condition cannot be cured by medication, but the painful, erosive lesions can usually be controlled with either topical or systemic corticosteroids. Also, topical application of retinoids has been shown to produce temporary resolution of reticular and papular oral lesions of lichen planus. Neither treatment can be justified, however, for most asymptomatic cases of lichen planus. Periodic clinical reevaluation to identify nonhealing ulceration, enlargement, and other features suggestive of carcinoma is warranted considering the increased oral cancer incidence among oral lichen planus patients.

Hyperplastic Candidiasis*

Definition. Superficial infection of the oral mucosa by the fungus *Candida albicans* and less common species of the same genus is a frequent occurrence among certain patient groups. This ubiquitous organism can be identified in the mouths of most patients, but infection generally does not occur unless one of several predisposing conditions exists. Most of these conditions compromise the resistance of the host to opportunistic candidal infection by altered local resistance, specific deficiencies of the immune system, or generalized physiologic debilitation of the patient. Table 15-1 provides a listing of common examples.

---

*The terms *candidosis* and *candidiasis* are both commonly used to refer to this superficial mycotic infection. Some authorities prefer *candidosis* because the *-osis* suffix is generally used in naming other fungal infections, such as blastomyc*osis* and coccidiomyc*osis*. The *-iasis* suffix may be less appropriate because it often reflects protozoan infection, as with leishman*iasis* and giard*iasis*. However, this suffix usage is hardly absolute, and *candidiasis* is the more commonly preferred term. For this reason and for consistency, *candidiasis* will be used in this text.

Table 15-1   Conditions associated with increased vulnerability or oral candidiasis

Category and condition	Mechanism
ALTERED LOCAL RESISTANCE TO INFECTION	
Poor oral hygiene (especially tongue)	Promotes organism adherence and colonization
Xerostomia	Absence of antimicrobial and flushing effects of saliva
Recent antibiotic treatment	Inhibits competitive oral bacteria, especially *Lactobacillus* species
Dental appliance	Isolates mucosa from saliva and functional cleansing; serves as an organism reservoir
COMPROMISED IMMUNE SYSTEM FUNCTION	
Early infancy	Immune competence has not completely developed
Genetic immune deficiency	Specific humoral or cellular immune defects
AIDS	Deficient cellular immune response
Corticosteroid therapy	Inhibition of immune function
Pancytopenia	Depletion of circulating leukocytes caused by chemotherapy, aplastic anemia, and similar hemopoietic disorders
GENERALIZED PATIENT DEBILITATION	
Anemia, malnutrition, malabsorption	Epithelial thinning and altered maturation; poor tissue oxygenation
Diabetes mellitus (especially with poor control)	Recurring hyperglycemia and mild ketoacidosis
Advanced systemic diseases	Metabolic toxicity or limited blood perfusion of tissues

The dentist should be alert to the possibility of causing oral candidiasis secondary to the treatment of other conditions. The most common example is antibiotic therapy to control bacterial infections. This alters or suppresses the normal oral flora, which allows opportunistic overgrowth of the fungal organisms. *Lactobacillus* species appear to be particularly important in this regard. A common sequela of topical corticosteroid therapy to control ulcerative oral conditions is the emergence of oral candidiasis. Placement of dentures in combination with poor hygiene can provide a barrier to the normal frictional removal of superficial organisms and result in infection.

Candidiasis can produce lesions of such diversity that it must be considered in the differential diagnosis of most diffuse and multifocal lesions of the oral mucosa that do not exhibit enlargement. *Hyperplastic candidiasis* is a chronic "yeast" infection included in this section because it produces white lesions of epithelial thickening that do not rub off. *Pseudomembranous candidiasis*, also known as *thrush*, is characterized by acute progression of thickened white lesions that do rub off and will be described later in this chapter. *Atrophic candidiasis* is a chronic infection that produces patchy red, thinned surfaces and will be considered with other red lesions in Chapter 16. Both the atrophic and pseudomembranous forms can produce pain, burning, and thinned areas suggesting loss of epithelial integrity. This may direct the clinician's differential diagnosis into the ulcerative lesion category. Patients with intraoral candidiasis often develop

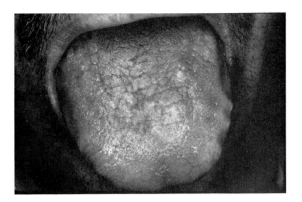

Fig. 15-12 Hyperplastic candidiasis. The white appearance of the dorsum of the tongue would not wipe off with lateral pressure using a gauze sponge. Microscopic examination of material scraped from the surface demonstrated filamentous organisms with features consistent with *Candida albicans.*

extraoral infection at the labial commissures characterized by nonhealing fissures that is referred to as *angular cheilitis.* Finally, careful examination of a patient with candidiasis often demonstrates the concurrence of two, three, or even all four lesion forms.

Clinical features. Hyperplastic candidiasis produces multiple or diffuse white lesions that appear variably thick, patchy, and do not rub off with lateral pressure. The borders are often vague, which mimics the appearance of epithelial dysplasia if the multifocal distribution of lesions is not apparent. The tongue (Fig. 15-12) is most commonly affected but lesions can develop on most oral surfaces. Examination usually reveals erythematous or atrophic areas peripheral to the white lesions, a hairy tongue appearance, white areas that rub off suggestive of the pseudomembranous lesions, or angular cheilitis in addition to the hyperplastic white lesions. In most cases, the medical history or clinical examination findings suggest a condition of diminished host resistance to infection. Many women with oral candidiasis also report symptoms of vaginal itching and discharge indicative of vaginal candidiasis.

Differential diagnosis. The combination of multifocal lesions, variable appearance of the lesions, focal white areas that rub off, and an underlying condition of diminished host resistance is strong evidence that the condition is candidiasis. Lichen planus may appear similar, but the characteristic striated appearance, the presence of skin lesions, the absence of a compromised host condition, and inability to wipe off any of the white lesions can usually be relied on to distinguish it from candidiasis. Oral candidiasis and hairy leukoplakia of AIDS often coexist. Hyperplastic candidiasis improves with antimycotic treatment, while hairy leukoplakia remains unchanged or progresses. Diagnostic confusion of hyperplastic candidiasis with other lesions of epithelial thickening is unlikely.

Management decisions. A working diagnosis of candidiasis should be confirmed by exfoliative cytology or by culture. When a definitive diagnosis of candidiasis is made, the patient may be treated with topical antifungal agents as described in Chapter 13. Topical treatment should continue at least 1 week after resolution of the clinical lesions. However, the clinician should be confident of the diagnosis before initiating topical antimycotic treatment because the drug is likely to interfere with any attempt to later culture or demonstrate the organisms by exfoliative cytology. Systemic administration of antimycotic agents such as fluconazole may be required for resistant infections. Effective cleaning of mucosal surfaces by brushing or scraping with a spoon promotes resolution of the infection by physical removal of superficial accumulations of keratin, organisms, and other materials that provide a reservoir. This is particularly important if the dorsum of the tongue is thickened or the papillae appear elongated or matted. Dentures also act as a reservoir for organisms. Therefore the dentures must be treated along with the patient. One treatment that is usually effective is to soak the dentures overnight in a solution of 1/2 teaspoon of household bleach in 1 cup of water or in the topical antimycotic agent for the duration of the treatment.

The priority clinical issue for patients with oral candidiasis and no history of a diminished host resistance condition is to determine if such a condition may be undiagnosed. Oral candidiasis is generally explained by changes in the oral environment, administration of broad spectrum antibiotics, or a common disease such as anemia or diabetes. However, oral candidiasis can be the initial manifestation of AIDS or other serious illness. Medical referral is justified if this opportunistic infection cannot be explained by known conditions.

Hairy Leukoplakia

Definition. Hairy leukoplakia is a relatively unique white lesion of the tongue that is common among patients with AIDS. The lesion is caused by an opportunistic Epstein-Barr virus infection in the immunocompromised AIDS patient. Why the lesion occurs in the characteristic location is unclear. Hairy leukoplakia has also been reported in immunocompromised patients who are HIV-seronegative.

Clinical features. The lesion is an asymptomatic white patch that does not rub off that usually affects the lateral border of the tongue. Symmetric involvement of both tongue borders is typical, as illustrated in Fig. 15-13, and prominent examples may cover much of the dorsal surface and extend to the ventral surface. Other oral surfaces are much less commonly affected. The surface texture is grainy, rough, corrugated, or "shaggy" in appearance. The borders of the lesion are usually irregular or jagged in contour and sharply delineated. Hairy leukoplakia commonly develops before other clinical features of AIDS, and oral candidiasis may be concurrent.

Differential diagnosis. The differential diagnosis of lesions exhibiting the features of hairy leukoplakia should include physiologic hyperkeratosis, idiopathic leukoplakia, lichen planus, and hyperplastic candidiasis. Physiologic hyperkeratosis caused by rough tooth

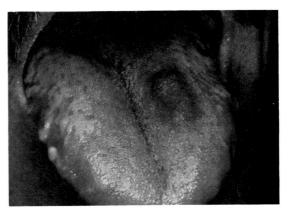

Fig. 15-13 Hairy leukoplakia. The patchy white lesions of the lateral borders of the tongue would not rub off. This patient was HIV seropositive and presented clinical features of AIDS including recurring respiratory infections, weight loss, necrotizing ulcerative gingivitis, and skin lesions of Kaposi's sarcoma. The dark, sessile enlargement of the dorsum of the tongue is typical of Kaposi's sarcoma.

surfaces or a tongue biting habit is usually less prominent and less symmetric than hairy leukoplakia. In addition, the habit will be reported by the patient or the rough tooth surfaces will be apparent. Idiopathic leukoplakia is usually a single, less delineated lesion, a tobacco habit can be identified, the patient is typically older, and risk factors for HIV infection may not be elicited. Prominent reticular lesions of lichen planus are unusual on the lateral borders of the tongue without peripheral striations and lesions of other surfaces. Hyperplastic candidiasis can also affect the tongue and appear similar to hairy leukoplakia, but the lesions are more diffuse and are characterized by atrophy, erythema, and removable pseudomembranous plaques in different sites. In many cases candidiasis will also be present when hairy leukoplakia is identified.

Management decisions. Incisional biopsy may be justified if the diagnosis is in doubt or if HIV infection has not been demonstrated. However, HIV serum testing will provide es-

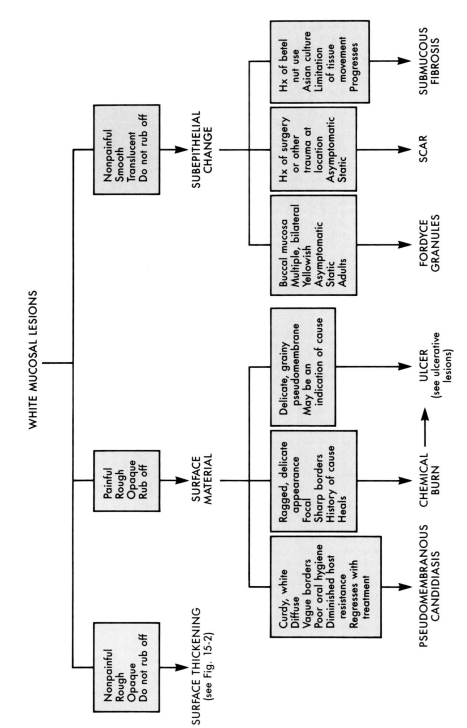

Fig. 15-14 Differential diagnosis of mucosal white lesions characterized by surface material or submucosal changes.

sentially the same diagnostic conclusion and should be the priority if undiagnosed HIV infection is a possibility. Hairy leukoplakia has been shown to resolve following treatment with antiviral agents such as acyclovir. There seems to be little justification for treating these asymptomatic, self-limited lesions in most cases. The clinical priority should be medical referral for diagnosis and management of the illness.

WHITE LESIONS OF SUPERFICIAL MATERIAL

Oral white lesions of superficial material are similar to white lesions of epithelial thickening in that the surface texture is grainy or rough and the white lesions appear opaque. White lesions caused by superficial material are distinguished because the majority of the white appearance can be removed by gentle lateral pressure with a cotton gauze or a blunt instrument. This usually reveals an erythematous or ulcerated mucosal surface. The other significant diagnostic feature of these lesions is that the patient reports pain because of the underlying ulcer. The only conditions that produce white lesions of superficial material are pseudomembranous candidiasis, several types of mucosal burns, and accumulation of a fibrinoid coagulum over some mucosal ulcers. Patients with very poor oral hygiene may also exhibit a white appearance of mucosal surfaces consisting of bacterial plaque and food, but when wiped away the mucosa appears normal. These lesions are compared in Fig. 15-14.

Pseudomembranous Candidiasis

Definition. The definition and significant clinical factors described for hyperplastic candidiasis apply in general to pseudomembranous candidiasis. The most significant difference is that pseudomembranous candidiasis is an *acute* superficial mucosal infection as compared with the *chronic* clinic course typical of hyperplastic and atrophic candidiasis. The most commonly infected individuals are in-

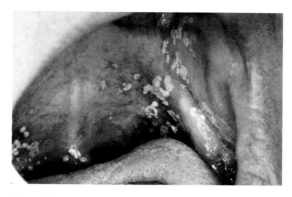

Fig. 15-15 Pseudomembranous candidiasis. These gelatinous white plaques could be easily removed to expose the underlying erythematous mucosa. This patient had been treated for AIDS during the preceding 8 months.

fants before the development of immune system competence and patients affected by a sudden loss of immune competence. This can be caused by systemic corticosteroid therapy, chemotherapy, AIDS, or acute debilitating illness.

Clinical features. Diffuse, patchy, or globular white thickened plaques such as those shown in Fig. 15-15 are present on multiple mucosal surfaces. The tongue, soft palate, and buccal mucosa are most often affected but most of the oral cavity may be covered in severe cases. The material appears opaque with a rough or gelatinous surface texture and can be easily wiped off with lateral pressure exposing erythematous, atrophic, or ulcerated mucosa. Patients frequently describe relatively mild burning pain that becomes more severe when the superficial coagulum is scraped away.

Differential diagnosis. The presence of a removable white surface coagulum affecting multiple sites and evidence of diminished host resistance to infection should leave little doubt about the diagnosis. This is particularly true with infants and with patients who report a recent change in their health status. The superficial white material of chemical burns of the mucosa usually appears thin and delicate as compared with the thickened nature of pseudomembranous candidiasis, and the patient history usually reveals the exposure of a caustic chemical to the oral mucosa. Ulcers with a white fibrinoid surface also appear thinner than the white lesions of candidiasis, and the ulcers with white fibrinoid surfaces are usually more focal.

Management decisions. The clinical features of pseudomembranous candidiasis usually provide the basis for a definitive diagnosis. This means that confirmation by culture or exfoliative cytology is unnecessary in most cases. Treatment is detailed in Chapter 13. Pseudomembranous candidiasis is the form of the infection most likely to spread to oropharyngeal and esophageal mucosal surfaces. This in addition to the patient's complaints of discomfort necessitates prompt and effective treatment. Medical referral to clarify possible conditions of compromised health may be indicated.

Chemical Mucosal Burns

Definition. Mucosal burns caused by corrosive chemicals are uncommon because most individuals are aware enough of the danger to avoid putting these substances in the mouth. The dentist occasionally encounters a patient who has placed an aspirin tablet on the buccal alveolar surface near a tooth in the mistaken belief that this will relieve a toothache. Iatrogenic mucosal burns by acids used to etch tooth surfaces may occur if rubber dam placement is ineffective. Chemical burns of the oral mucosa can result when children mistakenly drink household chemicals and with suicide attempts by ingestion of caustic materials, but the oral burns are usually a low-priority problem for these patients.

Clinical features. Chemical burns of the oral mucosa exhibit the appearance of a delicate, thin, homogeneous white film (Fig. 15-16). Gentle lateral pressure causes the white material to slide away exposing an ex-

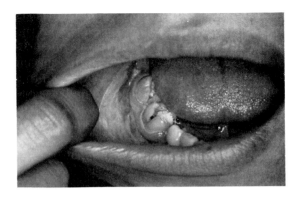

Fig. 15-16 Chemical burn caused by aspirin. Throbbing pain of the mandibular right molars prompted the patient to place an aspirin tablet in the buccal vestibule. The white superficial membrane could be removed easily, and the surface was extremely painful.

quisitely painful central ulceration and more adherent patches of white material at the periphery. Aspirin burns are focal with sharply delineated borders, although more diffuse burns are possible when caused by more extensive chemical exposure. The patient will usually admit to placing aspirin against the tooth if that is the cause. Infants and mentally compromised patients who have ingested caustic chemicals may not be able to clarify the source of chemical injury.

Differential diagnosis. Oral burns caused by aspirin or iatrogenic chemical injury usually do not represent a differential diagnostic problem when the source of chemical exposure is clear and the delicate, removable white surface is present. The thin, membranous appearance of the chemical burn is unlikely to be confused with the diffuse and multifocal lesions of candidiasis. The lesion may be categorized as ulcerative rather than white if the superficial white material has been abraded away before examination, but the acute onset, pain, and focal area of involvement usually provide adequate evidence of the physical nature of the injury.

Management decisions. Palliative care with a topical anesthetic or a bland coating suspension is the limit of the available treatment. Fortunately, these painful lesions heal quickly. The patient with an aspirin burn should be encouraged in the future to swallow the aspirin and obtain clove oil or a commercial topical anesthetic for temporary relief of oral pain.

Ulcers

Definition. Many oral ulcers may initially appear as white lesions because of a superficial fibrinoid coagulum that forms as a part of the repair process. Aphthous ulcers are a common example. Bulla formation, which is separation of the epithelium from the connective tissue that is characteristic of several oral ulcerative conditions, can also produce a thin, white "filmy" appearance. The ulcerative nature of these lesions, as with chemical burns, is evident when the ulcer is exposed by abrading away the superficial white material with gentle lateral pressure. The differential diagnostic issue is to appreciate that the superficial white appearance of some ulcerative lesions is *not* the primary manifestation of the condition. Differential diagnostic categorization of these lesions based on the feature of ulceration will yield a more accurate diagnosis. Chapter 17 is devoted to the discussion of oral ulcerative conditions.

Clinical features. Ulcers covered by white superficial material are painful and removal of the white material increases the discomfort. The white appearance associated with ulcers appears thin in contrast to many of the thickened, rough white lesions previously described. The white surface is homogeneous or mildly grainy with sharply delineated peripheral margins and a surrounding halo of erythema. Depending on the cause, more than one lesion may be present and the patient may report a history of healing and recurrence.

Differential diagnosis. The presence of pain and the removal of the white surface material should limit the diagnostic possibilities to ulcers, candidiasis, and chemical burns. Most white lesions of epithelial thickening are painless, will not rub off, and do not exhibit an erythematous halo. Candidiasis can be distinguished by identification of a condition associated with diminished host resistance, the diffuse distribution of lesions, and the mixture of different forms of fungal lesions. Aspirin burns and other chemical injuries will be clarified by history. Once the primary manifestation of the lesion is identified as ulceration, the differential diagnosis should proceed within that lesion category.

Management decisions. Management decisions require a specific diagnosis.

WHITE LESIONS OF SUBMUCOSAL CHANGE

White lesions of submucosal alteration appear pale because the normally vascular mucosal connective tissue has been replaced by less vascular tissue. These white lesions are distinguished by the smooth and translucent appearance of the normal epithelial surface as compared with the opaque, rough character of white lesions caused by epithelial thickening and superficial material. Also, white lesions of submucosal change do not rub off and are nonpainful. The common oral white abnormalities caused by submucosal change are Fordyce granules, scarring, and submucous fibrosis. The differential diagnosis of these lesions is illustrated in Fig. 15-14.

Fordyce Granules

Definition. Fordyce granules are ectopic sebaceous glands located within the oral mucosa. They increase in prominence with age and are usually located in the buccal mucosa region, although location in the labial mucosa is not unusual. Fordyce granules can be identified in the mouths of most older adults. These features support the attitude that this condition can be considered as a variation of normal tissues.

Clinical features. Small (1 to 2 mm) ovoid yellowish-white spots are present in a bilaterally symmetric distribution of the buccal surfaces (Fig. 5-1) and labial mucosa in some instances. They may appear slightly raised, but the smooth, translucent appearance of the surface indicates that the alteration is deep to the surface epithelium. Most patients with prominent Fordyce granules are older.

Differential diagnosis. No other condition is likely to be confused with the characteristic appearance of Fordyce granules. Pseudomembranous candidiasis can produce multiple granular fungal clumps, but they are readily removed by wiping with a cotton gauze.

Management decisions. No treatment or period of observation is indicated.

Scar

Definition. Healing and repair of soft tissue injuries with dense collagenous connective tissue or scar often produces a pale appearance as compared with adjacent, normal tissues. This is more apparent with loose mucosal tissues such as the soft palate, buccal mucosa, labial mucosa, and floor of the mouth. The hard palate and gingiva are normally composed of such dense fibrous connective tissue that scars may not be particularly noticeable.

Clinical features. The typical appearance is of a focal, homogeneous pale area with a smooth surface texture and sharply delineated borders. No pain, tenderness, or other symptoms are present. Pit or fissure depressions may be present if the injury or surgical procedure resulted in poor tissue apposition. One of the most commonly observed examples is a stellate pattern of pale lines radiating from the depression between the tonsillar pillars that represents healing following a tonsillectomy as shown in Fig. 15-17. The patient will usually remember a surgical procedure or traumatic injury if the suspected scar is large, but with smaller lesions the patient may not recall any specific incident.

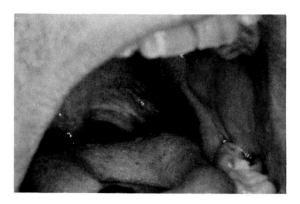

Fig. 15-17 Scar. The stellate pattern of sharply delineated pale lines in the tonsillar pillar region is characteristic of a tonsillectomy scar.

Differential diagnosis. The focal pale appearance with a smooth surface and a history of injury or surgery is adequate basis for a definitive clinical diagnosis. Submucous fibrosis is a much more generalized process and Fordyce granules are more numerous, much smaller, and more uniform in size. Traumatic lesions such as the traumatic fibroma can appear pale, but tissue enlargement is the more significant primary manifestation. Occasionally, the fissured or pitlike depression of an area of scarring is actually the orifice of a pathologic sinus. The mucosa near the depression will often be slightly erythematous. Probing reveals the tract and produces exudate in some cases. The most likely locations are near teeth affected by periapical inflammatory lesions and the extraction site of maxillary molars as a residual oroantral fistula.

Management decisions. Scars require no treatment. In some cases the diagnosis may be in doubt, but a period of observation will reveal the static nature of the abnormal appearance.

Submucous Fibrosis

Definition. Submucous fibrosis is generalized fibrosis of the connective tissue of the oral mucosa in response to habitual chewing of betel nut and frequent use of certain spices. This practice is common in certain regions of India and southeast Asia. The condition is rare in North America, except among individuals originally from these areas.

Clinical features. Generalized yellow-white discoloration of the oral mucosa with a smooth surface texture is present. The intensity of the color change may vary in different regions of the oral cavity. The loss of elasticity and firmness to palpation resulting from the generalized fibrosis is most apparent in the soft palate and buccal mucosa. Severe submucous fibrosis can cause trismus and eating difficulties. History reveals the use of betel nut or other oral habits of Asian cultural influence.

Differential diagnosis. The generalized oral mucosal fibrosis and history of the oral habit confirm the diagnosis. The autoimmune or collagen diseases, particularly systemic sclerosis, can also produce fibrosis, but tissues in addition to oral structures are affected. Chronic radiation fibrosis following radiotherapy of the head and neck may appear similar in some respects, but the superficial skin is also affected and the history clarifies the cause.

Management decisions. The patient should be encouraged to discontinue the habit, which will prevent progression of the process. Unfortunately, the fibrosis that has already occurred is irreversible. Stretching exercises and corticosteroid administration may be of limited benefit in severe cases. Frequent periodic clinical reexamination of individuals affected by submucous fibrosis is mandatory because approximately one third eventually develop squamous cell carcinoma.

SUMMARY

White lesions of the oral mucosa are characterized by the primary manifestation of an abnormally white or pale discoloration of the mucosa without enlargement or ulceration. The differential diagnosis of white lesions of the oral mucosa requires classification of an abnormality as a white lesion of epithelial thickening, surface material, or submucosal change. White lesions of epithelial thickening exhibit a rough surface texture, appear thickened, are opaque, will not rub off, and are not associated with pain. White lesions of superficial material are often painful, can be rubbed away, and also appear rough, opaque, and thickened. White lesions of submucosal change are pale and translucent, do not rub off, are asymptomatic, and do not appear thickened. The differential diagnosis within each group of white lesions is based on comparison of features such as the number of lesions, the sites affected, the duration, associated factors as possible causes, and age of onset.

BIBLIOGRAPHY

Bengel W and others: Differential diagnosis of diseases of the oral mucosa, Chicago, 1989, Quintessence.

Eversole LR: Clinical outline of oral pathology: diagnosis and treatment, ed 2, Philadelphia, 1984, Lea & Febiger.

Greenspan D and others: AIDS and the mouth: diagnosis and management of oral lesions, Munksgaard, 1990, Munksgaard.

Langlais RP and others: Oral diagnosis, oral medicine and treatment planning, Philadelphia, 1984, Saunders.

Lynch MA, Brightman VJ, Greenberg MS, editors: Burket's oral medicine: diagnosis and treatment, ed 8, Philadelphia, 1984, Lippincott.

Regezi JA, Sciubba JJ: Oral pathology: clinical-pathologic correlations, Philadelphia, 1989, Saunders.

Shafer WG, Hine MK, Levy BM: A textbook of oral pathology, ed 4, Philadelphia, 1983, Saunders.

Wood NK, Goaz PW: Differential diagnosis of oral lesions, ed 4, St Louis, 1991, Mosby-Year Book.

CHAPTER 16

Differential Diagnosis of Dark Mucosal Lesions

GARY C. COLEMAN

Dark lesions of the oral mucosa appear different from adjacent tissues because of dense melanin accumulation, aggregation of foreign pigmented material, or increased visibility of blood. Most dark discolorations of the oral mucosa are localized, limited reactions to incidental injury or physical irritation of the tissues. The reactive character of the lesions often becomes apparent when the lesions resolve after a short observation period. The clinician's differential diagnostic responsibility in evaluating focal dark mucosal discolorations is to identify the small proportion of lesions that may represent malignant neoplastic disease. Multifocal or diffuse dark lesions of the oral mucosa are clinically significant because they are often a manifestation of an underlying systemic condition. Bleeding disorders, hormonal abnormalities, and dietary deficiencies are a few examples of the conditions that can produce multiple dark mucosal discolorations. This differential diagnostic category specifically excludes dark oral

lesions that exhibit enlargement or ulceration as the primary manifestations of the condition.

DIAGNOSTIC FEATURES AND LESION CLASSIFICATION

The distinction between dark lesions caused by greater visibility of blood and those containing melanin or foreign pigmented material is based on the atypical color observed. Red or reddish-blue indicates increased visibility of blood, while brown, black, or bluish-black is caused by pigmentation that is either foreign or melanocytic in origin. The next distinction is based on whether the mucosal discoloration is focal and isolated or if the condition has produced multiple or diffuse dark lesions. This yields a differential diagnostic strategy based on four groups of dark lesions:

1. Isolated red lesions
2. Multiple or diffuse red lesions
3. Isolated pigmented lesions
4. Multiple or diffuse pigmented areas

Clinical Features of Isolated Red Lesions

The increased visibility of blood that explains the dark appearance of red and reddish-blue lesions results from:

1. An abnormally dense focal concentration of blood vessels
2. Abnormal enlargement or distention of blood vessels
3. Abnormal thinning of the surface epithelium
4. Bleeding into the loose connective tissue

Red lesions consisting of vascular distention or a dense accumulation of blood vessels become pale when pressure is applied because the pooled blood within the vessels is readily displaced from the area of discoloration. The red color quickly returns when pressure is released and the vessels refill. This phenomenon is referred to as *blanching*. Red lesions of epithelial thinning and bleeding into the connective tissue do not blanch significantly or as readily. The presence or absence of blanching is a dependable feature in distinguishing among isolated red lesions.

Clinical Features of Multiple and Diffuse Red Lesions

The initial differential diagnostic decision for nonisolated red lesions is whether the pattern of discoloration represents multiple, separate red areas or diffuse erythema limited to a single region. This distinction can be difficult at times because multiple red lesions often coalesce and appear as a single diffuse lesion. The presence or absence of blanching is a significant distinguishing feature for multiple red lesions, but it is less important in the differential diagnosis of diffuse erythema. Anatomic location, duration, and possible local or systemic factors support additional differential diagnostic decisions in the assessment of multiple and diffuse erythema.

Clinical Features of Isolated Pigmented Lesions

The initial distinction of pigmented oral lesions is based on color. Black and bluish-black lesions are usually caused by pigmented foreign materials. Brown lesions contain an abnormally dense accumulation of melanin. Melanocytic dark lesions are next categorized as either palpable or nonpalpable. Nonpalpable, isolated brown lesions of the oral cavity are in most instances a relatively insignificant clinical finding, whereas raised lesions must be carefully evaluated for the possibility that they represent malignant neoplasia of melanocytic origin.

Clinical Features of Multiple and Diffuse Pigmented Lesions

Multiple pigmented lesions of similar appearance and diffuse pigmentations of the oral cavity in most cases are a superficial manifestation of an underlying condition. The initial distinction can be based on whether the dark lesions were first noticed in infancy or are of relatively recent onset. The presence of characteristic brown oral lesions during infancy is characteristic of racial pigmentation or a developmental syndrome. Multiple oral brown lesions that develop later in life can be caused by certain drugs, hormonal abnormalities, and heavy metal intoxication. The clinical differential diagnosis relies on the identification of features indicative of the underlying condition.

ISOLATED RED LESIONS

Common isolated lesions characterized by red or reddish-blue discoloration without enlargement and their differential diagnostic features are schematically summarized in Fig. 16-1. The initial differential diagnostic distinction for isolated red lesions is whether or not the lesion blanches. Most of these conditions are common and are clinically inconsequential. The one exception is the erythroplakic appearance of epithelial dysplasia or early carcinoma.

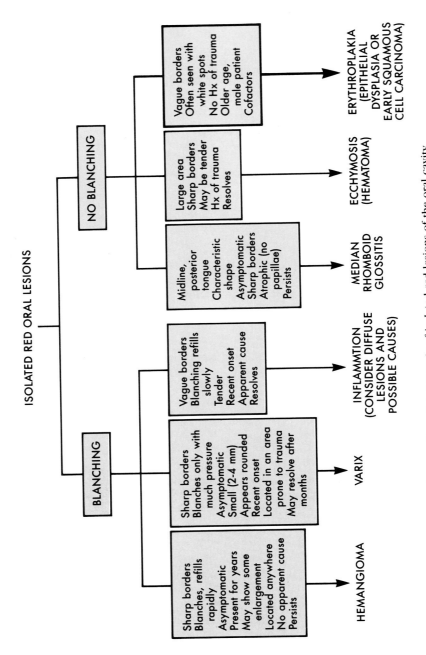

Fig. 16-1   Differential diagnosis of isolated red lesions of the oral cavity.

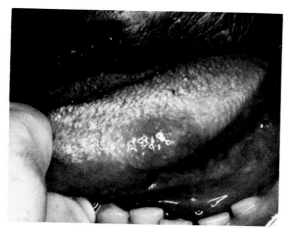

Fig. 16-2 Hemangioma. The patient had been aware of the dark reddish-blue area on the lateral border of the tongue since childhood. The prominence was spongy to palpation and blanched dramatically.

The differential diagnostic priority in the evaluation of all isolated red lesions should be the identification of these potentially serious lesions.

Hemangioma

Definition. Hemangiomas are developmental enlargements consisting of a focally dense concentration of blood vessels. They are present at birth and are first observed during infancy. Hemangiomas enlarge during childhood only in the sense of growth proportional to the growth of the individual and are static in size when observed in the adult. The lesion is most appropriately categorized with soft tissue enlargements, but this primary manifestation may not always be clinically apparent.

Clinical features. The bluish-red or purple color of a hemangioma is homogeneous and dark without alteration of the surface mucosa. The borders are sharply delineated, and sessile prominence compared with surrounding tissue contours is usually noted (Fig. 16-2). The lesion is spongy to palpation, blanches

dramatically with pressure, and refills quickly when decompressed. The lesion size is constant in the adult and the discoloration will be reported by the patient to have been present since childhood. Some patients may be unaware of an intraoral hemangioma because symptoms are unusual.

Differential diagnosis. Lesions of Kaposi's sarcoma and hereditary hemorrhagic telangiectasia may appear similar to hemangiomas, but these diseases produce multiple, enlarging lesions later in life. The vascular appearance of focal lesions such as peripheral giant cell granuloma, pyogenic granuloma, and inflammatory lesions can be confused with hemangiomas, but their recent occurrence and less dramatic blanching are helpful distinguishing features.

Sturge-Weber syndrome, also referred to as *encephalotrigeminal angiomatosis,* is characterized by a port-wine vascular discoloration referred to as *nevus flammeus* of the facial skin in the distribution of a branch of the trigeminal nerve. An associated hemangioma of the oral mucosa may be present. Additional manifestations of the related vascular malformations that are characteristic of this condition are described in Chapter 20.

The vascularity of *arteriovenous malformations,* also known as *A-V shunts or aneurysms,* may appear superficially similar to hemangiomas. These malformations contain numerous arteries that connect directly with venous channels of corresponding size without an intermediate capillary bed. The resulting clinical features of rapid enlargement, spontaneous hemorrhage, bruit during auscultation, and poor delineation of borders are diagnostic. A-V malformations must be approached with care because casual manipulations can lead to rapid exsanguination of the patient.

Management decisions. Biopsy is generally not justified because definitive diagnosis of hemangiomas can usually be made on the basis of the clinical features and history. Excision is generally not required because these lesions are nonprogressive. Occasionally, small facial hemangiomas will be removed for cosmetic reasons. Evidence of recent spontaneous hemorrhage warrants suspicion of an A-V malformation, which qualifies as a medical emergency requiring prompt evaluation in a hospital setting.

Varix

Definition. A varix is a commonly observed focal collection of dilated blood vessels that probably forms by organization and repair of a superficial mucosal "blood blister." The typical location of varices in areas prone to pinching trauma supports this hypothesis. The term *varix* should not be confused with *varicosity* as used in reference to venous distention, which is frequently observed on the ventral tongue surface.

Clinical features. A varix is usually small (2 to 4 mm) with sharply delineated borders and a smooth, rounded surface contour (Fig. 16-3, *A*). The color is uniformly dark reddish-blue, and blanching is typical but it may be difficult to demonstrate with small lesions (Fig. 16-3, *B*). The varix is of recent onset, although this is difficult to confirm because it is painless and the patient is usually unaware of its presence. Typical locations are sites prone to pinching injury such as the lateral border of the tongue and buccal mucosa. The lesion usually resolves after several months. This may be difficult to evaluate, however, since a new varix often develops in the region of a prior lesion. Several varices often occur independently.

Differential diagnosis. The features of varices usually allow a definitive clinical diagnosis. Hereditary hemorrhagic telangiectasia (Rendu-Osler-Weber syndrome) may produce lesions similar in appearance, but they are multifocal, hemorrhagic, larger, and widely distributed. A varix can be confused with some focal pigmented lesions, particularly the blue nevus because of the similarity of color. The usual brown color, failure to blanch, and the palpable nature of most nevi provide diagnostic distinction.

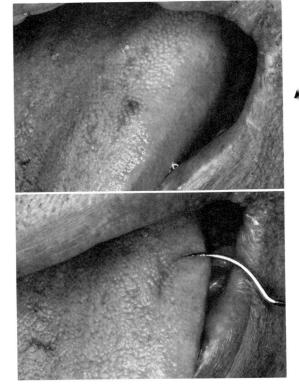

Fig. 16-3 Varix, although an unusually small hemangioma would exhibit the same features. **A,** The patient was unaware of the small blue discoloration near the lateral border of the tongue. **B,** Use of the lateral surface of the explorer tine to apply pressure demonstrated blanching.

Management decisions. Varices require no treatment. The suspicion of a nevus or other pigmented lesion cannot be completely excluded in some cases in which the most probable diagnosis is a varix. Clinical reevaluation of the lesion within 4 to 6 weeks is a reasonable approach. However, excision should be considered if the suspicion of a nevus persists.

Inflammation

Definition. Inflammation resulting from numerous origins can yield a focal red or red-blue lesion of the oral mucosa. The redness or erythema is produced by dilation of blood vessels as an elemental manifestation of the inflammatory process. Gingivitis is a common example that demonstrates the appearance of inflammatory erythema and its blanching response to pressure.

A detailed description of the possible inflammatory lesions is not practical in this section because there are so many possible causes and variations in the features of resulting lesions. The most common lesions of this type observed clinically are abrasions attributable to mild, focal trauma. Denture irritation without ulceration also fits into this category. The primary diagnostic requirement is the identification of a direct cause.

Clinical features. The focal erythematous area typically exhibits some variation in the degree of redness and gradually fades near the periphery. The area blanches with pressure, and erythema returns more slowly than a hemangioma when the pressure is removed. Inflammatory lesions are tender to palpation, and the patient is generally aware of its presence and duration. A cause is usually identified, which may be as obvious as poor adaptation of an appliance or as subtle as ingestion of abrasive foods before the onset of tenderness. The lesions quickly resolve following removal of the irritation.

Differential diagnosis. Ecchymoses and hematomas can be similar in superficial appearance, symptoms, and possible traumatic causes, but these dark lesions of extravasated blood do not blanch. Both focal inflammations and dark lesions of extravasated blood physiologically resolve relatively quickly, leaving the precise diagnosis as a secondary issue in most cases. The varix is asymptomatic and sharply delineated in contrast to inflammatory mucosal lesions. Hemangiomas blanch more readily, are asymptomatic, have been present since childhood, and do not resolve. Ulceration may be present if focal trauma has abraded the surface epithelium. Traumatic ulcers also resolve quickly with removal of the cause. If ulceration persists, then the differential diagnosis must be

expanded to include the chronic ulcerative lesion category.

Management decisions. The pain and tenderness of red inflammatory mucosal lesions are frequent sources of patient complaint. Removal of the probable source of inflammation should be the treatment goal. Persistence of the erythema beyond a few days after removal of the suspected cause requires reconsideration of the diagnosis.

Median Rhomboid Glossitis

Definition. Median rhomboid glossitis (MRG) is a common atrophic lesion located at the midline of the posterior dorsum of the tongue. The name is derived from the midline location and the typical geometric shape of the abnormality. Some confusion exists concerning the pathogenesis of MRG. It was once thought to represent a developmental deficiency of papillae in the tuberculum impar region, but the prevailing current opinion is that MRG is a superficial, focal candidiasis.

Clinical features. The atrophic, smooth appearance of the lesion is attributable to the absence of papillae in the tuberculum impar area of the dorsum of the tongue. The uniformly reddish-pink area does not blanch with pressure and no pain or tenderness to pressure is present. The borders are sharply delineated and the lesion often exhibits an angular or geometric shape. The size of the lesion seldom extends more than half the distance to the lateral border of the tongue. The atrophic patch is typically of long duration.

Differential diagnosis. The location, shape, color, and absence of papillae of MRG are adequately characteristic that a definitive diagnosis can be made based on the clinical appearance in most cases. Benign migratory glossitis typically produces multiple, asymptomatic, atrophic tongue lesions with a slightly elevated white, annular peripheral border. Multiple atrophic tongue lesions associated with complaints of pain or burning suggest more generalized atrophic candidiasis or mucosal atrophy caused by a dietary deficiency or

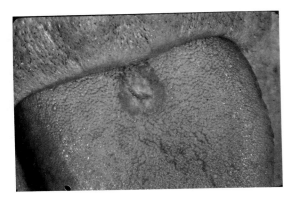

Fig. 16-4 Median rhomboid glossitis. This smooth, painless patch was located in the midline of the posterior dorsum of the tongue. A fissure with a peripheral white appearance was present in the center of the atrophic lesion.

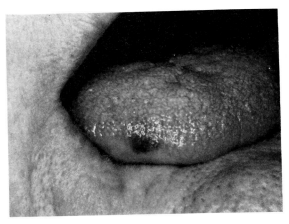

Fig. 16-5 Ecchymosis. This sharply delineated, homogeneous red macule was observed when the patient returned for adjustment 1 week after insertion of a maxillary complete denture and a mandibular partial denture. The nontender discoloration did not blanch and was not present when the dentures were inserted.

anemia. Some examples of MRG may appear somewhat lobulated or fissured (Fig 16-4), but the most frequently observed surface texture is uniformly smooth.

Management decisions. Biopsy is not required for diagnosis in most cases. Identification of mycotic organisms by culture or exfoliative cytology may not be effective with median rhomboid glossitis, and it is usually not indicated. An effort should be made to identify yeast if atrophic lesions are seen in other areas and the patient history supports the suspicion of generalized oral candidiasis. No treatment is normally indicated because the condition is asymptomatic and seldom progresses to symptomatic candidiasis.

Ecchymosis

Definition. The term *ecchymosis* applies to macular discolorations resulting from bleeding into the connective tissue. The immediate cause among patients with normal hemostatic function is traumatic injury, and ecchymosis of the oral mucosa is a common incidental observation during intraoral examinations. The term *petechiae* also refers to discoloration from connective tissue bleeding, but the smaller, pinpoint areas of petechial hemorrhage often indicate some form of bleeding tendency. *Purpura* is a term to describe any disease process that produces an abnormal bleeding tendency.

Clinical features. Soon after injury ecchymosis appears homogeneously red with relatively sharp peripheral borders (Fig. 16-5). The discoloration does not blanch and may be slightly tender. The bruise eventually exhibits variable alterations in color during the healing process and resolves within 1 to 2 weeks, depending on the extent of the discoloration. The patient may describe a traumatic injury that explains the bruise. Ecchymosis is also frequently present after surgical manipulation. Injury to a large vessel can produce hemorrhagic enlargement referred to as a *hematoma*, especially in areas of loose submucosal tissue and large vessels.

Differential diagnosis. Resolution of these lesions within 2 weeks and a history of trauma should allow exclusion of MRG and erythroplakia from diagnostic consideration. The presence of multiple petechiae without an indication of traumatic injury proportional to the discoloration requires consideration of a bleeding disorder. The absence of blanching allows exclusion of inflammatory erythema.

Management decisions. Biopsy of lesions with these features before a reevaluation period is not indicated. Reevaluation of suspected ecchymosis at 1 to 2 weeks is adequate for confirmation of the diagnosis. Pain and antiinflammatory medication may be indicated depending on the severity of the injury. Occasionally, evaluation of the patient's hemostatic mechanisms is indicated if bleeding is multifocal or appears disproportionate to the injury.

Erythroplakia

Definition. *Erythroplakia* refers to an atrophic, nonenlarged red lesion of the oral mucosa that does not appear to be primarily reactive to physical, infectious, or other inflammatory conditions. The term is descriptive and not a specific diagnosis. The significance of this term is that a relatively high proportion of persistent lesions of this appearance are eventually demonstrated by biopsy to be either precancerous or early squamous cell carcinoma. In other words, this term is best used when reactive and inflammatory factors do not adequately explain the features of the red lesion. Much of the differential diagnostic significance of assessing isolated red lesions in general is to identify this premalignant or malignant lesion.

Clinical features. The heterogeneous red discoloration of erythroplakia results from variable epithelial thinning as suggested by the lesion in Fig. 16-6. Therefore these lesions do not blanch. In addition to the variation in redness, spots or borders of the lesion often appear white. This appearance is referred to as *speckled erythroplakia.* Focal ulcerations may also be present and they seldom heal as would be expected for reactive lesions. These lesions exhibit vague peripheral borders and a rough or ragged surface texture. The patient is usu-

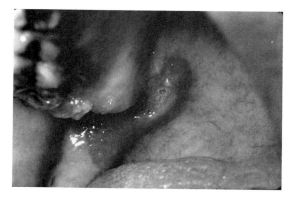

Fig. 16-6 Erythroplakia. This nonblanching red lesion was identified in the lateral soft palate, anterior tonsillar pillar region of a 45-year-old alcoholic with a cigarette smoking history of more than 50 pack-years. The margins appeared well delineated but the lesion exhibited subtle variation in the degree of redness and several white foci that would not rub off. Two incisional biopsies yielded a pathologic diagnosis of mild dysplasia. The clinician remained suspicious when the lesion did not resolve after a 1-month period. A third incisional biopsy led to the definitive diagnosis of superficially invasive squamous cell carcinoma.

ally unaware of the area since the lesion is typically nonpainful. Little or no indication of a direct cause can be identified, although the patient history often reveals habitual tobacco and alcohol use. Older males are most often affected.

Differential diagnosis. Many chronic reactive red lesions appear similar in one or more respects to erythroplakia. Identification of a direct cause and resolution of the lesion after removing the suspected cause is the primary differential diagnostic finding in distinguishing reactive red lesions from erythroplakia. *Squamous cell carcinoma must be the primary diagnostic suspicion for any nonblanching red mucosal lesion that fails to resolve after removal of a suspected cause.* Multiple lesions of separate oral mucosal surfaces are unusual for erythroplakia and should direct the differential diagnosis into the multiple red lesion category. However, the development of multiple independent erythroplakic lesions in the same general anatomic region in response to similar carcinogenic influences has been described as *field cancerization.* The suspicion that multiple erythematous lesions may be separate foci of erythroplakia must be based on the history of cofactors, heterogeneous appearance of the lesions, and persistence after removal of a possible cause.

Management decisions. *Any lesion demonstrating the diagnostic features listed above must be managed as squamous cell carcinoma until proven otherwise.* Reevaluation within a week to 10 days of the initial presentation is justifiable if there is a reasonable possibility that the lesion is reactive. This is particularly true with young adults and children for whom squamous cell carcinoma would be an unusual development.

Failure to resolve or progression after removal of a suspected cause necessitates excisional or incisional biopsy, depending on the lesion size and location. This should be accomplished by a clinician skilled in managing oral cancer. A tertiary care environment generally provides more expedient treatment if the erythroplakia is eventually determined microscopically to be advanced epithelial dysplasia or early squamous cell carcinoma. Delaying definitive diagnosis and treatment beyond a few weeks after discovery may adversely affect the prognosis and is unjustified. Exfoliative cytology is generally equivocal in the diagnostic evaluation of erythroplakic lesions and may unnecessarily delay treatment.

MULTIPLE AND DIFFUSE RED LESIONS

Multiple and diffuse red lesions appear red for all of the same basic reasons as isolated red lesions but the discoloration is likely to be caused by an underlying condition if large or multiple sites are affected. Most infections, for example, affect regions rather than appearing as isolated erythematous foci. As with focal lesions, an important feature is whether or not the lesions blanch with pressure. Additional considerations in the differential diagnosis of these lesions are illustrated in Fig. 16-7.

Hereditary Hemorrhagic Telangiectasia

Definition. Hereditary hemorrhagic telangiectasia or *Rendu-Osler-Weber syndrome* is a rare genetic condition characterized by multiple macular or papular vascular lesions of the skin, mucosal surfaces, and other tissues. Most of the symptoms associated with the disease relate to the tendency of these abnormal vessels to hemorrhage. The condition is usually noted early in life, although occasionally the telangiectatic lesions do not become pronounced until late adolescence.

Clinical features. When first identified, the lesions of hereditary hemorrhagic telangiectasia are small (2 to 6 mm) and sharply delineated at their periphery and they blanch with pressure. Multiple telangiectasias of the skin (Fig. 16-8) and mucosa can be observed in most cases. A common bleeding complaint of these patients is epistaxis. Other complaints depend on the locations of lesions. Blood loss from gastrointestinal lesions, for example, can produce blood in the stools and hemorrhagic anemia. Other members of the patient's family will usually be affected by the condition because the genetic mechanism is autosomal dominant transmission.

Differential diagnosis. Demonstration of multiple small, blanching vascular lesions and a history of similarly affected family members are an adequate basis for a definitive diagnosis. The adult patient will be aware of the diagnosis in most cases. Venous varices either of the ventral tongue surface or as encountered on the skin of an alcoholic may appear similar but are linear in shape and usually nonhemorrhagic.

Management decisions. Incidental trauma to the vascular lesions during examina-

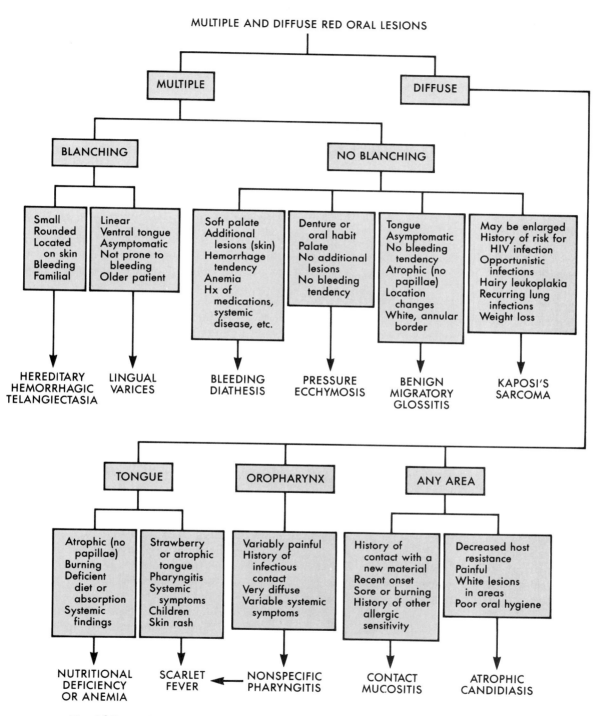

Fig. 16-7 Differential diagnosis of multiple and diffuse red lesions of the oral cavity.

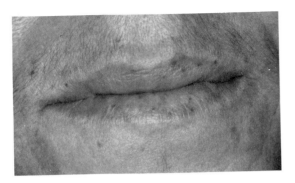

Fig. 16-8 Hereditary hemorrhagic telangiectasia. Several small, blanching bluish-red lesions were present on the exposed lip surfaces of this 17-year-old male. He denied any bleeding problems but was aware of the condition because his father and uncle were similarly affected.

tion and treatment procedures should be minimized to avoid hemorrhage. Control of bleeding can occasionally be a problem, but local hemostatic methods are usually effective.

Lingual Varices

Definition. Lingual varices are such a common observation among adult patients that the condition can be considered a normal anatomic variation. This distention or varicosity of the superficial veins of the ventral tongue surface occurs for unknown reasons. The common opinion that the prominence of the distended veins corresponds to the severity of the patient's hypertension can be a misleading generalization.

Clinical features. Lingual varices are blue or reddish-blue linear structures immediately subjacent to the mucosa of the ventral tongue surface. Blanching with pressure and the symmetric, branching distribution indicate the vascular nature of the discoloration. Occasionally, a similar but less pronounced venous distention may be observed in other areas such as the tonsillar pillar region. Patients are asymptomatic and unaware of the condition. Normal functional trauma is unlikely to cause hemorrhage, but laceration can cause persistent bleeding.

Differential diagnosis. Lingual varices are characteristic in appearance and diagnostic uncertainty is unusual. Enlargement or asymmetry warrants differential diagnostic consideration of vascular soft tissue enlargements. Hemangiomas may appear superficially similar, but the focal density of vessels, mild enlargement, and the asymmetry of hemangiomas are unlikely to be confused with the uniform, symmetric distribution of lingual varicosities.

Management decisions. No treatment or clinical reevaluation period is necessary.

Bleeding Diatheses

Definition. Disproportionate bleeding into the connective tissue following minor surface abrasion or injury is one of the earliest manifestations of a bleeding diathesis. *Petechial hemorrhage* of the soft palate is a common oral feature of a hemorrhagic condition. The vulnerability of the soft palate to minor functional trauma and its nonkeratinized epithelial surface make this a probable location in which to observe capillary hemorrhage. The concomitant observation of ecchymosis affecting skin surfaces is confirmational of a bleeding tendency but the observation of palatal petechiae alone is adequately characteristic to require further diagnostic evaluation. Congenital bleeding disorders such as classic hemophilia will be promptly reported by the patient. The more common acquired bleeding diatheses will also be revealed by the patient history in most instances. High doses of aspirin, therapeutic coagulation suppression with coumarin, hemopoietic suppression by antimetabolic drugs, and hepatic cirrhosis are common examples.

Clinical features. Multiple, small red spots are present on the nonkeratinized mucosal surfaces, particularly the soft palate. The small and uniform size (1 to 4 mm) of the red areas indicates capillary bleeding (Fig. 16-9). The larger, macular discolorations of ecchymosis suggest bleeding from larger vessels or focal injury. The red foci do not blanch and are asymptomatic. Skin petechiae and ecchymosis in areas

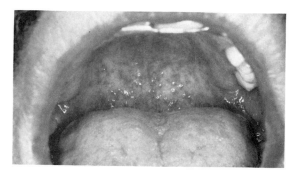

Fig. 16-9 Petechial hemorrhage of the soft palate suggestive of a bleeding tendency.

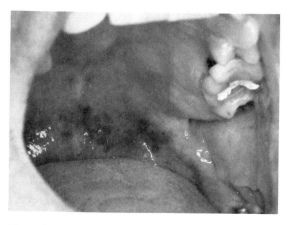

Fig. 16-10 Pressure ecchymosis, caused by fellatio. A 38-year-old woman requested treatment for pain of a maxillary molar. The illustrated symmetric distribution of diffuse, nonblanching red discoloration of the soft palate was an incidental observation. She confided that she frequently engaged in oral sexual activity as a prostitute.

vulnerable to incidental trauma are usually observed in addition to the oral discolorations. The patient history provides evidence of a possible cause and also reveals symptoms of other forms of bleeding, such as epistaxis and hematuria. Anemia is often a concurrent finding.

Differential diagnosis. Distinguishing ruptured vesicles of the soft palate caused by a viral infection from petechial hemorrhage can be difficult in some cases. Pain and tenderness to palpation at the site should direct the differential diagnosis into the ulcerative lesion category. Infectious mononucleosis, for example, commonly causes palatal petechia, but the fever, malaise, and serum tests provide a basis for the differentiation. Ecchymosis caused by most injuries is a larger, macular discoloration and the source of injury is apparent, whereas petechiae indicative of a bleeding disorder are smaller and cannot be as directly related to injury.

Management decisions. The suspicion of an undiagnosed bleeding problem requires referral for medical evaluation. This evaluation usually includes laboratory screening tests such as bleeding time, prothrombin time, and partial thromboplastin time. Dental procedures expected to cause bleeding should be delayed until the diagnosis is clarified. Dental treatment of a patient with a known bleeding problem should be initiated only after consultation with the patient's physician.

Pressure Ecchymosis

Definition. Diffuse ecchymosis of the palate can result from a blunt injury or recurring frictional trauma in patients with normal hemostatic function. This is analogous to the discoloration of "bruised" skin. Oral sexual activity and the negative pressure exerted by an ill-fitting denture retained by excessive reliance on denture adhesive products produce this effect.

Clinical features. The nonblanching discoloration of ecchymosis generally affects a relatively large area that has been subjected to injury. The area of discoloration may be mildly tender and either chronic or acute in onset, depending on the cause. Nonblanching redness of denture-bearing tissues may be associated with poor denture fit and use of a denture adhesive or with wearing the appliance 24 hours a day. Symmetric redness of both the posterior hard and anterior soft palates is the characteristic appearance of bruising produced by fellatio as illustrated in Fig. 16-10. No additional skin or oral discolorations are present, indicating normal hemostatic function. An admission of recent oral sexual activity may be difficult to obtain and must be approached tactfully. The lesion resolves rapidly after the removal of the denture or discontinuation of oral sexual activity.

Differential diagnosis. Identification of the cause is the most essential element in the diagnosis of pressure ecchymosis. Atrophic candidiasis commonly affects the denture-bearing tissues in cases of poor denture hygiene. Superficial fungal infection is more erythematous and patchy in distribution, and white superficial material that rubs off is present. Pressure ecchymosis, atrophic candidiasis, and diffuse inflammation caused by constant shifting of a loose denture are often concurrent processes and the combined effect is often referred to by the nonspecific phrase *denture stomatitis.*

Recently inserted dentures can induce a contact mucositis, particularly if the resin of the denture base is inadequately cured as may occur with some chairside reline materials. The onset of the erythema and a burning sensation shortly after the placement of a new denture or a relined denture is the most reliable indication of contact mucositis to the denture acrylic. Wearing an ill-fitting denture for years can cause a condition known as *inflammatory papillary hyperplasia* of the palate and *inflammatory fibrous hyperplasia* of the alveolar mucosa. These conditions are distinguished by soft tissue mobility and enlargement.

Management decisions. Ecchymosis and erythema of the denture-bearing tissues indicates the need to improve the adaptation either by remaking or relining the denture. Patients frequently resist this suggestion if the condition is asymptomatic. To minimize progression to inflammatory papillary hyperplasia, inflammatory fibrous hyperplasia, and atrophy of the alveolar bone, it is important to improve denture adaptation.

Topical treatment of candidiasis has previ-ously been described. Both the fungal colonization of the denture itself and the associated oral tissues must be treated to eliminate the infection. The ecchymosis associated with fellatio requires no particular treatment. However, when seen in association with pharyngitis or oral ulcerations, the possibility of an oral venereal infection must also be considered.

Benign Migratory Glossitis

Definition. Benign migratory glossitis, also called *geographic tongue,* produces relatively characteristic patchy atrophy of lingual papillae. The condition is common and of unknown pathogenesis. The process is chronic, asymptomatic, and results in no adverse effects, although the lesions can appear dramatically abnormal when initially identified. With the recent appreciation that other areas of the oral mucosa can be similarly affected, the terms *benign migratory stomatitis* and *geographic stomatitis* have been used to indicate lesions of oral sites other than the tongue.

Clinical features. Benign migratory glossitis is characterized by multiple reddish-pink, smooth patches of the dorsum of the tongue. These smooth areas result from atrophy or loss of the papilla. Fig. 16-11 illustrates the dull white, annular band often present at the periphery of the atrophic areas. Adjacent areas of the tongue appear normal in all respects. The condition is typically asymptomatic with no hemorrhagic tendency. The lesion configuration appears to change during an observation period of weeks or months. Fissured tongues often demonstrate lesions of benign migratory glossitis within the fissures. Similar atrophic lesions may affect other oral surfaces of some patients.

Differential diagnosis. Any indication of ulceration or discomfort should redirect the differential diagnosis into the ulcerative lesion category. Atrophic glossitis caused by vitamin B deficiency, anemia, dietary zinc deficiency, and candidiasis may appear similar to benign migratory glossitis, but the lesions of atrophic

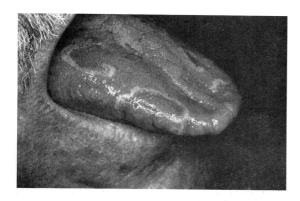

Fig. 16-11 Benign migratory glossitis. These atrophic red patches of the tongue were nonpainful, and the patient reported that the unusual appearance affected different areas of the tongue but were always present. The pale, bandlike borders of the atrophic lesions are particularly prominent in this example.

glossitis are nearly always tender, painful, or burning. In addition, evidence of diminished host resistance to fungal infection or gastrointestinal abnormality can generally be identified. Median rhomboid glossitis may also appear similar, but this condition is confined to a single midline location.

Management decisions. No treatment or additional evaluation is indicated. The patient should be advised of the benign nature of the condition.

Kaposi's Sarcoma

Definition. Kaposi's sarcoma is a malignant neoplasm of vascular origin that is characterized by multiple lesions affecting the skin, oral mucosa, and other sites. Most cases of Kaposi's sarcoma develop during the later stages of AIDS as an apparent consequence of ineffective suppression of the neoplastic process by the patient's compromised immune system. This malignancy must be included in the differential diagnosis of dark mucosal lesions without enlargement because the early lesions of Kaposi's sarcoma often appear flat.

Clinical features. Smaller lesions of Kaposi's sarcoma appear bluish or reddish-blue in color without enlargement or alteration of the superficial mucosal or skin surface texture. The discoloration is nonpainful, nonblanching, and is often homogeneous with relatively well delineated borders. The most frequently affected intraoral sites are the palate and gingiva, although other surfaces may also be affected. The facial skin is a frequent site of extraoral lesions. Larger, advanced lesions (see Fig. 15-13) appear darker red in color, manifest nodular enlargement, may cause ulceration, and are firm to palpation. Additional clinical indications of AIDS include hairy leukoplakia, oral candidiasis, progressive periodontitis, other opportunistic infections, weight loss, and exposure to the HIV virus.

Differential diagnosis. The combination of the various oral, extraoral, and historical findings typically identified among AIDS patients usually presents little diagnostic difficulty. The early lesions of Kaposi's sarcoma may resemble multiple sites of ecchymosis, but evidence of direct injury, a bleeding diathesis, and other findings typical of multifocal ecchymosis are lacking. Also, the discoloration of ecchymosis resolves within a week, in contrast to the progression of Kaposi's lesions. Kaposi's sarcoma can affect HIV-seronegative patients, although the occurrence is rare.

Management decisions. Medical referral for definitive diagnosis and management of the suspected AIDS patient is necessary. Palliative control of Kaposi's sarcoma enlargements is accomplished by radiotherapy. Treatment of other oral manifestations of AIDS should be approached in consultation with the patient's primary care physician.

Atrophic Glossitis

Definition. Atrophic glossitis is generalized or multifocal erythematous atrophy of the lingual papilla caused by vitamin B deficiency, some forms of anemia, gastrointestinal malabsorption conditions, or chronic debilitation of

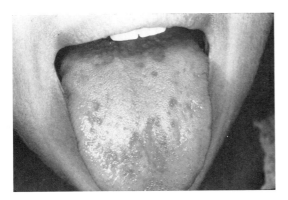

Fig. 16-12 Atrophic glossitis resulting from malabsorption. This 35-year-old woman reported that severe pain and burning from these red tongue lesions and similar areas of the soft palate had interfered with eating and sleeping for 3 months. During that time she reported a 20 pound weight loss, epigastric pain diagnosed as a stress induced ulcer, and episodic bouts of diarrhea. Endoscopic biopsy revealed giardiasis, a protozoan infection of the upper gastrointestinal tract.

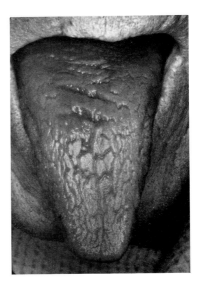

Fig. 16-13 Atrophic glossitis resulting from malnutrition. This smooth, erythematous appearance has been described as "beefy tongue." The patient was a 63-year-old man with alcoholism who appeared older than the stated age and cachectic. He reported that he had not eaten regularly since losing his job 4 months previously.

the patient. The oral lesions rapidly improve if the underlying illness can be effectively treated.

Clinical features. The dorsum of the tongue appears diffusely erythematous with patchy or generalized atrophy of the filiform and fungiform papillae (Figs. 16-12 and 16-13). The generalized atrophy has been described as "balding" or a "beefy red" tongue. Affected patients usually describe pain or a burning sensation that can be so severe as to interfere with eating. Anemia, a deficient diet, or abnormality of gastrointestinal absorption may be suggested by historical and examination findings such as unexplained weight loss, lethargy, facial pallor, pallor of the nails, epigastric pain, or lower gastrointestinal symptoms. Laboratory findings may demonstrate anemia or a hemostasis deficiency.

Differential diagnosis. A similar balding of the tongue may be present in the latter stages of scarlet fever, but the characteristic skin rash, fever, and rapid onset demonstrate

the acute nature of this infection. Chemotherapy and radiotherapy induce similar tongue lesions, but the cause of the mucosal atrophy in these cases is obvious. Evidence of multifocal tongue ulceration in addition to ulcers of other mucosal surfaces should direct the differential diagnosis into the ulcerative disease category. The atrophic tongue lesions of geographic tongue appear similar but are usually painless in contrast to the discomfort reported with atrophic glossitis. Atrophic candidiasis of the tongue can also cause papillary atrophy of the tongue, but the pattern is usually more patchy and at least a few focal white areas that rub off are present.

Management decisions. Blood studies including a complete blood count, hemoglobin concentration, hemoglobin indices, and serum levels of B vitamins are methods of determining anemia and nutritional deficiency. Specific test for dietary zinc deficiency, pernicious anemia, and low serum iron are also available. Evaluation and treatment are usually most effectively arranged by medical referral. Atrophic candidiasis often coexists with atrophic glossitis since vitamin deficiency may predispose the patient to opportunistic infection. Mycotic culture or exfoliative cytology may be required to make a definitive diagnosis.

Scarlet Fever

Definition. Scarlet fever, also known as *scarlatina,* is a communicable, seasonal bacterial infection that typically affects children. The most serious complications of the disease are progression to rheumatic fever and acute glomerulonephritis.

Clinical features. The characteristic oral finding in the early stage of the scarlet fever is the "strawberry tongue." This "spotty" appearance is produced by erythema and edema of the scattered fungiform papilla while the filiform papilla background appears relatively normal. A whitish pseudomembranous coating of the tongue may develop, and it is often sloughed in the latter stages of the disease, yielding a generalized smooth, erythematous appearance of the dorsal surface. Concurrent pharyngitis and tonsillitis are manifested by pain and bright red erythema of the oropharynx. Severe infection can also produce suppurative bacterial tonsillitis. Skin rash, fever, malaise, cephalgia, and lymphadenopathy are the systemic signs and symptoms of scarlet fever. The infection lasts approximately 4 to 7 days.

Differential diagnosis. β-Hemolytic streptococcal pharyngitis, colloquially known as *"strep throat,"* does not typically produce a skin rash and the pharyngitis is usually more painful. Also, a history of contact with another strep throat sufferer can often be identified. Viral infection or erythema multiforme can be excluded on the basis of a throat culture to demonstrate β-hemolytic streptococci, and the strawberry tongue appearance is unusual with viral infections. The acute onset, fever, skin rash, and pharyngitis allow exclusion of more

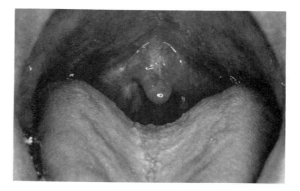

Fig. 16-14   Streptococcal pharyngitis.

chronic conditions such as vitamin deficiency or anemia.

Management decisions. Medical referral is indicated for definitive diagnosis and treatment. Antibiotic therapy is usually prescribed to minimize the possibility of complications such as rheumatic fever or disseminated infection. Supportive treatment includes analgesics, fluids, and bed rest.

Pharyngitis

Definition. Pharyngitis can be caused by a number of organisms and is commonly observed by the dentist. The diagnostic limitation with pharyngitis is that most forms of pharyngeal infection have more features in common than distinguishing characteristics. The clinician can usually offer little more than the nonspecific clinical designation of pharyngitis until microbial laboratory studies demonstrate the responsible organism. Therefore throat cultures are usually required to making a specific diagnosis. Scarlet fever is an exception in this regard because the skin rash and tongue changes aid the diagnosis.

Clinical features. Diffuse erythema of the tonsillar pillars and the posterior pharyngeal wall are the primary manifestations of pharyngitis (Fig. 16-14). The patient's awareness of pain during swallowing allows determination of the condition's duration, which is a contributory diagnostic feature. Fever, malaise, headache, and regional lymphadenopathy are frequent concurrent signs and symptoms, although mild forms of pharyngitis without these findings are also common. A history of infectious contact may suggest the specific infection. The most common examples are β-hemolytic streptococcal pharyngitis, infectious mononucleosis, and several forms of venereal pharyngitis.

Differential diagnosis. Purulent exudate, rapidly progressive swelling, fiery erythema of the oropharynx, and high fever are features of bacterial infections. Streptococcal pharyngitis should be considered the most probable diagnosis with these features based on frequency of occurrence and communicability of the organism. Scarlet fever is indicated by erythematous skin rash and tongue changes affecting a child. Development of multiple joint pain (polyarthritis) indicates rheumatic fever. A pseudomembranous coating of the throat is typical of diphtheria and infectious mononucleosis. Intact vesicles or multiple, herpetiform ulcerations and less severe fever suggest a viral infection. Herpangina, primary herpetic stomatitis, and infectious mononucleosis are the most common conditions and are discussed in Chapter 17.

Relatively mild, localized symptoms and a history of oral sexual activity may suggest a venereal pharyngitis, particularly if multiple partners or infected partners are involved. Gonococcal, trichomonal, chlamydial, and candidal organisms can all cause a mild, clinically nonspecific pharyngitis. More characteristic venereal diseases such as syphilis and primary herpes simplex infection present with their typical disease features in addition to pharyngitis.

Chronic exposure to sources of irritation can also produce oropharyngeal erythema and a mild sore throat. Smoking, nasal drainage, and mouth breathing are common sources of chronic pharyngeal erythema.

Management decisions. The most astute and experienced clinicians incorrectly identify the organism responsible for pharyngitis more than 25% of the time on the basis of clinical findings alone. *It is, therefore, essential to rely on throat cultures for the definitive diagnosis of pharyngitis.* This usually requires referral of patients to their primary care physician. Empiric antibiotic treatment of pharyngitis risks ineffective treatment and alters subsequent microbial culture results and antibiotic sensitivity tests. Treatment by the dentist can also be complicated by the difficulty in evaluating the extent and severity of possible complications such as otitis media. Referral to the patient's physician is the most prudent course.

Atrophic Candidiasis

Definition. Atrophic candidiasis is one clinical presentation of the oral fungal infection caused principally by *Candida albicans.* The frequent oral presence of the organism and the role of diminished host resistance in the development of infection have been discussed in Chapter 15. Whether oral candidiasis assumes the hyperplastic, atrophic, or pseudomembranous clinical form depends on differences in oral environmental factors among individuals and the condition causing diminished resistance to the infection.

Clinical features. Atrophic candidiasis produces multiple, vaguely-delineated, and erythematous mucosal lesions with a thinned but not ulcerated appearance. The patient usually describes vague pain or a burning sensation. If the discomfort is not spontaneous, pain can be elicited by mild abrasive pressure with a cotton gauze. The patchy distribution usually involves the tongue and tissues underlying an appliance, but any oral surface can be infected. Careful examination frequently reveals a few white, thickened foci (Fig. 16-15) that rub off leaving a painful surface, as well as other evidence of candidiasis such as angular cheilitis.

Features suggesting diminished host resistance are often identified. Examples include recent antibiotic therapy, systemic steroid medi-

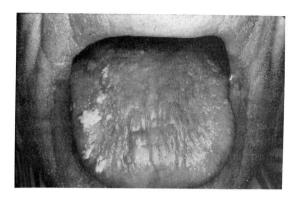

Fig. 16-15   Atrophic candidiasis. The patient reported burning pain and difficulty eating associated with the smooth, atrophic, and erythematous dorsal tongue surface. The white, gelatinous material near the lateral border was readily wiped away with a cotton gauze.

cation, immune system deficiency, xerostomia, anemia, diabetes, and poor oral hygiene. One of the more common sites to identify atrophic candidiasis is on the denture-bearing mucosa supporting a maxillary denture that the patient wears 24 hours a day. Women with intraoral candidiasis may also report symptoms of vaginal candidiasis.

Differential diagnosis. Atrophic candidiasis lesions can appear similar to those caused by nutritional deficiencies and oral allergic responses. Identification of a condition causing diminished host resistance is a reliable differential diagnostic feature of atrophic candidiasis in most cases. Occasionally, the patient will suffer from candidiasis superimposed on the atrophic mucosa caused by anemia or vitamin deficiency. In such cases ineffective treatment often suggests that one of the conditions has been controlled while the other has not. Atrophic candidiasis produces patient complaints similar to those of burning mouth syndrome. However, mucosal lesions are usually associated with a yeast infection in contrast to the normal mucosal appearance of burning mouth syndrome.

Management decisions. Culture or exfoliative cytology is usually necessary for diagnostic confirmation if candidiasis is suspected. Referral for blood studies and other tests may be indicated to identify a suspected diminished host resistance condition. Treatment of the candidiasis with topical antifungal agents in the form of a rinse is usually effective. Antimycotic treatment of a removable appliance worn by the patient is also necessary to eliminate this as a source of recurring infection. Systemic antimycotic therapy with agents such as fluconazole may be required for cases not controlled by topical treatment alone.

From the perspective of the patient's general health, identification of a condition causing diminished host resistance to the infection may be more important than controlling the oral yeast infection. Also, eliminating the underlying condition achieves more sustained control of the candidiasis in most instances than the reliance on topical antifungal therapy alone. In other situations, such as with chronic corticosteroid therapy, this is not possible and the only treatment course is to attempt to control this opportunistic infection with antimycotic agents.

Contact Mucositis

Definition. A variety of foreign substances can stimulate an allergic hypersensitivity response referred to as contact mucositis, which is analogous to contact dermatitis. Examples of frequently identified allergenic stimulants include metallic nickel, the flavoring agent cinnamic aldehyde, and the preservative benzoic acid.

Clinical features. Mucosal erythema and mild burning discomfort are the predominant features of a contact hypersensitivity. A "velvety" or finely granular surface texture of the erythematous areas has been described as relatively characteristic of mucosal contact hypersensitivity. Desquamation of the superficial epithelium and more severe pain may develop in severe cases. The lesion distribution depends on the mucosal surfaces exposed to the material. Hypersensitivity to nickel contained in the alloy of a fixed restoration, for example, causes erythema of the gingiva within 1 cm of the restoration. Contact mucositis to cinnamic aldehyde in a "tartar control" toothpaste assumes a more generalized distribution affecting the gingival and alveolar mucosa. The response is usually noted within hours or days of the exposure and the lesions resolve within a few days of discontinued use of the material.

Individuals prone to allergic diseases in general are more likely to develop oral contact mucositis. Therefore the patient reporting a history of hay fever, penicillin allergy, or frequent episodes of contact dermatitis is more likely to develop oral manifestations or similar reactions to other substances. This allergenic tendency may be suggested by additional manifestations such as a macular skin rash or nasal congestion.

Differential diagnosis. A hypersensitivity response should be suspected when diffuse or multifocal erythema develops shortly after initial exposure to a foreign substance. Resolution of the lesions following removal of the suspected cause is an adequate basis for a definitive diagnosis in most cases. This can be confirmed by patch testing the skin or by intentionally reexposing the patient to the suspected material. Ulceration caused by contact mucositis is unusual and its presence should redirect the differential diagnosis into the ulcerative lesion category.

Patients frequently report the suspicion of a contact allergy to a new restoration when in most cases they are experiencing inflammation caused by injury during the procedure, trapping of plaque by poorly adapted margins, or nonallergic tissue irritation of composite materials. Resolution of the erythema following adequate healing time, improvement of margins, improved hygiene, or replacement of a composite with a more tissue compatible material demonstrates the nonallergic nature of the inflammation.

The search for the specific allergenic stimulant can be frustrating. Cinnamon flavoring agents in "tartar-control" dentifrices, mouth rinses, and chewing gum are commonly implicated in contact mucositis reactions. Hypersensitivity to metallic nickel in restorative alloys is also relatively common and is suggested by an erythematous, pruritic skin reaction to contact with jewelry. Denture resins occasionally cause contact mucositis, but in most suspected cases the inflammation associated with the denture is atrophic candidiasis, irritation caused by poor adaptation, or a combination of the two.

Management decisions. The primary clinical goals are identification of the causative material and discontinuation of the patient's exposure to it. Patch testing of the skin for contact hypersensitivity reaction to specific materials in consultation with a dermatologist or allergist is often helpful. Incisional biopsy results of erythematous lesions often suggest an allergic response by demonstration of a large proportion of plasma cells in the inflammatory infiltrate. However, microscopic examination will not reveal the specific allergenic stimulant. Testing for anemia, nutritional deficiency, and atrophic candidiasis may be indicated in some cases since contact hypersensitivity can become a diagnosis of exclusion.

ISOLATED PIGMENTED LESIONS

Isolated dark lesions of the oral mucosa typically contain abnormal concentrations of melanin. One exception is the first item in the discussion, the tattoo, which contains pigmented foreign material. The primary intent in the clinical evaluation of isolated pigmented lesions is to rule out the possibility that the lesion is a melanoma. Early diagnosis of an oral melanoma is one of the few positive factors in the effective treatment of this aggressive malignancy. The differential diagnosis strategy for isolated, multifocal, and diffuse pigmented lesions is summarized in Fig. 16-16.

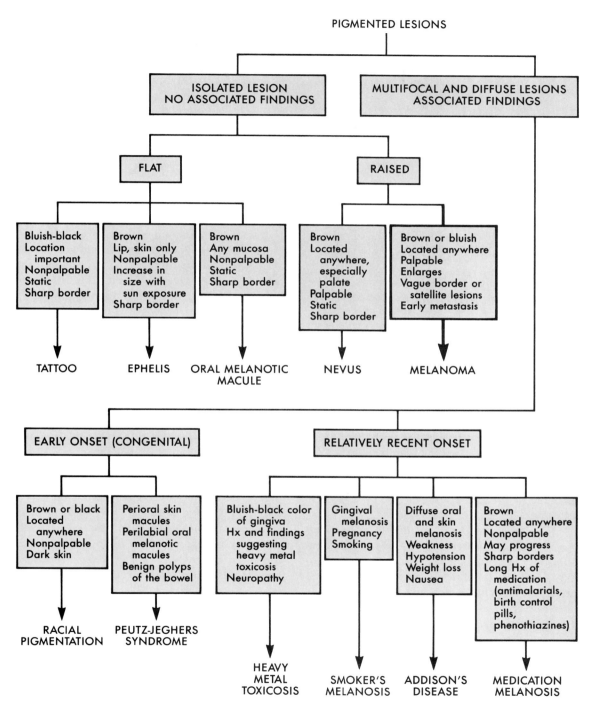

Fig. 16-16 Differential diagnosis of pigmented lesions.

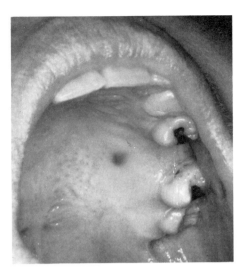

Fig. 16-17 Tattoo. The patient was aware of the round, sharply delineated, and nonblanching blue macule of the palatal alveolar surface. She first noticed the nontender discoloration several months after the tooth was endodontically treated. A metallic foreign body was demonstrated radiographically in the area.

Tattoo

Definition. Tattoo is tissue stained by a pigmented foreign material. The most common foreign material to cause an oral tattoo is dental amalgam, although graphite from pencils and other foreign materials are occasionally implicated.

Clinical features. The mucosal discoloration is well delineated in most cases, nonpalpable, and remains unchanged during an observation period of months or years. The mucosal surface is smooth, intact, and unaffected other than the abnormal homogeneous black or bluish-black color as illustrated in Fig. 16-17. Tattoos are located where impaction of a foreign material is likely. For amalgam this will be the alveolar ridge and occasionally the buccal mucosa adjacent to a buccal restoration. Metallic fragments of amalgam tattoos or other metallic materials can be demonstrated radiographi-

cally at the pigmented site in most cases. Graphite tattoos from puncture injuries by a pencil point usually appear on the hard palate.

Differential diagnosis. Many tattoos appear to enlarge slightly soon after the impaction of the material as the pigment diffuses within the connective tissue. This can give the clinical impression of enlargement and progression, which appropriately raises the suspicion of a melanoma. However, the injury or dental procedure that caused the tattoo should have occurred recently enough that the patient will recall the incident. Also, the tattoo is nonpalpable in contrast to the raised, palpable character of most melanomas. The black or bluish-black color of tattoos is unlikely to be confused with the brown color of isolated pigmented lesions containing melanin. The blue nevus is an exception, but that lesion rarely occurs in the oral cavity. The varix is somewhat similar in color, but the varix is usually round and blanches whereas the tattoo does not blanch and is less regular in shape.

Management decisions. No treatment is indicated if a definitive diagnosis can be made. Suspicion of melanoma based on enlargement, vague margins, or focal ulceration warrants excision and histopathologic examination.

Ephelis

Definition. The aggregation of melanin pigmentation known formally as an ephelis is commonly called a *freckle*. This focal melanosis becomes pronounced in response to sunlight exposure and is, therefore, not seen in the mouth. Ephelides are occasionally identified on the exposed lip surface.

Clinical features. The pigmentation is a small, focal homogeneous brown macule with sharp borders. Ephelides are nonpalpable and are located on the skin and the exposed lip mucosa. Freckles of the lip surfaces are much more likely if the person has numerous skin ephelides. The size and prominence of pigmentation increases with sun exposure and pales during the winter months.

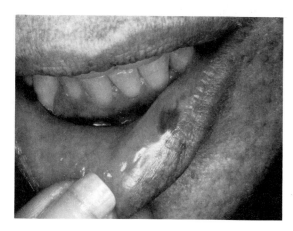

Fig. 16-18 Oral melanotic macule. This 38-year-old woman reported that the flat, sharply delineated brown macule located on the intraoral mucosal surface of the lower lip had been present since childhood.

Differential diagnosis. The ephelis is characteristic in appearance and is unlikely to be confused with other lesions.

Management decisions. No treatment or clinical reevaluation period is necessary.

Oral Melanotic Macule

Definition. The oral melanotic macule is a pigmented lesion of the mouth with the appearance of a large ephelis. This similarity in appearance does not imply that the two lesions are identical because oral melanotic macules, in contrast to ephelides, are unrelated to sunlight stimulation. Individuals with fair skin and numerous "freckles" are, however, more likely to exhibit an oral melanotic macule.

Clinical features. These lesions are a homogeneous brown color with sharply delineated borders (Fig. 16-18). They are typically ovoid in shape and less than 1 cm in diameter. Oral melanotic macules are nonpalpable and do not significantly enlarge with time.

Differential diagnosis. Ephelis is the correct term for these macular pigmentations on sun-exposed surfaces, while an intraoral loca-

tion is correctly referred to as an oral melanotic macule. The raised appearance of nevi serves to distinguish them from the nonpalpable oral melanotic macules. Occasionally, there may be difficulty in determining if a small lesion is palpable. Palpability, vague borders, and heterogeneous variation in pigmentation of melanomas are the most helpful features in differentiating them from oral melanotic macules. Color, history of injury, and radiographic findings are usually adequate to exclude tattoo from the diagnostic consideration of lesions with the features of an oral melanotic macule.

Management decisions. No treatment or period of clinical observation is indicated if the definitive diagnosis can be made on the basis of clinical features. As with other focal pigmented lesions, any suspicion that the lesion may be palpable or increasing in size justifies excision and histopathologic examination to achieve a definitive diagnosis.

Nevus

Definition. A melanocytic nevus is a developmental aggregation of melanocytes commonly referred to as a "mole." The average person has more than 30 nevi of the skin and occasionally a nevus may develop in the mouth.

Clinical features. The pigmentation is isolated and appears round or ovoid in shape with sharply delineated borders (Fig. 16-19). Homogeneous brown color is typical, although the rare intraoral *blue nevus* is an exception. Nevi are also palpable and appear slightly raised. A nevus has been present since infancy, although the patient may not be aware of it because it is asymptomatic. A patient who reports recent development of a nevus may have just become aware of the pigmentation, but it should still be viewed with suspicion.

Differential diagnosis. Identification of the homogeneous brown color and palpability of a nevus usually distinguishes it from other focal pigmentations of the oral cavity. The only other palpable isolated pigmentation is the

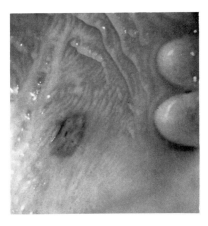

Fig. 16-19 Blue nevus. The 37-year-old man was aware of this palatal discoloration but was unsure of the duration. The ovoid, blue lesion of the hard palate was flat and nontender, and it exhibited variation in the darkness of pigmentation with gradual fading of the peripheral borders. This rare type of nevus is characteristically flat in contrast to most nevi.

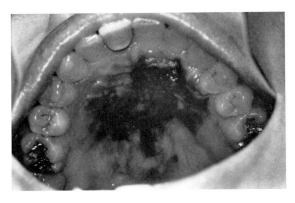

Fig. 16-20 Melanoma. This diffuse, nonblanching dark lesion of the anterior hard palate is characterized by vague peripheral borders, thickening in areas, and separate or satellite lesions. (Courtesy Dr John M Wright, Baylor College of Dentistry, Dallas, Texas.)

melanoma, which should be suspected when heterogeneous pigmentation, vague borders, and evidence of enlargement are observed. A blue nevus can appear similar to a tattoo or varix. The designation of nevi by types such as compound nevi and junctional nevi is based on the cellular arrangement of the melanocytes. Therefore this diagnostic distinction must be made by histopathologic features rather than clinically.

Management decisions. The constant frictional stimulation of the oral environment is believed to promote the transformation of junctional nevus cells into a melanoma. Even though this may be an unlikely event, the threateningly poor prognosis of melanoma and the inability to clinically identify which nevi are the junctional type provides justification for excision and histopathologic examination of *all* palpable intraoral pigmented lesions.

Melanoma

Definition. Melanoma is malignant neoplasia of melanocytic origin, and it is the primary diagnostic concern in the differential diagnosis of isolated oral pigmentations. All other focal oral pigmentations are benign abnormalities that are clinically inconsequential except that they might be a melanoma. The prognosis of melanomas is poor unless total excision is accomplished while the lesion is small and superficial. The phrase "malignant melanoma" is often used for this neoplasm to emphasize the threatening nature of the lesion, but addition of the word "malignant" is considered redundant. Melanomas commonly occur on sun-exposed skin, while oral melanomas are rare.

Clinical features. Melanomas may appear brown, bluish, or pale and may be located anywhere in the mouth, although the palate is the most frequently affected region (Fig. 16-20). Features suggesting malignancy include rapidly progressive growth, heterogeneous pigmentation, poorly delineated peripheral borders, and the presence of separate discolorations called *satellite lesions* adjacent to the primary enlargement. Foci of ulceration may also be present. The lesion is palpable except in the early, superficial-spreading phase of enlargement. Palpation of the regional lymph nodes may reveal metastatic enlargement.

Differential diagnosis. The clinical suspicion of melanoma is based on identification of an isolated pigmented lesion exhibiting one or more features of malignant growth noted above. Nevi are the only other palpable isolated oral pigmented lesions and they are generally homogeneous in color with sharply delineated borders and no evidence of progressive enlargement. The same features suggesting suspicious growth listed above apply to melanomas located on sun-exposed skin.

Management decisions. Excision and histopathologic examination of palpable, isolated intraoral pigmented lesions is mandatory. An observation period of a few weeks may confirm the clinical suspicion of melanoma by demonstrating enlargement, but this is not justified in most cases because the delay in definitive treatment can adversely affect the prognosis. A pathologic diagnosis of melanoma warrants immediate referral to a tertiary oncology care center for staging and definitive treatment.

DIFFUSE AND MULTIFOCAL PIGMENTED LESIONS

The occurrence of diffuse and multifocal pigmentations implies a generalized or systemic causative mechanism as contrasted with the pathogenesis of isolated pigmentations. Certain developmental syndromes, metabolic conditions, and medications can produce this effect. One approach to categorizing diffuse or multiple oral pigmentations relies on whether the abnormal color has been present since birth or is a recent development. Identification of additional clinical features (Fig. 16-16) provides further direction to the differential diagnosis. The primary clinical importance of multiple and diffuse pigmented lesions is the clinical implication of the underlying condition rather than the superficial pigmentation.

Racial Pigmentation

Definition. Individuals of racial groups characterized by dark skin often exhibit pigmentation of the oral mucosa. This should be considered as a variation of healthy tissue appearance rather than as an abnormality.

Clinical features. Racial pigmentation of the oral mucosa is brown to black in color, diffuse, and nonpalpable. The most conspicuous intraoral areas of racial pigmentation are near the mucogingival border and the hard palate. The mucogingival pigmentation may appear to blend into the normal pink or red color of the alveolar mucosa or it may be sharply delineated. The pigmentation is symmetric, has been present since infancy, and remains unchanged.

Differential diagnosis. The intraoral appearance of racial pigmentation can be similar to other pigmentations of the oral mucosa, but symmetry and the patient's dark skin strongly supports the diagnosis. Distinguishing racial pigmentation of these patients from mucosal melanosis caused by Addison's disease or medications can be difficult. Review of the history, physical findings, and evidence of changes in oral pigmentation support the suspicion of these conditions.

Management decisions. No treatment or reevaluation period is indicated.

Peutz-Jeghers Syndrome

Definition. Perilabial melanotic macules and perioral ephelides are features of Peutz-Jeghers syndrome that are likely to be observed by the dentist. The additional developmental abnormality of this rare syndrome is polyposis of the large bowel. Additional aspects of this condition are discussed in Chapter 20.

Clinical features. Excessive pigmentation consists of multiple ephelides of the perioral skin and multiple, perilabial intraoral melanotic macules. The pigmentation is first noted in childhood. The skin pigmentations tend to increase in size and darkness with sun exposure. Multiple polyps of the small bowel eventually develop. Familial occurrence of this autosomal dominantly inherited condition is typical. These polyps are considered to have significant potential for malignant transformation, but this development is less frequent than the consistent malignant transformation of the intestinal polyps in Gardner syndrome. Clinical manifestations of the polyposis include gastrointestinal bleeding, anemia, abdominal cramps, and recurring diarrhea.

Differential diagnosis. Many healthy patients have freckles and many patients eventually develop benign polyps of the bowel. The individual with Peutz-Jeghers syndrome exhibits exceptionally prominent perioral pigmentation and the intestinal polyps are more numerous and appear at an earlier age than the common intestinal polyp. No other condition is likely to be confused with Peutz-Jeghers syndrome.

Management decisions. Treatment of the perioral pigmented lesions is not indicated. Referral is indicated to establish periodic evaluation of the intestinal polyps and for the management of any gastrointestinal symptoms, which are variable.

Heavy Metal Toxicosis

Definition. Heavy metal toxicosis caused by ingestion or inhalation of materials containing lead, bismuth, or other heavy metals produces a pathognomonic pigmentation of the gingiva. Gingival inflammation appears to play a role in the degree of tissue pigmentation because the discoloration is minimal in the absence of inflammation even with significant tissue concentration of the heavy metal. The systemic toxicity suggested by the oral pigmentation is the primary clinical issue rather than the oral lesions.

Clinical features. Linear gray to black discoloration is noted either along the cervical margin of the gingiva or near the mucogingival junction (Fig. 16-21). The degree of the pigmentation is proportional to the heavy metal concentration, duration of the intoxication, and the severity of gingival inflammation. The patient history often reveals a source of heavy metal intake. This may be occupational exposure to vapors or particulate material. Children

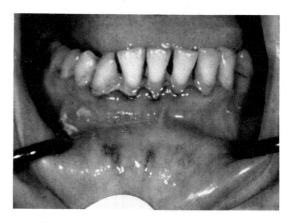

Fig. 16-21 Heavy metal toxicosis, bismuth. The linear band of bluish-black pigmentation follows the contour of the marginal gingival and gingival inflammation is indicated by the edematous appearance and the obvious plaque accumulation. Pigmentation of the mucosal lip surface is also present. (Courtesy Dr Lester W Burket.)

with *pica,* an unusual behavioral compulsion to eat inedible materials, may exhibit this gingival pigmentation after ingesting lead-based paint chips. Symptoms of neurologic and gastrointestinal dysfunction develop with advanced heavy metal intoxication.

Differential diagnosis. The presence of intraoral pigmentation is an advanced finding of this condition and a rare clinical observation. Neurologic signs of heavy metal toxicity usually prompt medical evaluation long before oral pigmentation develops. Diffuse or multifocal oral pigmentation caused by Addison's disease and certain drugs produce macular lesions rather than the linear pattern of the gingiva caused by heavy metal toxicity. Racial pigmentation is usually a broader band of pigmentation. Smoker's melanosis resulting from smoking is more diffuse, and the patient history allows clinical distinction.

Management decisions. Referral for medical evaluation is important if the condition is suspected. Neurologic examination and laboratory testing for serum concentrations of heavy metals are diagnostic of the intoxication.

Addison's Disease

Definition. Addison's disease, also called *primary adrenal cortical insufficiency,* produces multifocal pigmentation in addition to the systemic effects of cortisol deficiency described in Chapter 7. Low serum cortisol concentration stimulates pituitary production of ACTH in response to the cortisol insufficiency and, for unknown reasons, excessive pituitary production of melanocyte stimulating hormone (MSH) also occurs. Visible increases in skin and mucous membrane pigmentation are the pathophysiologic consequence of the excessive MSH production.

Clinical features. Multiple brown macular lesions are present on the skin and occasionally on the oral mucosa. There is also a generalized, diffuse increase in skin pigmentation. Systemic features of adrenal insufficiency include weakness, weight loss, nausea, vomiting, and hypotension. History may reveal a recent serious infection or autoimmune condition to explain adrenal degeneration although the condition is often idiopathic.

Differential diagnosis. The combination of hyperpigmentation and features of cortisol deficiency are characteristic of Addison's disease. Definitive diagnosis is based on serum electrolyte imbalance and hormonal studies. Patients taking medications known to cause hyperpigmentation and who are also suspected of having Addison's disease can present a diagnostic problem. Serum studies generally provide a definitive diagnosis.

Management decisions. Referral for definitive diagnosis and management is indicated. The oral pigmented lesions are of no particular significance other than as evidence of the endocrine deficiency.

Smoker's Melanosis

Definition. Smoker's melanosis is multifocal pigmentation of oral tissues caused by exposure to tobacco smoke. This condition is apparently potentiated by elevated serum hormone concentrations.

Clinical features. Vague brown pigmentation affects areas exposed to high concentrations of tobacco smoke such as the labial gingiva, hard palate, and lips. The borders of the hyperpigmentation are vague. Female smokers with elevated serum estrogen and progesterone concentrations resulting from pregnancy or high-dose birth control pills are most frequently affected. The more commonly prescribed low-dose birth control pills are less likely to cause excessive pigmentation. Males who smoke heavily are occasionally affected. The pigmentation typically disappears with the removal of one or both of the contributing factors.

Differential diagnosis. The combination of smoking, a condition suggesting hormonal imbalance, and hyperpigmentation is diagnostic of the condition. This can be easy mistaken for racial pigmentation if the patient is dark-skinned. Other forms of adult-onset oral pigmentation are generally focal or macular. Disappearance of the melanosis at the end of pregnancy or after smoking is discontinued is convincing evidence of the cause. This melanotic pigmentation of the tissues should not be mistaken for simple staining of the tissues by the tobacco tars, which fade when wiped with a cotton gauze.

Management decisions. No treatment is indicated. The patient should be advised to discontinue smoking, especially in view of the known relationship of smoking with adverse fetal effects.

Medication Melanosis

Definition. Medication melanosis is a well-known side effect of certain medications. The exact mechanism is not apparent, but use of the medication for years is usually required to produce the hyperpigmentation.

Clinical features. Brown, homogeneous, macular lesions with sharply delineated bor-

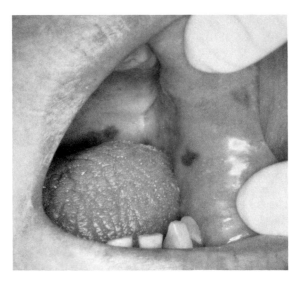

Fig. 16-22 Medication melanosis. This 56-year-old woman reported that the brown discoloration of her mouth had developed within the last 6 months and that her skin had become darker recently. Two nonraised, nontender brown macules were present on the buccal mucosa and a third lesion of the soft palate can be seen beyond the dorsum of the tongue. Medical consultation including laboratory studies revealed no evidence of Addison's disease. The patient had taken thioridazine, a phenothiazide, to manage a nonspecified mental problem for the preceding 14 years.

ders of recent onset are present on the skin and oral mucosa as shown in Fig. 16-22. The lesions may progress during a period of clinical observation. The patient has usually been taking a drug known to produce skin and mucosal pigmentation for several years. Some examples include antimalarials, birth control pills, phenothiazides, cis-platinum, minocycline, and cyclophosphamide. The pigmentation may progress if the medication is continued or regress with discontinuation of the drug.

Differential diagnosis. The medication history clarifies the cause of the pigmentation changes. Addison's disease should also be considered in the differential diagnosis since the

brown macules of the two conditions are indistinguishable. Serum laboratory studies may be required to achieve a definitive diagnosis.

Management decisions. The pigmented lesions require no treatment. The patient should be reassured of the benign nature of the abnormality.

SUMMARY

The differential diagnostic strategy for dark mucosal lesions is based on classification of the lesion by the color and the extent of the abnormal appearance into one of the following groups:

1. Isolated red lesions
2. Multifocal and diffuse red lesions
3. Isolated brown and black pigmentations
4. Multifocal and diffuse pigmentations

The dark appearance of isolated red lesions is produced by increased visibility of blood within the connective tissue. The observation of blanching with pressure indicates that blood is contained within vessels. Absence of blanching suggests the blood is extravasated into the connective tissue or is more visible because the superficial epithelium is thinned. Identification of isolated heterogeneous red lesions known as erythroplakia is the differential diagnostic priority in the assessment of isolated red lesions. A high proportion of nonblanching erythroplakic lesions results from irregular surface thinning caused by premalignant epithelial dysplasia or early squamous cell carcinoma.

Multifocal and diffuse red lesions appear abnormal for the same reasons as isolated red lesions, but the more extensive distribution suggests a generalized process. The differential diagnosis of multifocal and diffuse red lesions based on the presence or absence of blanching, sites affected, and additional clinical features is directed to the identification of the underlying abnormality responsible for the visible lesions.

Isolated pigmented lesions of the oral cavity are caused by pigmented foreign material impacted into the tissue or by focally dense accumulations of melanin. The differential diagnostic priority for isolated pigmented lesions of the oral mucosa is the identification of palpable pigmented lesions that could represent the rare occurrence of an intraoral melanoma.

Multifocal and diffuse pigmentations can be caused by a variety of developmental, metabolic, and hormonal abnormalities. Developmental conditions produce unusual melanin pigmentations shortly after birth, while appearance of multifocal pigmentations later in life suggests an acquired disease. The combination of the age of onset and additional clinical findings is the basis for identifying the underlying condition.

BIBLIOGRAPHY

Bengel W and others: Differential diagnosis of diseases of the oral mucosa, Chicago, 1989, Quintessence.

Buchner A, Hansen LS: Melanotic macule of the oral mucosa: a clinicopathologic study of 105 cases, Oral Surg Oral Med Oral Pathol 48:244-249, 1979.

Buchner A, Hansen LS: Pigmented nevi of the oral mucosa: a clinicopathologic study of 32 new cases and review of 75 cases from the literature. Part I. A clinicopathologic study of 32 new cases, Oral Surg Oral Med Oral Pathol 48:131-142, 1979.

Buchner A, Hansen LS: Pigmented nevi of the oral mucosa: a clinicopathologic study of 32 new cases and review of 75 cases from the literature. Part II. Analysis of 107 cases, Oral Surg Oral Med Oral Pathol 49:55-62, 1980.

Eversole LR: Clinical outline of oral pathology: diagnosis and treatment, ed 2, Philadelphia, 1984, Lea & Febiger.

Langlais RP and others: Oral diagnosis, oral medicine and treatment planning, Philadelphia, 1984, Saunders.

Lynch MA, Brightman VJ, Greenberg MS, editors: Burket's oral medicine: diagnosis and treatment, ed 8, Philadelphia, 1984, Lippincott.

Rapini RP and others: Primary malignant melanoma of the oral cavity, a review of 177 cases, Cancer 55:1543-1551, 1985.

Regezi JA and Sciubba JJ: Oral pathology: clinical-pathologic correlations, Philadelphia, 1989, Saunders.

Shafer WG, Hine MK, Levy BM: A textbook of oral pathology, ed 4, Philadelphia, 1983, Saunders.

Wood NK, Goaz PW: Differential diagnosis of oral lesions, ed 4, St Louis, 1991, Mosby-Year Book.

CHAPTER 17

Differential Diagnosis of Oral Ulcers

STEVEN D. VINCENT
MICHAEL W. FINKELSTEIN

Ulcerative diseases of oral mucosa represent a therapeutic challenge for the dentist because patients are eager for relief from discomfort. Effective treatment relies on an accurate diagnosis, which is often difficult because ulcerative lesions resulting from different conditions can be similar in clinical appearance. Because most oral ulcers are painful, patients can usually provide an accurate history of their discomfort. The history of symptoms is one of the most contributory diagnostic findings. Some important historical features to determine in all cases of oral ulceration are the following:

1. Onset of the lesions as acute or gradual. Ulcers of acute onset form within 1 to 2 days.
2. Duration of the lesions as limited versus protracted. Lesions of limited duration heal within 2 to 4 weeks.
3. Recurrence or progression of the lesions. Recurrent conditions are characterized by lesions that heal completely and by new ulcers appearing at variable intervals. An individual who suffers different ulcerative episodes of the same locations and with comparable healing time is probably affected by a single condition that is recurrent rather than by different conditions. Progressive lesions do not heal but gradually worsen.
4. The presence of vesicles preceding the ulcers suggests a viral infection in most cases, although vesicles can be caused by immune-mediated diseases. Vesicles in the oral cavity may not be noticed because they rapidly rupture to form ulcers. Thus the absence of vesicles does not mean that they were not present. The presence of vesicles excludes aphthous ulcers, ulcers caused by bacteria, infectious mononucleosis, and injury from diagnostic consideration.
5. The presence of skin, eye, or genital lesions suggests certain diseases and excludes others as diagnostic possibilities.
6. The concurrence of oral ulcers and sys-

temic manifestations such as fever, malaise, and lymphadenopathy also allows the clinician to exclude certain diseases.

7. Many medications taken by the patient can cause oral ulcers.

PRIMARY CLINICAL FEATURES AND LESION CLASSIFICATION

Four critical factors to consider in classifying oral vesiculoulcerative diseases are the lesion onset, ulcer duration, presence of vesicles, and presence of systemic manifestations. Oral ulcers can initially be separated into two groups based on onset and duration. Acute or abrupt onset with the healing of the lesions within several weeks usually represents injury, systemic viral infection, or a localized bacterial infection. The lesions that do not heal or heal but then recur can be caused by genetic defects, chronic infections, recurring trauma, autoimmune or immune disorders, and malignant neoplasms. A few ulcerative conditions are idiopathic. The clinical course and suspected cause of ulcerative lesions can be combined to form a differential diagnostic classification as follows:

1. Oral ulcerations with acute onset and short duration
   a. Bacterial infections or injury
   b. Generalized viral infections
2. Oral ulcerations with chronic or recurrent course
   a. Genetic diseases
   b. Recurrent viral and idiopathic diseases
   c. Autoimmune diseases
   d. Granulomatous diseases and malignancy

This differential diagnostic strategy for oral ulcers is illustrated in Fig. 17-1.

In addition, several conditions characterized by mucosal atrophy as indicated by a diffuse erythematous appearance can cause oral ulcers in severely affected patients. This probably results from increased vulnerability of the thinned mucosal epithelium to functional abra-

sion or incidental injury because ulcers are not generally a primary manifestation of these conditions. The most common examples are atrophic candidiasis, atrophic glossitis, and allergic reactions. The differential diagnosis of ulcerative lesions should include these conditions on the basis of the clinical features and associated findings described in Chapter 16. Also, chemotherapy and radiotherapy can produce dramatic oral ulcers, but this is more of a therapeutic challenge, as discussed in Chapter 13, than a diagnostic issue.

ORAL ULCERATIONS OF ACUTE ONSET AND SHORT DURATION

This group of lesions consists of some of the most common ulcers observed by the dentist. The primary diagnostic features for these lesions are the demonstration of a direct cause and the resolution of the lesion following removal of the cause. In most cases the diagnosis is not difficult if the clinician recognizes the acute onset and short duration of the lesion. The comparative diagnostic features of these conditions are illustrated in Fig. 17-2.

Traumatic Ulcer

Definition. Traumatic ulcers result from physical injury and are probably the most common form of oral ulceration. The causative injury is usually evident or can be determined by history and clinical examination. Examples include cheek biting, denture sores, irritation from a rough tooth or restoration, and injury during dental treatment.

Clinical features. The ulcer is usually solitary, covered by a white or tan fibrin clot, and located in an area subject to injury such as the lateral border of the tongue or the buccal mucosa near the occlusal plane. The lesion can be painful, especially soon after the injury. An ulcer caused by recurring trauma may exhibit firmness to palpation with an elevated, rolled border. The ulcer resolves within 1 to 2 weeks after removal of the cause.

Differential diagnosis. Solitary ulcers of

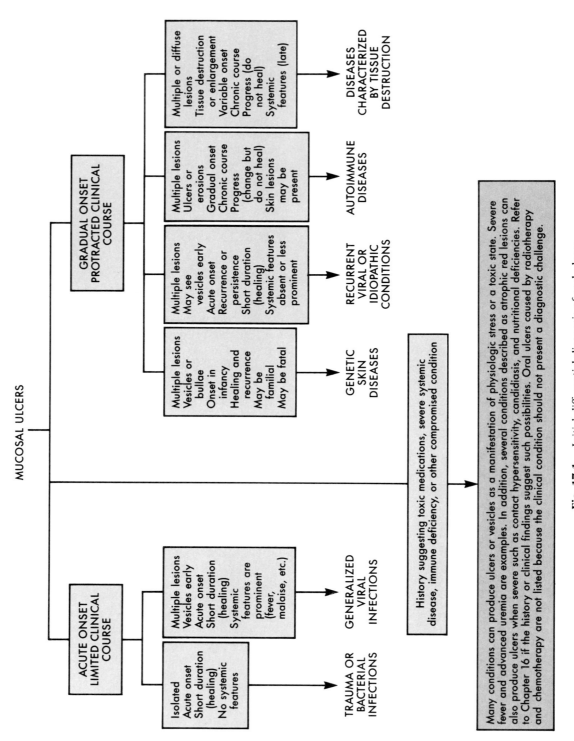

Fig. 17-1   Initial differential diagnosis of oral ulcers.

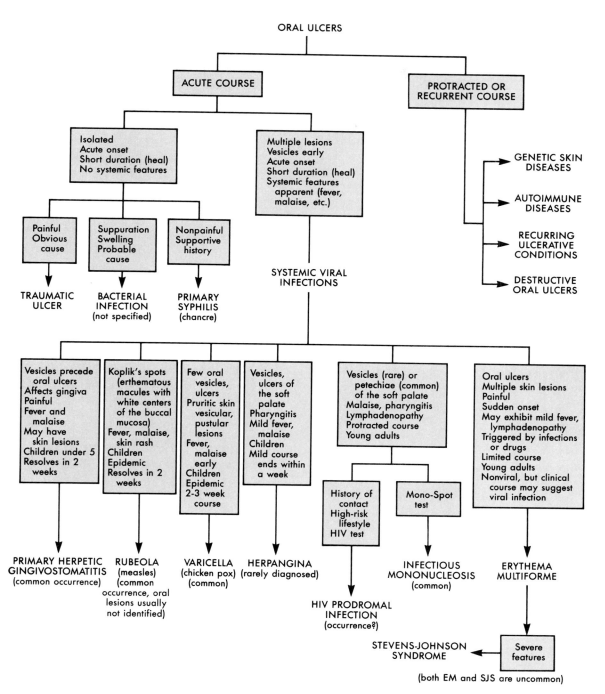

Fig. 17-2 Differential diagnosis of acute oral ulcers.

bacterial origin are typically suppurative. The syphilitic chancre is usually painless, has an indurated border, and is associated with cervical lymphadenopathy. The patient with a syphilitic chancre may relate an infectious contact. A history of a specific traumatic event is helpful in making a diagnosis of traumatic ulcer. However, a history of injury cannot be accepted as absolute proof that the lesion is traumatic because patients often relate ulcers caused by other conditions to incidental injuries. The most definitive diagnostic feature of a traumatic ulcer is rapid resolution of the lesion after removal of the suspected cause.

Management decisions. The patient should be reevaluated in 1 to 2 weeks after removal of the possible cause. Persistence of the ulcer after the suspected cause is eliminated forces the clinician to reevaluate the diagnosis. Biopsy is indicated if a malignant neoplasm remains in the differential diagnosis.

Localized Bacterial Infections

Definition. Periapical and periodontal abscesses cause most oral ulcerations that are related to a localized bacterial infection. A common example is the *pathologic sinus* that forms as an epithelial-lined drainage channel from a periapical or periodontal abscess. A sinus is not a true ulcer, but it is included in this section because it can resemble an ulcer.

Clinical features. The opening of the sinus is associated with underlying edematous enlargement, peripheral erythema, and a white or yellow center (Fig. 17-3). Gentle probing of the apparent ulcer often produces pus and may cause pain. The lesion is usually located in the mucosa overlying the alveolar process, but occasionally it opens on the skin of the lower face or neck.

Differential diagnosis. The release of pus from the lesion indicates the bacterial infection. Radiographic and clinical examination of the teeth in the area usually confirms the diagnosis. Systemic or diffuse bacterial infections rarely cause isolated oral ulcers and are typi-

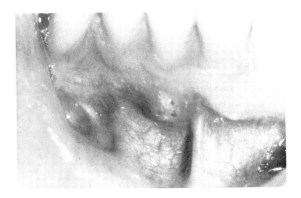

Fig. 17-3 Sinus track. This erythematous, fluctuant, asymptomatic nodule was located near an incisor unresponsive to pulp testing.

cally accompanied by fever, malaise, and lymphadenopathy.

Management. The tooth associated with bacterial infection should be treated periodontally, endodontically, or by extraction to eliminate the infection. If the lesion is well delineated and systemic manifestations are absent, then antibiotic therapy in addition to dental treatment is usually not necessary.

Chancre of Primary Syphilis

Definition. The chancre occurs at the site of inoculation, which is usually the genitalia. The oral mucosa can be the site of primary infection following oral sexual contact with an infected individual.

Clinical features. The chancre is a nonpainful, solitary ulcer that can measure up to 2 cm in diameter. The surrounding tissue is indurated and mildly elevated and has smooth, rolled borders. Painless cervical lymphadenopathy is usually concurrent with the chancre. The ulcer develops several weeks or months after sexual contact with an infected partner and resolves spontaneously 3 to 6 weeks after appearance.

Differential diagnosis. A history of sexual contact with an infected individual supports a diagnosis of chancre. Squamous cell carcinoma can produce an indurated, painless ulcer with elevated borders similar to that of a chancre. However, carcinoma increases in size and is associated with cervical lymphadenopathy only in advanced stages. Chronic traumatic ulcers are usually painful, small, and quickly resolve once the cause is removed. Aphthous ulcers can be large and indurated but are quite painful and heal when treated with corticosteroids. Chronic granulomatous infections can be large and ulcerated, but they are painful and do not spontaneously resolve.

Management decisions. Chancres are literally teeming with spirochetes and are highly infectious. Examination without gloves is associated with risk of infection. The patient should be referred for definitive diagnosis including laboratory tests and treatment. Penicillin is the antibiotic of choice unless the patient is allergic to the drug.

GENERALIZED VIRAL INFECTIONS

Generalized viral infections are characterized by acute onset and systemic manifestations including fever, malaise, tender lymphadenopathy, and lymphocytosis. They can produce multiple oral vesicles that quickly rupture to form painful ulcers. The ulcers heal within several weeks. Generalized viral infections are more common in children, but they can occur in adults who have not been previously exposed to the virus or who have not been vaccinated.

Several exceptions to these generalizations exist. Erythema multiforme is not a viral infection, but it is included in this category because its clinical course and features are similar to those of viral diseases. Infectious mononucleosis does not produce vesicles, and the duration of symptoms is more protracted. Also of clinical significance is the observation that most generalized viral infections produce few symptoms other than vague malaise in some patients or the infection may be completely unapparent to the patient. The only evidence of the infection in these individuals is serologic

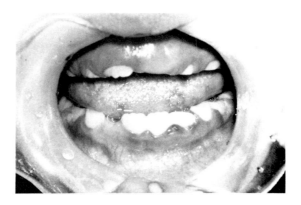

Fig. 17-4 Primary herpetic gingivostomatitis. Malaise, 39° C fever, and decreased appetite of 3 days duration affected this 7-year-old boy. Intraoral examination revealed multiple, nonindurated, well demarcated ulcers on buccal, labial, glossal, gingival, and palatal mucosa.

demonstration of an immunologic response to the organism.

Primary Herpetic Gingivostomatitis

Definition. The initial infection with herpes simplex virus (HSV) can result in primary herpetic gingivostomatitis. Both type 1 and type 2 HSV can infect the oral mucosa, although most cases are believed to represent type 1 HSV infections. Most adults produce antibodies to the virus, which indicates that the infection is common. The infrequent clinical observation of the characteristic features of the generalized infection suggests that most cases are subclinical.

Clinical features. Primary herpetic gingivostomatitis is characterized by the abrupt onset of fever, malaise, and tender lymphadenopathy of the cervical chains. Lesions consist of vesicles that rapidly rupture forming painful ulcers (Fig. 17-4). The lesions can be found on any oral mucosal or skin surface. The fluid-filled vesicles contain many virions and are highly infectious. The gingiva is often diffusely enlarged, erythematous, and ulcerated. The lesions usually resolve spontaneously within 10 to 14 days.

Herpes simplex infection of the finger is known as *herpetic whitlow.* The primary infection causes erythema, edema, vesicles, ulcers, and pain in the infected finger and can prevent the clinician from practicing for several weeks.

Differential diagnosis. Primary herpes produces systemic manifestations similar to other generalized viral infections, but it can usually be distinguished from these diseases by the characteristic oral lesions. Recurrent or secondary herpetic lesions are identified by the absence of systemic manifestations and the limitation of lesions to keratinized surfaces such as the lips and gingiva.

Management decisions. Primary herpes can be diagnosed on the basis of clinical features. Therefore additional diagnostic procedures are not necessary. Management consists of bed rest and analgesics. Younger patients should be encouraged to maintain adequate fluid intake since dehydration can develop rapidly. Systemic acyclovir is usually of little value in treating primary herpetic gingivostomatitis unless the drug is initiated during the first few days of the disease. Acyclovir is beneficial in limiting the severity and complications of primary herpes in immunocompromised patients.

Varicella

Definition. Varicella, also known as *chickenpox,* and *herpes zoster (shingles)* are caused by the varicella zoster virus, which is structurally similar to the herpes simplex virus. Varicella is extremely common, highly contagious, and usually epidemic in occurrence.

Clinical features. Varicella begins with mild fever and malaise that is soon followed by an exanthem or skin rash consisting of extremely pruritic papules (Fig. 17-5), vesicles, and ulcers. Successive crops of lesions begin on the trunk and progressive involvement eventually includes the face and extremities. Oral vesicles and ulcers resembling primary herpetic lesions occasionally develop.

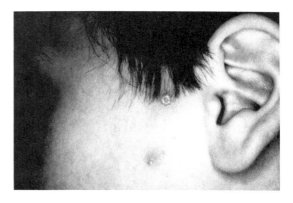

Fig. 17-5 Varicella. Mild fever and malaise of 24 hours duration was associated with multiple erythematous pruritic vesicles affecting an 8-year-old boy. Lesions were originally noticed on the trunk and later appeared on the face. Note the collapsed vesicle near the hairline.

Differential diagnosis. Varicella can be distinguished from other viral infections by the skin rash and its pattern of spread from the trunk to the face and extremities, as well as by the history of exposure to an infected individual.

Management decisions. Treatment is palliative and aimed at reducing pruritus. Varicella usually has a mild clinical course, and complications are rare, except in neonates, the elderly, and immunocompromised patients. Salicylates should not be administered to children with varicella and influenza because of the risk of toxic complications known as *Reye's syndrome.* This condition should be suspected if a patient with these viral infections becomes agitated, confused, and experiences severe vomiting after taking aspirin.

Rubeola

Definition. Although most adults have had rubeola or *red measles* and most children have been immunized, outbreaks of the disease occasionally occur. The major clinical significance of rubeola is the rare possibility of serious complications including pneumonia and encephalitis.

Clinical features. Rubeola begins with fever, conjunctivitis, photophobia, cough, and nasal discharge. Erythematous macules and vesicles with white centers, known as *Koplik's spots,* may be observed on the buccal mucosa early in the infection. An erythematous, maculopapular skin rash appears several days after the Koplik's spots. The rash first affects the face then spreads to the trunk and extremities. The skin rash and other features gradually resolve in approximately 1 week.

Differential diagnosis. Rubeola can be distinguished from other viral infections by the pattern of spread of the skin rash and history of exposure to an infected individual. The Koplik's spots involve only the buccal mucosa, as opposed to the diffuse distribution of ulcers in primary herpetic gingivostomatitis. *Rubella* or *German measles* is a milder infection than rubeola and does not produce oral lesions.

Management decisions. Rubeola is usually a benign, self-limited disease. In addition to supportive care, the patient should be observed for rare complications such as bacterial pneumonia, otitis media, and encephalitis.

Herpangina

Definition. Herpangina is caused by a group A coxsackievirus. It is rarely identified clinically because the systemic features are generally subclinical.

Clinical features. Herpangina most commonly affects children. Systemic manifestations such as fever, malaise, lymphadenopathy, and anorexia are exceptionally mild. The oral lesions consist of vesicles and ulcers that are confined to the soft palate and tonsillar pillars. These lesions may lead to complaints of sore throat, but they are usually discovered incidentally. The manifestations of herpangina typically last less than 1 week.

Differential diagnosis. Rubeola and varicella can be eliminated from the differential diagnosis by the absence of a skin rash. Primary

herpetic gingivostomatitis produces more diffusely distributed oral lesions. Aphthous ulcers are not confined to the soft palate, no vesicles form, and systemic manifestations do not develop.

Management decisions. Treatment is usually not required because the mild symptoms of the disease resolve spontaneously and complications are rare.

Infectious Mononucleosis

Definition. Infectious mononucleosis is caused by the patient's initial exposure to Epstein-Barr virus. "Mono" is a common infection among adolescents and young adults.

Clinical features. The clinical severity of mononucleosis varies, but a more gradual onset and longer course is observed as compared with other generalized viral infections. Systemic manifestations include fever, malaise, generalized lymphadenopathy, and splenomegaly, as well as hepatomegaly in some instances. Pharyngitis is usually present and may cause considerable discomfort. The most common oral lesions are palatal petechiae. Oral ulcers may develop, but they are not preceded by vesicles.

Differential diagnosis. Mononucleosis can be difficult to distinguish from other viral infections initially, but the infection should be considered if general "viral" symptoms of mild fever, malaise, and lymphadenopathy persist more than 1 to 2 weeks. A definitive diagnosis requires serologic demonstration of antibodies to the Epstein-Barr virus. Serologic testing may be negative during the first week of symptoms. Streptococcal pharyngitis is characterized by more rapid onset and can be diagnosed by throat culture.

Management decisions. Treatment is supportive. The acute disease usually resolves within 2 to 4 weeks.

Erythema Multiforme

Definition. Erythema multiforme is a nonviral condition, but it is included in this sec-

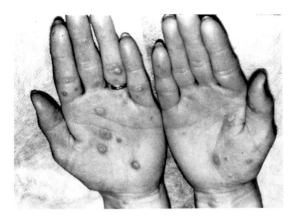

Fig. 17-6 Erythema multiforme. Acute onset ulcerative stomatitis was associated with the characteristic maculopapular "target" lesions of the skin.

tion because its acute onset and other features are similar to generalized viral infections. The cause of erythema multiforme is unknown, but the disease involves deposition of immune complexes in walls of blood vessels in the skin and mucosa. Approximately one half of the cases of erythema multiforme appear to be triggered by infections such as herpes simplex viruses or drug administration, primarily antibiotics.

Clinical features. Erythema multiforme can affect the skin and oral mucosa independently or simultaneously. The most characteristic feature is the "iris" or "target" lesion of the skin, which appears as a central vesicle surrounded by concentric erythematous and skin-colored rings (Fig. 17-6). Painful oral ulcers are most commonly located on the lips, buccal mucosa, and tongue. Headache, fever, and malaise may accompany skin and oral mucosal lesions. The onset of erythema multiforme is typically acute followed by spontaneous resolution within several weeks. In some circumstances the manifestations may be observed in a recurrent or chronic course.

Stevens-Johnson syndrome is a severe, debilitating form of erythema multiforme that pro-duces more generalized and serious manifestations. Conjunctivitis develops in addition to severe skin and mucosal lesions of the anal, genital, and oral regions.

Differential diagnosis. The diagnosis of erythema multiforme is straightforward when the characteristic "target" skin lesions are present. In the absence of skin lesions, the systemic features and oral ulcers suggest primary herpetic gingivostomatitis as a diagnostic possibility. Primary herpes usually produces lymphadenopathy, which is unusual with erythema multiforme.

Management decisions. Mild cases of erythema multiforme require only palliative treatment, and a good prognosis is expected, although recurrences may develop. Stevens-Johnson syndrome is a serious condition that may progress rapidly and can be fatal. Systemic corticosteroid administration and hospitalization may be necessary.

ORAL ULCERATIONS WITH A CHRONIC OR RECURRENT COURSE

These conditions are distinguished by recurrent episodes of oral ulceration or reactivation of a past infection. The distribution, duration, and appearance of the lesions usually allows a definitive diagnosis. This group includes two of the most common oral ulcerative conditions, aphthous stomatitis and recurrent herpes simplex infection. The differential diagnostic approach to these conditions is illustrated in Fig. 17-7.

Epidermolysis Bullosa

Definition. The most illustrative genetic skin disease that produces recurring oral ulcers is epidermolysis bullosa. This condition is described in Chapter 20.

Clinical features. Adult patients are nearly always aware of the diagnosis because recurring ulcers since infancy have prompted diagnostic evaluation. Skin lesions are invariably present and consist of bullae that rupture to form ulcers. They are most commonly located

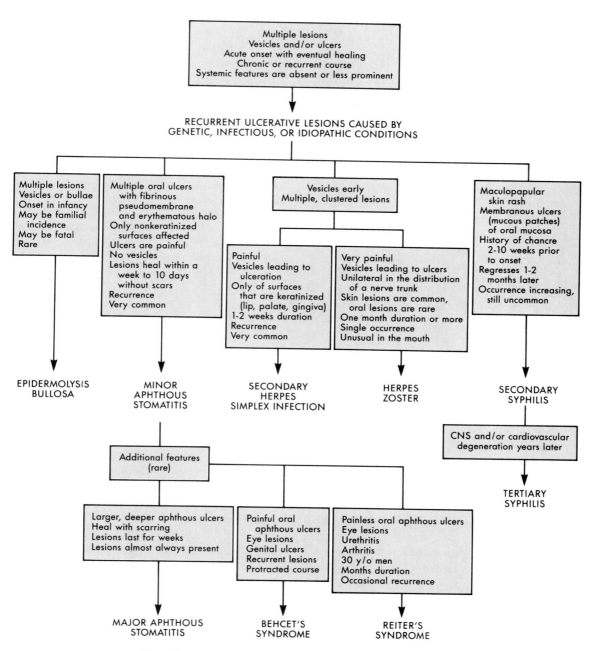

Fig. 17-7 Differential diagnosis of recurring oral ulcers.

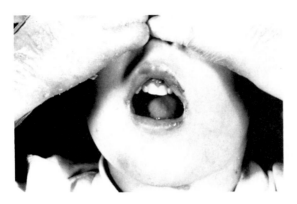

Fig. 17-8 Epidermolysis bullosa. This 4-year-old boy has experienced epidermal blistering, scarring, and oral ulcers recurrently since birth.

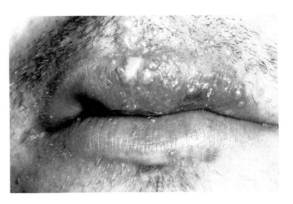

Fig. 17-9 Herpes zoster. These painful, fluid filled vesicles and ulcers of the skin and mucosa of the upper lip that are limited to the patient's left side appeared 3 days previously. Unilateral oral mucosal ulcers were also present on the hard palate and gingiva. (Courtesy of Dr. Catherine M. Flaits, University of Texas at Houston.)

in areas of friction or pressure such as the hands, feet, scalp, elbows, and buttocks. Scarring may cause limitation of movement and contraction. Oral blisters and ulcers (Fig. 17-8) vary in frequency and severity. Scarring, restricted oral opening, and ankyloglossia are complications of the more dramatic forms of the condition. Teeth are usually normal in appearance, although hypoplastic enamel has been observed.

Differential diagnosis. Epidermolysis bullosa is readily diagnosed because skin lesions are continually present from childhood and a familial occurrence is a frequent feature. Most patients are aware of the diagnosis of their disease by the time they appear for dental treatment.

Management decisions. Epidermolysis bullosa cannot be cured or effectively controlled. Treatment is supportive and may include administration of palliative coating preparations, analgesics for pain, and antibiotics to prevent secondary bacterial infections.

Herpes Zoster

Definition. Herpes zoster, also known as *shingles,* is a secondary or latent infection caused by the varicella zoster virus. The primary varicella infection usually occurs in childhood. The virus becomes latent after infecting one or more sensory ganglia, and it is clinically undetectable until reactivated.

Clinical features. Herpes zoster most often affects middle age or older adults. The reactivation is often a consequence of immune system compromise by medications or another illness. Skin lesions are common, while oral lesions are relatively unusual.

The initial symptom is prodromal pain, paresthesia, or burning lasting several hours or days in the distribution of one or more sensory nerves. Patients may complain of odontalgia during the prodrome if the maxillary or mandibular divisions of the trigeminal nerve are affected. The clusters of clear, fluid-filled vesicles that eventually form are limited in distribution to the skin or mucosa innervated by the affected sensory nerve(s) as shown in Fig. 17-9. The vesicles rupture and coalesce, which results in ulcers that heal within 2 to 3 weeks. Secondary bacterial infections may complicate and prolong the healing. Persistence of pain of the same nerve branch lasting several weeks or months following healing of the ulcers is referred to as *postherpetic neuralgia* (Chapter 9). The duration and severity of pain tends to be greatest among elderly patients.

Differential diagnosis. The prodromal pain of herpes zoster involving the maxillary and mandibular trigeminal branches may be difficult to differentiate from the odontalgia of irreversible pulpitis. Once the vesicles form, the historical features and unilateral sensory nerve distribution usually allow a definitive diagnosis.

Management decisions. If the clinical features are insufficient to diagnose the disease, exfoliative cytology usually reveals multinucleated epithelial giant cells characteristic of herpes virus infections. Although severely immunocompromised individuals may benefit from systemic antiviral therapy with acyclovir or vidarabine, most patients suffering from herpes zoster are best managed with supportive therapy only.

Recurrent Herpes Simplex

Definition. Recurrent herpes simplex is a secondary or latent infection caused by the herpes simplex virus type 1 or type 2. Most type 1 infections involve the orofacial region and most type 2 infections involve the genitals, although this generalization is less than absolute in view of the possibility of infection from oral-genital contact. Introduction of the virus into the trigeminal ganglion occurs during primary herpes simplex infection. After resolution of the acute infection, the virus then remains latent and clinically undetectable until reactivated.

Clinical features. Recurrent episodes of oral herpes simplex activation can affect any age group. Episodes may be "triggered" in different individuals by a variety of exogenous or endogenous factors such as physical injury, systemic disease, or emotional stress. Each episode usually begins with prodromal tingling or discomfort of several hours duration that is

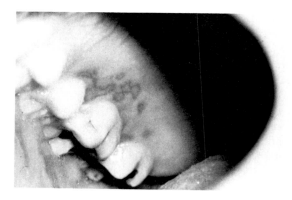

Fig. 17-10 Recurrent herpes simplex. These coalescing, painful ulcers were focally located on palatal mucosa adjacent to the right second premolar and first molar. The area has been painful for 48 hours.

localized to the site of eventual lesion formation. Multiple clear, fluid-filled vesicles less than 3 mm in diameter form in a cluster located most often on the lip vermilion, perioral skin, gingiva, or palatal mucosa. The vesicles are transient, usually lasting no more than a few hours before rupturing to form multiple ulcers that frequently coalesce (Fig. 17-10). Healing is usually complete within 2 weeks.

Differential diagnosis. The oral ulcerative disease most commonly confused with recurrent herpes is aphthous stomatitis. In most cases, however, the clinical and historical features are sufficient to differentiate these two conditions. Recurrent aphthous stomatitis is characteristically found only on nonkeratinized oral mucosa, whereas recurrent herpes affects keratinized surfaces such as the exposed lip surface, gingiva, and palate. Aphthous stomatitis has no vesicular stage, and recurrent episodes seldom involve clustering of 1 to 2 mm diameter ulcers. Exfoliative cytology of newly ruptured herpetic vesicles reveals epithelial giant cells indicative of viral infection. Generalized viral infections can be differentiated from recurrent herpes simplex by greater distribution of oral ulcers and concurrent fever, malaise, and lymphadenopathy.

Management decisions. Management for most episodes of recurrent herpes simplex is supportive. Some patients have found topical application of acyclovir to be of value in reducing the symptoms and overall healing time, but this is only effective if applied immediately after the onset of the prodromal symptoms. Prophylactic use of systemic acyclovir can be effective in reducing the number of recurrent episodes for immunocompromised patients, but this is seldom indicated for otherwise healthy individuals.

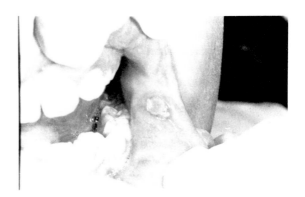

Fig. 17-11 Aphthous stomatitis.

Aphthous Stomatitis

Definition. Aphthous stomatitis is an idiopathic, noninfectious inflammatory disease characterized by recurrent ulcers involving nonkeratinized oral mucosa. The typical clinical course consists of unpredictable exacerbations and remissions, and familial occurrence is often observed. While the cause of aphthae is unknown, many patients report citrus fruits, spicy foods, and mild tissue injury as exacerbating factors.

Three forms of aphthous stomatitis have been traditionally described. *Minor aphthous stomatitis* is the common form that produces recurrent outbreaks of one or more relatively small ulcers that heal without scarring within 7 to 10 days. *Major aphthous stomatitis,* also known as *periadenitis mucosa necrotica recurrens* and *Sutton's disease,* produces ulcers of similar appearance except that they are larger, require a longer healing period, heal with scarring, and at least one lesion is nearly always present. *Herpetiform aphthae* usually present as multiple, exceptionally painful ulcers 1 to 2 mm diameter that affect nonkeratinized mucosa. Clinical observations reveal, however, that many patients exhibit features intermediate between these characteristic forms. Also, the severity of different episodes affecting an individual can appear typical of more that one form of aphthous stomatitis. This supports the hypothesis that aphthous stomatitis is a single pathologic process with variably severe manifestations. In addition, aphthouslike oral lesions are a diagnostic feature of *Reiter's syndrome* and *Behçet's syndrome,* which are briefly described below.

Clinical features. Aphthae present as one or more ulcers on nonkeratinized oral mucosal surfaces. Minor aphthae are typically less than 1 cm in diameter while herpetiform aphthae are 1 to 2 mm in size and major aphthae can be greater than 1 to 2 cm in diameter. These subclassifications are somewhat arbitrary and many patients with aphthae present with a wide range of lesion size at initial examination or during subsequent episodes. The ulcers (Fig. 17-11) are superficial, well delineated with an erythematous halo, nonindurated, and painful. Healing time ranges from 7 to 10 days for small aphthae to 3 to 4 weeks or more for larger lesions.

Differential diagnosis. A definitive diagnosis of aphthous stomatitis can be based on the clinical and historical findings in most cases. A biopsy reveals only nonspecific ulceration. The chronic, recurrent pattern of the episodes without systemic manifestations eliminates generalized viral infections such as primary herpes simplex and acute onset diseases such as erythema multiforme from the differential diagnosis. The location of lesions on nonkeratinized mucosal surfaces is inconsistent with recurrent herpes simplex infection.

Management decisions. Most patients who suffer from infrequent aphthous attacks are best managed by palliative treatment with topical anesthetic preparations. Patients who suffer from numerous episodes of aphthae or who are seldom aphthae-free have been successfully treated with initial burst therapeutic regimens of systemic corticosteroid therapy followed with prophylactic use of a topical steroid preparation. As with most chronic or recurrent oral ulcerative conditions, patients should be counseled that the therapeutic goals are to control symptoms and reduce the frequency of recurrences because no cure is available for these conditions. This promotes the development of reasonable treatment expectations by the patient.

Reiter's Syndrome

Reiter's syndrome is an uncommon immune-mediated disease identified most often among young adult males. The diagnostic elements of the syndrome are oral aphthouslike ulcers, polyarthritis, urethritis, and conjunctivitis or uveitis. The manifestations can last weeks or months and may recur. The diagnosis is based on the recognition of the signs and symptoms since no laboratory tests directly contribute to the diagnosis. Manifestations usually follow an antigenic stimulation by an enteric or genitourinary infection, and most affected individuals exhibit the specific histocompatibility antigen HLA-B27. This suggests Reiter's syndrome is a form of *reactive arthritis* analogous to rheumatoid arthritis. The symptoms are usually managed with nonsteroidal antiinflammatory medications.

Behçet's Syndrome

Behçet's syndrome is an idiopathic disorder characterized by oral, ocular, and genital lesions. The syndrome has at times been reported to have a genetic component. The ocular features include uveitis, retinitis, and conjunctivitis. Genital features usually include ulcerations of skin or mucosa and oral features include aphthouslike ulcers. No laboratory or biopsy features are of value in confirming a diagnosis of Behçet's syndrome. Therefore the diagnosis is usually based on recognition of the syndrome's clinical features. Systemic corticosteroids have been prescribed for management of Behçet's syndrome with varying success.

Secondary Syphilis

Definition. Secondary syphilis is a mucocutaneous ulcerative disease that develops several weeks after the initial infection by *Treponema pallidum* in the absence of antibiotic treatment.

Clinical features. This widely disseminated infection causes malaise, fever, a variably intense skin rash, and multiple mucosal ulcers called *mucous patches.* Slightly raised, broad-based ulcers known as *condyloma latum* may develop and persist for 5 to 10 weeks if not treated. A course of multiple exacerbations and remissions may be observed before the infection enters a period of latency lasting months or years. The latent period is followed in many untreated patients by development of *tertiary syphilis.* This stage of the infection is characterized by the development of destructive lesions called *gummas* affecting multiple organs including the central nervous system and heart.

Differential diagnosis. The mucous patches appear somewhat similar to aphthous ulcers except that they are mildly thickened and are usually painless. Systemic features including persistent or recurrent lymphadenopathy, fever, malaise, and mucosal ulceration suggest the need for serologic studies to identify the infection. The diagnosis of syphilis is usually based on clinical features, history of infectious contact, and positive serologic results as described in Chapter 11.

Management decisions. The patient should be referred for definitive diagnosis and

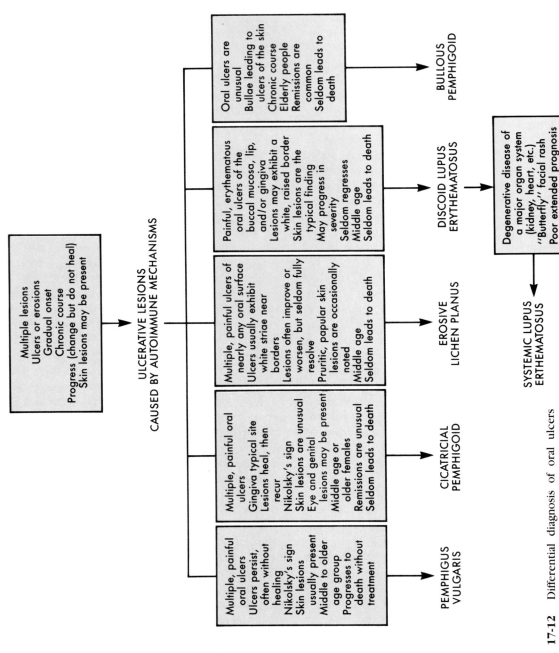

Fig. 17-12   Differential diagnosis of oral ulcers caused by autoimmune diseases.

treatment. The treatment of choice for syphilis continues to be 2.4 million units of benzathine penicillin. Tetracycline or erythromycin is effective for patients allergic to penicillin.

AUTOIMMUNE DISEASES

Autoimmune diseases that cause oral ulcerations have a gradual onset and a chronic, progressive course with exacerbations and partial remissions. Multiple ulcers of oral mucosa are limited to the superficial mucosal surface in contrast to chronic ulcerative diseases characterized by tissue destruction, which are described later in this chapter. In addition, autoimmune conditions that produce oral ulcers can also affect the skin or other mucosal surfaces. Differential diagnostic comparisons are summarized in Fig. 17-12.

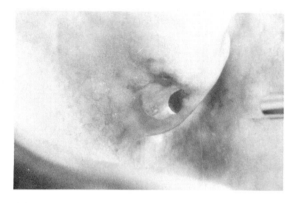

Fig. 17-13 Cicatricial pemphigoid. A Nikolsky's sign was noted during tangential air syringe blast to the left retromolar pad of a 64-year-old male with a history of intermittent oral ulcers for the preceding 6 years.

Cicatricial Pemphigoid

Definition. Cicatricial pemphigoid is an autoimmune condition that is also known as *benign mucous membrane pemphigoid.* The autoantibody appears targeted to a substance in the lamina lucida of the epithelial basement membrane.

Clinical features. Cicatricial pemphigoid is most often first identified in persons over 50, and women are affected more often than men. Mucous membranes including oral and conjunctival surfaces develop lesions earlier and more extensively than the skin. Individual lesions consist of transient vesicles and bullae that rupture leaving a superficial ulcer. Ulcers of cicatricial pemphigoid tend to heal with more scarring than do the ulcers of bullous pemphigoid. If present, skin lesions are usually located on the head or extremities. Oral lesions can be widespread or involve only the gingiva, which presents as "desquamative gingivitis." A Nikolsky's sign can be demonstrated in affected individuals by epithelial separation and bulla formation following gentle lateral pressure on an apparently normal mucosal surface (Fig. 17-13).

Differential diagnosis. The clinical and historical features of cicatricial pemphigoid are similar to pemphigus, bullous pemphigoid, and lichen planus. In contrast to pemphigus and bullous pemphigoid, circulating antibodies are not detectable in most cases. The definitive diagnosis is made by microscopic and immunopathologic analysis of a representative biopsy specimen. Deposition of immunoglobulin, usually IgG, in a linear pattern along the basement membrane is a distinguishing diagnostic feature in many cases.

Management decisions. An incisional biopsy specimen fixed and evaluated both by routine and immunofluorescent techniques is necessary to achieve a definitive diagnosis in most instances. Long-term management of cicatricial pemphigoid usually requires topical or systemic corticosteroids or other immunosuppressive agents. The major morbidity of many cases is conjunctival ulceration, adhesion, and scarring that can produce corneal opacification and blindness. For this reason, all patients diagnosed with oral cicatricial pemphigoid should be referred to an ophthalmologist for evaluation.

CORTICOSTEROID THERAPY

The management of noninfectious, ulcerative diseases of the oral cavity such as aphthous stomatitis, lichen planus, and cicatricial pemphigoid often requires the use of topical or systemic antiinflammatory medications such as corticosteroids. Other immunosuppressive agents have also been used with varying degrees of success. Of primary importance is to educate the patient as to the nature and goals of therapy. These diseases are currently considered incurable and are characterized by a prolonged clinical course of unpredictable exacerbations and remissions. Therapy is rendered in an attempt to promote healing of current lesions and to minimize the formation of future lesions with the expectation that treatment will be required at least occasionally for the life of the patient.

The initial therapeutic regimen should be a topical corticosteroid preparation for most patients. Modification of topical corticosteroid application is necessary to determine the minimal amount of medication necessary to prevent lesion recurrence. Intraoral topical steroids such as triamcinolone are only effective when extended contact with the mucosa is maintained. Therefore the suspension or ointment should be applied after meals and, if necessary, just before bed at night. When using a rinse, the patient must expectorate rather than swallow the residual suspension to minimize systemic absorption.

Failure of topical corticosteroid preparations to control the lesions indicates the need to establish lesion control with a systemic "burst therapy" of prednisone. Once controlled, the lesions can usually be kept in remission through prophylactic use of topical steroid application "as needed." Intralesional injection of a corticosteroid preparation may promote healing of ulcers if both topical and systemic regimens have failed to attain initial control of the disease.

Therapeutic use of corticosteroids should be initiated only after a complete review of the patients current medical status and medical history. Use of systemic corticosteroids is contraindicated for patients with a history of tuberculosis, clinical evidence of current acute infections, symptoms suggestive of peptic ulcerative disease, and other conditions. Consultation with the patient's primary care physician will be appropriate in most instances requiring systemic corticosteroid therapy.

The following therapeutic regimens are appropriate for most adults:

Oral Rinse
Rx: Triamcinolone acetonide 0.1% aqueous suspension*
Disp: 200 ml
Sig: 5 ml oral rinse and expectorate QID AM and HS, NPO 1 hr

Ointment
Rx: Triamcinolone acetonide 0.1% or 0.2% ointment
Disp: 15 gm or 20 gm tube
Sig: Apply thin film to lesion QID NPO 1 hr

Systemic Steroid (Burst Therapy)
Rx: Prednisone 5 mg, 10 mg, or 20 mg tabs (professional judgment)
Disp: (professional judgment)
Sig: 40 mg to 60 mg AM (1 hour after arising) × 5 days followed by 10 mg to 20 mg AM (1 hour after arising) QOD (every other day)

Intralesional Steroid Injection
Rx: Triamcinolone injectable 40
Dilute 10 mg to 20 mg into sterile water for injection or local anesthetic solution.

*Directions to the pharmacist: Dilute injectible triamcinolone 40 into 200 ml of water for irrigation and add 5 ml of 95% ethanol.

Bullous Pemphigoid

Definition. Bullous pemphigoid is an autoimmune disease characterized by autoantibodies directed against a 220 Kd protein found within the lamina lucida of the epithelial basement membrane.

Clinical features. The disease is usually first identified in persons over 50 years old, and it affects women more often than men. The skin is the primary site of involvement, while oral lesions are usually absent or comparatively mild. Transient, clear fluid-filled vesicles and bullae affect the surface and a Nikolsky's sign is usually evident. The trunk and extremities are the typical locations of lesions. Oral lesions are usually widely distributed.

Differential diagnosis. The clinical and historical features of bullous pemphigoid are similar to cicatricial pemphigoid, pemphigus, and lichen planus. Serologic analysis will usually reveal titers of circulating basement membrane autoantibodies. The definitive diagnosis is made by microscopic and immunopathologic analysis of a biopsy specimen. Immunofluorescence of the surgical pathology specimen will characteristically reveal a linear band of immunoglobulin, usually IgG, at the level of the basement membrane.

Management decisions. Initial therapeutic management of bullous pemphigoid consists of topical corticosteroid application, although systemic corticosteroids may be required and some clinicians report good results using dapsone. Long-term steroid therapy may be necessary and can result in significant side effects or complications.

Pemphigus Vulgaris

Definition. Pemphigus vulgaris is an autoimmune, vesiculobullous disease that primarily affects the skin and mucous membranes. The characteristic autoantibody target is the epithelial desmosome complex. Autoantibody interaction with these structures yields disruption of cellular adhesion and epithelial separation. A genetic component has been related to the disease, and association with other autoimmune diseases such as rheumatoid arthritis and Sjögren's disease is occasionally observed.

Clinical features. Epidermal and mucosal features of pemphigus vulgaris include transient, clear, fluid-filled vesicles and bullae that rupture leaving an ulcer partially covered by a fragile membrane. A Nikolsky's sign can be demonstrated in most instances and the ulcers usually heal within 2 weeks. The disease course is characterized by a chronic onset followed by a progressive, unpredictable admixture of exacerbations and remissions. Most individuals are middle-aged or older at the time of diagnosis, although children and young adults can also be affected.

Differential diagnosis. The clinical and historical features of pemphigus vulgaris may be indistinguishable from other pemphigus variants including the vegetans and foliaceous forms. Other diseases that can mimic pemphigus include cicatricial pemphigoid, bullous pemphigoid, and lichen planus. Serologic analysis for circulating pemphigus autoantibodies can provide a comparative indication of the disease severity, progression of the condition, and treatment effectiveness during the disease course. The definitive diagnosis of pemphigus vulgaris relies on microscopic analysis including immunofluorescence of a representative biopsy specimen.

Management decisions. As with most autoimmune diseases, therapy relies on immunosuppressive agents including topical and systemic corticosteroids. The prognosis is guarded, because of the progressive nature of the disease and the side effects of chronic corticosteroid therapy.

Lupus Erythematosus

Definition. Lupus erythematosus is an autoimmune disease in which autoantibodies form to various tissues including skin and oral mucosa. The lesions of *discoid lupus erythematosus* are confined to the skin and mucosa, whereas *systemic lupus erythematosus* is a serious multisystemic disease that usually produces renal damage as well as surface lesions.

Clinical features. Discoid lupus causes skin lesions of the face, scalp, ears, and other sun exposed regions. The lesions are erythematous, scaly, and hyperpigmented patches. Older lesions often heal by central atrophic scarring and hyperkeratosis of the periphery. Vitiligo and alopecia are also common. Skin lesions are exacerbated by sun exposure.

Oral lesions of discoid lupus are uncommon in the absence of skin lesions. A white, rough plaquelike appearance with peripheral ulcers or erythema is typical. A border zone of white striae similar to that of lichen planus lesions may be present.

The classic skin lesion of systemic lupus is a symmetric erythematous rash of the malar re-

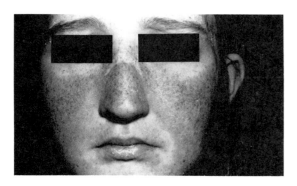

Fig. 17-14 Discoid lupus erythematosus. The typical erythematous "butterfly" rash affecting the midface region of a 21-year-old woman was exacerbated by sun exposure.

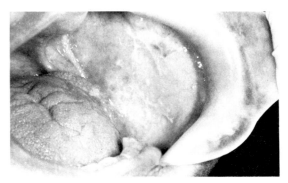

Fig. 17-15 Lichen planus. A 59-year-old man complained of intermittent oral pain described as "burning" for the past 15 years. Clinical findings revealed white, hyperkeratotic striations overlying erythematous buccal and labial mucosa bilaterally.

gions known as the "butterfly rash" (Fig. 17-14). Other skin lesions and oral lesions of systemic lupus are identical in appearance to those of discoid lupus. Systemic manifestations of systemic lupus include arthritis, vasculitis, pericarditis, seizures, and psychoses. The most common cause of death is renal disease leading to secondary hypertension. Numerous laboratory abnormalities may be present, but circulating immunoglobulins to DNA referred to as *antinuclear antibodies* or ANA are of greatest diagnostic significance. Oral candidiasis secondary to corticosteroid therapy is a common complication for lupus patients.

Differential diagnosis. Oral lesions of lupus can resemble lichen planus, but the relatively symmetric, bilateral distribution of lesions affecting the buccal mucosa distinguishes the reticular form of lichen planus. Also, the skin lesions of lupus are unlikely to be confused with the erythematous papules and plaques of lichen planus. Carcinoma in situ and early squamous cell carcinoma of oral mucosa should be considered if localized lesions fail to respond to therapy as expected.

Management decisions. Administration of topical or systemic corticosteroids is effective treatment for most patients. Referral to a dermatologist is required because of the skin involvement and to evaluate for the possibility of renal or other organ system lesions. The prognosis for discoid lupus is good, whereas the prognosis for systemic lupus depends on the extent of systemic damage at the time of diagnosis.

Lichen Planus

Definition. Lichen planus is a noninfectious, inflammatory disease characterized by T-cell destruction of the basal layer of surface epithelium. The target antigen is unknown but similar findings have been reported in some forms of allergic drug reaction and graft versus host disease. The designation *erosive lichen planus* is appropriate if ulcers are the primary manifestation of the disease.

Clinical features. Lichen planus is identified most often during middle age without gender predilection. The oral features consist of two distinct manifestations. Areas of mucosa show hyperkeratosis arranged in plaques or a reticular pattern similar to Wickham's striae of the skin. Adjacent areas of mucosa are erythematous and atrophic (Fig. 17-15). Ulcers form if the mucosal atrophy is pronounced, and bullae occasionally develop. These oral features can be localized but most patients are affected by lesions of several oral mucosal surfaces. Erosive lichen planus is a common cause of the clinical presentation known as "desquamative gingivitis" when ulcers are limited to the gingiva. The lesions undergo dynamic changes in appearance and arrangement. The disease course is characterized by unpredictable exacerbations and remissions. Skin lesions of lichen planus appear as pruritic, erythematous macular-papular patches with superficial fine white striae, or Wickham's striae (see Fig. 15-11).

Differential diagnosis. Most cases of oral

lichen planus can be diagnosed based on the clinical and historical features alone. The "desquamative gingivitis" presentation may be clinically indistinguishable from cicatricial pemphigoid. A medication-related lichenoid reaction and graft versus host disease in transplant patients may be considered if supported by the patient history. Dysplastic surface epithelial lesions, carcinoma in situ, and early invasive squamous cell carcinoma should be considered for focal lesions atypical of lichen planus. Features suggesting dysplasia or neoplasia include heterogeneous hyperkeratosis and erythema associated with induration, tissue fixation, and failure to respond to corticosteroid therapy.

Management decisions. Incisional biopsy is indicated if the clinical diagnosis is in doubt. Lichen planus is most often controlled with topical or systemic corticosteroids. During periods of symptomatic remission, the hyperkeratotic plaques and striations seldom resolve completely. Thus the goals of therapy are relief of symptoms, healing of ulcers, and a reduction in tissue erythema. Opportunistic candidiasis may develop due to corticosteroid therapy.

ORAL ULCERATIVE CONDITIONS CHARACTERIZED BY TISSUE DESTRUCTION

The conditions in this group are, fortunately, relatively rare. All are characterized by the destruction of tissue and superficial ulceration as the principal disease manifestations. The tissue alteration may appear as cavitation or a granulomatous enlargement, but the distinct clinical impression is one of tissue destruction. The differential diagnostic approach to these lesions is summarized by Fig. 17-16. Acute bacterial infections and other previously discussed ulcerative lesions can be distinguished either by the presence of pus and edematous enlargement, or by the superficial limitation of the ulcers.

Granulomatous Infections

Definition. Fungal organisms and tuberculosis that cause oral ulcers usually infect the lung primarily and then spread to oral mucosa by infected sputum. The initial infection is generally acquired by inhalation of the organisms as an aerosol. Infections caused by mycotic organisms include histoplasmosis, coccidioidomycosis, cryptococcosis, and blastomycosis, and the organisms responsible for these infections are generally endemic to specific geographic regions. A superficial oral mycotic or tubercular infection can progress without evidence of lung infection in rare instances. This usually affects patients with conditions of compromised host resistance. These infections are considered as a group because they exhibit few distinguishing clinical features.

Clinical features. The initial manifestations are usually related to the pulmonary infection and include fever, night sweats, chest pain, and hemoptysis. Oral infection is indicated by one or more nonhealing, indurated, slightly raised ulcerations. Chronic lesions may eventually develop cavitation.

Differential diagnosis. The oral manifestations of fungal infections and tuberculosis are often difficult to distinguish from primary malignant neoplasms or large, chronic aphthous ulcers. The definitive diagnosis requires histopathologic evaluation of an adequate biopsy specimen stained by special techniques to demonstrate the organisms. Microbial cultures may be contributory in some instances.

Management decisions. Treatment of deep mycotic infections depends on chemotherapeutic agents including ketoconazole, fluconazole, and amphotericin B. The oral ulcers will usually resolve concurrent with control of the systemic infection, although resection of large, necrotic lesions or primary closure of chronic ulcers may be required in some cases.

Noma

Definition. Noma is a rare form of gangrene localized to the orofacial region; it affects patients with compromised resistance to infection caused by immunosuppression, malnutrition, or debilitating systemic illness. Tissue necrosis progresses after infection by anaerobic bacteria, including spirochetes and

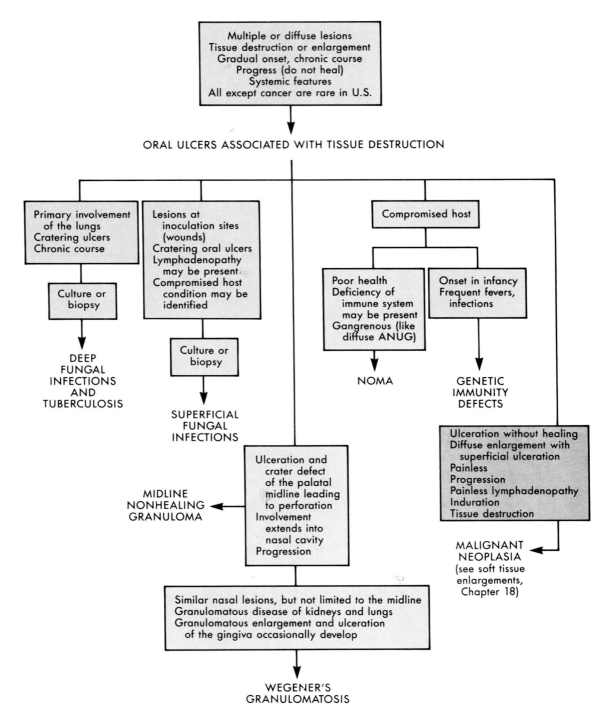

Fig. 17-16 Differential diagnosis of oral ulcers characterized by tissue destruction.

fusiforms. This extensive, destructive bacterial infection can be considered similar in many respects to the more commonly observed infection known as acute necrotizing ulcerative gingivitis (ANUG). The designation *necrotizing stomatitis* has been applied to the progression of necrotizing gingivitis and periodontitis to gangrenous deterioration of adjacent tissues among patients with AIDS.

Clinical features. Noma usually begins as a nonspecific ulcer of the buccal or alveolar mucosa. The ulcer fails to heal and progressive necrosis eventually destroys underlying tissues, producing cavitation (Fig. 17-17). The peripheral edema, erythema, and purulence of the inflammatory response appears disproportionally mild compared with lesion size.

Differential diagnosis. The diagnosis is usually evident in cases of progressive, diffuse tissue necrosis affecting a debilitated patient. Microbial cultures and a biopsy are indicated to exclude specific mycotic and other granulomatous conditions.

Management decisions. Local tissue debridement, therapeutic doses of broad spectrum antibiotics such as penicillin, and treatment of any underlying systemic conditions are indicated. Antibiotic sensitivity tests may reveal a particularly effective antimicrobial agent if the specimen was obtained before the initiation of empiric antibiotic therapy.

Genetic Immune System Deficiencies

Definition. The inherited immunodeficiencies are a diverse group of rare diseases with the unifying feature of dysfunction involving one or more components of the cellular or humoral immune systems. *Chronic granulomatous disease* is an x-linked autosomal recessive disorder characterized by dysfunction of macrophages and neutrophils. *Bruton's disease* or *x-linked agammaglobulinemia* results from impaired B-lymphocyte function. *DiGeorge's syndrome* features thymic hypoplasia and a decrease in cellular immune function. *Wiskott-Aldrich syndrome* is an x-linked disorder of T-lymphocytes. Many other hereditary immunologic deficiencies exist.

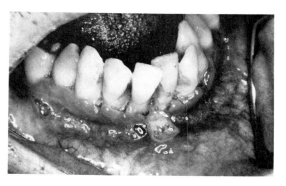

Fig. 17-17 Necrotizing stomatitis. A 29-year-old HIV seropositive man was affected by the advanced manifestations of AIDS including pneumocystis carinii pneumonia and skin lesions of Kaposi's sarcoma. Generalized destruction of gingival papilla, exudate, and fetid breath indicative of necrotizing ulcerative gingivitis were present. The ulcer of the alveolar mucosa labial to the mandibular central incisors was associated with underlying gangrenous tissue destruction.

Clinical features. The manifestation common to most of these diseases is the unexplained recurrence of viral, mycotic, or bacterial infections during infancy and childhood. Oral lesions characteristically present as multiple ulcerations that recur or persist. Biopsy specimens reveal nonspecific granulomatous inflammation. The combination of clinical features and historical pattern of infections and the emergence of opportunistic infections such as oral candidiasis indicates an elemental deficiency of the immune system.

Differential diagnosis. The diagnosis of these conditions relies on sophisticated laboratory tests. Specific neutrophil function tests are available to confirm the diagnosis of chronic granulomatous disease. Serologic testing for congenital HIV infection is indicated. The primary clinical issue is the suspicion of diminished resistance to infection with onset in infancy.

Management decisions. In general, no treatment is available beyond efforts to prevent infection and antimicrobial therapy with supportive care after specific infections develop.

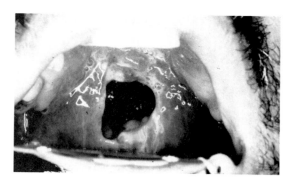

Fig. 17-18 Palatal perforation caused by midline nonhealing granuloma.

Midline Nonhealing Granuloma

Definition. This disease is an idiopathic inflammatory process that affects the maxilla by producing ulceration, eventual perforation of the palate, and destruction of nasal cartilage and bone. Before the development of effective treatment methods, the condition was known as *midline lethal granuloma.*

Clinical features. Lesions initially appear as single or multiple, indurated, slightly raised ulcers near the midline of the palate. The ulcers progress to destruction of the underlying tissues and cavitation, which can eventually perforate the palate if untreated (Fig. 17-18). The lesion may progress and destroy the midface before causing death by exsanguination after erosion of large blood vessels.

Differential diagnosis. The clinical and historical features of midline nonhealing granuloma are similar to Wegener's granulomatosis, which is distinguished by evidence of lung or renal lesions. Other diseases characterized by tissue destruction such as noma, chronic infections such as tuberculosis or syphilis, deep mycoses, or malignant neoplasms may produce similar findings. The diagnosis of midline nonhealing granuloma is based on location, clinical features, and exclusion of other destructive conditions by biopsy and serologic tests. The histopathologic features are nonspecific, revealing only inflammation and tissue necrosis.

Management decisions. Biopsy is necessary to exclude conditions such as granulomatous infections and malignancy. The treatment approach varies depending on lesion extent and other factors but usually consists of radiotherapy to the lesion site or corticosteroid administration.

Wegener's Granulomatosis

Definition. Wegener's granulomatosis is an idiopathic, chronic inflammatory condition that typically affects the upper respiratory tract, lungs, and kidneys.

Clinical features. The disease is most often identified among middle aged patients. The process initially produces upper respiratory lesions in most cases. Patients present with chronic nasal congestion, sinus pain, and epistaxis. Systemic manifestations may include fever and arthralgia. Initial oral lesions are ulcerative with granular appearing erythema of the alveolar or palatal mucosa. Nasal septum perforation commonly develops, but palatal perforation is unusual. Lower respiratory lesions may result in chronic respiratory failure, and kidney involvement produces gradual renal failure.

Differential diagnosis. The diagnosis is based on the finding of chronic granulomatous inflammation focally involving the respiratory system and kidneys. No clinical laboratory tests have proven diagnostic. Other chronic granulomatous diseases such as tuberculosis and deep mycotic infections, as well as lymphomas, must be excluded by pathologic examination.

Management decisions. Biopsy of affected tissues is indicated to confirm the diagnosis. Systemic steroids and other chemotherapeutic agents such as cyclophosphamide have proven effective management for this disease if therapy is initiated early in the disease course.

Malignancy

An ulcer or a "sore that does not heal" is a frequently described feature of malignancy affecting skin and mucosal surfaces. The disrupted epithelial growth and maturation of epithelial dysplasia or superficial squamous cell carcinomas generally produces intermixed white areas of epithelial thickening and red foci of epithelial thinning. In some instances small ulcers are a part of this heterogeneous pattern. Surface ulceration caused by advanced neoplasms is generally the result of secondary trauma or ischemic necrosis of superficial tissues. These destructive processes are caused by a tumor enlargement that has achieved substantial size. The ulceration causes secondary inflammation that may be painful and prompt the patient to seek care. Therefore while ulceration is a frequent manifestation of oral malignancy, the primary feature of malignant neoplasia is either heterogeneous appearance of a superficial lesion or obvious clinical enlargement. This will generally direct the differential diagnosis of such lesions to the white lesion, dark lesion, or tissue enlargement categories.

SUMMARY

Numerous conditions are capable of producing ulcerations of the oral mucosa. The diagnostic priority is to determine the onset, distribution, duration, and clinical course of the lesions as the most effective indication of the diagnosis. The diagnostic strategy is to categorize the patient's condition in one of the following groups:

1. Oral ulcerations with acute onset and short duration
   a. Bacterial infections and injury are indicated by pus or an apparent source of injury.
   b. Generalized viral infections are suggested by fever and other systemic manifestations.
2. Oral ulcerations with chronic or recurrent course
   a. Genetic diseases will have affected the patient since infancy.
   b. Recurrent viral or idiopathic diseases are characterized by appearance and distribution.
   c. Autoimmune diseases are indicated by superficial, sloughing ulcers and demonstration by biopsy of immunologic abnormalities.

d. Granulomatous diseases and malignancy are indicated by tissue destruction.

Within each category the differential diagnosis relies on comparison of the clinical features to eliminate as many of conditions as possible from diagnostic consideration. A diagnosis of acute lesions, genetic diseases, and recurrent or idiopathic ulcers is usually possible on the basis of clinical findings. Autoimmune and destructive ulcerative conditions usually require biopsy to achieve a definitive diagnosis.

BIBLIOGRAPHY

Ahmed A and Hombal S: Cicatricial pemphigoid, Int J Dermatol 25:90-96, 1986.

Cotran RS, Kumar V, Robbins SL, editors: Robbins pathologic basis of disease, ed 4, Philadelphia, 1989, Saunders.

Daniels TE, Quadra-White C: Direct immunofluorescence in oral mucosal disease: a diagnostic analysis of 130 cases, Oral Surg Oral Med Oral Pathol 51:38-47, 1981.

Hanson R, Olsen K, Rogers R: Upper aerodigestive tract manifestations of cicatricial pemphigoid, Ann Otol Rhinol Laryngol 97:493-499, 1988.

Laskaris G, Sklavounou A, Stratigos J: Bullous pemphigoid, cicatricial pemphigoid, and pemphigus vulgaris: a comparative clinical survey of 278 cases, Oral Surg Oral Med Oral Pathol 54:656-662, 1982.

Lozada-Nur F, Gorsky M, Silverman S Jr: Oral erythema multiforme: clinical observations and treatment of 95 patients, Oral Surg Oral Med Oral Pathol 67:36-40, 1989.

Nelson J and others: Midline "nonhealing" granuloma, Oral Surg Oral Med Oral Pathol 58:554-560, 1984.

Regezi JA, Sciubba JJ: Oral pathology: clinical-pathologic correlations, Philadelphia, 1989, Saunders.

Sedano HO, Gorlin RJ: Epidermolysis bullosa, Oral Surg Oral Med Oral Pathol 67:555-563, 1989.

Spruance S and others: The natural history of recurrent herpes labialis, N Engl J Med 279:69-75, 1977.

Venning V and others: Mucosal involvement in bullous and cicatricial pemphigoid: a clinical and immunopathologic study, Br J Dermatol 118:7-15, 1988.

Vincent SD and others: Oral lichen planus: the clinical, historical and therapeutic features of 100 cases, Oral Surg Oral Med Oral Pathol 70:165-171, 1990.

Wilson JD and others, editors: Harrison's principles of internal medicine, ed 12, New York, 1991, McGraw-Hill.

Vincent SD: Diagnosing oral lichen planus, JADA 122:93-96, 1991.

CHAPTER 18

Differential Diagnosis of Oral Soft Tissue Enlargements

CATHERINE M. FLAITZ

Soft tissue enlargements of the oral cavity often present a diagnostic challenge because a diverse group of pathologic processes can produce such lesions. An enlargement may represent a variation of normal anatomic structures, inflammation, cysts, developmental anomalies, and neoplasms. The goal of the differential diagnosis is to determine the nature of the enlargement as a basis for formulating a rational treatment approach. The symptoms, growth rate, palpation characteristics, surface morphology, and location generally allow categorization of a soft tissue enlargement into one of five lesion groups as illustrated in Fig. 18-1. These descriptive categories consist of papillary enlargements of the surface epithelium, acute inflammatory enlargements, reactive hyperplasias, benign submucosal neoplasms and cysts, and malignant neoplasms. Following this initial categorization, the characteristics of the lesion can then be compared with those of the diagnostic possibilities within that category.

The distinctive features of papillary enlargements of the surface epithelium, inflammatory lesions, and reactive hyperplasias generally allow a straightforward clinical diagnosis. Microscopic examination of excised tissue is necessary to reach a definitive diagnosis of suspected cysts and neoplasms.

PAPILLARY ENLARGEMENTS OF THE SURFACE EPITHELIUM

Most papillary enlargements of the surface epithelium are exophytic, pale, and firm with a pebbly or rough surface texture. These lesions are generally painless, slow-growing with a limited enlargement potential, and well delineated. A viral infection is implicated as the primary etiologic agent of most of these lesions, although additional factors may be contributory. No systemic manifestations are associated with these enlargements, although multiple oral lesions and similar lesions of distant body sites may result from separate infections by the

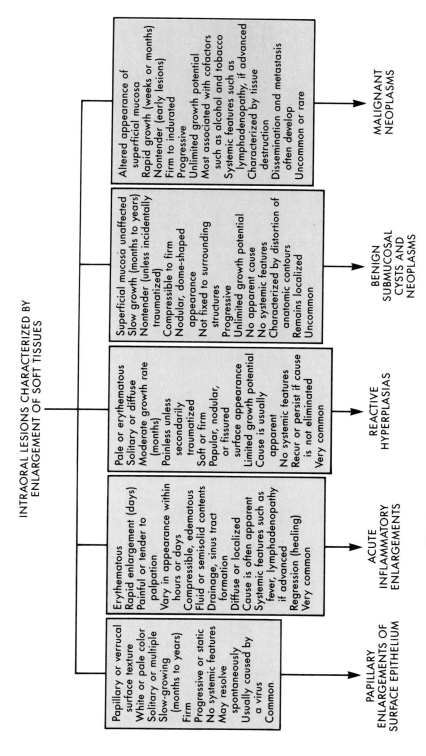

Fig. 18-1   Initial differential diagnosis of soft tissue enlargements.

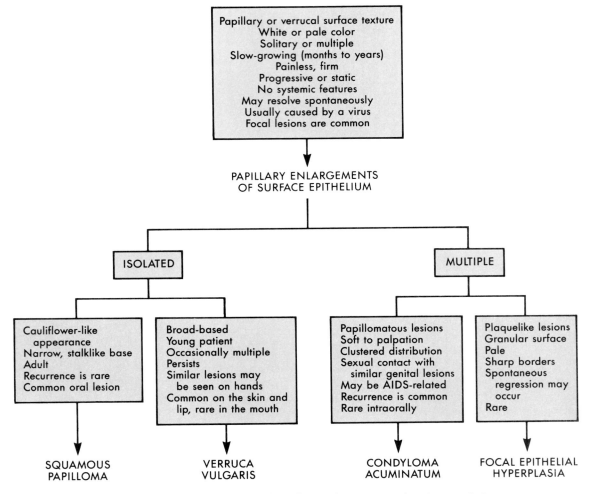

Fig. 18-2 Differential diagnosis of papillary enlargements of surface epithelium.

same virus. The diagnostic approach to papillary enlargements of the surface epithelium is illustrated in Fig. 18-2.

Squamous Papilloma

Definition. The squamous papilloma is a benign proliferation of the surface epithelium usually caused by the human papillomavirus. It is the most common papillary lesion affecting the oral mucosa and is related to verruca vulgaris.

Clinical features. The squamous papilloma is a pale, solitary lesion that occurs primarily among adults. A cauliflower-like shape results from the larger size of the exophytic portion of the lesion relative to the narrow base (Fig. 18-3). The papilloma is firm, rough, and nontender to palpation. A limited growth potential of less than 1 cm in diameter is generally observed. The palate, tongue, and lips are the most common sites of involvement.

Differential diagnosis. The diagnosis of

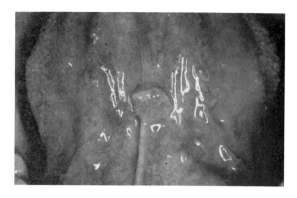

Fig. 18-3 Papilloma. This pink, pedunculated and papillary lesion on the lingual frenum was present for 1 year with minimal change in size.

squamous papilloma is usually uncomplicated. The suspected squamous papilloma must be differentiated from the verruca vulgaris, condyloma acuminatum, and focal epithelial hyperplasia. Verruca vulgaris usually forms with a broad or sessile base, in contrast to the narrow, stalklike attachment of the squamous papilloma. In addition, verruca vulgaris develops primarily on the skin of children and rarely occurs intraorally. Both the condyloma acuminatum and focal epithelial hyperplasia are unlikely possibilities unless multiple papillary lesions develop.

Management decisions. Excision with histopathologic examination is the recommended treatment for the squamous papilloma. Recurrence is unlikely, if the excision includes the base of the lesion.

Verruca Vulgaris

Definition. Verruca vulgaris or the *common wart* is an exophytic skin lesion caused by the human papillomavirus. The oral mucosa is rarely affected, although lesions of the vermilion border of the lip and adjacent skin are occasionally observed.

Clinical features. This lesion is clinically similar in most respects to the squamous papil-

loma. Warts appear sharply delineated from adjacent tissues and pale with a pebbly surface texture. The lesions are painless and firm to palpation. The verruca vulgaris is slow-growing and is usually less than 1 cm in size. The exophytic portion of the lesion is narrow in comparison with the broad base. This viral infection primarily affects the hands and fingers of children and young adults. Warts of the oral and perioral regions typically develop on the vermilion border of the lips or palate. Oral involvement usually results from direct viral contact with hand lesions.

Differential diagnosis. The location and comparative size of the lesion base are distinguishing features between verruca vulgaris and squamous papilloma and are discussed in the differential diagnosis section for papillomas. Multiple verrucae of the lip may suggest the possibility of condyloma acuminatum or focal epithelial hyperplasia, but these multifocal conditions are typically limited to "wet" mucosal surfaces.

Management decisions. Excision of intraoral lesions is the treatment of choice for the oral verruca. Contact with surrounding tissues should be avoided during removal to minimize the possibility of viral inoculation. Referral for the removal of cutaneous lesions is appropriate if the cosmetic appearance of the site is a concern. These viral lesions occasionally regress without treatment.

Condyloma Acuminatum

Definition. Multiple papillomatous lesions characterize the clinical presentation of condyloma acuminatum or *venereal warts.* The human papillomavirus causes this sexually transmitted disease and the anogenital mucosa is usually affected. The viral inoculation that produces the less common oral lesions results from direct contact.

Clinical features. Condylomas of the oral mucosa are relatively soft, pale, and papillomatous enlargements of mucous membranes. The lesions are usually sharply delineated and may

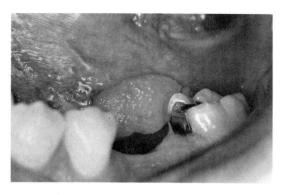

Fig. 18-4 Condyloma acuminatum. Coalescing soft, pink, broad-based lesions with finely stippled surfaces were located on the ventral tongue. History was positive for venereal warts of the penis.

appear sessile or pedunculated (Fig. 18-4). The typical locations are the labial mucosa and tongue. Multiple separate lesions often develop in a cluster pattern and may eventually coalesce to produce enlargements significantly larger than 1 cm in diameter. A history of oral contact with similar anogenital lesions of an infected partner is a typical finding. An increased incidence of venereal warts occurs among HIV seropositive individuals.

Differential diagnosis. Focal epithelial hyperplasia is the only other condition of the oral mucosa to routinely produce multiple papillomatous lesions. The finely granular surface texture and plaquelike shape of the enlargements produced by this condition can be distinguished in most cases from the cauliflower-like appearance of condylomas. Also, focal epithelial hyperplasia tends to affect younger Native Americans. Multiple verruca may be a diagnostic possibility when the lips are affected, but the occurrence of multiple intraoral verrucae is rare.

Management decisions. Excision of all lesions is the recommended treatment. The procedure should be accomplished with care to avoid inoculation of adjacent tissues. A medical referral is indicated to accomplish removal of genital lesions from both partners in order to prevent reinfection. Diagnosis of condyloma acuminatum in a child is suggestive of sexual abuse and must be reported to appropriate agencies.

Focal Epithelial Hyperplasia

Definition. Focal epithelial hyperplasia or *Heck's disease* is caused by a human papillomavirus subtype. The condition is rare among white individuals, whereas it is relatively common among certain Native American groups. The ethnic predilection of this condition may be related to a genetic cofactors that increase the vulnerability of the individual to the viral infection.

Clinical features. Multiple soft, papular or plaquelike lesions that occur in clusters characterize the presentation of focal epithelial hyperplasia. The mucosal surface of the lip, buccal mucosa, and tongue are the most commonly affected sites. The lesions are nontender and usually appear slightly pale. Drying the lesions reveals a finely granular surface texture. Focal epithelial hyperplasia is typically observed among children, although this condition may affect a wide age range.

Differential diagnosis. Condyloma acuminatum is the condition with the greatest similarity to focal epithelial hyperplasia. The differences in surface texture and affected age groups have been described in the differential diagnosis discussion of condyloma. Several rare genetic conditions such as tuberous sclerosis, Darier's disease, and multiple hamartoma syndrome may cause similar oral lesions. These conditions can usually be excluded from consideration in the absence of other anomalies such as cutaneous lesions.

Management decisions. Confirmation of the clinical diagnosis may require microscopic examination of excised tissue. Otherwise, no treatment is indicated. Many of these lesions will eventually regress without treatment.

ACUTE INFLAMMATORY ENLARGEMENTS

Acute inflammatory enlargements are characterized by abrupt onset, rapid progression, compressible tissue distention, erythema, pain, and tenderness to pressure. Systemic manifestations such as fever, malaise, and lymphadenopathy may develop if the inflammation progresses from a localized to a regional process. These features of acute inflammation provide a reliable basis for differentiating these common lesions from other soft tissue enlargements. A definitive diagnosis can generally be reached on the basis of these features and the cause of the acute inflammation, which is apparent in most instances, as summarized in Fig. 18-5. Eliminating the source of inflammation generally produces rapid resolution of the lesion. However, recurring cycles of partial resolution and acute exacerbation often result if this is not accomplished. Effective treatment of these enlargements is a clinical priority to prevent serious disseminated infections.

Soft Tissue Abscess

Definition. The soft tissue abscess is a focal collection of pus in response to a noxious stimulus. This lesion is the most common entity in the category of acute inflammatory enlargements. Most oral examples are a sequela of advanced periodontitis or pulpal necrosis, although tissue impaction of a foreign body can elicit a similar response. An alveolar abscess is occasionally referred to as a *parulis* or *gum boil*.

Clinical features. The gingiva and alveolar mucosa are the typical sites of occurrence. These tender, compressible swellings may appear erythematous or yellowish-white in color. Palpation often produces a purulent exudate (Fig. 18-6). Careful probing in many cases reveals a sinus tract that extends from the surface to the source of the bacterial infection. Abscesses associated with a sinus tract are generally less painful because this passage allows release of inflammatory pressure. The appearance of regional lymphadenopathy indicates that the infection is no longer localized and some patients, especially children, will become febrile. Radiographs contribute to the identification of the source of most odontogenic abscesses.

The clinical course of oral abscesses is unpredictable. Most dental abscesses are actually an acute exacerbation of a chronic dental infection. The acute infection usually subsides when the purulence drains. Removal of the source of the infection produces dramatic reduction of the swelling within hours or days. If the source of infection remains untreated, however, the acute infection eventually recurs. This "waxing and waning" of dental abscesses is frequently seen among patients who refuse definitive treatment of the infection.

Differential diagnosis. Demonstration of purulence and a source of the infection associated with an alveolar enlargement is an adequate basis for a definitive diagnosis. Cystic lesions of the jaws occasionally become secondarily infected and can exhibit many of the features of an alveolar abscess. Radiographic features and pulp testing generally clarify whether or not the infection is related to the teeth. Several alveolar enlargements such as the pyogenic granuloma are compressible and appear erythematous, but these lesions can be distinguished from abscesses by the absence of pain and purulence. The mucous retention phenomenon may appear superficially similar to the soft tissue abscess. These lesions are generally less painful than an abscess, and the drainage from the mucous retention phenomenon appears watery or slightly cloudy in contrast to the creamy white or cheesy appearance of purulence.

Management decisions. Effective treatment requires the removal of the source of the infection. Most alveolar abscesses resolve following periodontal or endodontic procedures or the extraction of the tooth. Incision and drainage may be appropriate if focal fluctuance has developed. Antibiotic therapy is not a rou-

Fig. 18-5 Differential diagnosis of acute inflammatory soft tissue enlargements.

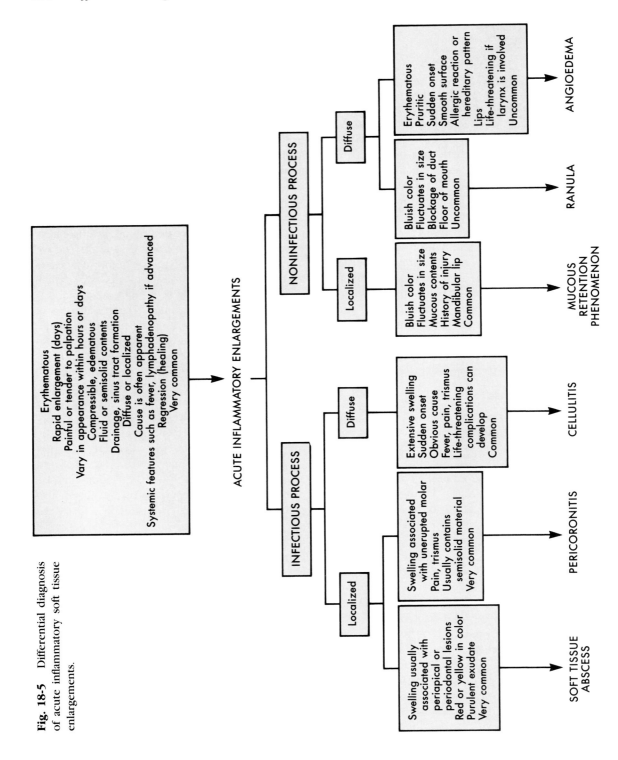

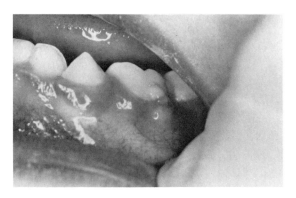

Fig. 18-6 Gingival abscess. Purulent exudate was expressed from this tender, pale nodule of the attached gingiva. Entrapment of a foreign body in the gingival sulcus was suspected. The lesion resolved following curettage.

tinely recommended treatment for localized abscesses unless systemic features such as fever are apparent or the patient is immunocompromised. Penicillin is the antibiotic of choice for nonallergic patients. Bacterial culture and antibiotic sensitivity testing are indicated for abscesses that persist after elimination of the source of infection and empiric antibiotic therapy.

Pericoronitis

Definition. Pericoronitis or *acute operculitis* is a common inflammatory lesion of the gingiva surrounding partially erupted molars. The infection is caused by entrapment of bacteria, plaque, and food material in the pericoronal space as described in Chapter 8. The likelihood of developing pericoronitis increases with longer duration of the incomplete eruption.

Clinical features. Pericoronitis produces edema, erythema, and tenderness of the gingival tissues surrounding the crown of a partially erupted tooth (see Chapter 8, Fig. 8-14). The tenderness is usually localized but may radiate to the face and ear. Trismus is a common feature of more severe examples and the soft tissue swelling is frequently aggravated by trauma from the opposing tooth. Patients usually describe a foul taste, and regional lymph nodes are palpable and tender during acute episodes. Careful probing or lavage produces purulent exudate or granular, semisolid material from the pericoronal space.

The patient usually describes a cyclic clinical course of exacerbation interspersed with remission as the eruption of the tooth proceeds. Cellulitis is a common complication of this infection because of the proximity of the buccinator and masseter muscle spaces.

Differential diagnosis. A definitive diagnosis of pericoronitis is usually straightforward with the identification of the offending tooth associated with inflammation and purulence. Myofascial pain secondary to temporomandibular joint dysfunction is a common cause of similar trismus and pain among adolescents and young adults. However, this condition is not associated with focal tissue inflammation of tissues near a partially erupted tooth unless the progression of pericoronitis has triggered myofascial symptoms.

Management decisions. Lavage of the inflamed lesion by the dentist and antibiotic therapy usually lead to rapid resolution of the acute infection. Definitive treatment depends on the eruption status of the causative tooth. If eruption of the molar appears likely, then a gingivectomy may be necessary. The removal of gingival tissue prevents recurrences by promoting eruption and minimizing the entrapment of debris. Extraction is appropriate if eruption is unlikely. Delaying extraction until the acute infection has resolved decreases the risk of subperiosteal abscess or cellulitis following removal of the tooth.

Cellulitis

Definition. Cellulitis is the extension of a localized inflammatory process into adjacent soft tissue spaces that produces a regional soft tissue infection and enlargement. Chronic dental infections are a common source of cellulitis

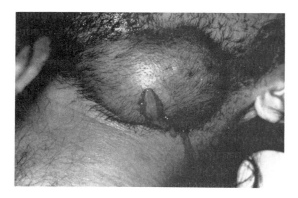

Fig. 18-7 Cellulitis. A diffuse, painful, submandibular swelling developed suddenly, secondary to a chronically infected molar. Copious purulent exudate was drained from the site. (Courtesy of Dr Brian R Smith, University of Texas Health Science Center at San Antonio.)

of the face and neck. Group A, β-hemolytic streptococcus is the causative microorganism in most cases because this bacteria elaborates hyaluronidase. This enzyme alters the connective tissue integrity, which destroys the normal protection barriers to infection and promotes suppurative infiltration.

Clinical features. Extensive edema, erythema, pain, and facial asymmetry are the predominant features of cellulitis as illustrated by the dramatic example in Fig. 18-7. The enlargement feels warm when palpated and the compressibility of the affected tissues varies from indurated and rigid to soft and fluctuant. Onset is sudden and dramatic progression within hours is typical. Fever, malaise, and lymphadenopathy are prominent and consistent features of cellulitis. Spontaneous formation of an intraoral or extraoral sinus tract with drainage of a purulent exudate may develop or the infection may continue to spread into adjacent tissue spaces. Clinical and radiographic examinations usually demonstrate a periapical lesion secondary to pulpal necrosis, pericoronitis, or other dental infection. Patients often describe a history of cyclic episodes of dental

pain interspersed with asymptomatic periods.

Differential diagnosis. The combination of clinical and systemic findings is characteristic of an extensive, acute inflammatory condition. The diagnostic challenge usually relates to determining the severity and extent of the infection. Ranula, angioedema, and emphysema may also produce diffuse, fluctuant enlargements of acute onset. *Emphysema* is entrapment of air within soft tissues that is usually iatrogenically produced during dental procedures. Characteristic features of this condition include crepitus during palpation and the expression of bubbly, clear fluid rather than a purulent exudate from the site. Angioedema produces rapid enlargement, but the swelling is less painful than that of acute bacterial infections. The ranula develops within a longer time period and is characterized by more mild, episodic tenderness. All three of these conditions are distinguishable from cellulitis by the absence of purulence, lack of a source of the infection, and absence of systemic features such as fever.

Management decisions. Cellulitis is a serious infection capable of rapid progression. The condition demands immediate attention in order to prevent potentially life-threatening complications. These include progression to septicemia and compromised airway from submandibular enlargement known as *Ludwig's angina.* Also, anterior maxillary infections can spread via the venous channels into the cavernous sinus of the brain and cause intravascular coagulation referred to as *cavernous sinus thrombosis.* Marked periorbital swelling, difficulty breathing, or dramatic fever, in addition to other signs of cellulitis, warrants immediate hospitalization and intravenous antibiotic therapy. Less severe examples of cellulitis can be managed on an outpatient basis but frequent clinical reevaluation is mandatory. Noncompliance with treatment or development of resistance to the prescribed antibiotic can allow rapid progression of the infection.

A broad spectrum antibiotic and the establishment of drainage are the recommended treatment of cellulitis. Incision and drainage should not be attempted, however, unless a soft, fluctuant site can be identified. The exudate obtained from the drainage site should be submitted for culture and sensitivity testing. Treatment of the local source of infection is necessary following improvement of the regional infection.

Mucous Retention Phenomenon

The mucous retention phenomenon is a common soft tissue enlargement that is also known as a *mucocele* and *mucous extravasation phenomenon.* This lesion is noninfectious in contrast to the previously described lesions of this group. It is caused by traumatic injury to a salivary duct, which results in the release of mucin into the surrounding connective tissue. This accumulation of mucin induces a localized inflammatory reaction and organization of a peripheral tissue border surrounding the extravasated fluid.

The term *ranula* refers to a mucous retention phenomenon that forms in the floor of the mouth. It is usually associated with the sublingual gland, whereas the submandibular gland is less commonly involved. Ranulas tend to be significantly larger than the mucous retention phenomena of minor salivary glands. A *plunging ranula* refers to the herniation of mucoid material from a ranula through the mylohyoid muscle and into the fascial spaces of the neck.

Clinical features. The lesions are compressible, dome-shaped, and bluish to translucent in appearance with mild peripheral erythema. The superficial mucosa appears smooth and intact unless secondary injury has caused ecchymosis or ulceration. The mandibular labial mucosa is the most common location (see Fig. 11-6, *A*), although the mucous retention phenomenonn can occur wherever minor salivary glands are present. A ranula exhibits similar features but is larger and located lateral to the midline of the floor of the mouth (Fig. 18-8).

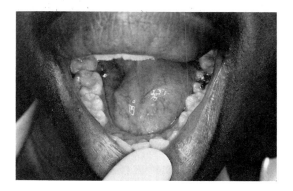

Fig. 18-8 Ranula. This unilateral, compressible, tender swelling appeared suddenly in the floor of the mouth. This fluid-filled mass reached its maximum size in the morning, slowly decreasing in size during the day.

Mild tenderness to pressure is typical. Superficial lesions appear localized in contrast to deeper lesions that are less delineated. These lesions tend to fluctuate in size because of resorption of the mucoid contents or release of the fluid through a minor injury to the surface epithelium. Patients complain of a salty flavor when this fluid escapes. The accumulation of fluid recurs once the surface epithelium heals. Children and adolescents are most often affected by this inflammatory enlargement. A history of facial injury usually coincides with the location and onset of the lesion.

Differential diagnosis. The fluctuation in size of the mucous retention phenomenon is similar to the cyclic course of many abscesses. However, the erythematous to yellowish-white color and greater tenderness of the abscess indicates the greater degree of inflammation. In addition, the purulent content of abscesses can usually be expressed with minimal digital pressure. The translucent bluish color of mucous retention phenomena may resemble vascular enlargements. Both of these lesions are compressible, and both are common in the pediatric age group. Vascular lesions are usually darker, blanch when compressed, and are constant in size. When the clinical features are less distinctive, aspiration may help the dentist to distinguish between these lesions by demonstrating their contents.

Ranulas may in some instance enlarge relatively rapidly similar to cellulitis. However, the absence of fever and minimal tenderness support the diagnosis of ranula. Mucoepidermoid carcinoma and adenocarcinomas occasionally contain a significant fluid component that is similar to a mucous retention phenomenon or ranula. Although these malignant neoplasms may be compressible, they produce persistent enlargement without fluctuation in size. Also, an older patient population is affected.

The ranula can also be confused with ductal dilation and sialoadenitis caused by obstruction of the submandibular duct by a sialolith or mucus plug. This condition usually causes progressive glandular pain and enlargement during secretory stimulation while eating or drinking. An occlusal radiograph may be helpful in identifying a ductal salivary stone. Dermoid cysts and thyroglossal tract cysts are uncommon enlargements of the floor of the mouth that are distinguished by their midline location in contrast to the lateral location of most ranulas.

Management decisions. Excision is the preferred treatment for the mucous retention phenomenon. The excision must include the associated minor salivary gland, or recurrence is predictable. Incision and drainage is seldom effective. Marsupialization is the recommended treatment for most ranulas. If the lesions recur, then surgical extirpation of the associated submandibular or sublingual gland is indicated.

Angioedema

Definition. Angioedema produces rapid tissue enlargement by immune mediated mechanisms. The acquired form accounts for the majority of cases and is an IgE-mediated allergic reaction that is usually triggered by a specific food or drug. The hereditary variant of

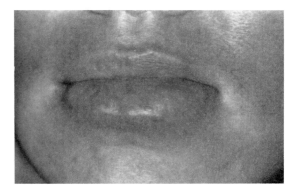

Fig. 18-9 Angioedema. This adolescent boy developed a diffuse pruritic swelling of the mandibular lip following the ingestion of an aspirin product. Note the amount of edema with subsequent loss of normal vertical wrinkling of the vermilion border.

angioedema is an autosomal dominant trait related to both a qualitative and quantitative deficiency of C1 esterase inhibitor. Traumatic injury may be a triggering factor in the hereditary form of angioedema.

Clinical features. Angioedema produces a diffuse, soft, painless swelling that results from the accumulation of edematous fluids within the affected tissues (Fig. 18-9). The upper lip is the most common site of occurrence, although other areas of the face, oral cavity, and pharynx may be affected. A prodromal pruritus often precedes the sudden onset of the swelling. The enlargement regresses within several hours to 1 or 2 days. Urticaria frequently accompanies the enlargement, and recurrences are common. Airway obstruction may occur in severe cases that affect the tongue, uvula, and larynx.

Differential diagnosis. The diffuse, rapid enlargement of angioedema is similar to that of cellulitis, but the erythema, pain, and purulence of a bacterial infection are absent in angioedema. Also, a source of infection in the anterior maxilla would be expected with cellulitis and absent with angioedema.

Management decisions. The allergen affecting the hypersensitive individual should be identified, if possible, to decrease the risk of recurrences and development of more severe hypersensitive reactions. Because tissue trauma can trigger episodes in the hereditary form of angioedema, dental procedures should be accomplished so as to minimize tissue injury. Systemic antihistamines are used to manage most episodes of angioedema, although mild cases may require only observation. Corticosteroids are administered in severe cases of respiratory distress. A rare, serious complication of angioedema is progression to anaphylactic shock.

REACTIVE HYPERPLASIAS

Most reactive hyperplasias develop in response to a chronic, recurring tissue injury that stimulates an exuberant or excessive tissue repair response. These inflammatory enlargements are characterized by a moderate growth rate, absence of discomfort, and lack of systemic symptoms. The superficial mucosa is usually intact but the surface may appear pale or erythematous in color with a smooth, bosselated, or fissured texture. Most of these enlargements are localized and sessile or pedunculated in shape. A generalized or multifocal lesion distribution is observed when these reactive lesions are caused by medications, hormonal imbalances, or ill-fitting dentures. The degree of vascularity and edema of the enlargement determines the color and compressibility of the mass. Reactive hyperplasia slowly develops within several months and exhibits a limited growth potential. Partial regression of the enlargement may occur after removal of the source of tissue injury. The differential diagnosis of reactive hyperplasias is summarized in Fig. 18-10.

Traumatic Fibroma

Definition. The traumatic fibroma is one of the most common soft tissue enlargements of the oral cavity. The term *fibroma* is a misnomer for this reactive lesion because it is not a true neoplasm of fibrous connective tissue. The pathologist often uses the designation *localized fibrous hyperplasia,* which more accurately describes the nature of the lesion. Most traumatic fibromas represent exuberant scar formation caused by recurring tissue injury.

Clinical features. The traumatic fibroma is a localized, slow-growing, dome-shaped to polypoid enlargement with a smooth surface. This lesion is generally firm, uniformly pale to normal in color, and painless unless recent injury has occurred. The traumatic fibroma has limited growth potential and most examples remain static in size for many years. The patient ordinarily cannot specifically associate the lesion with a traumatic incident. The lesions are most often located where masticatory injury is likely such as the gingiva, tongue, and buccal mucosa (Fig. 18-11).

Differential diagnosis. The clinical features of a traumatic fibroma are not unique. These submucosal enlargements resemble other lesions in this category and benign mesenchymal and salivary gland neoplasms. The location at a site prone to injury and the static size of the traumatic fibroma are the most reliable features in distinguishing this reactive lesion from neoplasms that typically exhibit progressive enlargement.

Differentiation of traumatic fibromas of the gingiva and alveolar mucosa from other reactive gingival enlargements in this lesion group can be difficult. These include the peripheral ossifying fibroma, the peripheral giant cell granuloma, and the pyogenic granuloma. The peripheral ossifying fibroma and traumatic fibroma are both pale, firm, and nontender. The peripheral ossifying fibroma may be firmer because of calcified material within the stroma. In addition, the peripheral ossifying fibroma exhibits a tendency to displace adjacent teeth. The pyogenic granuloma and the peripheral giant cell granuloma generally appear more vas-

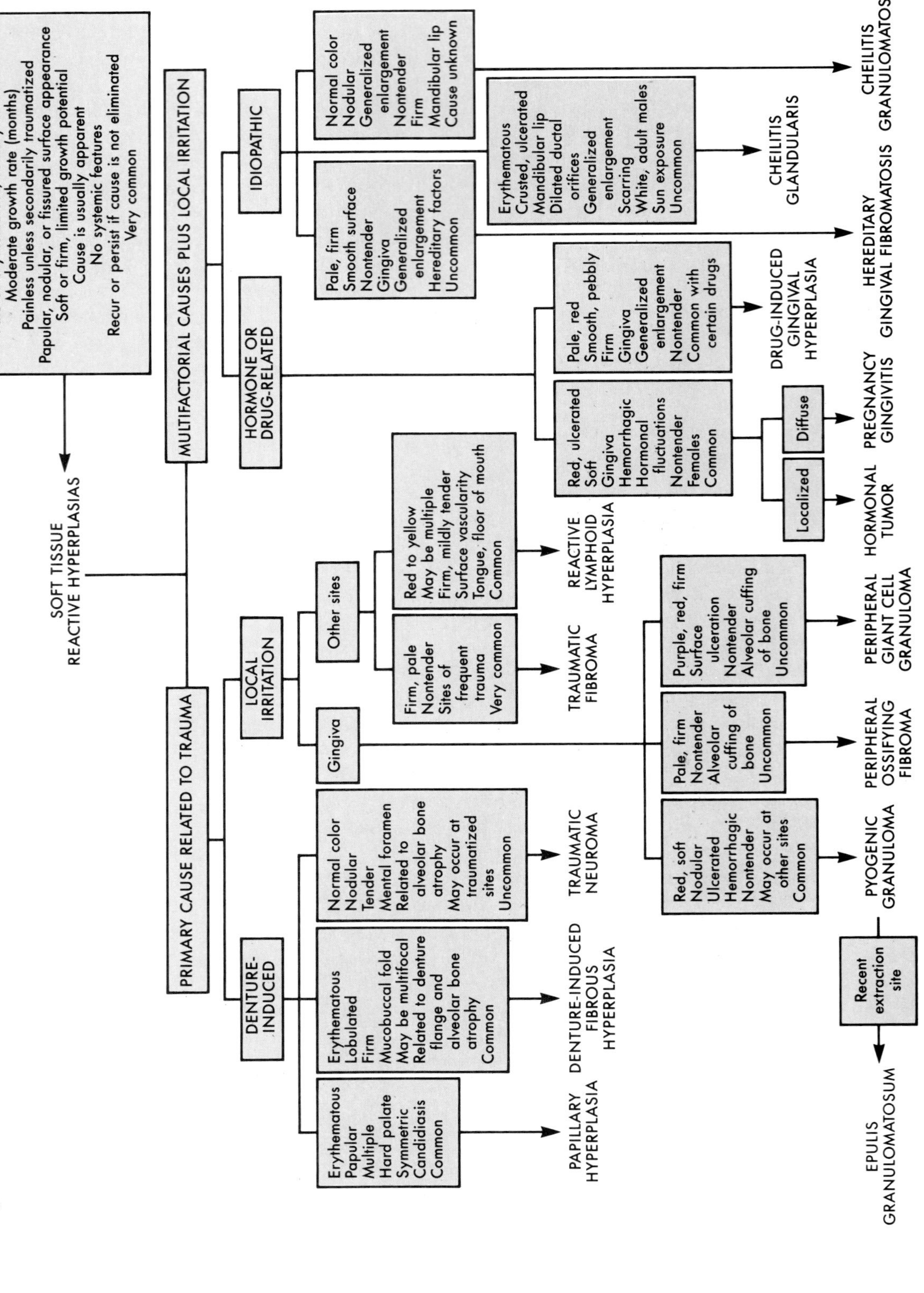

Fig. 18-10   Differential diagnosis of soft tissue reactive hyperplasias of the oral cavity.

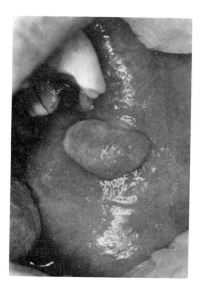

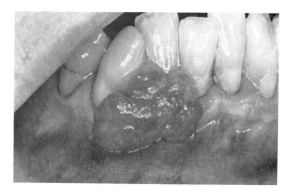

Fig. 18-12 Pyogenic granuloma. This vascular, bosselated lesion of the attached gingiva bled when manipulated. Previous placement of multiple composite resin restorations with poorly contoured margins was a contributing factor.

Fig. 18-11 Traumatic fibroma. Firm, pedunculated mass of the buccal mucosa slowly increased in size over a period of many years. Surface erythema is related to habitual biting of the lesion.

cular and may bleed when palpated or probed.

Management decisions. Excisional biopsy is the treatment of choice for many traumatic fibromas since they are difficult to distinguish from benign neoplasms. Also, many patients function more comfortably after removal of larger traumatic fibromas. If possible, the source of recurring injury should be eliminated to minimize the probability of recurrence. Documentation and periodic reexamination of the suspected traumatic fibromas may be justified in some cases of asymptomatic lesions that exhibit static growth.

Pyogenic Granuloma

Definition. The pyogenic granuloma is a reactive enlargement that is an inflammatory response to a local irritation such as calculus, a fractured tooth, rough dental restorations, and foreign materials. This lesion differs from the other reactive hyperplasias because it usually has an ulcerated, friable surface. These surface changes result from a cyclic pattern of second-ary irritation by oral fluids and microorganisms. A hormonal imbalance is a contributing factor to the development of some pyogenic granulomas. For this reason, this lesion is occasionally referred to as a *pregnancy* or *hormonal tumor.*

Clinical features. The pyogenic granuloma is a nontender nodule with either a pedunculated (Fig. 18-12) or sessile base. These lesions usually appear deep red with yellowish-white foci. Palpation does not produce blanching but frequently causes hemorrhage. Friable ulceration of the surface is typical and pronounced examples may exhibit a variegated red and white pattern. The gingiva is the primary oral site of occurrence, although pyogenic granulomas may develop on the lower lip, buccal mucosa, and tongue. Most pyogenic granulomas are solitary, but development of multiple lesions is not uncommon when hormonal imbalance is a contributory factor. In particular, the hormonal fluctuations during pregnancy and puberty can account for this exaggerated proliferative response to focal irritation. Pyogenic granulomas occur more frequently among females, and a wide age range is affected.

Differential diagnosis. The peripheral giant cell granuloma and the peripheral ossifying fibroma are reactive hyperplasias that should be included in the differential diagnosis of a suspected pyogenic granuloma. These enlargements are firm to palpation and only occur on the gingiva and alveolar mucosa. The peripheral ossifying fibroma is pale unless incidentally traumatized, whereas the peripheral giant cell granuloma has a purplish-red appearance. Both of these lesions may demonstrate radiographic evidence of superficial cuffing of the alveolar bone in contrast to the pyogenic granuloma. Many pyogenic granulomas fibrose with time and appear identical to the traumatic fibroma. Lack of pain and absence of purulence allow distinction of pyogenic granulomas from soft tissue abscesses.

The vascular appearance of a pyogenic granuloma is suggestive of a capillary hemangioma. Most hemangiomas are congenital lesions that blanch with pressure. Injury and surgical manipulation produce moderate to brisk hemorrhage. Nodular lesions of Kaposi's sarcoma are purplish-red enlargements that are indistinguishable from pyogenic granulomas in appearance, but lesions of Kaposi's sarcoma are usually multifocal and are manifestations of AIDS.

Management decisions. Excisional biopsy is the recommended treatment for a suspected pyogenic granuloma. The associated source of local irritation must be eliminated or recurrence is likely. Occasionally, small hemorrhagic lesions will significantly regress after the removal of the cause.

Epulis Granulomatosum

Definition. Epulis granulomatosum is a reactive hyperplasia that develops within a tooth socket after the extraction or exfoliation of a tooth. The majority of these lesions are caused by bone spicules or root fragments retained within the healing socket.

Clinical features. Epulis granulomatosum is exuberant, dark red granulation tissue extruding from a tooth socket. This nonpainful lesion can occur at almost any age and it be-

comes apparent within 2 weeks after the loss of a tooth. The enlargement is soft and hemorrhagic with an erythematous to white, smooth surface. A small radiopacity suggestive of a root or bone fragment may be demonstrated within the tooth socket.

Differential diagnosis. A pulp polyp, an antral polyp, or, rarely, an intrabony malignancy can resemble an epulis granulomatosum. The pulp polyp is a chronic hyperplastic pulpitis associated with severe decay that has exposed the dental pulp of a molar tooth. Extensive crown destruction by decay may allow the pulp polyp to essentially cover the remaining roots, which are revealed radiographically. Extrusion of an antral polyp through an oroantral fistula into a recent extraction site of a maxillary posterior tooth may appear similar to epulis granulomatosum. However, the sinus wall defect is usually demonstrated either radiographically or by requesting the patient to blow air through the nose while the nostrils are occluded.

Management decisions. Curettage to remove the granulation tissue and smoothing the socket borders is indicated. If unusual radiographic alterations of the socket suggest the possibility of a central lesion of bone, an excisional biopsy is appropriate.

Peripheral Ossifying Fibroma

Definition. The peripheral ossifying fibroma has also been referred to as the *peripheral odontogenic fibroma, peripheral fibroma with ossification,* and *peripheral fibroma.* Although specific microscopic differences are associated with each of these designations, no significant clinical differences distinguish these entities. As with other reactive hyperplasias, the peripheral ossifying fibroma develops in response to a chronic inflammatory irritant.

Clinical features. The peripheral ossifying fibroma is a slow-growing, pale enlargement with a pedunculated or sessile base. The surface is smooth or bosselated with foci of ulceration in some cases. This abnormality is non-

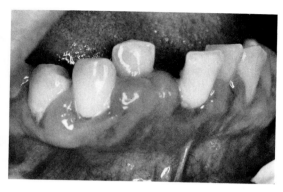

Fig. 18-13 Peripheral ossifying fibroma. Firm, smooth-surfaced, gingival enlargement resulted in the lingual displacement of the mandibular lateral incisor.

tender and firm to palpation, and occasionally it feels gritty to bony hard, depending on the proportion of calcified material within the lesion.

Peripheral ossifying fibromas develop in most cases from the gingiva or alveolar mucosa mesial to the first molar. The peripheral ossifying fibroma occurs more frequently among young adult women. The slow, persistent growth of this reactive lesion may cause gradual displacement of the adjacent teeth, as suggested in Fig. 18-13. Occasionally, an intraoral radiograph will demonstrate superficial erosion of the underlying alveolar bone and varying amounts of calcified material within the lesion.

Differential diagnosis. This lesion should be differentiated from other localized gingival enlargements, in particular the pyogenic granuloma and the peripheral giant cell granuloma. These latter conditions are characterized by greater vascularity that is reflected by their red or reddish-blue color and tendency to bleed. In contrast, the peripheral ossifying fibroma is pale and firmer to palpation and radiographic evidence of focal opacities may be present.

Management decisions. Surgical excision is the recommended treatment for this reac-

tive lesion. The excision should extend deep to include the affected periodontal ligament. Recurrences may develop after incomplete removal of the lesion and failure to eliminate the source of irritation.

Peripheral Giant Cell Granuloma

Definition. The peripheral giant cell granuloma is the least common of the reactive gingival hyperplasias. This lesion is thought to arise from the periodontal ligament or periosteal tissues in response to chronic irritation. This reactive enlargement should not be confused with the central giant cell granuloma that originates within the cortices of the mandible and maxilla.

Clinical features. The peripheral giant cell granuloma is a slightly compressible, broad-based enlargement that appears red to purplish-red in color. This nontender lesion exhibits a smooth surface that may become ulcerated as a consequence of incidental injury. Slight pressure or probing usually induces hemorrhage. Location is limited to the gingiva or alveolar mucosa and most examples occur anterior to the first molar.

This reactive hyperplasia increases in size within several weeks and then tends to remain static with an average size of approximately 1 cm. Females are more commonly affected, and the incidence involves a wide age range. Radiographic evidence of a depression or cuffing of the alveolar bone may be apparent when the lesion occurs on an edentulous site.

Differential diagnosis. This reactive gingival lesion is clinically indistinguishable from the pyogenic granuloma in most cases. Therefore the same differential diagnosis developed for that lesion is applicable for the peripheral giant cell granuloma.

Management decisions. Excisional biopsy and elimination of any source of chronic irritation in the area are the recommended treatments. Recurrences are uncommon if complete excision of the lesion is accomplished.

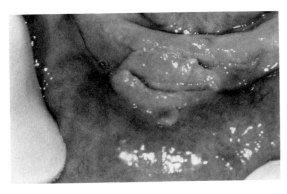

Fig. 18-14 Denture-induced fibrous hyperplasia. Lobulated, firm mass of the mandibular mucobuccal fold was associated with a poorly fitting denture. Note the deep, ulcerated fissure where the denture flange traumatized the tissue.

Denture-Induced Fibrous Hyperplasia

Definition. Denture-induced fibrous hyperplasia is synonymous with the terms *inflammatory fibrous hyperplasia* and *epulis fissuratum*. This reactive tissue enlargement is caused by recurring injury to alveolar tissue by the flange of a denture or other appliance and by loss of alveolar ridge height. Dense scar tissue forms in response to chronic pressure from a denture that is unstable during function or from an overextended flange.

Clinical features. Denture-induced fibrous hyperplasia is a firm, pale to erythematous enlargement of the alveolar mucosa, mucobuccal fold, or the floor of the mouth. This lesion has an elongated, elliptical shape with deep folds or fissures as shown in Fig. 18-14. The denture flange often fits into a prominent fold when the enlargement is located near the peripheral extent of the prosthesis. Usually this redundant tissue is nontender unless the pressure from the denture is excessive. Several lesions may correspond to the denture border and the alveolar crest because these lesions are usually caused by generalized osseous atrophy of the entire alveolar ridge.

Differential diagnosis. The direct relationship of this lesion with an ill-fitting denture and alveolar atrophy usually justifies a definitive diagnosis. Dramatic examples may suggest the possibility of a benign neoplasm. However, neoplastic lesions slowly displace the denture by progressive enlargement rather than conforming to the contours of the prosthesis.

Management decisions. Discontinuation of use of the ill-fitting denture may yield partial regression of this reactive enlargement, especially when the tissue is inflamed and edematous. Surgical removal of denture-induced fibrous hyperplasia is usually required to restore optimal tissue contours for prosthetic adaptation. The offending prosthetic appliance must be adjusted, relined, or reconstructed to avoid recurrence.

Papillary Hyperplasia

Definition. Papillary hyperplasia is also known as *palatal papillomatosis* and *inflammatory papillary hyperplasia*. This reactive lesion is usually associated with a removable prosthetic appliance that is worn continuously. A superimposed candidiasis of the mucosa supporting the denture is the stimulus for this hyperplastic tissue response of the hard palate. This tissue reaction is occasionally observed in individuals with a narrow, prominent palatal vault who do not wear an appliance.

Clinical features. This reactive lesion is characterized by numerous small, papillary enlargements of the hard palate. These pebbly to nodular thickenings of the mucosa (Fig. 18-15) tend to cluster in the palatal vault and are less prominent or absent on the alveolar mucosa. Papillary hyperplasia varies from pale to brightly erythematous in color. This granular to papillary surface texture may be firm or compressible depending on the severity of the inflammation.

Differential diagnosis. Papillary hyperplasia is unlikely to be confused with other conditions because of the characteristic appearance and location and the association with continu-

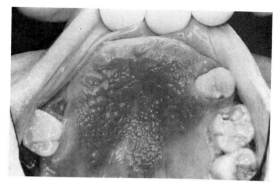

Fig. 18-15 Papillary hyperplasia. Multiple erythematous papules were observed in the hard palate under an ill-fitting denture.

ous wearing of a denture. The association of candidiasis with this hyperplastic lesion suggests the possibility that other oral tissues may be infected.

Management decisions. Initial treatment includes wearing the denture as little as possible and using a topical antimycotic agent. The denture must also be soaked to destroy the fungus because the appliance serves as an organism reservoir. In many cases this is adequate treatment. If mucosal thickening persists after resolution of the infection and inflammation, removal of the enlargement by a superficial surgical stripping procedure may be necessary. This usually requires relining of the denture or fabrication of a new prosthesis.

Traumatic Neuroma

Definition. The traumatic neuroma is a reactive enlargement that consists of disorganized repair and scarring of a peripheral nerve after traumatic injury. Surgical procedures, lacerations, and recurring compression by a denture are the most common sources of oral injury. Injury to the nerve stimulates a proliferation of nerve fibers, but the presence of scar tissue, reinjury, or adjacent bone interferes with normal reinnervation and repair.

Clinical features. The traumatic neuroma usually appears initially as a firm, pale nodule with a smooth surface. A linear scar or depression is often evident in the area of tissue injury. Manipulation of the lesion produces tenderness or pain in more than one half of the cases. A reflex neuralgia is associated with some traumatic neuromas, and this neuralgia produces referred pain to a distant site of the face. Pain relief after injection of an anesthetic solution into the traumatic neuroma demonstrates it as the source of the referred pain.

A traumatic neuroma can occur in any area subjected to traumatic injury, but most intraoral examples develop near the mental foramen. They are usually caused by atrophy of the edentulous alveolar bone, which subjects the mental nerve to recurring impingement by the denture flange. The tongue, mandibular lip, and the buccal mucosa are additional sites that are occasionally affected.

Differential diagnosis. A tender, firm enlargement near the mental foramen is strongly suggestive of a traumatic neuroma. Presence of a reflex neuralgia with referred pain is also a feature of myofascial pain, atypical facial pain, and trigeminal neuralgia. Both the traumatic neuroma and trigeminal neuralgia exhibit well-defined trigger points, whereas this pattern is not a consistent finding in the other two conditions. Enlargement and pain control with anesthetic injection are unusual with trigeminal neuralgia in contrast to a traumatic neuroma. An intrabony or soft tissue abscess may mimic the pain of a traumatic neuroma. The signs and symptoms of acute inflammation, such as erythema, edema, and purulence, and a source of infection are not consistent with a the features of a traumatic neuroma.

Management decisions. Excision is optimal treatment for the traumatic neuroma, and recurrences are unlikely. Modification of the denture base with a soft lining material may provide temporary pain relief. Significant hemorrhage and paresthesia or anesthesia are potential complications of surgery in the area of the mental nerve.

Generalized Gingival Hyperplasia

Definition. Generalized gingival hyperplasia is a diffuse enlargement of the gingival tissues that can be stimulated by several conditions. The most common cause of gingival enlargement is chronic inflammation from plaque and calculus formation. Conditions associated with hormonal changes such as pregnancy and specific drugs may cause generalized gingival overgrowth. Phenytoin was the first drug associated with this gingival response and more recently cyclosporine and calcium channel blockers such as nifedipine have also been implicated. The mechanism of this drug-induced fibrous hyperplasia is not completely understood, but the reaction is not directly related to the duration or dosage of the drug. However, this hyperplastic response of the gingiva is aggravated by the inflammation associated with poor oral hygiene.

An idiopathic form of gingival hyperplasia known as *hereditary gingival fibromatosis* or *fibromatosis gingivae* is another well-recognized condition. This form of gingival hyperplasia begins in childhood with no apparent local or systemic factors. However, a hereditary pattern of this condition has been observed in some cases.

Clinical features. Generalized enlargement of both the free and attached gingiva is present with the greatest tissue expansion involving the interdental papillae. The overgrowth is so dramatic in some cases that the gingiva covers the entire anatomic crowns of the teeth. Delayed eruption or displacement of teeth may result in some instances. The mucosal surface is usually smooth or pebbly in texture. The gingival contours are bulbous with a rolled, blunted appearance. Palpation of these hyperplastic lesions reveals spongy to firm, nontender tissue. The color varies from pale pink to deep red depending on the degree of inflammation caused by plaque and calculus accumulations.

Differential diagnosis. The generalized gingival enlargement combined with a history

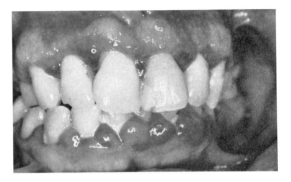

Fig. 18-16 Hormone-induced gingival hyperplasia. Pregnant woman was concerned about generalized, hemorrhagic enlargement of the gingival tissues. Gross accumulation of plaque and calculus were aggravating factors.

of pregnancy or drug therapy known to cause this side effect are adequate to make a definitive diagnosis. Hormonal-induced gingival enlargement is typically more edematous, erythematous, and hemorrhagic (Fig. 18-16) than the drug-induced lesions (Fig. 18-17). The enlargement of hereditary gingival fibromatosis is indistinguishable in appearance from the drug-induced lesions. This condition is suggested by onset at a young age, familial occurrence, and a negative history for drugs known to cause this response.

Acute leukemia is the most important disease to exclude in cases involving sudden onset of generalized gingival enlargement. Leukemic infiltration produces gingival tissues that are edematous and dramatically hemorrhagic with focal areas of petechiae. Additional features suggestive of leukemia include areas of ecchymosis, anemic pallor, halitosis, and lymphadenopathy. Malaise, fever of unknown origin, and recent unexplained weight loss are other findings suggestive of malignant disease.

Management decisions. Effective oral hygiene and frequent professional prophylaxes have been shown to minimize the enlargement in many susceptible individuals. Surgical excision is often necessary in cases of extensive en-

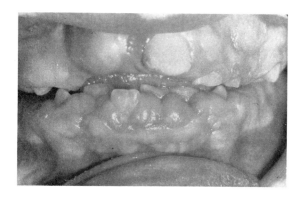

Fig. 18-17 Phenytoin-induced gingival hyperplasia. Severe generalized enlargement of the gingival tissues was observed in this mentally retarded child with a seizure disorder. This fibrous overgrowth resulted in delayed eruption and displacement of teeth.

largement. Consultation with the patient's physician may result in the substitution of an alternative medication that is less likely to cause this complication. However, most physicians are reluctant to alter an effective drug regimen to control this rather minor side effect.

Reactive Lymphoid Hyperplasia

Definition. Ectopic lymphoid tissues, also known as accessory oral tonsils, are common exophytic structures of the posterior oral cavity. These tissues may become enlarged in response to inflammatory stimulation, which results in reactive lymphoid hyperplasia. A related developmental lesion is the *lymphoepithelial cyst* (see Fig. 18-21). This lesion is clinically identical to ectopic lymphoid aggregates, but it is distinguished by microscopic demonstration of a central cystic space.

Clinical features. The nodular enlargements of reactive lymphoid hyperplasia appear edematous with a glistening, smooth surface and are yellowish-pink to brightly erythematous in color. A prominent, telangiectatic or vascular appearance of the surface may be observed. The enlargement is usually firm, movable, less than 1 cm in diameter, and nontender except during episodes of active inflammation.

Reactive lymphoid hyperplasia is a benign condition that most frequently occurs in young adult males. These lesions are widespread with a predilection for the ventral and posteriolateral tongue, floor of the mouth, anterior tonsillar pillars, and soft palate.

Differential diagnosis. The yellowish-pink, nodular appearance of a hyperplastic lymphoid aggregate is similar to that of a soft tissue abscess, lipoma, or dermoid cyst. These lesions are generally more compressible and soft to doughy when palpated. The soft tissue abscess is tender to manipulation, whereas both the superficial lipoma and the dermoid cyst are freely movable. These features are in contrast to the nontender, attached character of the reactive lymphoid aggregate.

Management decisions. No specific management is required for reactive lymphoid hyperplasia. Some lesions resolve after elimination of the source of inflammation. Excisional biopsy is appropriate if progressive enlargement suggests the possibility of a neoplasm.

Cheilitis Glandularis

Definition. Cheilitis glandularis is an uncommon inflammatory enlargement of the lips that results from chronic inflammation of the minor salivary glands. Although the exact cause of this condition is not known, several factors contribute to its progression. Chronic exposure to environmental extremes, including excessive sunlight, and bacterial infection, poor oral hygiene, tobacco use, and stress have been implicated.

Clinical features. Diffuse, firm, multinodular enlargement of the mandibular lip with subsequent eversion of the labial mucosa is the primary manifestation of this condition. This process develops within a period of several weeks to a few months. The lip surface varies from normal appearance to a white, scaly, and crusted character. Dilation of multiple ductal orifices of the minor salivary glands of the labial mucosa is a prominent feature. Occasionally, a thick exudate can be expressed from the ductal orifices. Healing with scarring is a consistent feature of this process. White men are most frequently affected.

Differential diagnosis. Cheilitis granulomatosa, sarcoidosis, angioedema, and labial cellulitis can produce diffuse swelling of the lip that is similar to that of cheilitis glandularis. Angioedema and cellulitis can usually be excluded on the basis of sudden onset, edematous compressibility, and rapid resolution. The erythema of multiple dilated ductal orifices is characteristic of cheilitis glandularis and is the most reliable feature for differentiating this condition from cheilitis granulomatosa and sarcoidosis.

Management decisions. Definitive diagnosis of this condition requires incisional biopsy and histopathologic examination of the tissue. Protection from sun exposure, improvement in oral hygiene, and topical corticosteroid application may minimize the progression of mild cases. Surgical reduction of the enlarged lip may be necessary to restore facial contours once the enlargement has been arrested. Cases of squamous cell carcinoma associated with cheilitis glandularis probably represent concurrent actinic damage to the surface epithelium rather than a premalignant tendency associated with this inflammatory process.

Cheilitis Granulomatosa

Definition. Cheilitis granulomatosa is a chronic granulomatous condition that results in diffuse lip enlargement. The cause is unknown but speculation includes the possibility of a localized form of sarcoidosis, an atypical allergic reaction to an unidentified antigen, or an unusual manifestation of regional enteritis. In some cases dental infections have been implicated as possible triggering mechanisms.

Clinical features. This condition produces

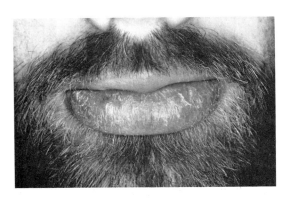

Fig. 18-18 Cheilitis granulomatosa. This diffuse, firm, mildly tender enlargement of the mandibular lip slowly increased in size within the preceding month. Intralesional steroid injections resulted in significant regression of the lesion.

a diffuse, persistent enlargement of the entire lip (Fig. 18-18) within a period of several months. The lower lip is the most common site of occurrence, although the upper lip or both lips may be affected. In rare instances the buccal mucosa, palate, and gingiva may exhibit a similar increase in size. The enlargement is firm and nontender to palpation. The mucosal surface exhibits normal color with a nodular irregularity of contour. Cheilitis granulomatosa may occur as an isolated condition or in association with fissured tongue and facial nerve paralysis. This unusual triad is referred to as *Melkersson-Rosenthal syndrome.*

Differential diagnosis. Differential diagnosis of cheilitis granulomatosa includes the same possibilities as those listed for cheilitis glandularis.

Management decisions. Incisional biopsy and histopathologic examination are required to demonstrate the granulomatous character of the enlargement. However, a definitive diagnosis of cheilitis granulomatosa requires exclusion of a chronic mycotic infection and sarcoidosis. This may include culture of tissue, serologic testing, pulmonary evaluation, and a Kveim test for sarcoidosis. Dental infections should be identified and treated to eliminate them as contributory factors.

Intralesional corticosteroid injections within a period of several weeks may control the enlargement or produce some size reduction. Surgical recontouring of the lip may eventually be necessary to achieve a satisfactory cosmetic result, but recurrence is not unusual.

BENIGN SUBMUCOSAL CYSTS AND NEOPLASMS

Benign submucosal cysts and neoplasms of the oral cavity are uncommon compared with the epithelial enlargements, acute inflammatory lesions, and reactive hyperplastic conditions previously discussed. Submucosal neoplasms and cysts are generally characterized by more similar clinical features than distinctive differences. Therefore a confident diagnosis on the basis of clinical findings alone is seldom possible. For this reason, surgical removal and histopathologic examination is required for a definitive diagnosis.

The lesions in this group are usually nodular to dome-shaped, well delineated, and freely movable enlargements with the normal appearance of the superficial mucosal surface. Palpation characteristics of these lesions vary from soft to rubbery or firm depending on the tissue composition. The slow and persistent growth of these enlargements is usually apparent within a period of months to years. These lesions are painless unless they are incidentally injured or impinge on neural structures. No evidence of a direct cause or associated systemic feature is present. These enlargements appear to cause an alteration or distortion of the normal tissues rather than tissue destruction.

The differential diagnosis strategy for the numerous entities in this lesion category is illustrated in Fig. 18-19. For manageability, these submucosal lesions are subdivided and dis-

cussed as soft tissue cysts, benign mesenchymal tumors, and salivary gland neoplasms.

Soft Tissue Cysts

Definition. Soft tissue cysts are epithelial lined sacs that contain either fluid or a semisolid material. These cysts can be categorized by origin as either odontogenic or nonodontogenic. The odontogenic cysts of soft tissues are the gingival cyst, dental lamina cyst, and eruption cyst. Nonodontogenic cysts of soft tissues include the cyst of the incisive papilla, nasolabial cyst, dermoid cyst, lymphoepithelial cyst, thyroglossal tract cyst, Epstein's pearls, and Bohn's nodules.

Clinical features. Cystic enlargements are consistently well delineated and movable within loose connective tissue. They are nontender to palpation and the compressibility depends on the contents of the pathologic cavity. Fluid-filled cysts tend to be soft and fluctuant, whereas semisolid contents produce a doughy response to palpation. The surface mucosa appears smooth with a degree of discoloration that depends on the cystic contents and the depth of the lesion relative to the surface. Superficial lesions appear translucent and the color of the reflected light is generally pale blue with serous fluid content, white for proteinaceous materials, yellow in cases of high lipid content, and red if blood is present. The appearance of deeper cysts is partially masked by the overlying stroma, which yields no color change or a pale pink hue. The single most significant diagnostic feature once the cystic character of the lesion has been identified is the location of the enlargement.

Most intraoral soft tissue cysts are odontogenic and are located within the gingiva or alveolar mucosa. *Dental lamina cysts* develop as multiple pale papules aligned along the alveolar surface of neonates and usually regress spontaneously within 3 months. These lesions are also known as *gingival cysts of the newborn. Eruption cysts* are childhood lesions that

Fig. 18-19   Differential diagnosis of benign submucosal cysts and neoplasms.

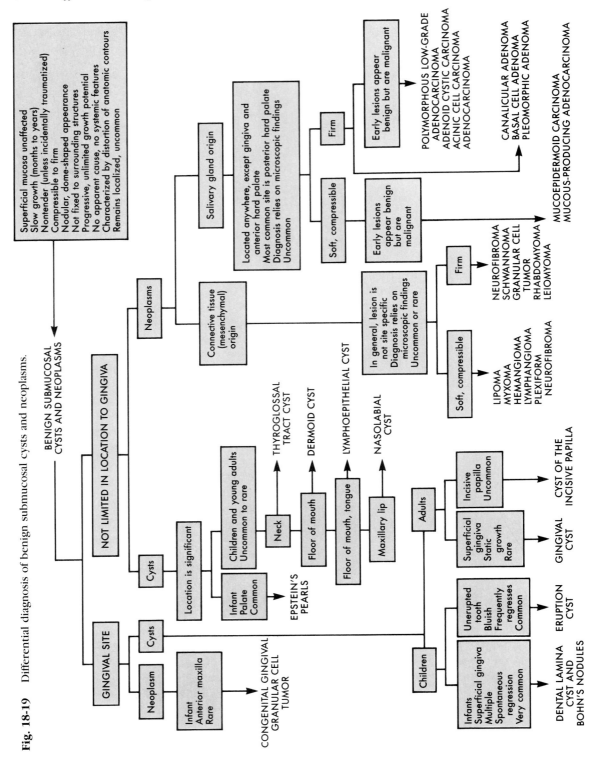

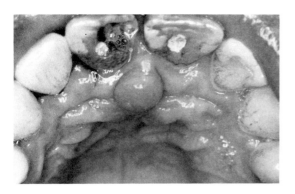

Fig. 18-20 Incisive papilla cyst. A well-circumscribed, compressible, dome-shaped mass of the anterior hard palate had not changed in size for several months. Although a dentoalveolar abscess was initially suspected, lack of pain, static growth rate, and normal radiographic findings did not support an acute inflammatory process.

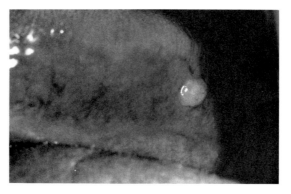

Fig. 18-21 Lymphoepithelial cyst. Well-circumscribed, soft nodule of the posterior lateral border of the tongue was found during a routine dental examination. Note the pale surface areas with evidence of superficial vascularity.

are often purplish-blue in color and develop in the site of an erupting tooth. The *gingival cyst* is typically a small, clear or pale pink enlargement of long duration on the gingiva of an adult.

Nonodontogenic soft tissue cysts are suspected when an enlargement with cystic features is located away from the gingiva and alveolus. *Epstein's pearls* are firm cystic lesions that appear similar to dental lamina cysts, but they are located at the midline of the hard palate of neonates. They develop from epithelial inclusions along this junction and spontaneously regress during infancy. Bohn's nodules are also similar to dental lamina cysts but are found along the buccal and lingual apsects of the dental ridges. The *cyst of the incisive papilla* (Fig. 18-20) initially appears as a compressible enlargement of the incisive papilla of adults. The superior extent of the labial vestibule near the maxillary canine eminence is the location of the *nasolabial cyst*. This lesion is usually the color of the surrounding tissues and affects middle-aged adults. The midline of the floor of the mouth is the most common lo-

cation of an intraoral *dermoid cyst*, which is a pale, doughy enlargement of adults. The *thyroglossal tract cyst* is usually a midline enlargement of the neck, although the posterior tongue is a possible intraoral site of occurrence. This cyst generally develops before age 30 and exhibits the color of the adjacent normal tissues. The *lymphoepithelial cyst* is most often located in the floor of the mouth or the ventral surface of the tongue (Fig. 18-21). This lesion appears pale yellow or yellowish-pink and is most common among young adults.

Differential diagnosis. The patient's age and the site and color of gingival and alveolar cysts provide an adequate basis on which to make a definitive diagnosis from among the three possible odontogenic cysts. The primary consideration is the exclusion of compressible, inflammatory dental lesions such as pericoronitis and chronic periodontal abscesses on the basis of pain, tenderness, and exudate.

Nonodontogenic cysts that occur in areas other than the gingiva and alveolar process may resemble a number of lesions that are compressible including hemangiomas, lymphangiomas, lipomas, and mucous retention phenomena, depending on the lesion location.

Hemangiomas can be distinguished by blanching during palpation and the less delineated character of the lesion margins. Mucous retention phenomena are mildly tender, fluctuate in size, and are often related to a traumatic injury in contrast to cysts.

The features of a dermoid cyst are similar to those of a lymphoepithelial cyst, lipoma, ranula, salivary gland tumor, or superiorly located thyroglossal tract cyst. All these lesions occur in the anterior floor of the mouth or submental region. However, the thyroglossal tract cyst and dermoid cyst are typically midline structures, while the other lesions are likely to be located laterally. The thyroglossal tract cyst is difficult to differentiate from the dermoid cyst if it is located inferior to the mylohyoid muscle. Movement of the mass with swallowing or extension of the tongue favors a diagnosis of thyroglossal tract cyst because of its usual indirect attachment to the hyoid bone. The yellowish color, compressibility, and distinct delineation of the lymphoepithelial cyst make it difficult to distinguish from a lipoma.

The nasolabial cyst may be difficult to differentiate from other compressible lesions that develop in the labial vestibule near the canine. These include salivary gland neoplasms, lipomas, and an odontogenic infection that has perforated the cortical bone. An infection can usually be eliminated as a possible cause in the absence of pain, purulence, and an obvious dental source of inflammation.

Management decisions. Aspiration of a cyst may provide contributory information concerning the contents of the lesion and aid in the differential diagnosis. A watery, straw colored fluid is typical of nonkeratotic cysts. A thyroglossal tract cyst yields a dark amber fluid. In contrast, a thick, yellowish, granular aspirate is characteristic of the dermoid cyst. Unproductive aspiration suggests that the lesion is composed of solid tissue, which in combination with compressibility during palpation indicates a lipoma, salivary gland neoplasm, or myxoma as more likely diagnostic possibilities.

Excisional biopsy is the recommended treatment and basis for a definitive diagnosis of suspected cysts in most but not all cases. Eruption cysts usually resolve without surgical intervention when the tooth perforates the gingiva. However, "unroofing" the lesion usually expedites the eruption process and controls discomfort. Dental lamina cysts, Epstein's pearls, and Bohn's nodules usually slough spontaneously in infancy and require no treatment. Surgical excision may be inadvisable for a cystic lesion if the clinical impression is a thyroglossal tract cyst. In some cases tissues associated with the cyst at the base of the tongue may represent the patient's only functional thyroid tissue. Surgery should be deferred until functional thyroid tissue is demonstrated in the typical location of the neck.

Recurrences are unusual after total excision of soft tissue cysts. Periodic clinical reexamination is required following a histopathologic diagnosis of thyroglossal tract cyst because remnants of these lesions occasionally undergo malignant transformation.

Benign Mesenchymal Neoplasms

Definition. This group of soft tissue lesions are benign neoplasms that originate from connective tissue, muscle, fat, vascular structures, and peripheral neural elements. These lesions individually and collectively occur much less frequently in the oral cavity than papillary enlargements of the surface epithelium, acute inflammatory enlargements, reactive hyperplasias, and oral cysts. The designations of the neoplasms relate to their tissue of origin:

Fibrous connective tissue:	Myxoma
Vascular tissue:	Hemangioma, lymphangioma
Neural tissue:	Neurofibroma, schwannoma, granular cell tumor
Muscular tissue:	Rhabdomyoma, leiomyoma, congenital gingival granular cell tumor
Adipose tissue:	Lipoma

Although this listing is not complete, these are the more common examples of benign mesenchymal neoplasms that develop in the oral and facial region.

Clinical features and differential diagnosis. The lesions in this group develop as an isolated enlargement with a nodular, sessile, or polypoid shape. The lesion periphery is well delineated and the superficial mucosa appears smooth and intact. These neoplasms are usually painless, and the clinical course is characterized by slow, progressive increase in size. In general, these enlargements are unattached and freely movable, but this may be difficult to demonstrate unless the lesion develops in loose connective tissue. These lesions occur most often, but are not limited to, specific sites of predilection.

Lesion compressibility depends on the tissue composition. The lipoma, myxoma, some neurofibromas, and the congenital gingival granular cell tumor (congenital epulis of the newborn) are somewhat soft or moderately compressible. The hemangioma and lymphangioma are spongy because of their fluid content. Most neural and muscular lesions are rubbery or firm to palpation. The remainder of this section describes the clinical characteristics and differential diagnosis that are specific for each lesion.

Lipoma. The lipoma (Fig. 18-22) is an uncommon oral lesion that is usually observed in adults. This benign neoplasm of fat tissue is distinctly soft to palpation. The pale yellowish-white color with fine surface vascularity is partially masked by connective tissue for lesions that are more deeply situated within the soft tissues. The enlargement is well circumscribed and freely movable. The most common sites of occurrence include the buccal mucosa, ventral tongue, and floor of the mouth.

A traumatic fibroma with a fibrofatty stroma is the most common lesion to resemble the color and painless compressibility of lipomas. Less common lesions that are well circumscribed, pale but firmer to palpation, are the lymphoepithelial and dermoid cysts. The myx-

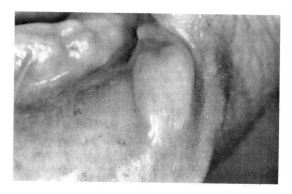

Fig. 18-22 Lipoma. Soft, compressible, sessile mass was located on the labial mucosa of an elderly woman. This slow-growing, asymptomatic lesion had a smooth, yellowish-pink surface.

oma, plexiform neurofibroma, and lymphangioma are also moderately compressible, but they are not as well circumscribed as most lipomas.

Myxoma. The myxoma is a rare benign neoplasm of connective tissue origin that occurs in adults. This infiltrative lesion can develop anywhere in the oral cavity but the palate is the favored location.

The myxoma resembles the myxomatous degeneration of some traumatic fibromas both clinically and microscopically. Other moderately compressible lesions that resemble myxomas include the lipoma, plexiform neurofibroma, lymphangioma, and mucous retention phenomenon.

Granular cell tumor. The granular cell tumor is an uncommon lesion of the oral cavity that originates from the Schwann cells of peripheral nerves. The granular cell tumor is a firm, infiltrative enlargement that is dome-shaped and usually develops on the tongue (Fig. 18-23). The mucosal surface overlying approximately one half of granular cell tumors appears rough, white, and thickened. This unique feature of this neoplasm is a reactive response of the surface epithelium that is referred to as *pseudoepitheliomatous hyperplasia*.

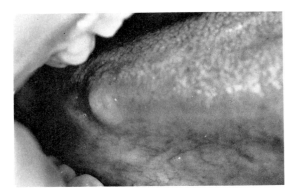

Fig. 18-23 Granular cell tumor. This firm, fixed nodule of the posterior lateral border of the tongue had a white, rough surface. It is important to exclude early squamous cell carcinoma, when this location is involved.

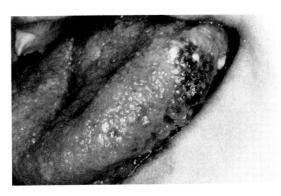

Fig. 18-24 Lymphangioma. This diffuse, compressible, congenital lesion of the tongue had a pebbly, variegated pink to reddish-brown surface. No blanching with pressure was observed with this exophytic mass.

Granular cell tumors with thickening of the superficial epithelium must be distinguished from an early exophytic squamous cell carcinoma, which is difficult if the peripheral borders of the granular cell tumor are indistinct. Other firm, benign lesions such as the neurofibroma, schwannoma, and traumatic fibroma resemble the features of granular cell tumors without pseudoepitheliomatous hyperplasia.

Hemangioma and lymphangioma. Both of these lesions are congenital, developmental abnormalities rather than true neoplasms. Therefore hemangiomas and lymphangiomas are first identified during infancy and do not enlarge except in proportion to the growth of the individual. These lesions are poorly delineated and spongy to palpation. The red color of hemangiomas (see Fig. 16-2) blanches readily during compression, and they quickly refill with blood when the pressure is released. The lymphangioma (Fig. 18-24) appears pale pink or bluish-red in color and does not blanch because the lymphatic vessels do not contain blood. The superficial surface associated with deeper, diffuse hemangiomas and lymphangiomas appears smooth with normal color. Both

lesions occur most frequently on the lips, tongue, and buccal mucosa. Lymphangiomas also develop in the neck and can cause a dramatic, diffuse enlargement shortly after birth that is referred to as a *cystic hygroma.*

The initial identification of the abnormality during infancy, the spongy consistency, and the absence of progressive increase in size is an adequate basis for a definitive clinical diagnosis. The blanching of hemangiomas is a dependable identifying feature. Some intraoral hemangiomas and lymphangiomas may resemble mucous retention phenomena, ranulas, or soft tissue cysts.

Neurofibroma and schwannoma. The solitary neurofibroma and schwannoma (Fig. 18-25) are firm, well delineated, and painless enlargements with a nodular shape that exhibit slow, gradual increase in size. The tongue, palate, and buccal mucosa are the typical sites of occurrence. The *plexiform neurofibroma* is the more diffuse and compressible variant of neurofibroma associated with *neurofibromatosis,* which is discussed in Chapter 20. Multiple lesions develop in this condition and they vary in shape from nodular enlargements to poorly

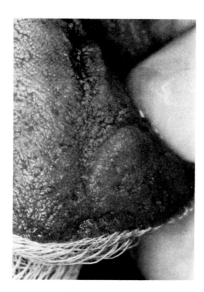

Fig. 18-25 Schwannoma. Firm, localized, sessile nodule of the anterior dorsal tongue had increased in size within a 2-year period.

delineated, lobular, or pendulous tissue masses. Most intraoral examples are the same color as surrounding tissues. A significant difference between solitary neurofibromas and the lesions of neurofibromatosis is that plexiform neurofibromas may undergo malignant transformation with advancing patient age.

The features of solitary neurofibromas and schwannomas are similar to those of traumatic fibromas, other firm benign mesenchymal neoplasms, and firm salivary gland tumors. The palpation characteristics of plexiform neurofibroma is suggestive of lymphangiomas and lipomas, but additional manifestations of neurofibromatosis such as skin pigmentation are present. Sudden onset of rapid enlargement of a plexiform neurofibroma in an older patient with neurofibromatosis must be considered the emergence of a malignant neural tumor until proven otherwise.

Rhabdomyoma and leiomyoma. These rare benign neoplasms originate from striated muscle and smooth muscle, respectively. Both are characterized by rubbery to firm, painless enlargement without alteration of the overlying mucosal surface. These tumors occur most frequently in adults and the favored intraoral sites include the tongue, palate, and buccal mucosa. The differential diagnosis for these lesions is similar to that described for solitary neural neoplasms.

Congenital gingival granular cell tumor. This benign mesenchymal neoplasm is also known as the *congenital epulis of the newborn*. It is first noticed in early infancy as a sessile to pedunculated gingival enlargement that ranges from a few millimeters to several centimeters in diameter with a smooth, pink surface. The congenital gingival granular cell tumor usually occurs on the anterior alveolus with a predilection for the maxillary ridge.

Differential diagnosis of lesions with these features includes dental lamina cyst, eruption cyst, and neonatal alveolar lymphangioma. A rare benign tumor that also affects this region shortly after birth known as the *neuroectodermal tumor of infancy* must also be considered. Lack of radiographic findings and absence of pigmentation excludes the eruption cyst and the typically pigmented neuroectodermal tumor of infancy. Dental lamina cysts are distinguished by a multiple presentation, whitish color, and small size.

Management decisions. The treatment of choice for most benign mesenchymal neoplasms is excision with histopathologic examination. Recurrences are not expected after complete removal of the lesions in this group. Surgical removal of the multiple neurofibromas associated with the syndrome is not justified unless rapid enlargement of an individual lesion is noticed. Congenital vascular anomalies usually require observation only, unless they present a cosmetic concern or their progressive growth interferes with normal function. Recurrences are common with some vascular enlargements because of the poor peripheral delineation of these progressive lesions.

Salivary Gland Neoplasms

Definition. The category of salivary gland neoplasms encompasses numerous benign and malignant neoplasms that produce a wide range of clinical features, rates of enlargement, and prognostic implications. The parotid gland is the most common site of salivary neoplasm occurrence; and in decreasing order of frequency, the intraoral minor salivary glands, submandibular glands, and sublingual glands are less likely sites. The benign salivary gland tumors that occur most frequently in the oral cavity are the pleomorphic adenoma, canalicular adenoma, and basal cell adenoma. Intraoral malignant salivary gland neoplasms include the mucoepidermoid carcinoma, polymorphous low-grade adenocarcinoma, adenoid cystic carcinoma, acinic cell carcinoma, and adenocarcinoma, not otherwise specified.

Clinical features. Most small benign and malignant salivary gland tumors are painless, nodular to dome-shaped enlargements with smooth contours and normal appearance of the overlying mucosa. Incidental traumatic injury or progressive expansion may cause thinning and ulceration of the mucosal surface. Ulceration is also a later feature of malignant tumors, and it is not a feature of benign salivary neoplasms unless traumatized. These lesions tend to be relatively well localized and the compressibility varies from soft to firm. Those with higher mucous or myxoid tissue content such as some mucoepidermoid carcinomas, pleomorphic adenomas, and mucous-producing adenocarcinomas are most likely to be compressible. Other salivary gland neoplasms with a greater proportion of cellular tissue are rubbery or firm to palpation. Poorly differentiated adenocarcinoma and adenoid cystic carcinoma are exceptional in comparison to most salivary neoplasms because they cause pain and dysesthesia by their tendency to invade peripheral nerves.

The most common intraoral site of occurrence for salivary gland neoplasms is lateral to the midline of the posterior hard palate as

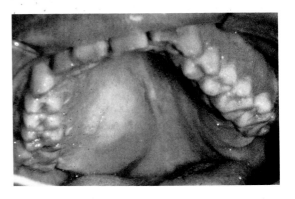

Fig. 18-26 Pleomorphic adenoma. This firm, smooth-surfaced exophytic mass of the hard palate was present for 5 years. Note that the slow growth of this benign submucosal neoplasm has not significantly altered the surface appearance. (Courtesy of Dr Brian R Smith, University of Texas Health Science Center at San Antonio.)

shown in Fig. 18-26. Other sites of predilection include the upper lip, buccal mucosa, and the retromolar region. Radiographic features may contribute to the diagnosis of larger tumors that develop adjacent to bone. Benign lesions tend to cause a cuffing depression by remodeling of bone, while malignant lesions are more likely to produce poorly delineated radiolucencies suggestive of bone lysis. Salivary gland neoplasms as a group develop over a wide age range with no greater occurrence by gender.

Differential diagnosis. Salivary gland neoplasms must be considered in the differential diagnosis of painless, well-delineated enlargements of all intraoral surfaces, excluding the anterior hard palate and gingiva because no salivary glands are present in these sites. The differential diagnosis for enlargements that are firm also includes the traumatic fibroma and firm benign mesenchymal neoplasms. Additional diagnostic possibilities in the posterior palatal region are reactive lymphoid hyperplasia and lymphoma. Most compressible enlargements must be compared with such possibilities as the mucous retention phenomenon, lipoma, myxoma, and soft tissue cysts.

The diagnostic challenge of evaluating suspected salivary gland neoplasms is that several salivary gland malignancies tend to appear clinically benign. Low-grade mucoepidermoid carcinomas, many adenoid cystic carcinomas, acinic cell carcinomas, and polymorphous low-grade adenocarcinomas exhibit well-delineated borders and normal appearance of the overlying mucosa. The association of the enlargement with ulceration and other surface alterations is more suggestive of malignancy. When these features are present, the differential diagnosis must broaden to include squamous cell carcinoma, lymphoma, a palatal abscess, granulomatous lesions, and an unusual degenerative condition of palatal salivary glands known as *necrotizing sialometaplasia.* Pain or tenderness is a less reliable feature in distinguishing inflammatory lesions from salivary gland neoplasms because these tumors can produce pain by perineural invasion.

Management decisions. Excisional biopsy with wide surgical margins is the treatment of choice for salivary gland neoplasms in general. This more aggressive approach is justified by the frequent recurrence of many benign salivary gland neoplasms such as the pleomorphic adenoma and by the possibility of a slowly progressive salivary gland malignancy. Also, recurrence of benign lesions, particularly the pleomorphic adenoma, is associated with a slight risk for malignant transformation.

Higher grade malignant neoplasms require referral for staging and definitive treatment. Regional metastasis is typically to the cervical lymph nodes, and the lung is the most frequent distant site. Definitive treatment usually includes additional surgery in combination with radiotherapy and chemotherapy. The 5-year survival rates for the more common intraoral salivary gland malignancies appears relatively favorable. However, the poor prognosis of these persistent, slowly-progressive tumors is reflected by the substantially lower survival percentages at 10 or more years after treatment.

SOFT TISSUE MALIGNANCIES

Cancer statistics compiled by the National Cancer Institute predict that more than 30,000 new cases of oral cancer occur in the United States annually. These figures are based on surveys that include malignancies of the lips, tongue, floor of the mouth, salivary glands, pharynx, and other unspecified sites within the oral cavity. Although the numbers are small in comparison to other forms of cancer, approximately 10,000 people die of oral and oropharyngeal cancer each year. Approximately 90% of all oral cancers are squamous cell carcinoma. The remaining oral cancers are malignant salivary gland tumors, lymphomas, metastatic disease, and a variety of rare sarcomas.

Most oral cancers with the specific exception of salivary gland malignancies exhibit rapid, progressive growth that is apparent clinically within a period of weeks to months. This rapid increase in size in many cases alters the overlying mucosa. The surface changes include asymmetric, bosselated to lobulated contours and crateriform ulcers with poorly delineated, rolled margins. The exophytic portion of most oral malignancies is indurated to palpation as a consequence of dense cellularity. The base is diffuse with fixation to surrounding structures because of infiltrative growth.

Unfortunately, discomfort is rarely produced during the early growth of most soft tissue malignant neoplasms of the oral cavity. Pain and hemorrhage are more likely features of large tumors. Aberrant neural sensation such as persistent tingling, numbness, or referred pain associated with a firm enlargement is strongly suggestive of malignancy. The typical clinical course is enlargement and tissue destruction by local invasion. This is followed by regional metastasis to cervical lymph nodes and eventually distant metastasis, usually to the lung or liver. Systemic manifestations are an ominous indication of widely disseminated dis-

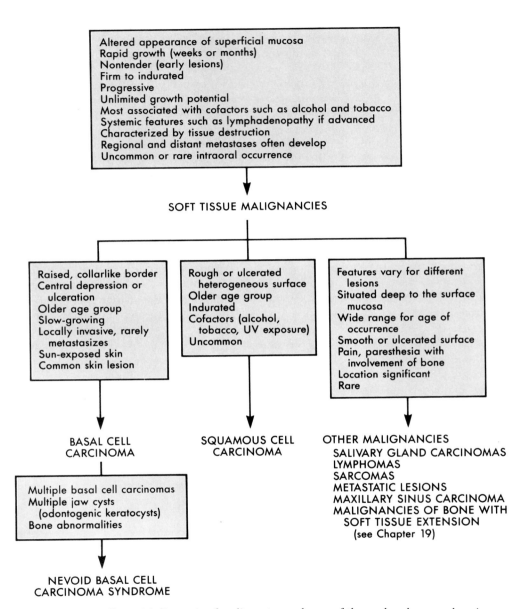

Altered appearance of superficial mucosa
Rapid growth (weeks or months)
Nontender (early lesions)
Firm to indurated
Progressive
Unlimited growth potential
Most associated with cofactors such as alcohol and tobacco
Systemic features such as lymphadenopathy if advanced
Characterized by tissue destruction
Regional and distant metastases often develop
Uncommon or rare intraoral occurrence

SOFT TISSUE MALIGNANCIES

Raised, collarlike border
Central depression or
    ulceration
Older age group
Slow-growing
Locally invasive, rarely
    metastasizes
Sun-exposed skin
Common skin lesion

Rough or ulcerated
    heterogeneous surface
Older age group
Indurated
Cofactors (alcohol,
    tobacco, UV exposure)
Uncommon

Features vary for different
    lesions
Situated deep to the surface
    mucosa
Wide range for age of
    occurrence
Smooth or ulcerated surface
Pain, paresthesia with
    involvement of bone
Location significant
Rare

BASAL CELL
CARCINOMA

SQUAMOUS CELL
CARCINOMA

OTHER MALIGNANCIES
    SALIVARY GLAND CARCINOMAS
    LYMPHOMAS
    SARCOMAS
    METASTATIC LESIONS
    MAXILLARY SINUS CARCINOMA
    MALIGNANCIES OF BONE WITH
        SOFT TISSUE EXTENSION
        (see Chapter 19)

Multiple basal cell carcinomas
Multiple jaw cysts
    (odontogenic keratocysts)
Bone abnormalities

NEVOID BASAL CELL
CARCINOMA SYNDROME

Fig. 18-27   Differential diagnosis of malignant neoplasms of the oral and paraoral regions.

ease. The differential diagnosis of oral and perioral malignancies is illustrated in Fig. 18-27.

Basal Cell Carcinoma

Definition. Basal cell carcinoma is a common, low-grade epithelial malignancy of the skin. This tumor arises from the basal cells of the epidermis or from the external root sheath of hair follicles. Although oral lesions with microscopic features of basal cell carcinoma have been reported, they are rare, isolated occurrences. Therefore the inclusion of this malignancy in the differential diagnosis of oral lesions is seldom justified.

The most significant contributory factor in the development of basal cell carcinomas is actinic damage of the skin by the ultraviolet spectrum of sunlight. Fair-skinned individuals with outdoor vocations or hobbies are at greatest risk. Other contributory factors for basal cell carcinoma include radiotherapy, severe burns, and a genetic predisposition associated with developmental syndromes. The most common syndrome is the *nevoid basal cell carcinoma syndrome,* which is discussed in Chapter 20. Basal cell carcinomas have little potential for metastasis but can cause disfiguring destruction by local invasion.

Clinical features. Small basal cell carcinomas initially appear as firm papules or nodules with smooth surfaces. The enlargement may be translucent white, fleshy pink, or brownishblack in color. Telangiectatic distention of blood vessels of the overlying or adjacent skin is a frequent observation. As the tumor enlarges, a central depression within the nodule develops, causing an elevated, rolled appearance of the lesion periphery (Fig. 18-28). This central depression eventually becomes ulcerated and crusted. Basal cell carcinomas are characterized by slow, progressive growth that produces a thickened, ulcerated area of tissue destruction. The midface is the most common location and the patient is usually older than age 50.

Differential diagnosis. Basal cell carcino-

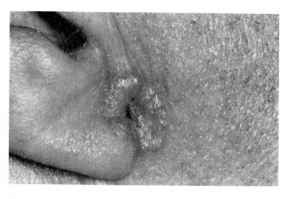

Fig. 18-28   Basal cell carcinoma. Firm, nodular lesion with a depressed center and surface telangiectasia was located anterior to the ear in an elderly man. History of chronic, unprotected sun exposure.

mas resemble and are often indistinguishable from small squamous cell carcinomas. Pigmented basal cell carcinomas suggest the possibility of melanoma and seborrheic keratosis. Both of these lesions frequently occur on the face and are related to sun exposure. Seborrheic keratosis is a plaquelike thickening with a fissured or pebbly surface texture, homogeneous pigmentation, and sharply delineated borders.

Management decisions. Surgical excision with wide margins of apparently normal tissue is indicated for lesions with the described features. Patients should be referred to a dermatologist for treatment and follow-up in view of the facial location of most examples.

Squamous Cell Carcinoma

Definition. Intraoral squamous cell carcinoma originates in most cases from the surface epithelium and is the most common malignancy of the oral cavity. The most significant risk factor in the development of this intraoral malignancy is the habitual use of tobacco and alcohol. Exposure to ultraviolet radiation is a significant contributing factor to squamous cell carcinomas located on the exposed mucosa of the lower lip. Other influences implicated in oral squamous cell carcinoma include genetic predisposition and common viruses including the family of herpesviruses and the human papillomavirus group.

Verrucous carcinoma is an uncommon oral malignancy of surface epithelial origin that accounts for approximately 5% of all intraoral squamous cell carcinomas. The primary causative factor of this malignancy in the oral cavity is use of tobacco products, especially smokeless tobacco.

Clinical features. Oral squamous cell carcinoma produces a variety of primary clinical manifestations at different stages of the lesion's clinical course. Early, superficial squamous cell carcinoma is described in Chapter 15 as a white lesion, in Chapter 16 as an erythroplakia, and in Chapter 17 as a cause of ulceration. The more advanced, exophytic lesions are described here in the context of soft tissue enlargements.

The exophytic form is a nodular to polypoid elevation that is firm or indurated to palpation and fixed to underlying structures. The surface texture is rough, granular, or papillary with a heterogeneous appearance that may include areas of white, pink, or red discoloration (Fig. 18-29). The bosselated surface usually exhibits irregular contours with focal sites of ulceration. The margins are diffuse and difficult to delineate. Increase in size is usually noticeable within weeks or months and large lesions (Fig. 18-30) may cause pain, other abnormal sensations, or hemorrhage. The most common oral sites of squamous cell carcinoma are the exposed lower lip surface, the lateral border of the tongue, and floor of the mouth. However, any mucosal surface may be affected. Essentially the same general features apply to squamous cell carcinoma of the facial skin.

Regional metastasis to the cervical lymph nodes at the time of discovery is a frequent observation with diffuse, ulcerative, and invasive forms of oral squamous cell carcinoma. Me-

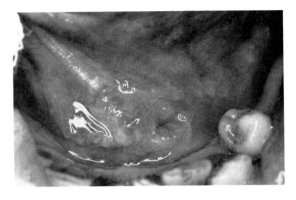

Fig. 18-29 Squamous cell carcinoma. Firm, fixed, exophytic mass with a red and white granular surface developed in the floor of the mouth of a 60-year-old male. History included cigarette smoking and alcohol abuse of long duration.

tastasis is less likely with early, well-localized, and exophytic carcinomas that are eventually characterized as well differentiated on the basis of microscopic findings. Skin and lower lip squamous cell carcinomas that are related to ultraviolet radiation seldom spread to regional lymph nodes by the time they are identified. This probability of regional metastasis generally corresponds to the patient's prognosis.

Differential diagnosis. The papillary squamous cell carcinoma is indistinguishable on the basis of clinical features from verrucous carcinoma. Histopathologic examination of representative tissue with proper orientation is necessary to achieve an accurate diagnosis. Exophytic squamous cell carcinomas may resemble granular cell tumors, malignant salivary gland neoplasms, granulomatous enlargements, sarcomas, and metastatic disease. Many of these lesions are relatively rare in comparison with squamous cell carcinoma. The suspicion of squamous cell carcinoma is supported by the presence of induration and vague peripheral borders, in addition to a history of habitual tobacco and alcohol use. Also, squamous cell carcinoma of the oral cavity is unusual before

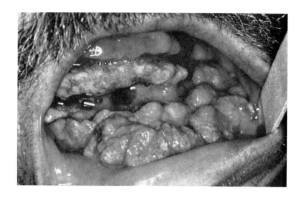

Fig. 18-30 Squamous cell carcinoma. Fungating, indurated mass of the floor of the mouth was rapidly growing in this 50-year-old male. Massive destruction of the underlying structures was associated with cutaneous extension and distant metastasis. (Courtesy of Dr Brian R Smith, University of Texas Health Science Center at San Antonio.)

age 50, whereas more common reactive and benign neoplastic lesions usually occur among young adults. One exception is the granular cell tumor with pseudoepitheliomatous hyperplasia, which is often indistinguishable from an early nodular squamous cell carcinoma on the basis of clinical features.

The rare occurrence of other forms of oral cancer favors squamous cell carcinoma as the diagnosis if convincing features of a malignant neoplasm are present. One exception to this generalization is that rare sarcomas of the facial region usually occur during childhood and adolescence.

Management decisions. Incisional biopsy of large lesions and excisional biopsy of relatively small lesions that are suggestive of squamous cell carcinoma are justified to achieve a definitive diagnosis. However, a combination of features that are strongly suggestive of squamous cell carcinoma warrants referral for oncologic treatment without the delay associated with accomplishing a biopsy. Treatment depends on the clinical staging and the microscopic features of the lesion. Small, well-differentiated lesions are usually amenable to surgical excision with wide margins. Larger lesions are managed by surgery, radiotherapy, or a combination of both modalities. Neck dissection of regional lymph nodes is recommended for suspected or apparent regional metastasis. Chemotherapy is advocated as adjunctive therapy in advanced cases. Dental management of complications associated with such treatment is described in Chapter 13.

Other Oral Malignancies

Other possible malignancies of the oral cavity include salivary gland carcinomas, lymphomas, various sarcomas, metastatic lesions, maxillary sinus carcinoma, and malignancies of bone. As indicated in the discussion of squamous cell carcinoma, these lesions rarely occur in the oral cavity with the exception of malignant salivary gland tumors. Squamous cell carcinoma is the favored clinical impression for lesions with features of malignancy in middle-aged and older patients. However, a similar lesion affecting a child, adolescent, or young adult suggests the possibility of one of the more unusual lesions described briefly below. Pertinent clinical features of these rare lesions are discussed.

Salivary gland malignancies. Most malignant neoplasms of salivary gland origin occur in the major salivary glands. Sublingual tumors are almost always malignant, while parotid enlargements are more likely to be benign. Minor salivary gland malignancies occur most commonly in the posterior hard palate and soft palate region. As discussed in the section concerning benign salivary gland neoplasms, mucoepidermoid carcinomas, adenoid cystic carcinomas, polymorphous low-grade adenocarcinomas, and acinic cell carcinomas can present misleadingly benign clinical features. These findings include slow growth, well-delineated borders, and normal appearance of the overlying mucosa in many cases.

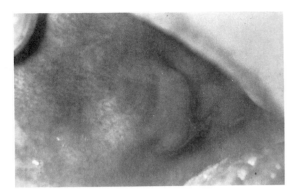

Fig. 18-31 Non-Hodgkin's lymphoma. Firm, fixed, bosselated mass with poorly delineated borders developed in the buccal mucosa of this elderly woman. Note that surface epithelium has a normal appearance, which is characteristic of early submucosal malignancies.

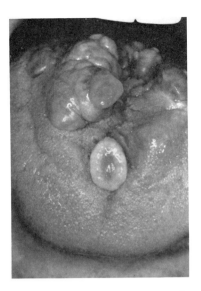

Fig. 18-32 Kaposi's sarcoma. Vascular, fixed, multinodular enlargement was observed on the dorsal tongue of a homosexual man with AIDS. Foci of ulceration coincided with areas of rapid growth.

Lymphomas. Intraoral enlargement caused by a lymphoma (Fig. 18-31) is usually but not necessarily associated with the lymphoid tissues of the oropharynx or the submandibular lymph nodes. A diffuse soft tissue enlargement of the hard palate is the typical intraoral presentation. In most instances, distant enlargement of one or more lymph nodes is a much more dramatic feature of the lymphoma than the oral lesion. The nodes are most often painless without evidence of an infection or other inflammatory process to explain the lymphadenopathy.

Sarcomas and leukemias. Many sarcomas and leukemias typically affect children. Oral incidence is rare, but the observation of a rapid enlargement can be dramatic. The most common oral indication of leukemias is a bleeding tendency and boggy, generalized enlargement of the gingiva that appears disproportionately severe in comparison to gingivitis. The differential diagnosis for leukemic infiltration of the gingiva is discussed under generalized gingival hyperplasia.

Kaposi's sarcoma. The appearance of Ka-posi's sarcoma is relatively characteristic and the oral cavity is often affected. The flat, dark red lesions of early Kaposi's lesions are described in Chapter 16. The multiple, reddish-blue, nodular enlargements of more advanced lesions (see Figs. 15-13 and 18-32) appear somewhat similar to those of hemangiomas and pyogenic granulomas. The appearance of Kaposi's sarcoma is a manifestation of AIDS. Approximately 20% of all AIDS patients eventually develop Kaposi's sarcoma. Other oral lesions such as hairy leukoplakia, candidiasis, and necrotizing periodontitis support the clinical impression of AIDS.

Metastatic neoplastic lesions. Metastatic lesions of the oral cavity from distant primary tumors are quite variable in appearance. Most examples originate in bone during the late stages of a previously diagnosed and treated malignancy. Therefore a history of a malignant neoplasm and radiographic evidence of diffuse bone destruction should alert the clinician to the possibility of a metastatic lesion. This is becoming an increasingly frequent diagnostic consideration for dentists because of the greater number of patients in remission after the treatment of what were previously terminal diseases. On the other hand, the jaws are an unlikely site of metastasis for most common malignancies until the terminal stages of the condition. Metastatic lesions rarely develop in the oral soft tissues unless a bone lesion has infiltrated into the adjacent soft tissues.

Carcinoma of the maxillary sinus. Carcinoma of the maxillary sinus is a rare tumor that originates from the lining mucosa. Most examples are poorly differentiated squamous cell carcinomas that have metastasized to the regional lymph nodes before symptoms of the primary tumor develop. Enlargement of the alveolus, extrusion of posterior maxillary teeth, diffuse pain in this region, and altered movement of the eye are typical features of this condition.

Central malignant neoplasms of the jaws. The radiographic features of central jaw malignancies are described and illustrated in Chapter 19. Diffuse enlargement of the jaw is typically the initial clinical indication of the lesion. Most malignancies of the jaws cause pain as a consequence of neural compression and pressure against the resistance of rigid cortical bone. These features and many radiographic features mimic the much more common infectious jaw lesions that are confronted by the dentist. The nature of the discomfort described by the patient may be one of the more reliable distinguishing characteristics. Pain caused by inflammatory lesions tends to be episodic with dramatic variation in severity as the nature of the infection is affected by drainage, antibiotic therapy, or removal of a suspected cause. Bone pain produced by malignant neoplasms tends to be steady and progressive in severity without dramatic fluctuations in degree.

Differential diagnosis and management. The same general differential diagnostic and clinical management considerations apply for these conditions as were described in the preceding discussion of oral squamous cell carcinoma.

SUMMARY

Soft tissue enlargement as the primary clinical manifestation of an abnormality is produced by a diverse group of specific conditions. In the context of differential diagnosis, soft tissue enlargements of the oral cavity can be categorized in one of the following groups:

1. Papillary enlargements of the surface epithelium
2. Acute inflammatory enlargements
3. Reactive hyperplasias
4. Benign submucosal cysts and neoplasms
5. Malignant neoplasms

Once an abnormality is identified as a manifestation of one of these disease groups, the differential diagnosis can proceed more efficiently with consideration of specific diagnostic possibilities.

Papillary enlargements of the surface epithelium are painless, white or pale in color, and firm to palpation. They exhibit a rough or papillary surface texture and slow enlargement within a period of months or years. A viral infection is implicated as a cause for most of these lesions. An important distinguishing characteristic among these conditions is whether the abnormality occurs as an isolated lesion or as multiple enlargements.

Acute inflammatory enlargements are painful, compressible, and appear erythematous. Rapid increase in size within hours or days and the presence of purulence usually indicate bacterial infections. An obvious dental source of the infection can usually be identified with most orofacial examples.

Reactive hyperplasias of the oral cavity are caused by chronic irritation or mild recurring injury of tissues. The clinical features of these lesions are variable depending on whether or not the inflammatory process that caused the enlargement is currently active. In most instances, the diagnosis relies on identification of the direct cause, which is usually apparent. These lesions may be nontender, pale or erythematous in color, and soft or moderately firm to palpation. The growth rate may yield enlargement within months but the growth potential is limited. Therefore reactive hyperplasias eventually become static in size.

Benign submucosal cysts and neoplasms exhibit slow growth within a period of months or years, but the growth potential of these lesions is generally unlimited. No apparent inflammatory cause or source of injury is related to these nontender lesions. The overlying mucosa typically appears smooth and intact and in most cases the borders of the lesion are well delineated. Excision and histopathologic examination are necessary to achieve a definitive diagnosis for these lesions.

Most oral examples of malignant neoplasms are squamous cell carcinomas, which usually affect older patients with a history of tobacco and excessive alcohol use. Rapid increase in size within weeks or months, altered appearance of the superficial mucosa, poor delineation of peripheral borders, and a general impression of tissue destruction are clinical features of malignant neoplasms. Oral malignancies other than squamous cell carcinoma are uncommon, but they should be considered if these features affect younger patients, are present in certain locations, or are associated with a previous history of a distant malignancy.

BIBLIOGRAPHY

Boring CC, Squires TS, Tong T: Cancer statistics, 1991, CA-Cancer J Clin 41:19, 1991.

Bouquot JE, Gundlach KKH: Oral exophytic lesions in 23,616 white Americans over 35 years of age, Oral Surg Oral Med Oral Pathol 62:284, 1986.

Ellis GL, Auclair PL, Gnepp DR, editors: Surgical pathology of the salivary glands, vol 25, Major problems in pathology, Philadelphia, 1991, Saunders.

Gnepp DR, editor: Pathology of the head and neck, vol 10, Contemporary issues in surgical pathology, New York, 1988, Churchill Livingstone.

Mashberg A, Samit AM: Early detection, diagnosis, and management of oral and oropharyngeal cancer, CA-Cancer J Clin 39:67, 1989.

Neville BW and others: Color atlas of clinical oral pathology, Philadelphia, 1991, Lea & Febiger.

Regezi JA and Sciubba JJ: Oral pathology: clinical-pathologic correlations, Philadelphia, 1989, Saunders.

Scully C and others: Papillomavirus: the current status in relation to oral disease, Oral Surg Oral Med Oral Pathol 65:526, 1988.

Silverman S: Color atlas of oral manifestations of AIDS, Philadelphia, 1989, Decker.

Wood NK, Goaz PW: Differential diagnosis of oral lesions, ed 4, St Louis, 1991, Mosby-Year Book.

CHAPTER 19

Differential Diagnosis of Radiographic Abnormalities

GARY C. COLEMAN

Radiographs provide an essential source of diagnostic information concerning abnormalities that affect the jaws and related structures. The radiographic findings that are contributory to the diagnosis of dental disease are discussed separately in Chapter 8. The differential diagnostic approach to nondental lesions within the jaws and adjacent structures is presented here.

Most central lesions of the jaws cannot be directly visualized or palpated because the superficial mucosa and cortical bone are intact. Radiograph evaluation of jaw lesions essentially replaces the direct visual inspection and palpation used to evaluate soft tissue lesions. Unfortunately, radiographic limitations and the nature of bone lesions complicate the differential diagnosis of jaw lesions and must be considered during their interpretation:

1. The two dimensional radiographic representation of a three dimensional jaw lesion and adjacent structures can be misleading at times. Fig. 8-38 illustrates one example. In general, a single radiograph rarely provides adequate information to fully evaluate a bone lesion. Additional exposures are usually necessary to eliminate technical defects and to minimize superimposition of structures.

2. The differential diagnoses for bone lesions generally must include more conditions than those for mucosal and soft tissue abnormalities. Radiographic information often justifies limiting the differential diagnosis to a single lesion category, but confident exclusion of many lesions within that category is usually not possible.

3. Many jaws lesions exhibit different radiographic features during their clinical course. In general, the most characteristic radiographic features of bone lesions do not develop until the lesion is relatively advanced.

Table 19-1 Summary of radiographic features and their diagnostic significance

Radiographic feature	Interpretive alternatives	Interpretive implications
X-ray attenuation	Radiolucent (dark) Mixed radiolucent-radiopaque Radiopaque (light)	Reflects composition of the lesion. Radiolucency within bone implies replacement of normal bone with nonmineralized tissue or material. Radiopacity suggests greater density of mineralization than trabecular bone. A mixed appearance indicates the presence of both mineralized and nonmineralized tissues.
Pattern	Homogeneous (uniform attenuation) Heterogeneous (attenuation varies)	A homogeneous pattern reflects uniform lesion composition, while variation in attenuation is produced by a combination of different materials. The arrangement of heterogeneous components can indicate whether or not the tissue of the lesion is generating a mineralized product.

Location (extent)	Focal-anatomic location
	  1. Tooth-bearing bone
	  2. Non–tooth-bearing area
	Multifocal (multiple separate lesions)
	Generalized alteration of bone morphology
		Odontogenic lesions are located adjacent to teeth or in tooth-bearing bone. Location in bone that does not support teeth excludes odontogenic lesions in most instances. Non-odontogenic lesions can develop in bone that supports teeth, but they usually develop in nonalveolar bone. A number of conditions can produce multiple separate lesions. Generalized alteration of bone morphology suggests metabolic disorders or systemic disease.

Margins	Sharply delineated
	  1. Corticated bone reaction
	  2. Hyperostotic bone reaction
	  3. Absence of bone reaction
	Poorly delineated
		Sharply delineated margins generally indicate slow growth. Formation of cortical bone peripheral to the lesion is typical of cysts, most odontogenic lesions, and some benign nonodontogenic neoplasms. Many lesions of bone

INTERPRETATION OF RADIOGRAPHIC FEATURES

The goal of radiographic interpretation is to appreciate the alterations produced by the lesion as evidence of its pathologic characteristics. The *feature recognition method* approaches this task by the objective description of seven distinct radiographic features for any abnormality. This assessment should be accomplished as much as possible without the bias of a presumptive clinical diagnosis. The tendency to interpret the radiographic information to fit the clinical opinion is a common source of misdiagnosis. These features can sug-

gest possible origin, composition, and growth characteristics of the abnormality, which when combined with clinical findings justify differential diagnostic decisions.

Radiographic Features

The radiographic features useful in the interpretation of any bone lesion are summarized in Table 19-1. These features and the terms used to refer to their interpretation are used in the discussions of specific lesions in this chapter.

X-ray attenuation. X-ray attenuation is the proportion of an x-ray beam absorbed or scat-

Table 19-1 Summary of radiographic features and their diagnostic significance—cont'd

Radiographic feature	Interpretive alternatives	Interpretive implications
		or connective tissue origin stimulate a wider, sclerotic border referred to as hyperostosis. Absence of bone reaction or poor delineation of the lesional margins indicates rapid enlargement.
Shape	Unilocular (round or ovoid) Multilocular (scalloped borders or lobulated appearance) Irregular	Unilocular shape is usually produced by slow, uniform growth that is typical of cysts and many benign neoplasms. Multilocularity indicates slow growth from multiple independent sites of growth that is typical of some benign neoplasms and cysts. Irregular shape results from rapid, multifocal growth that is usually produced by inflammatory lesions or malignant neoplasms.
Size	Small size (less than 1 centimeter) Larger size (more than 1 centimeter)	Small size suggests early development of the lesion. Therefore more characteristic features such as multilocularity or appearance of a calcified product may not yet be apparent. Large lesion size implies unlimited growth potential in most instances and characteristic features of most lesions are more likely to be present.
Alteration of adjacent structures	Distortion of adjacent structure (e.g., cortical expansion, shifting of teeth) Destruction of adjacent structures (e.g., cortical perforation, extrusion of teeth)	Distortion of adjacent structures suggests slow growth that allows time for remodeling of the normal bone near the lesion. Destruction of adjacent structures usually indicates that the abnormality is enlarging faster than bone can remodel, which results in lysis of bone.

tered by the subject material before the primary radiation interacts with the film or other imaging medium. X-ray attenuation is determined by the thickness of the structure and the proportion of mineralized material present. The composition of an abnormality is reflected in contrast to normal tissue. The term *radiolucent* describes a structure within bone that appears darker radiographically because nonmineralized tissue has replaced normal bone. *Radiopaque* structures, conversely, appear lighter than normal bone because a greater mineral content attenuates more of the x-ray beam than the adjacent bone. *Mixed radiolucent-ra-diopaque* lesions contain both soft tissue and mineralized components. The lesion composition, which is suggested by relative radiopacity, is the dependable differential diagnostic feature that provides the basis for initial categorization of jaw lesions.

Pattern. The pattern of abnormality refers to the consistency of the x-ray attenuation within the lesion. A *homogeneous* appearance results from uniform mineral content and a *heterogeneous* pattern reflects variation in the degree of mineralization. Most radiolucencies and radiopacities appear homogeneous. Homogeneous radiopacities exhibit either a granular consistency referred to as a *"ground glass"* appearance or a filamentous character often described as a *"cotton-wool"* appearance. Inflammatory and malignant neoplastic lesions are likely to produce the intermixture of normal tissue and lesion tissue that yields heterogeneity of radiolucent lesions and radiopacities.

The pattern of a mixed radiolucent-radiopaque lesion refers to the proportion of radiopaque material to radiolucent material, distribution of radiopaque formations, and whether or not toothlike arrangements are present. A central radiopacity or a "speckled" arrangement of radiopaque foci surrounded by a radiolucent zone suggests that mineralized material has been generated by the soft tissue of the lesion. This is referred to as a *productive lesion.* A predominant proportion of radiopaque material suggests advanced progression or "maturity" of these productive lesions. Mixed lesions that contain toothlike radiopacities and a thin peripheral radiolucent component are odontogenic. A haphazard intermixture of radiolucent and radiopaque components generally reflects alteration of bone by chronic inflammation or malignant neoplasms.

Location. Lesion location is stated in specific anatomic terms and includes recognition of multiple, separate lesions with similar characteristics, if that is the case. Lesion location may suggest the origin of an abnormality, and many abnormalities tend to occur in certain anatomic regions. Multiple similar lesions generally represent multifocal manifestations of a generalized disease process.

Margins. The growth rate of the lesion may be suggested by the radiographic characteristics of the interface between the abnormality and normal bone. The slow, uniform remodeling of bone caused by cysts and many benign neoplasms yields sharp marginal delineation and a cortexlike radiopaque border. The rapid lysis of bone produced by malignant neoplasms and inflammatory lesions creates a marginal admixture of normal and abnormal tissues that appears vaguely delineated radiographically. The most accurate radiographic representation of the lesional margin is observed at the interface between the lesion and trabecular bone. Teeth roots, the cortex, and other anatomic structures located near the margins can misrepresent the radiographic characteristics. In general, the marginal delineation of a radiographic lesion is the best single radiographic indication of growth rate.

Several chronic, slow-growing lesions are exceptional in that they exhibit less distinct margins for reasons independent of growth rate. For example, chronic inflammatory lesions that have oscillated between progression and healing often exhibit indistinct borders. Many benign lesions of connective tissue origin induce a peripheral sclerosis called *hyperostosis.* These lesions appear localized but their margins often appear vague or "fuzzy" compared with the sharpness of cortical borders.

Shape. The shape of a lesion is described in geometric terms if possible. *Unilocular* refers to a round or ovoid shape that is usually produced by distention from a central point— analogous to inflating a balloon. Most cysts and benign neoplasms appear unilocular. Other benign enlargements characteristically develop multiple independent centers of growth that yield a "lumpy" or "soap-bubble" appearance referred to as a *multilocularity.* Multilocularity can also be suggested by a scalloped peripheral lesion contour. Acute inflammatory and malignant neoplastic lesions grow by rapid extension into anatomic structures that offer minimal resistance and produce an irregular lesion shape.

Size. Lesion size is determined by measuring the radiograph and specifying the dimensions in metric units as diameter, mesial-distal width, or superior-inferior extent. The comparison of a current lesion size with a previously exposed radiograph or one exposed at a later date may provide a qualitative estimate of growth rate. Lesion size greater than 1 to 2 cm in diameter indicates that additional growth potential is likely. Large lesion size alone does *not* suggest rapid growth rate because many jaw lesions are asymptomatic and the current size may reflect years of enlargement.

Some lesions have characteristic features that are more likely to become visible radiographically as larger size is attained (e.g., multilocularity or production of a calcified component). Considered another way, a small lesion generally exhibits few distinctive radiographic features and its differential diagnosis must include more diagnostic possibilities.

Changes in adjacent structures. Alterations in adjacent structures by an abnormality are interpreted as either *distortion* or *destruction* of normal tissues. Distortion is caused by the slow growth of cysts and benign neoplastic lesions, whereas tissue destruction suggests rapid bone lysis caused by inflammatory or malignant neoplastic conditions. Observations indicative of distortion include shifting of teeth, sharply delineated external resorption of teeth, altered course of an intact inferior alveolar canal, expansion of the contours of the bone, and uniform thinning of cortical bone. Destruction is indicated radiographically by extrusion of teeth, irregular perforation of cortical bone, "punched-out" radiolucencies without peripheral hyperostosis, and "ragged" external resorption of teeth.

To avoid the temptation to focus on prominent features and overlook other features, the dentist should independently interpret all seven features (x-ray attenuation, pattern, location, margins, shape, size, and changes in adjacent structures). A disciplined, thorough method for recognizing radiographic information is to prepare a written description of the lesion that specifically addresses all seven features. This is usually redundant in a dental setting because the radiographs accompany the patient record. However, interpreting the radiograph with the attitude of preparing a report promotes a more complete assessment.

Interpretation of Radiographic Findings

Integrating the seven specific radiographic features into a composite interpretation of an abnormality requires formulating opinions about the biologic behavior of the lesion and the response of surrounding tissues. Decisions must be made concerning the lesion's composition, probable origin, possible formation of a calcified product, growth rate, and potential for continued growth. Table 19-2 lists these interpretive issues and the radiographic features that support different conclusions. The differential diagnosis of the abnormality is based on these conclusions as modified by clinical information.

Radiographic features are occasionally contradictory, equivocal, or inconsistent with the clinical signs and symptoms. The differential diagnosis in such cases often includes many lesions because indefinite interpretive conclusions may not justify confident exclusion of disease categories. Supplemental diagnostic information as provided by additional radiographs or clinical tests may help resolve such contradictions. The definitive diagnosis of most jaw lesions eventually requires surgical removal and histopathologic evaluation.

Classification of Radiographic Abnormalities

The possibility that an unusual radiographic appearance may not represent a disease process at all must be considered based on the interpretation of radiographic features. Unusual radiographic appearances unrelated to disease can be technical image artifacts or prominent anatomic structures. Technical artifacts can be demonstrated when the abnormality disappears in a new radiograph that has been exposed to avoid the artifact. Normal anatomic structures are characterized by occurrence in expected locations and bilateral symmetry. If these possibilities cannot be excluded, then the abnormal appearance is approached as a disease process.

The differential diagnosis of radiographic lesions commonly encountered by the dentist is most effectively approached by classifying abnormalities based on the tissues or anatomic structures affected. Fig. 19-1 represents the di-

Table 19-2 Interpretative conclusions concerning bone lesions and the supportive radiographic features

Interpretative issue	Options	Indicative features
1. *Composition*	Nonmineralized material or tissue	Homogeneous radiolucency
	Mixture of mineralized and nonmineralized materials	Heterogeneous mixture of radiolucency and radiopacity
	Formation of a mineralized product	Central radiopacity with peripheral radiolucency or scattered foci of radiopacity ("speckled" appearance)
	Predominance of mineralized tissue	Radiopacity, granular ("ground glass") or filamentous ("cotton-wool") appearances
2. *Origin*	Odontogenic	Associated with teeth or located in tooth-bearing regions
	Nonodontogenic	Usually centered away from teeth, but occasionally develop near teeth
3. *Growth rate*	Nonenlarging (static)	Sharp, corticated borders, no alterations of adjacent structures
	Slow growth	Sharp borders, round or multilocular shape, distortion of adjacent structures
	Rapid growth	Vague borders, irregular shape, destruction of adjacent structures
4. *Pattern of growth*	Unicentric	Round or ovoid shape
	Multicentric	Multilocular shape, scalloped borders, or irregular intermixture of radiolucency and radiopacity
	Multifocal	Multiple separate lesions with similar features
	Generalized	Alteration of morphologic arrangement of trabecular and cortical bone in all areas
5. *Growth potential*	Limited growth	Small lesion size, features suggesting that the lesion is not enlarging
	Unlimited growth	Large lesion size, expansion of cortical contours

agnostic classification strategy consisting of focal lesions within bone, generalized bone conditions, abnormalities of the maxillary sinus, soft tissue calcifications, and alterations of the temporomandibular joint. The focal bone lesions are further classified as radiolucencies, mixed radiolucent-radiopaque lesions, and radiopacities. The radiolucent lesions are divided on the basis of lesion shape and the delineation of borders into unilocular radiolucencies, multilocular lesions, and irregularly shaped radiolucencies.

UNILOCULAR RADIOLUCENCIES OF THE JAWS

The differential diagnostic strategy for radiolucencies of the jaws is schematically represented in Fig. 19-2. Unilocular shape with corticated borders is so typical of the unicentric growth of cysts that the term *cystic* is often used to describe this radiographic appearance. Some benign neoplasms also enlarge from a central focus and appear cystic.

Small radiolucencies represent an interpretive challenge because many lesions have char-

Fig. 19-1 Initial differential diagnostic categorization of radiographic abnormalities.

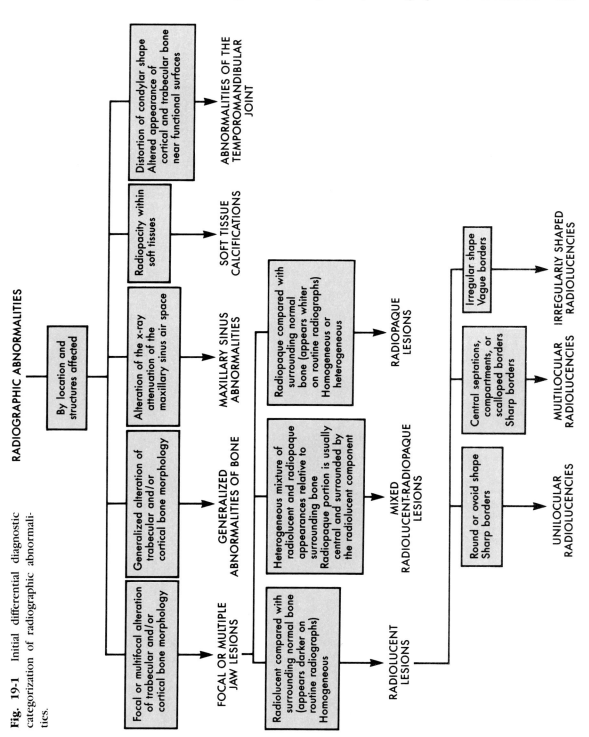

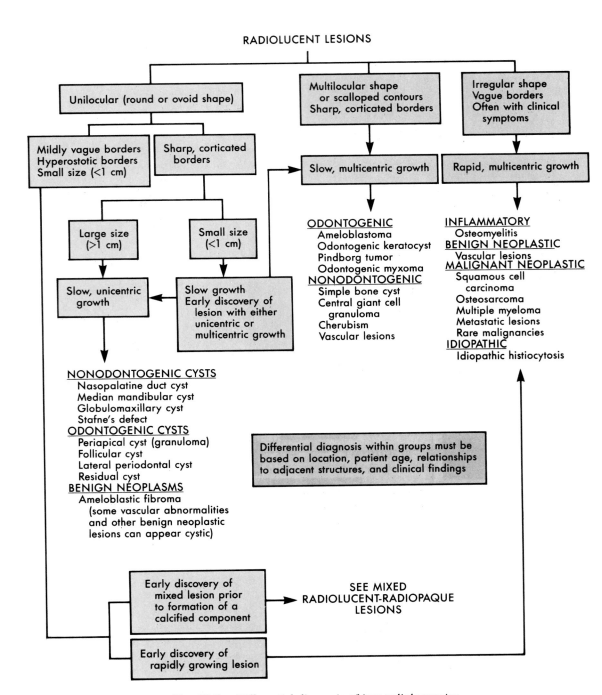

Fig. 19-2   Differential diagnosis of jaw radiolucencies.

acteristic radiographic features that are not apparent early in lesion development. Many multilocular lesions, rapidly enlarging radiolucencies, and mixed radiolucent-radiopaque lesions less than 1 cm in diameter can appear as unilocular radiolucencies. As Fig. 19-2 suggests, the presence of sharply delineated, corticated borders around small radiolucencies is evidence that the lesions can safely be considered slow-growing and that they may be listed among either the unilocular or multilocular lesions. When a small radiolucency exhibits irregular shape and vague borders without peripheral radiopacity, an inflammatory or malignant neoplastic process is suggested. Peripheral hyperostosis of a small radiolucency suggests the possibility of the existence a productive mixed lesion before the calcification of the mineralized tissue component.

Fissural Cysts

Definition. Fissural cysts are nonodontogenic, epithelial-lined lesions that originate at embryonic junction sites from epithelial remnants. The *nasopalatine duct cyst,* also referred to as *incisive canal cyst,* develops at the anterior maxillary suture near the apices of the central incisors. This is the most common fissural cyst, and the remaining fissural cysts that form within the jaws are rare. The *median palatal cyst* occurs at the midline of the hard palate posterior to the incisive foramen. The *median mandibular cyst* forms at the midline of the mandible near the apices of the central incisors, and the *globulomaxillary cyst* occurs between the maxillary lateral incisor and canine teeth.

Radiographic features. Fissural cysts exhibit unilocular shape, homogeneous radiolucency, and sharply delineated, cortical borders as illustrated by the example shown in Fig. 19-3. Slow, symmetric enlargement is typical. Even if the radiolucency is somewhat asymmetric, the center of the lesion is near the developmental junction. The nasopalatine duct cyst may appear heart-shaped in some projec-

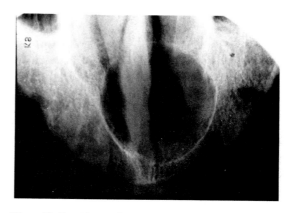

Fig. 19-3 Nasopalatine duct cyst. The round shape and sharply delineated, cortical borders are characteristic of cystic lesions in general.

tions because the anterior nasal spine is superimposed over the superior margin. Divergence of adjacent tooth roots is a common finding, whereas sharply delineated external resorption and arrested root formation are less likely features.

Clinical features. Fissural cysts are asymptomatic lesions and are usually an incidental radiographic finding. Large examples may cause expansion of the jaw or the hard palate. Careful probing of the incisive papilla may reveal a sinus tract leading to the nasopalatine duct cyst and drainage of fluid via the sinus may explain the limited growth potential of some nasopalatine duct cysts.

Differential diagnosis. Location as listed in Table 19-3 is the primary feature that suggests a cystic radiolucency may be a fissural cyst. Several other cystic radiolucencies can occur in the alveolus near developmental junctions. They include chronic periapical inflammatory lesions secondary to pulpal necrosis and follicular cysts associated with unerupted teeth. Periapical cysts and granulomas secondary to pulpal necrosis are usually centered over an apex rather than between the teeth. Also, apical loss of periodontal ligament integrity and evidence of pulpal necrosis are

Table 19-3 Anatomic locations of lesions that typically produce unilocular radiolucency

Unilocular radiolucencies	Location
NONODONTOGENIC CYSTS	
Nasopalatine duct (incisive canal) cyst	Maxillary midline between the central incisors
Median palatal cyst	Midline of palate, posterior to incisive foramen
Median mandibular cyst	Midline of the mandible
Globulomaxillary cyst	Between the roots of the maxillary canine and lateral incisor
Stafne's defect	Adjacent to the inferior border of the mandible near the angle
ODONTOGENIC CYSTS	
Periapical cyst (and granuloma)	Near apex, loss of periodontal ligament integrity
Follicular (eruption and dentigerous) cyst	Surrounding the crown of an unerupted tooth
Lateral periodontal cyst	Between roots of teeth, usually in the mandibular premolar region
Residual cyst	Site of an extracted tooth, usually at the apical level
BENIGN NEOPLASMS	
Ameloblastic fibroma	Pericoronal, associated with failure of tooth to erupt

present in most instances. A toothlike radiopacity located near the periphery of the cystic radiolucency is typical of a follicular cyst. Radiographically prominent incisive canals may suggest the possibility of a small nasopalatine duct cyst. This anatomic structure is usually most prominent among children, the radiolucency is less than 5 mm in diameter, and trabecular bone is superimposed over the radiolucency. Also, the cortical border fades near the crest of the alveolar ridge. Other cystic odontogenic lesions and benign nonodontogenic neoplasms (Fig. 19-2) are also possible in these locations.

Management. Surgical excision is indicated and recurrence is unusual.

Stafne's Defect

Definition. Stafne's defect, which is also called the *static bone cyst* and *developmental salivary gland defect,* is a concavity in the lingual surface of the mandible (Fig. 19-4). The depression contains lobules of normal submandibular salivary gland tissue, which suggests indentation of bone or partial enclosure of sub-

mandibular gland tissue within bone during development. Similar entrapment of sublingual gland tissue in the anterior mandible and premolar region, referred to as an *anterior lingual mandibular salivary gland defect,* is less common.

Radiographic features. The Stafne's defect is located below the inferior alveolar canal near the angle of the mandible, and it exhibits homogeneous radiolucency, unilocular shape, and sharply delineated borders. The radiolucency is surrounded by a radiopaque cortical border that is often significantly wider (Fig. 19-4, *A*) than the thin cortical rim adjacent to most cystic radiolucencies. Comparisons of radiographs representing an extended time interval reveal no change in size. Radiographs exposed following injection of a radiopaque contrast medium into the Wharton's duct demonstrates that these defects contain submandibular tissue. Cortical enlargement or other alterations of adjacent structures are unusual.

Anterior lingual mandibular salivary gland defects are located mesial to the mandibular

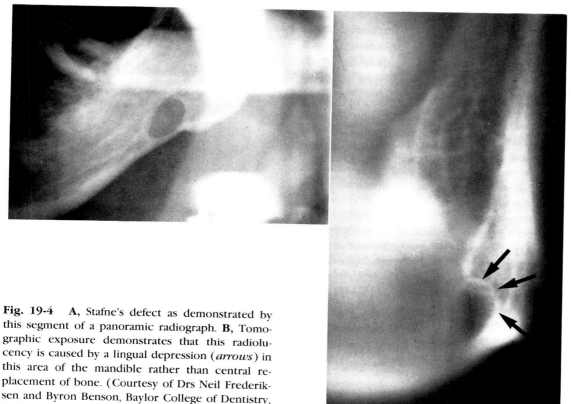

Fig. 19-4   A, Stafne's defect as demonstrated by this segment of a panoramic radiograph. **B,** Tomographic exposure demonstrates that this radiolucency is caused by a lingual depression (*arrows*) in this area of the mandible rather than central replacement of bone. (Courtesy of Drs Neil Frederiksen and Byron Benson, Baylor College of Dentistry, Dallas, Texas.)

first molar near the apices of the teeth. The radiographic features are similar in all other respects to those of Stafne's defect.

Clinical features. Both Stafne's defects and anterior lingual mandibular salivary gland defects are asymptomatic without expansion.

Differential diagnosis. A unilocular radiolucency with wide, cortical borders located below the inferior alveolar canal near the angle of the mandible is pathognomonic of Stafne's defect. Comparison of radiographs showing no enlargement with time and sialographic demonstration of salivary ducts extending into the radiolucency are confirmational.

The differential diagnosis of anterior lingual mandibular salivary gland defects is more challenging because other cystic lesions also occur in this region. The absence of symptoms and expansion along with the presence of an unusually wide cortical border favor the diagnosis of anterior lingual mandibular salivary gland defect for a unilocular radiolucency in this region.

Management. No treatment is indicated.

Periapical Cyst and Granuloma

Definition. Periapical cysts and granulomas secondary to pulpal necrosis have been discussed in Chapter 8. These two chronic lesions are discussed jointly in the context of radiographic differential diagnosis because they are indistinguishable in most cases before surgical removal and histopathologic examination. The more general designations *radicular gran-*

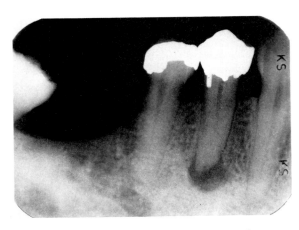

Fig. 19-5   Periapical radiolucency secondary to necrotic pulp disease. The increased radiopacity apical and lateral to the radiolucency represent chronic inflammatory sclerosis of bone referred to as condensing osteitis.

uloma and *radicular cyst* refer to inflammatory lesions secondary to pulpal necrosis near any root surface. Radicular granulomas and cysts are by far the most common unilocular radiolucent jaw lesions and are a diagnostic possibility for any cystic lesion located near root surfaces.

Radiographic features. A unilocular, homogeneous radiolucency located near the apex of a tooth is the typical appearance of these chronic inflammatory lesions. The margins are sharply delineated in most cases, but radiographic appearance of the bone adjacent to the radiolucency varies considerably. A thin, cortical margin indicates slow, chronic progression with minimal active inflammation, which suggests a periapical cyst. A broader hyperostotic or sclerotic periphery referred to as *condensing osteitis* as shown in Fig. 19-5 often results from cyclic episodes of acute exacerbation and chronic, asymptomatic inflammation. A peripheral border of trabecular bone with little evidence of hyperostosis is compatible with more progressive inflammation.

Most examples are less than 2 cm in diameter. Lesions of long duration may grow larger, and early lesions may appear as little more than an apical widening of the periodontal ligament (PDL) space. This alteration or destruction of the PDL (Fig. 19-5) is the most conclusive radiographic evidence that a periradicular radiolucency is a consequence of pulpal necrosis. Radiographs often reveal conditions likely to cause pulpal necrosis such as deep decay. External resorption of the root may also be present.

Clinical features. The numerous clinical findings indicative of pulpal necrosis and periapical inflammation are described in Chapter 8. Periapical cysts and granulomas are painless.

Differential diagnosis. The combination of periapical radiolucency, alteration of the PDL, and clinical evidence of pulpal necrosis is strong evidence that a cystic radiolucency near an asymptomatic tooth is either a periapical cyst or granuloma. Pain or tenderness to percussion associated with similar radiographic findings indicates a periapical abscess. Other cystic lesions must be considered as possible diagnoses for a unilocular periapical radiolucency in the absence of convincing evidence of pulpal necrosis and a normal periodontal ligament appearance. Location of these noninflammatory lesions (see Table 19-3) is the most helpful differentiating feature.

Management. Endodontic treatment of the tooth affected by pulpal necrosis leads to resolution of most periapical cysts or granulomas. Clinical and radiographic reevaluation following endodontic treatment is required to identify lesions that do not resolve or instances of noninflammatory cystic lesions misdiagnosed as secondary to pulpal necrosis.

Residual Cyst

Definition. The residual cyst is an odontogenic cyst that persists after the removal of the tooth originally associated with the lesion. Most examples originate as periapical cysts, although follicular cysts can also become residual.

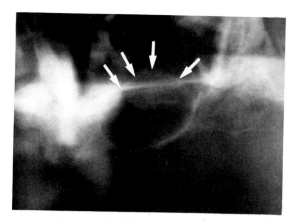

Fig. 19-6 Residual cyst of the maxillary premolar region. This segment of a panoramic radiograph demonstrates radiolucency that was originally considered to be a portion of the maxillary sinus until the thin cortical "roof" of the cystic lesion and the floor of the sinus (*arrows*) were identified.

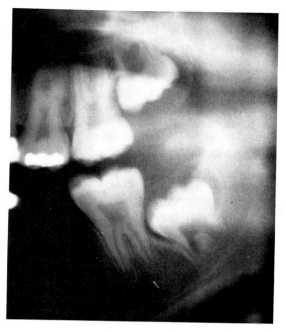

Fig. 19-7 Cystic enlargement associated with both unerupted third molars. Note that both pericoronal radiolucencies exhibit relatively uniform enlargement on all surfaces of the crown and that the radiolucency stops abruptly near the cementoenamel junction of the teeth.

Radiographic features. A homogeneous, unilocular radiolucency with sharply delineated, cortical borders located at an extraction site, as illustrated in Fig. 19-6, is the characteristic presentation of a residual cyst. Radiographs exposed before extraction reveal a similar lesion.

Clinical features. Residual cysts are usually asymptomatic and an incidental radiographic finding. A pathologic sinus draining the cyst or other residual effect of the original lesion may be present in some cases.

Differential diagnosis. The differential diagnosis is simplified if the presence of a similar cystic radiolucency before the extraction can be confirmed. If prior radiographs are unavailable, then the occurrence of cystic lesions unrelated to the extracted tooth should also be considered, depending on the location.

Management. Surgical enucleation is indicated and recurrence is unlikely. Prevention of residual cysts by enucleation of the original lesion at the time of extraction is recommended if feasible.

Follicular Cyst

Definition. Follicular cysts originate from the dental follicle and, therefore, always surround the crown of an unerupted tooth. Follicular cyst is a general designation for both the *eruption cyst,* if the emergence of the tooth into the oral cavity is imminent, and the *dentigerous cyst,* if normal eruption is unlikely.

Radiographic features. Follicular cysts exhibit homogeneous, unilocular radiolucency with sharply delineated, corticated borders. The earliest radiographic evidence of a follicular cyst is pericoronal radiolucency greater than 3 mm that surrounds the crown of an unerupted tooth (Fig. 19-7). Dentigerous cysts can demonstrate unlimited growth potential by achieving large size, although the growth rate is slow as indicated by the sharp delineation of the borders. Displacement of the unerupted tooth, shifting or external resorption of adjacent teeth, cortical expansion, and similar distortions of adjacent anatomic structures may be associated with follicular cysts.

Clinical features. Smaller dentigerous cysts are generally asymptomatic and an incidental radiographic finding. Larger lesions may produce alveolar enlargement and mild tenderness of adjacent teeth. Teeth prone to impaction such as the third molars and the maxillary canine are most commonly affected, but a dentigerous cyst can originate from any unerupted tooth. Dentigerous cysts can also form from the follicular tissue of unerupted supernumerary teeth such as mesiodens and odontomas.

Eruption cysts produce compressible enlargement of the alveolus, reddish-blue mucosal color, and the mild tenderness often associated with eruption. Most eruption cysts spontaneously resolve after the cystic epithelium fuses with the surface epithelium. The cystic epithelium of both eruption and dentigerous cysts can become continuous with the crevicular space of an adjacent tooth, which can allow entrapment of bacteria and food material within the follicular space. The resulting infection represents the combination of a periodontal abscess and pericoronitis that is the source of episodic pain and purulence.

Differential diagnosis. Most unilocular, pericoronal radiolucencies are eventually determined to be follicular cysts or enlargement of the follicular connective tissue referred to as *follicular hyperplasia.* However, other odontogenic cysts and neoplasms often develop as pericoronal radiolucencies. Evidence of multilocularity or scalloped peripheral borders and inclusion of a significant proportion of the tooth root within the radiolucency are features suggestive of these lesions rather than a follicular cyst. The ameloblastic fibroma is the odontogenic tumor most likely to produce pericoronal radiolucency among children, while odontogenic keratocysts and ameloblastomas usually affect adults. Several mixed radiolucent-radiopaque odontogenic lesions often develop adjacent to unerupted teeth and the calcified component of the lesion may not be apparent radiographically. Pericoronal location of a nonodontogenic lesion is unusual.

Management. Surgical removal of eruption cysts, commonly referred to as "unroofing," controls discomfort and facilitates eruption. Enucleation of dentigerous cysts during the removal of the impacted tooth is indicated and recurrence is unusual. A treatment option for large dentigerous cysts is *marsupialization,* which is the surgical creation of an opening between the cyst and the oral cavity. Maintaining this passage with frequent irrigation for a period of weeks or months allows gradual shrinkage of the cyst and a less complicated surgical removal.

Lateral Periodontal Cyst

Definition. The lateral periodontal cyst is a noninflammatory lesion that originates from odontogenic epithelial rests.

Radiographic features. Lateral periodontal cysts exhibit unilocular, homogeneous radiolucency with sharply delineated, cortical borders. Most examples are located near mandibular premolars (Fig. 19-8) and enlargement may cause slight divergence of the roots. The lamina dura of adjacent teeth appears intact or continuous with the cortical border of the cyst. A rare variant of the lateral periodontal cyst known as the *botryoid odontogenic cyst* produces a multilocular radiolucency.

Clinical features. Lateral periodontal cysts are asymptomatic and are discovered during routine radiographic examination of adults. The cyst is not directly related to pulpal necrosis or advanced periodontitis.

Differential diagnosis. Other odontogenic cysts and tumors can produce unilocular radiolucency unrelated to inflammation near the mandibular premolars of an adult, but the lateral periodontal cyst is a more likely possi-

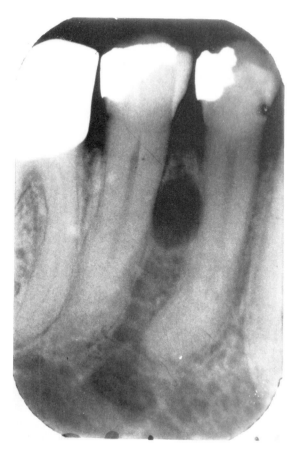

Fig. 19-8   Lateral periodontal cyst.

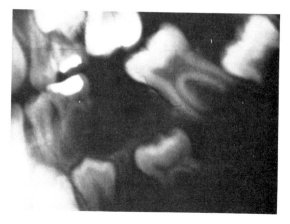

Fig. 19-9   Ameloblastic fibroma of a 7-year-old boy. The slow growth of this lesion is indicated by the relatively small size the lesion attained in the 4 years since the enlargement blocked the eruption of the second deciduous molar before age 2. (Courtesy of Dr Roger Wilson, Rapid City, South Dakota.)

bility in this region. A radicular cyst is the probable diagnosis if pulpal necrosis or advanced periodontitis is associated with the radiolucency.

Management. Recurrence is unusual following enucleation.

Ameloblastic Fibroma

Definition. The ameloblastic fibroma is a benign odontogenic neoplasm that usually forms near the crown of an unerupted tooth of a child or adolescent. Most examples develop near posterior mandibular teeth.

Radiographic features. Sharply delineated, cortical margins surrounding a homogeneous, unilocular radiolucency are the typical radiographic features of an ameloblastic fibroma. The development near the crown of an unerupted tooth often blocks eruption and causes apical tooth displacement. Comparison of the patient's age, the typically small lesion size, and the expected eruption age for the impacted tooth demonstrates the slow growth of most ameloblastic fibromas as shown by the example in Fig. 19-9.

Clinical features. This asymptomatic lesion is usually discovered during routine radiographic examination or suspected on the basis of failure of a tooth to erupt. Unusually large examples may cause mild alveolar expansion.

Differential diagnosis. The differential diagnosis of a pericoronal radiolucency with the features suggestive of an ameloblastic fibroma should include follicular cysts. Follicular cysts produce uniform, symmetric widening of the radiolucency around the entire crown of the tooth, while the radiolucency of ameloblastic fibromas may be less centered around the crown. A periapical inflammatory lesion from a deciduous mandibular molar can produce radiographic features identical to those of an ameloblastic fibroma and is a more likely possibility if clinical findings suggest pulp necrosis. Other odontogenic cysts and neoplasms such as odontogenic keratocysts and ameloblastomas are usually identified in adults.

Management. Conservative surgical removal is indicated. Unlike some other odontogenic tumors, ameloblastic fibromas seldom recur. Eruption of a displaced tooth usually proceeds if root formation is incomplete. Otherwise, the tooth should be removed with the ameloblastic fibroma.

MULTILOCULAR RADIOLUCENCIES OF THE JAWS

Multilocularity reflects slow growth from multiple, independent foci that is a typical feature of certain benign odontogenic and nonodontogenic lesions. This produces a loculated or "soap bubble" shape as larger size is attained. Patient age, lesion location, and the presence of expansion are the most contributory differential diagnostic features within this lesion category.

Ameloblastoma

Definition. The ameloblastoma is a benign odontogenic neoplasm that characteristically produces extension or "budding" of small nests of tumor cells into normal tissues at the lesion margin. This local invasiveness explains the frequent recurrence of ameloblastomas because these tumor buds are not removed by conservative excision. Subclassification of ameloblastomas by histopathologic features yields designations such as *plexiform* or *granular cell ameloblastoma.* However, little clinical significance is related to this subclassification in most instances. The *mural* or *cystic ameloblastoma* is an ameloblastoma that develops within an odontogenic cyst. The diagnostic features and probability of recurrence of a cystic ameloblastoma are those of the parent cyst in most cases rather than those of a solid ameloblastoma.

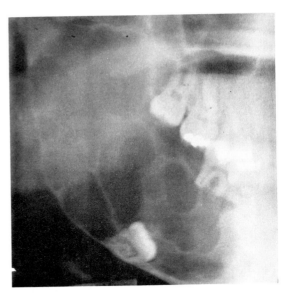

Fig. 19-10 Ameloblastoma. (Courtesy of Dr Gilbert Lilly, University of Iowa College of Dentistry, Iowa City, Iowa.)

Radiographic features. Homogeneous radiolucency and sharply delineated, corticated borders are consistent radiographic features. Unilocular shape is typical of small lesions, while scalloped or lobulated peripheral contours, radiopaque lines crossing the center of the radiolucency, or other features of multilocularity, as shown in Fig. 19-10, usually develop with ameloblastomas greater than 1 to 2 cm in diameter. Comparison of radiographs representing a time span of months or years demonstrates slow growth. Larger ameloblastomas produce cortical expansion as well as gradual displacement and external resorption of adjacent teeth.

Clinical features. Most ameloblastomas form in the alveolus of the posterior mandible of adults. Small ameloblastomas are encountered during routine radiographic examination, while painless expansion of the posterior mandible is the usual clinical presentation of larger lesions. Shifting and mobility of adjacent teeth may also develop.

Differential diagnosis. An ameloblastoma must be considered in the differential diagnosis of unilocular and multilocular radiolucencies of tooth-bearing bone. Other odontogenic cysts and tumors must be included in the differential diagnosis of a suspected ameloblastoma exhibiting unilocular shape with relative probability determined by patient age, location, and the relationship of the lesion to adjacent teeth. Multilocularity of the posterior alveolus limits the diagnostic possibilities to ameloblastoma and other odontogenic lesions because nonodontogenic multilocular lesions generally occur in the body of the mandible or in the anterior segment.

Management. Surgical removal of an ameloblastoma must include local tumor extensions into the bordering tissue to prevent recurrence. Therefore block excision, if it is surgically feasible, or vigorous curetting of surrounding bone after removal of the lesion is indicated with a working diagnosis of an ameloblastoma. Clinical reevaluation for recurrence is necessary following surgical removal.

Odontogenic Keratocyst

Definition. As the name implies, the odontogenic keratocyst is an odontogenic cyst characterized by central accumulation of keratin. The odontogenic keratocyst and ameloblastoma are similar in that independent foci of growth often yield multilocularity and local invasiveness with common recurrence. A *primordial cyst* is an odontogenic cyst that develops in place of a tooth, and these lesions usually exhibit the histopathologic features of odontogenic keratocysts. Multiple odontogenic keratocysts are a feature of *nevoid basal cell carcinoma syndrome* as described in Chapter 20.

Radiographic features. The odontogenic keratocyst produces homogeneous radiolucency with sharply delineated, cortical borders. The radiolucency may appear milky or hazy compared with radiolucent lesions of similar size because of the greater x-ray attenua-

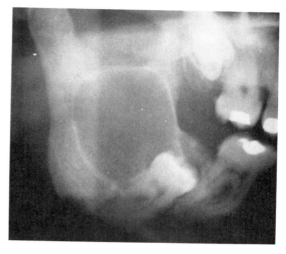

Fig. 19-11   Odontogenic keratocyst. The radiolucency exhibits no evidence of multilocularity, but the lesion appears less radiolucent than other radiolucent lesions of similar size because of the greater x-ray attenuation of the central keratin. Note that the relationship of the lesion to the unerupted molar lacks the uniform increase in follicular width (see Fig. 19-7) expected with a dentigerous cyst.

tion of the central keratin (Fig. 19-11). Unilocular shape may be noted with smaller lesions, but multilocular contours become apparent as larger size is attained.

Clinical features. The lesion is painless and may cause alveolar enlargement or displacement of teeth. Odontogenic keratocysts are more likely to develop among adults and the posterior mandible is the typical location. However, lesions may develop in any tooth-bearing bone and children are occasionally affected.

Differential diagnosis. Odontogenic keratocyst is a diagnostic possibility for all unilocular and multilocular radiolucencies of the alveolar bone of the mandible and maxillae. Certain features associated with a cystic or multilocular radiolucency such as replacement of a tooth by a multilocular radiolucency, a history of numerous basal cell carcinomas, or "milky" radiolucency of the lesion indicate greater probability of an odontogenic keratocyst.

Management. Removal of a suspected odontogenic keratocyst must be approached with the same concern for recurrence as with ameloblastomas. Discovery of yellow, cheesy material within a cyst during surgery indicates the need to remove bone from the borders of the lesion. Periodic reevaluation for recurrence after surgery is appropriate.

Odontogenic Myxoma

Definition. The odontogenic myxoma is a benign neoplasm dominated by gelatinous connective tissue. The lesion is uncommon and its recurrence rate of approximately 25% is explained in part by the surgical difficulty of totally removing this amorphous tumor substance.

Radiographic features. This slowly enlarging lesion produces sharply delineated, cortical borders with a scalloped contour. The central area is predominantly radiolucent with a relatively uniform reticular, lacy pattern of slender radiopaque lines (Fig. 19-12). This has been described as a "tennis racket" appearance. Divergence of roots and distortion of adjacent anatomic contours may be associated with larger lesions.

Clinical features. Localized, painless expansion of the alveolus affecting a young adult is the typical presentation. The posterior segments of the maxilla and mandible are the usual occurrence sites. Adjacent teeth may be displaced.

Differential diagnosis. The lacy, reticular pattern of multilocularity is relatively characteristic of odontogenic myxomas. Other multilocular lesions such as an ameloblastoma and odontogenic keratocyst should also be considered as possibilities.

Management. Curettage of the surrounding bone following removal should be accomplished to minimize the probability of recurrence and periodic reevaluation after surgery is warranted. More aggressive excision of adjacent tissues is usually not justified.

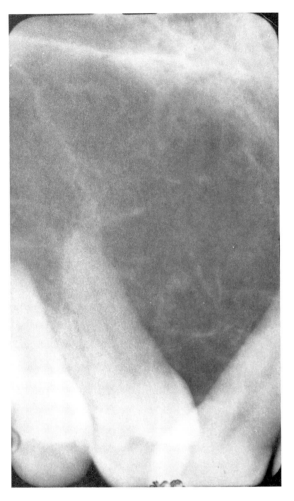

Fig. 19-12 This periapical radiograph demonstrates the slender, weblike radiopaque lines that are a characteristic feature of the central areas of an odontogenic myxoma.

Simple Bone Cyst

Definition. The simple bone cyst is a nonodontogenic lesion that is not a true epithelial-lined cyst. Surgical entry reveals an empty space, yellowish serous fluid, or serosanguineous material with a thin tissue lining of fibrous connective tissue. The most accepted pathogenesis of simple bone cysts is that traumatic injury produces a hematoma within bone,

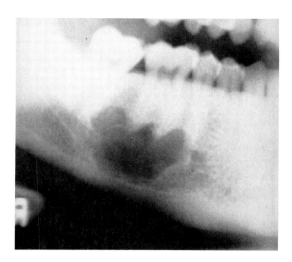

Fig. 19-13 Simple bone cyst. The tendency for extensions of the multilocular radiolucency to protrude between the roots of mandibular teeth without displacing them is characteristic of this lesion.

which promotes bone resorption in response to steady hydrostatic pressure. This proposed mechanism explains some of the synonyms for the lesion such as *traumatic bone cyst, hemorrhagic bone cyst,* and *extravasation cyst.*

Radiographic features. Multilocularity is demonstrated by the scalloped peripheral borders or lobulated shape of this homogeneous radiolucency. A periapical location in the body of the mandible is the typical location, and maxillary occurrence is unusual. Narrow, fingerlike extensions of the radiolucency between the roots of teeth without displacement (Fig. 19-13) is a characteristic effect produced by simple bone cysts. Sequential radiographs may reveal rapid enlargement in the early development of the lesion followed by slower progression or periods without significant change in lesion size. The borders are sharply delineated, but cortexlike radiopacity may not become apparent until after the early rapid growth phase.

Clinical features. Most simple bone cysts affect adolescents or young adults and are painless with little or no jaw enlargement. Ap-

proximately 50% of patients associate traumatic jaw injury with the lesion.

Differential diagnosis. The typical location of the lesion epicenter in the body of the mandible rather than the alveolus suggests that the lesion is nonodontogenic. Central giant cell granulomas are also multilocular and affect young adults, but obvious cortical expansion is a typical feature of this lesion. The frequent periapical location of the simple bone cyst can suggest a periapical inflammatory lesion secondary to pulpal necrosis, but the intact periodontal ligament apparatus and lack of evidence suggesting pulpal necrosis serve to exclude this possibility. Stafne's defect exhibits broader cortical borders and is located below the interior alveolar canal, whereas simple bone cysts originate superior to this region.

Management. The diagnosis usually becomes apparent with the discovery of minimal lesion contents during surgery. Curettage of surrounding bone to stimulate hemorrhage and closure provides a clot matrix for healing and repair.

Central Giant Cell Granuloma

Definition. The central giant cell granuloma is a relatively rapidly enlarging, nonodontogenic lesion with features suggestive of both a reactive lesion and a benign neoplasm. The central giant cell granuloma is unique to the jaws and is similar in some respects to the *aneurysmal bone cyst,* which commonly occurs in other bones but is unusual in the jaws. The pathogenesis of both enlargements may be variations of the same process involving hemorrhage within bone. The *peripheral giant cell granuloma* of the gingiva should not be confused with the central jaw lesion despite the similarity of their histopathologic features and designations because the location, course, and management of the two lesions are different.

Radiographic features. Central giant cell granulomas produce homogeneous radiolucency and multilocular shape anterior to the first molar of either the mandible or maxilla. The borders are sharply delineated, but the cortical rimming typical of most other benign radiolucencies is often less apparent. Relatively dramatic cortical enlargement and displacement of teeth are associated features.

Clinical features. The patient is usually younger than 30 years of age and aware of painless jaw enlargement within the preceding several months. Clinical examination of the area reveals pronounced expansion and overlying mucosa appears distended but intact.

Differential diagnosis. The central giant cell granuloma is the most likely diagnosis for a multilocular radiolucency of the anterior jaw segments that is associated with pronounced expansion and patient age less than 30. Odontogenic lesions that produce multilocularity such as ameloblastomas and odontogenic keratocysts must also be considered, but their expansion is usually less dramatic than that of central giant cell granulomas. Simple bone cysts can usually be excluded from the differential diagnosis since they seldom cause expansion. Aneurysmal bone cyst should be considered if pain and tenderness are present.

Management. Conservative surgical removal of central giant cell granulomas and aneurysmal bone cysts is adequate treatment since these lesions seldom recur.

Cherubism

Definition. Cherubism is an uncommon developmental condition that produces symmetric jaw enlargement of children. The familial occurrence of the condition indicates genetic pathogenesis, but the mechanism of transmission is not completely understood as a consequence of variable penetrance and expressivity.

Radiographic features. Homogeneous radiolucency with a multilocular shape and sharply delineated, cortical borders are typical features of cherubism at the initial diagnosis. Bilateral lesions of the mandibular ramus regions is the typical distribution, although any area of the mandible and maxillae may be affected. The slow growth of the lesions produces a general impression of distorted enlargement of the facial bones without cortical perforation. A mixed radiolucent-radiopaque appearance eventually develops as the lesions regress during adolescence and remodeling of bone predominates. A mottled or granular appearance suggestive of disorganized trabecular bone replacement of the lesions may persist into adulthood.

Clinical features. The symmetric fullness of the cheeks yields a cherublike appearance that characteristically affects younger children. Maxillary lesions may produce distortion of the orbital floor causing a superiorly directed gaze. Premature exfoliation of deciduous teeth adjacent to the lesions may also occur.

Differential diagnosis. The symmetric enlargement, characteristic facial appearance, age of onset, and radiographic features provide an adequate basis for a definitive diagnosis in most cases. Other conditions capable of producing multiple bone lesions among infants and small children such as polyostotic fibrous dysplasia and Letterer-Siwe disease are suggested by more diffuse radiolucent lesions, asymmetric enlargements, and addition lesions of other bones.

Management. The size and distribution of the lesions at the time of diagnosis usually precludes surgical excision, although incisional biopsy to confirm the diagnosis is usually justified. The lesions generally become static later in childhood and subsequent normal bone growth and remodeling yields normal facial contours in many cases. Cosmetic recontouring of the jaws following completion of skeletal growth may be beneficial in some instances.

IRREGULARLY SHAPED RADIOLUCENCIES OF THE JAWS

Acute inflammatory and malignant neoplastic conditions produce rapid lytic replacement of bone that follows multiple "paths of least resistance" rather than uniform outward expansion. This results in irregularly shaped radiolucencies and vague peripheral borders because time is not available for production of a cortical or hyperostotic response by normal peripheral bone. These radiographic features give the general impression of bone destruction rather than the anatomic distortion that is typical of slow growing lesions.

Acute Inflammatory Lesions of Bone Secondary to Dental Infections

Definition. Radiolucencies representing inflammation secondary to pulpal necrosis, advanced periodontitis, and other dental inflammatory lesions are the most common radiolucencies encountered by the dentist. As discussed in Chapter 8, most acute dental infections are exacerbations of chronic inflammatory lesions. Therefore the "chronic" radiographic features of periapical cysts and granulomas that are associated with the clinical abscess developed before the acute exacerbation. The bone lysis produced by a purely acute infection is less frequently demonstrated radiographically. In some cases, clinical signs and symptoms clearly indicate an acute infection while the radiograph reveals little evidence of abnormality. The conclusion from this is that clinical signs and symptoms provide more dependable diagnostic information concerning the immediate status of jaw infections than radiographs.

The diagnosis of jaw infections depends on the location and extent of the process. *Acute periapical abscess* refers to liquefaction, degeneration, and related inflammation secondary to pulpal necrosis confined to the immediate periapical region. *Acute periodontal abscess* indicates an identical radicular infection secondary to periodontitis. *Acute osteomyelitis* indicates spread of the infection into marrow spaces of adjacent bone. *Acute subperiosteal abscess* refers to extension of the infection between the cortex of the bone and the periosteum. *Cellulitis* is defined as spread of the bacterial infection into the fascial planes of the adjacent soft tissues.

Radiographic features. The periodontal ligament apparatus and bone may appear normal or only slight, focal widening of the periodontal ligament space may be apparent early in the course of acute dental infections. Deep axial decay extent, advanced periodontal bone loss, and other radiographic evidence of the causative infection are often present.

Vague radiolucency of the trabecular bone without peripheral delineation surrounding a focal interruption of the lamina dura may be present in cases of acute infection of several weeks duration. The degree of radiolucency is greatest immediately adjacent to the tooth and gradually fades to normal trabecular appearance. Acute exacerbation of a chronic inflammatory lesion is indicated by the unilocular, sharply delineated radiolucency typical of periapical cysts and granulomas or by a sclerotic, granular radiopacity peripheral to the radiolucency (Fig. 19-5).

Clinical features. The combination of spontaneous pain, tenderness to palpation, pain elicited by percussion, mucosal erythema, and compressible enlargement are all features of an acute dental infection. Fever, malaise, and regional lymphadenopathy may be present in severe cases. Additional clinical features of acute dental infections are described in Chapter 8.

Differential diagnosis. The combination of clinical features and radiographic findings provide a definitive diagnosis in most cases. The specific diagnosis from among those described above depends on the extent of tenderness to palpation and enlargement demonstrated clinically.

Management. Treatment of dental infections is described in Chapter 8.

Idiopathic Histiocytosis

Definition. Idiopathic histiocytosis, formerly called *histiocytosis X,* refers to three conditions with the common feature of destructive lesions composed of cells that resemble histiocytes. Table 19-4 summarizes and compares the three characteristic forms of id-

Table 19-4   Comparison of different clinical forms of idiopathic histiocytosis

Form of idiopathic histiocytosis		Age of occurrence	Lesion distribution	Clinical course
Current designation	Former designation			
Acute disseminated idioapthic histiocytosis	Letterer-Siwe disease	Infancy and early childhood	Multiple lesions affecting bone, skin, and other organs	Rapidly progressive, often fatal; considered by many to be malignant neoplastic disease
Chronic disseminated idiopathic histiocytosis	Hand-Schüler-Christian disease	Children	Multiple bone lesions and extrabony manifestations such as exophthalmos, diabetes insipidus, lymphadenopathy, splenomegaly, hepatomegaly, dermatitis	Gradual progression, lesions usually controlled by surgical removal and/or low-dose radiotherapy
Chronic localized idiopathic histiocytosis	Eosinophilic granuloma	Older children, adolescents, and young adults	Isolated or multiple lesions limited to bone	Manifestations considered as either idiopathic inflammatory or benign neoplastic disease; usually controlled by surgical removal, although progression to the chronic disseminated form can occur

iopathic histiocytosis, although individual cases may consist of features intermediate between these forms.

Radiographic features. The solitary or multiple bone lesions of idiopathic histiocytosis appear homogeneously radiolucent with irregular shape. The lesional margins appear well localized grossly, but close examination reveals a ragged or vague transition from the radiolucency to normal trabecular bone without peripheral sclerosis. This yields an impression of bone destruction that is described as a "punched out" appearance. Idiopathic histiocytosis can destroy the bone surrounding one or more teeth, which produces a "floating tooth" appearance.

Clinical features. Mobility, premature exfoliation of teeth, and pain are often related to the radiographic lesions. The associated gingival and alveolar tissues appear bulbous and erythematous, but enlargement proportional to the radiolucent lesion—as expected with many neoplastic and inflammatory lesions—is absent. The additional clinical manifestations listed in Table 19-4 may also be present.

Differential diagnosis. Premature loss of teeth caused by idiopathic histiocytosis may suggest juvenile periodontitis. The focal or multifocal lesions of idiopathic histiocytosis are intermixed with normal bone support of unaffected teeth in contrast to the generalized bone destruction of juvenile periodontitis. The absence of purulent exudate excludes acute bacterial infections.

Solitary chronic localized idiopathic histiocytosis lesions must be considered in the differential diagnosis of many isolated radiolucencies with a punched out appearance affecting a child or young adult. Multiple punched out bone lesions are also produced by multiple myeloma, but this disseminated neoplasm of plasma cell origin afflicts middle-aged and older adults.

The rapid progression and multiple lesions of bone, skin, lymph nodes, and other organs of acute disseminated idiopathic histiocytosis is indistinguishable from other disseminated malignancies of infancy and early childhood. The definitive diagnosis must be made based on histopathologic examination.

Management. The management of the acute disseminated form is by chemotherapy, and the prognosis must be considered guarded. The chronic forms are usually effectively controlled by surgical removal or radiotherapy. Frequent reexamination following treatment is required to identify recurrence and development of new lesions.

Central Vascular Lesions

Definition. Two developmental vascular lesions that occur within bone are the *central hemangioma* and the *arteriovenous malformation*. Central hemangiomas are dense collections of otherwise normal blood vessels that enlarge only in proportion to the growth of the individual. Unusual instances of progression may be explained by injury and intralesional bleeding analogous to the causative mechanism described for simple bone cysts. Arteriovenous malformation, also known as *arteriovenous fistula*, is a dense collection of vascular structures characterized by direct blood flow from arteries to veins without an intermediate capillary bed. The hydrostatic forces associated with this malformation produce rapid progression and potentially life-threatening hemorrhage. Fortunately, both lesions are rare in the jaws.

Radiographic features. The only consistent radiographic feature of central vascular lesions is that their replacement of trabecular bone yields radiolucency. Nearly any combination of lesion shape, location, and pattern can develop. Unilocularity, multilocularity, a "honeycomb" pattern, and heterogeneous degrees of radiolucency are all possible. The margins of hemangiomas are usually well delineated without peripheral hyperostosis, but some examples produce vague borders. Arteriovenous malformations are usually diffuse, irregularly shaped, and poorly delineated.

Clinical features. Central hemangiomas are usually asymptomatic and are discovered incidentally during routine radiographic examination. Arteriovenous malformations may be asymptomatic, but tenderness, enlargement, cortical perforation, and spontaneous hemorrhage eventually develop. The bleeding starts suddenly without apparent cause and can be difficult to control. A bruit caused by the rush of blood through large arterial-venous channels can occasionally be detected by auscultation. Elevated systolic blood pressure and an abnormally large pulse pressure are additional findings.

Differential diagnosis. Central vascular lesions of bone have been referred to as the "great mimics" of other radiolucent lesions because of the variety of possible lesion shapes and margin features they can produce. Therefore central vascular lesions should be considered a possibility in the differential diagnosis of nearly all radiolucencies. The progressive enlargement and spontaneous hemorrhage of arteriovenous malformations are characteristic and unlikely to be confused with other abnormalities.

Management. The possibility that most radiolucencies of the jaws could be central vascular lesions demands that aspiration of all radiolucent lesions be performed before surgical entry. Demonstration of free blood flow during aspiration requires that the surgical removal of the lesion be planned in anticipation of extensive hemorrhage. Alternatives to surgical removal of central vascular lesions include injection of sclerosing chemicals such as sodium morrhuate, laser ablation, and cryosurgery. Spontaneous oral hemorrhage associated with a diffuse radiolucency is a medical emergency requiring immediate hospitalization.

Malignant Neoplasms of the Jaws

Definition. Most cases of malignancy affecting the jaws are squamous cell carcinomas of mucosal origin that destroy bone by direct invasion. The appearance of the clinical enlargement usually leaves little doubt about the diagnosis. Radiographs contribute primarily to the determination of the lesion extent during the staging process. Squamous cell carcinoma, mucoepidermoid carcinoma, and various sarcomas that originate within the jaws are much less common. Metastatic jaw lesions from primary malignancies such as breast and prostatic carcinomas seldom develop before the end stage of the disease when metastasis is widespread and the diagnosis is well known. Jaw lesions of disseminated malignancies such as lymphomas can also develop, but these lesions are usually of minor diagnostic importance in comparison with the obvious clinical manifestations resulting from damage to other organ systems.

Radiographic features. Invasion of bone by malignant neoplastic lesions produces heterogeneous radiolucency with poorly delineated margins. The impression of bone destruction is indicated by areas of ragged cortical erosion and "pocked" radiolucency (Fig. 19-14, *A* and *B*), often described as a "moth-eaten" appearance. Other malignancies such as multiple myeloma produce multiple radiolucencies without peripheral alteration of bone, which is referred to as a "punched out" appearance (Fig. 19-15). Increase in lesion size may be demonstrated by comparing radiographs representing a duration of only a few weeks. Teeth in the area of bone invasion may exhibit ragged external resorption, but they are usually extruded by the tumor.

Clinical features. The mucosal carcinoma capable of producing bone destruction by lo-

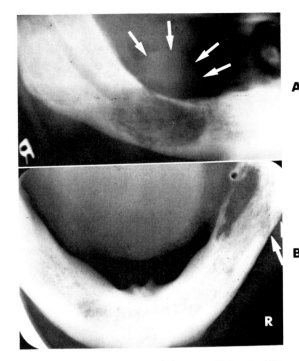

Fig. 19-14   Carcinoma of the mandible. **A,** This segment of a panoramic radiograph reveals poorly delineated radiolucency with a "pocked" appearance in the central areas of the lesion, which indicates multifocal destruction of the buccal and lingual cortical bone. A prominent soft tissue enlargement (*arrows*) was apparent clinically. **B,** Occlusal radiograph of the same lesion reveals the ragged, "moth eaten" destruction of bone. Note the vague thinning of the buccal cortex (*arrow*). This was metastatic carcinoma of the lung. (Courtesy of Dr Gilbert Lilly, University of Iowa College of Dentistry, Iowa City, Iowa.)

cal invasion will be conspicuous during clinical examination. The enlargement is indurated with a rough, heterogeneous surface appearance. Poorly localized bone pain is a frequent patient complaint associated with malignant neoplastic invasion of bone. Painless enlargement of regional lymph nodes indicating metastasis may be present. Intraoral squamous cell carcinoma is associated with age greater

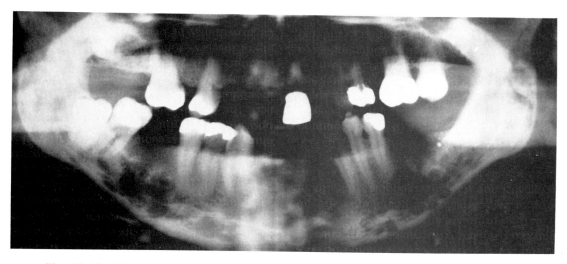

Fig. 19-15 Panoramic radiograph of a 47-year-old woman suffering from multiple myeloma. Numerous "punched out" radiolucencies are present in the mandible. Similar lesions of the skull were demonstrated by lateral skull projection. (Courtesy of Drs Gilbert Lilly and Steven Vincent, University of Iowa College of Dentistry, Iowa City, Iowa.)

than 50 and habitual use of tobacco and alcohol.

Differential diagnosis. The combination of pain, rapid enlargement, and radiographic features of bone destruction narrows the differential diagnosis to malignant neoplasia and inflammatory disease in most cases. Inflammatory bone disease is suggested by a source of infection and purulence as well as smooth surface texture, erythema, and compressibility of the enlargement. Malignant neoplasms lack these features and are indurated with a rough, heterogeneous superficial appearance.

Squamous cell carcinoma of mucosal origin invading bone is suggested by the patient's age, carcinogenic habits, and the large size of the clinical enlargement compared with the bone destruction. Malignancy that has originated within the jaws and perforated the superficial tissues is suggested by more extensive radiographic destruction of bone as compared with the clinical size of the lesion, younger patient age, and absence of tobacco or alcohol habits. Metastatic lesions involving the jaws may be suspected with a history of a distant primary malignancy.

Management. Referral to a tertiary care center for definitive diagnosis, staging, and treatment is indicated if malignancy is suspected.

MIXED RADIOLUCENT-RADIOPAQUE LESIONS OF THE JAWS

The differential diagnostic approach to mixed radiolucent-radiopaque jaw lesions is represented in Fig. 19-16. The three differential diagnostic categorizations within the mixed lesion group are based on the features of the radiopaque component, the arrangement of the components, and the delineation of peripheral borders:

1. Mixed lesions that contain toothlike radiopacities
2. Mixed lesions with central globular or speckled radiopacity and peripheral radiolucency
3. Mixed lesions with random admixture of radiolucent and radiopaque components

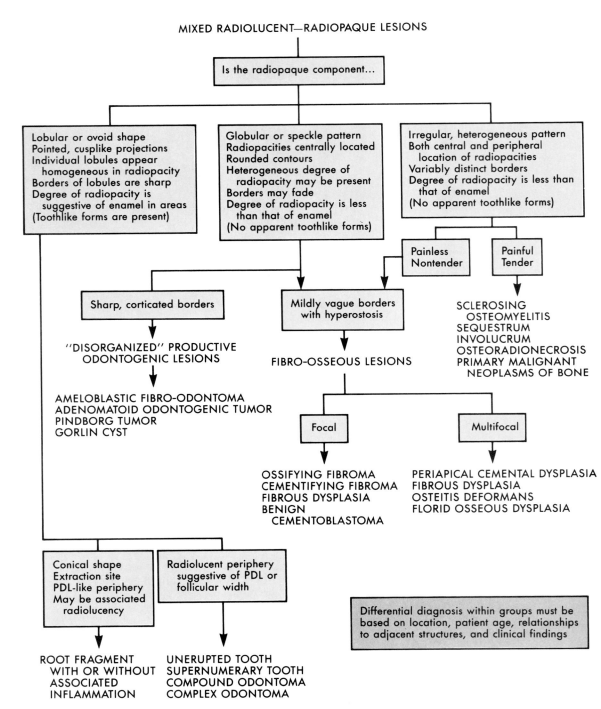

Fig. 19-16 Differential diagnosis of mixed radiolucent-radiopaque lesions.

Root Fragments and Unerupted Teeth

Definition. Dental structures that are contained within bone often appear radiographically as mixed radiolucent-radiopaque abnormalities. These formations include root fragments as well as supernumerary teeth and an unerupted tooth of the normal dental complement as described in Chapter 8.

Radiographic features. Root fragments exhibit conical shape, homogeneous radiopacity without enamel, and size typical of a tooth root. The radiolucency of the pulp canal may also be present. The supernumerary tooth exhibits a typical arrangement of dentin and enamel radiopacities but the formation is usually microdontic with a rudimentary coronal shape. However, some examples exhibit size and contours typical of normal teeth.

The radiolucency surrounding the root fragments and supernumerary teeth is comparable to normal periodontal ligament (PDL) or follicular width with a thin, cortical peripheral rim. Occasionally, a unilocular radiolucency with sharply delineated borders typical of a periapical cyst may be associated with a root fragment. Similarly, a dentigerous cyst and other odontogenic lesions may develop near a supernumerary tooth. Root fragments are located in the site of a past extraction, and deciduous root fragments are frequently identified in the mandibular premolar region.

Clinical features. Most dental formations within bone are asymptomatic and discovered during routine radiographic examination. Root tips enfolded by a chronic inflammatory lesion may become tender in some cases and a chronic pathologic sinus is occasionally identified.

Differential diagnosis. The combination of radiographic features is generally diagnostic.

Management. Removal of root fragments and unerupted teeth is warranted if a radiolucency significantly larger than the typical PDL or follicular width is present or if the root fragments and teeth are likely to interfere with prosthesis adaptation. Otherwise, periodic radiographic reevaluation is usually adequate management.

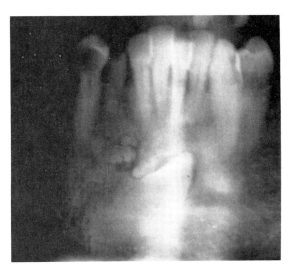

Fig. 19-17 Compound odontoma that has caused impaction of the mandibular canine.

Odontoma

Definition. The odontoma is not a "tooth tumor," as the literal derivation of the term implies. Considering the odontoma as a dental hamartoma that produces a poorly formed tooth or teeth more accurately reflects the nature of the abnormality. *Compound odontoma* is the more commonly encountered type and consists of multiple formations that resemble microdontic teeth. The *complex odontoma* also contains all of the tissue components of teeth, but the arrangement contains no recognizable teeth. The development of a follicular cyst from an odontoma produces a *cystic odontoma.*

Radiographic features. Odontomas are predominantly radiopaque, and the degree of radiopacity in some areas appears typical of enamel. Compound odontomas are usually located in alveolar bone anterior to the molars of either arch and are composed of multiple microdontic, rudimentary toothlike formations (Fig. 19-17). Conical crowns capped with enamel, roots, and central radiolucency of pulp tissue can be identified. Complex odontomas are usually located in the molar region. Radiopaque foci suggestive of enamel are present but the arrangement of calcified material appears globular, filamentous, or granular without morphologic features of teeth.

The radiopaque component of odontomas is surrounded by a thin band of radiolucency with a sharply delineated margin and a thin cortical rim. This arrangement is similar to the tissues normally associated with unerupted teeth. Impacted teeth are often located apical to odontomas. Increased width of the peripheral radiolucent component may suggest the development of a cystic odontoma or a non-mineralized odontogenic lesion.

Clinical features. Odontomas are usually discovered during routine radiographic examination of children and young adults. Delayed eruption of a tooth because its eruption is blocked by the odontoma is a common complication. Painless jaw expansion may be caused by larger lesions.

Differential diagnosis. Most odontomas present radiographic features that allow a definitive radiographic diagnosis. Some mixed radiolucent-radiopaque lesions may appear similar to complex odontomas, but these lesions either exhibit a greater proportion of radiolucency or the appearance of the margin lacks the follicular arrangement of the odontoma. A complex odontoma with cystic enlargement may be radiographically indistinguishable from other productive odontogenic lesions such as the ameloblastic fibro-odontoma.

Management. Surgical removal is often justified to facilitate eruption of blocked teeth or if follicular enlargement is present. Periodic radiographic reevaluation rather than surgical removal may be adequate management in the absence of complications.

Ameloblastic Fibro-Odontoma

Definition. The ameloblastic fibro-odontoma is a benign odontogenic enlargement that produces calcified dental tissues that are more "disorganized" than those of an odontoma. Some authorities consider this lesion to be the

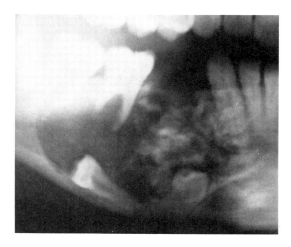

Fig. 19-18   Ameloblastic fibro-odontoma of a 15-year-old boy. The radiolucent component of the lesion and the sharply delineated lesional border are most evident in the molar region, whereas the radiopaque portion is most apparent in the premolar region.

early formation of a odontoma, whereas others believe it to be a distinct odontogenic lesion.

Radiographic features. The lesion is predominantly radiolucent, round or ovoid in shape, and located in the posterior alveolar segments. The radiopaque component consists of multiple round or elongated formations that are generally near the center of the radiolucency (Fig. 19-18). Some areas may be adequately calcified to exhibit radiopacity comparable to that of enamel. The peripheral margins are sharply delineated with a thin, cortical border. Slow growth is demonstrated by comparison of radiographs representing several years. Distorted enlargement and associated impacted teeth are often present.

Clinical features. The ameloblastic fibro-odontoma typically occurs in patients younger than age 20. Alveolar expansion, displacement of teeth, and failure of teeth to erupt often suggest the presence of the lesion.

Differential diagnosis. The location of the lesion in tooth-bearing areas, the corticated borders, and central radiopacities strongly suggest an odontogenic lesion. However, other "disorganized" productive odontogenic lesions (Fig. 19-16) can produce identical features. The adenomatoid odontogenic tumor generally occurs in the anterior segments rather than posterior areas. The calcifying epithelial odontogenic tumor and calcifying odontogenic cyst usually affect adults older than than 20.

Management. Surgical removal by enucleation is adequate treatment without significant probability of recurrence. This should not be confused with the high recurrence rate of ameloblastomas because of the term "ameloblastic" in this lesion's designation.

Adenomatoid Odontogenic Tumor

Definition. The adenomatoid odontogenic tumor is a rare benign neoplasm capable of producing calcified material in a "disorganized" pattern. The lesion is also known as the *odontogenic adenomatoid tumor* (OAT).

Radiographic features. Early lesions exhibit unilocular shape and homogeneous radiolucency with sharply delineated, cortical borders. Most adenomatoid odontogenic tumors form near the crown of an unerupted tooth in the anterior maxilla. This yields a radiographic appearance indistinguishable from that of a dentigerous cyst. Small radiopaque foci in a scattered or "speckled" distribution within the predominant radiolucency is the characteristic appearance of more advanced lesions.

Clinical features. Failure of an anterior maxillary tooth to erupt with painless alveolar expansion is the typical clinical presentation. The lesion affects adolescents and young adults.

Differential diagnosis. The radiographic appearance of the four "disorganized," productive odontogenic lesions (Fig. 19-16) is indistinguishable. The differential diagnosis of these lesions is based on location and age of occurrence as discussed for the ameloblastic fibro-odontoma. The adenomatoid odontogenic tu-

mor is a differential diagnostic possibility for a cystic radiolucency near the crown of an impacted anterior tooth.

Management. Surgical enucleation is effective treatment and recurrence is not to be expected.

Calcifying Epithelial Odontogenic Tumor

Definition. The calcifying epithelial odontogenic tumor, more commonly called a *Pindborg tumor,* is a rare lesion capable of producing a radiopaque component. The radiopacity is produced by mineralization of amorphous proteinaceous material generated by the tumor cells rather than the disorganized formation of dental tissues.

Radiographic features. The radiographic attenuation shown by calcifying epithelial odontogenic tumors ranges from totally radiolucent to mostly radiopaque (Fig. 19-19). Most lesions are predominantly radiolucent with a variably dense scattering of globular or filamentous radiopaque bodies near the center of the lesion. The peripheral margins are sharply delineated with a thin, cortical border. The slow growth of the calcifying epithelial odontogenic tumor can produce expansion and displacement of teeth. Approximately one half of Pindborg tumors are associated with an impacted tooth.

Clinical features. The Pindborg tumor is generally located in the molar region of adults. Small lesions may be an incidental radiographic finding, while painless enlargement or failure of a tooth to erupt may suggest the presence of larger examples.

Differential diagnosis. The calcifying epithelial odontogenic tumor must be considered in the differential diagnosis of both radiolucent and mixed radiolucent-radiopaque lesions of the alveolus with sharply delineated borders. The mixed presentation of Pindborg's tumor should be included in the differential diagnosis of lesions with radiographic features suggestive of complex odontomas, odontomas with cystic

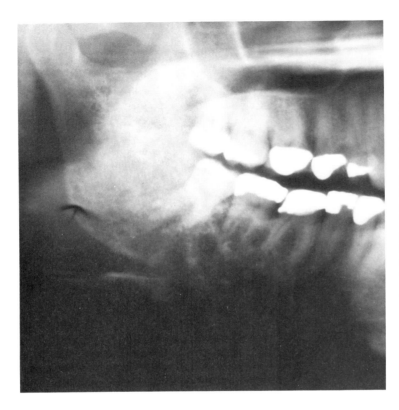

Fig. 19-19 Calcifying epithelial odontogenic (Pindborg) tumor of the posterior mandible. The sharp border of this exceptionally large and predominantly radiopaque example of this lesion is most evident near the sigmoid notch. The mixed radiolucent-radiopaque character is demonstrated in the periapical area of the second molar. (Courtesy of Dr Robert Schow, Baylor College of Dentistry, Dallas, Texas.)

enlargement, ameloblastic fibro-odontomas, and Gorlin cysts.

Management. Surgical removal should include a border of normal tissue if possible because Pindborg's tumors may recur after conservative enucleation. The recurrence rate is less than that for ameloblastomas and odontogenic keratocysts, but periodic reevaluation is warranted.

Calcifying Odontogenic Cyst

Definition. The calcifying odontogenic cyst is a rare lesion that has also been referred to as *Gorlin cyst* and the *keratinizing and calcifying odontogenic cyst.* As with the calcifying epithelial odontogenic tumor, the mineralization within Gorlin cysts is unrelated to the formation of dental tissues.

Radiographic features. Calcifying odontogenic cysts typically exhibit predominant radiolucency with unilocular shape and sharply delineated, cortical borders. Radiopacity may not be apparent within small lesions, but multiple "speckles" or globular radiopaque foci become visible as larger size is attained. The lesion is located in tooth-bearing bone, and an association with impacted teeth is common. The slow enlargement of this lesion may produce displacement of teeth and expansion.

Clinical features. Most calcifying odontogenic cysts affect young to middle-aged adults, and the painless lesion is often discovered during routine radiographic examination. Failure of a tooth to erupt or alveolar expansion are related findings in some cases.

Differential diagnosis. The calcifying odontogenic cyst should be considered a differential diagnostic possibility for most cystic radiolucencies near teeth. Observation of multiple radiopaque foci within the radiolucency increases the probability of a Gorlin cyst, but other "disorganized" odontogenic lesions (Fig. 19-16) must also be considered.

Management. Enucleation is adequate treatment. Recurrence is unusual.

Ossifying (Cementifying) Fibroma

Definition. The ossifying fibroma is a benign nonodontogenic neoplasm that is categorized as a *fibro-osseous lesion* (see Fig. 19-16). This term indicates the presence of a bonelike calcified product within a fibrous connective tissue stroma. The calcified material in some cases exhibits histopathologic features more suggestive of cementum, which yields the designation *cementifying fibroma.* The term *cementifying and ossifying fibroma* is applied if both osseous and cemental tissues are present. These distinctions are of little clinically importance because the morphology of the mineralized tissue is unrelated to occurrence, clinical course, or probability of recurrence.

Radiographic features. Approximately two thirds of ossifying fibromas are periapically located in the mandibular posterior segments. The typical radiographic presentation consists of round to ovoid, homogeneous radiopaque bodies surrounded by a peripheral radiolucent zone (Fig. 19-20). Ossifying fibromas may also produce homogeneous radiolucency with a unilocular or multilocular shape.

Ossifying fibromas produce well delineated margins suggestive of their slow growth, but they are less sharply demarcated than odontogenic lesions. The hyperostosis peripheral to the radiolucency has the appearance of a collar of dense trabeculation that is slightly wider and less radiopaque than the cortical border associated with odontogenic lesions. These marginal features of fibro-osseous lesions are demonstrated best at the interface of the lesion with trabecular bone. Borders near anatomic structures can falsely appear corticated.

Clinical features. The ossifying fibroma is

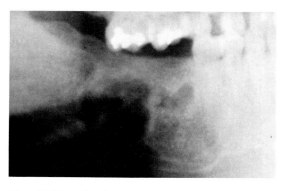

Fig. 19-20 Ossifying fibroma of the mandibular molar region. This example exhibits central radiopaque formations, multilocular shape, and hyperostotic borders that are most apparent at the superior and mesial margins of the lesion. Compare the appearance of the borders of this fibro-osseous lesion with the corticated borders of the cyst illustrated in Fig. 19-3.

painless, and it is usually discovered during routine radiographic examination of young and middle-aged adults. Larger lesions may produce expansion.

Differential diagnosis. Ossifying fibromas can present unilocular or multilocular radiolucency, a mixed appearance, and predominant radiopacity. This range of possible presentations demands consideration of an ossifying fibroma as a differential diagnostic possibility for many jaw lesions. The wide hyperostotic "collar" and less sharp marginal delineation are often an adequate basis on which to distinguish ossifying fibromas from most odontogenic lesions. Chronic inflammation associated with retained root tips and chronic osteomyelitis can produce a similar mixed radiolucent-radiopaque appearance with vague margins. However, these inflammatory lesions usually cause episodic pain.

An ossifying fibroma can be distinguished from other nonodontogenic lesions in most instances based on the patient's age and the location and number of lesions present. Periapical cemental dysplasia and florid osseous dysplasia produce multiple periapical lesions, whereas the ossifying fibroma is isolated. Fibrous dysplasia and osteitis deformans can appear similar, but fibrous dysplasia affects adolescents, and osteitis deformans is identified among older adults. The benign cementoblastoma is usually painful and produces a heterogeneous, striated, or radial appearance of the radiopaque component rather than the lack of pain and homogeneous radiopacities typical of ossifying fibromas. The multilocular radiolucent presentation of the ossifying fibroma can appear identical to that of simple bone cysts and central giant cell granulomas. Simple bone cysts generally produce little jaw expansion, and central giant cell granulomas cause rapid expansion in the anterior region.

Management. Conservative surgical removal by enucleation is adequate treatment because most ossifying fibromas do not recur.

Benign Cementoblastoma

Definition. The benign cementoblastoma is a nonmalignant neoplasm that originates from cementoblasts. This rare lesion has also been called a *true cementoma,* although use of the term *cementoma* in any context is currently considered confusing and inappropriate.

Radiographic features. The benign cementoblastoma is usually centered around the root of a posterior mandibular tooth and consists of central radiopacity surrounded by a variably wide radiolucent zone. The central radiopacity appears heterogeneous in a mottled or radial striated pattern, and it is continuous with the tooth root in at least one area. The tooth root and the lesion are bordered by continuity of the lamina dura.

Clinical features. Adolescents and young adults are usually affected and occurrence in locations other than the posterior mandible are also possible. The patient may complain of dull pain and alveolar expansion may result from larger lesions. Tests reveal pulp vitality unless the pulp is coincidentally necrotic.

Differential diagnosis. The radiographic features are adequately characteristic to allow a definitive diagnosis in most cases. Other mixed lesions may appear superimposed radiographically over a tooth root. However, the periodontal ligament and lamina dura exhibit normal continuity around the tooth root rather than surrounding the lesion, as with the benign cementoblastoma.

Management. Conservative surgical removal of the lesion including the attached tooth is adequate treatment since recurrence is unusual. Simple extraction of the tooth usually fails because the attached cemental mass cannot pass through the socket.

Periapical Cemental Dysplasia

Definition. Periapical cemental dysplasia is a common fibro-osseous condition of poorly understood pathogenesis. Multiple lesions develop, progress gradually for a period of years, and then become static. This course suggests a reactive process, but no specific cause has been proven. The frequent occurrence among black women suggests that genetic and other influences contribute to a predisposition for the abnormality, but the mechanisms are unclear. The lesions are nonprogressive and nondestructive.

Radiographic features. Periapical cemental dysplasia typically produces multiple lesions located near the apices of mandibular teeth without evidence of attachment to the roots. The incisor and first molar regions are the typical sites. Maxillary lesions and an isolated mandibular lesion are less common occurrences. Lesions are totally radiolucent in the early *osteolytic stage* of development. The *intermediate* or *mixed stage* is indicated by the appearance of central homogeneous radiopacity surrounded by a peripheral radiolucent band (Fig. 19-21) as central areas of the lesions mineralize. The *mature* or *radiopaque stage* is indicated by homogeneous radiopacity with minimal peripheral radiolucency and little additional increase in lesion size.

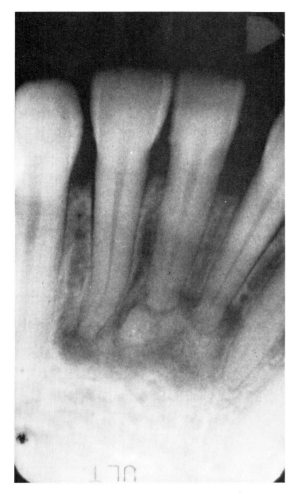

Fig. 19-21 Periapical cemental dysplasia.

The margins of the lesions are well delineated with peripheral hyperostosis. Because growth potential is limited in periapical cemental dysplasia, lesions are generally less than 1 cm in diameter, although several adjacent lesions may appear to coalesce, suggesting a larger size. Significant alterations of adjacent structures do not develop.

Clinical features. The lesions of periapical cemental dysplasia are painless without enlargement and are discovered during routine radiographic examination. Pulpal vitality of adjacent teeth is demonstrated by pulp testing unless coincidental pulpal necrosis has occurred. The condition is generally observed among middle-aged, black women.

Differential diagnosis. The combination of radiographic features, absence of clinical findings, and demographic characteristics of the patient usually allow a definitive diagnosis. The isolated lesion is indistinguishable radiographically from the ossifying fibroma except that a series of radiographs demonstrates that periapical cemental dysplasia eventually attains a static size, whereas ossifying fibromas usually progress. Similar lesions of larger size that produce expansion suggest florid osseous dysplasia or osteitis deformans.

Management. Pulp testing is indicated to exclude the possibility of periapical inflammatory lesions secondary to pulpal necrosis. Surgical removal of one or more lesions to confirm the diagnosis of this nonprogressive, nondestructive condition is unwarranted.

Florid Osseous Dysplasia

Definition. Florid osseous dysplasia is similar in most respects to periapical cemental dysplasia except that (1) the lesions are larger, (2) maxillary lesions often form, and (3) mild expansion may develop. The condition is also known as *gigantiform cementoma, sclerosing cemental masses of the jaws, diffuse cementosis,* and by several other designations. The relatively avascular mineralized tissue is predisposed to bacterial infection, which occurs so frequently that florid osseous dysplasia was formerly considered primarily inflammatory and was referred to as *chronic diffuse sclerosing osteomyelitis.* Despite the use of the term "osseous," the mineralized tissue is mostly abnormal cementum. Florid osseous dysplasia might reasonably be considered an exuberant form of periapical cemental dysplasia.

Radiographic features. Multiple mixed lesions with a dominant central radiopaque component and a variably wide radiolucent pe-

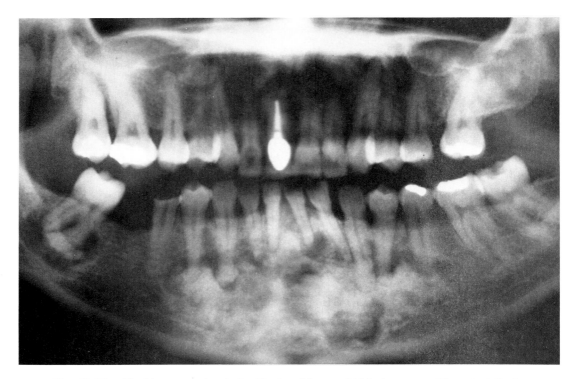

Fig. 19-22 Florid osseous dysplasia affecting 54-year-old black woman. Characteristic features include multiple mixed radiolucent-radiopaque lesions with a "cotton-wool" appearance located in both the mandible and maxillae. In addition, radiographic evidence of expansion was confirmed by clinical examination. (Courtesy Drs Neil Frederiksen and Paul Goaz, Baylor College of Dentistry, Dallas, Texas.)

riphery occupy a large proportion of the alveolar process and adjacent bone of the posterior mandibular segments. Similar lesions occasionally develop in the maxilla and the anterior mandibular region. The radiopaque masses exhibit either a homogeneous, granular pattern suggestive of sclerotic bone or a filamentous, "cotton-wool" appearance. The margins are generally well delineated and may be rimmed by sclerotic hyperostosis. Large lesions or the continuity of several lesions can produce altered appearance of the majority of the mandibular and maxillary alveolar processes as shown in Fig. 19-22. Cortical enlargement and elevation of the maxillary sinus floor may occur.

Clinical features. Most affected patients are black women beyond the age of 30. Early lesions may be an incidental radiographic observation, whereas larger lesions may be associated with diffuse alveolar enlargement. Chronic dull pain, tenderness, and drainage indicate a chronic osteomyelitis associated with these lesions.

Differential diagnosis. Multiple, large mixed radiographic lesions with jaw expansion confined to or near the alveolar bone of a middle-aged black woman is adequate for a definitive diagnosis in most situations. Osteitis deformans can be distinguished by the demonstration of similar lesions within other bones and elevated serum alkaline phosphatase concen-

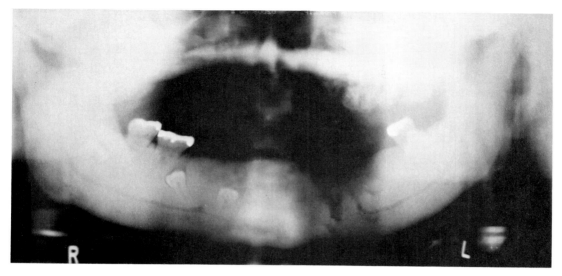

Fig. 19-23   Osteitis deformans or Paget's disease of bone. A mixed "cotton-wool" lesion is present in the maxillary left quadrant, whereas the majority of the mandible exhibits homogeneous, granular radiopacity. Note the narrow width of the inferior alveolar canals. (Courtesy Dr Paul Goaz, Baylor College of Dentistry, Dallas, Texas.)

tration. Polyostotic fibrous dysplasia and cherubism can produce similar radiographic features, but these conditions develop during childhood. Smaller lesions confined to the mandible without jaw enlargement are more typical of periapical cemental dysplasia.

Management. Incisional biopsy to confirm the diagnosis is usually not necessary and surgical removal of the lesions even when feasible is not justified. Complication by chronic osteomyelitis requires antibiotic therapy, surgical debridement, and other infection control measures. Prevention of jaw infections by avoiding dental extractions and by prompt treatment of dental infections is appropriate.

Osteitis Deformans

Definition. Osteitis deformans or *Paget's disease of bone* produces gradual alteration of bone morphology by the concurrence of abnormal bone resorption and deposition. Multiple lesions are usually present and the axial

skeleton including the skull, spine, and sacrum is generally affected. Dramatic elevation of serum alkaline phosphatase concentration is characteristic of the process.

Radiographic features. As observed for most fibro-osseous conditions, the lesions of Paget's disease of bone progress through an early radiolucent stage, a mixed radiolucent-radiopaque period, and a radiopaque or mature phase. Different lesions of a patient are usually in different stages, which is indicated by different proportions of radiopaque to radiolucent content (Fig. 19-23). Early lesions exhibit localized homogeneous, granular radiolucency with disappearance of adjacent cortical bone including the lamina dura. The mixed stage lesion may initially consist of linear radiopaque striations or a "speckled" appearance. Eventually, filamentous radiopacities with a "cotton-wool" appearance develop. The proportion of radiopacity to radiolucency continues to increase until only a thin rim of radiolucency remains or granular radiopacity predominates. The lesions are generally localized, but the margins are not sharply delineated and coalescing lesions may suggest a generalized osseous abnormality. Cortical expansion, separation of teeth, and generalized hypercementosis are associated with the disease.

Clinical features. Patients are over 40 years of age and early lesions may be an incidental radiographic finding. Patient complaints and the physical findings relate to bone enlargement, which may feel warm because of increased vascularity. Expansion may cause dull pain, headache, inability to insert appliances, altered facial appearance, spinal deformity, and neuropathy from constriction of neural canals.

Differential diagnosis. The radiographic features, multiple lesions, age of onset, and gradual enlargement are characteristic of the disease. The association with elevated serum alkaline phosphatase provides the definitive diagnosis. The lesions of florid osseous dysplasia are radiographically similar but are limited to the jaws. Fibrous dysplasia also produces similar radiographic features but children rather than adults are affected.

Management. Serum enzyme testing is preferable to incisional biopsy in making the definitive diagnosis of Paget's disease. Administration of calcitonin appears to slow the progression of lesions. Surgical decompression of entrapped nerves may become necessary. Periodic clinical reevaluation is indicated because an increased incidence of osteosarcoma among older adults is associated with preexisting osteitis deformans.

Fibrous Dysplasia

Definition. Fibrous dysplasia is an uncommon fibro-osseous enlargement of bone that affects children and adolescents. Most cases affect a single bone and are referred to as *monostotic fibrous dysplasia. Polyostotic fibrous dysplasia* affects multiple bones and is described in Chapter 20. The enlargement progresses slowly during adolescence and

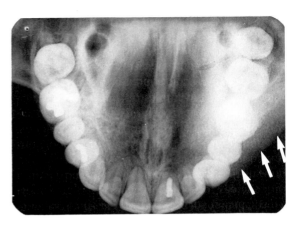

Fig. 19-24 Fibrous dysplasia of the maxilla. The diffuse, fusiform enlargement (*arrows*) is poorly delineated and exhibits a characteristic granular, "ground glass" radiopacity. Note the absence of cortical bone in the area of the lesion.

ceases at the end of normal skeletal growth, which suggests a developmental pathogenesis.

Radiographic features. Fibrous dysplasia appears either as a granular, homogeneous radiolucency or a mottled, mixed lesion at the time of discovery. More advanced lesions exhibit a granular, homogeneous radiopacity that has been described as a "ground glass" or "orange peel" appearance (Fig. 19-24). All lesions of fibrous dysplasia exhibit poorly delineated margins that appear to gradually blend into the normal trabecular pattern of adjacent bone. Diffuse expansion and alteration of normal anatomic contours, such as the course of the inferior alveolar canal, produce the overall impression of distortion rather than destruction. Teeth may be displaced or their eruption may be blocked. Cortical bone adjacent to the lesion becomes indistinguishable within the homogeneous radiopacity.

Clinical features. The patient's parents usually describe gradual, asymmetric enlargement of several months or years duration. The enlargement is fusiform in shape and firm to palpation without alteration of the overlying mucosa. The lesions are usually identified among older children and early adolescents, and altered occlusal relationships may develop. Mild tenderness may be associated with the region, but most lesions are painless.

Differential diagnosis. The combination of chronic enlargement, absence of pain, radiographic features, and age generally allows a definitive diagnosis. Identification of café-au-lait macules of the skin indicates the possibility of the polyostotic form of the disease.

Management. Incisional biopsy to confirm the diagnosis may be necessary for early lesions and in unusual cases. Excision of fibrous dysplasia is not feasible in most cases. The accepted approach is to delay surgical treatment until the end of adolescence and then accomplish cosmetic recontouring. Cases involving compression of vital structures such as the orbit may require surgical reduction before the cessation of growth.

Chronic Osteomyelitis

Definition. Chronic osteomyelitis of the jaws usually results from bacterial infections of dental origin. The specific form of chronic osteomyelitis that develops depends on the duration of the infection, the principal organism, the location, and host resistance. Bone vascularity is a major infection resistance factor. This explains the predominant occurrence of chronic osteomyelitis in the mandible rather than in the more vascular maxilla. Conditions that produce diminished vascularity such as florid osseous dysplasia and osteitis deformans predispose to progression of relatively minor, superficial infections into chronic osteomyelitis. Radiotherapy to the jaws produces vascular sclerosis of the bone tissue that can cause a severe form of chronic osteomyelitis known as *osteoradionecrosis.*

The morphologic abnormalities of chronic osteomyelitis result from a chronic course of alternating episodes of inflammatory bone lysis during progression and peripheral bone repair during relative quiescence. This has been de-

scribed as a "smoldering" infection as contrasted with the "wild fire" progression of acute osteomyelitis.

Chronic focal sclerosing osteomyelitis, also called *condensing osteitis,* is the most common form of chronic osteomyelitis identified by the dentist. The typical example is localized sclerosis of bone associated with a periapical dental infection. *Chronic diffuse sclerosing osteomyelitis* is an extensive, regional infection of bone by anaerobic pathogens that is characterized by duration of several months or more and variably severe discomfort. *Garré's osteomyelitis,* which is more formally called *chronic osteomyelitis with proliferative periostitis,* is a diffuse, progressive infection that causes fusiform bone expansion by stimulating the formation of successive layers of peripheral cortical bone. Proliferative periostitis is usually observed among children and young adults. These forms of osteomyelitis are summarized and compared in Table 19-5.

Radiographic features. Chronic osteomyelitis produces a mixed radiolucent-radiopaque pattern of x-ray attenuation with variation in the proportion and arrangement of the components. The epicenter of most lesions is in the periapical region of the mandible and can be related to a chronic dental infection. The peripheral borders are poorly delineated in most instances.

The radiographic appearance of chronic focal sclerosing osteomyelitis consists of a radiolucency surrounded by a variably wide zone of granular radiopacity that blends peripherally with normal trabeculation (Fig. 19-5). Chronic diffuse sclerosing osteomyelitis produces a heterogeneous or mottled admixture of poorly delineated radiolucent foci and granular radiopaque areas. The entire superior-inferior width of the mandible is usually affected and diffuse expansion often develops. Necrotic bone or a *sequestrum* is suggested by an irregularly shaped central radiopacity with ragged borders surrounded by radiolucency and a peripheral rim of sclerosis. Garré's osteomyelitis exhibits

Table 19-5 Comparison of the radiographic and clinical features of different forms of osteomyelitis

Form of osteomyelitis	Symptoms	Occurrence (age; frequency)	Radiographic appearance	Treatment response	Additional features
Acute suppurative osteomyelitis	Acute onset of severe pain and purulence	Any age; common	Bone may appear normal, diffusely radiolucent, or peripheral sclerosis may be present	Rapid resolution in most cases with antibiotic therapy and removal of the source of infection	Usually represents acute exacerbation and progression of a chronic dental infection
Chronic focal sclerosing osteomyelitis (condensing osteitis)	Usually asymptomatic and identified incidentally; history often reveals a chronic course of past episodes of tenderness and pain	Any age; common	Radiolucency centered around the source of inflammation with a peripheral zone of granular radiopacity that blends with surrounding normal bone	Rapid resolution in most cases with removal of the source of infection; the radiopaque bone changes persist as focal sclerosis after resolution of the inflammation	Usually represents limited extent and chronic duration of inflammatory bone lysis and peripheral sclerotic healing of bone associated with an untreated dental infection
Chronic diffuse sclerosing osteomyelitis	Pain, tenderness, enlargement, and drainage of long duration; symptoms may vary in intensity, but course is progressive	Usually older than 20; uncommon	Heterogeneous admixture of radiolucency and radiopacity with expansion and poorly delineated peripheral borders	Symptoms may be controlled by a combination of antibiotics, debridement, and hyperbaric oxygen therapy of extended duration	Represents diffuse extent and chronic duration of bone infection secondary to dental infection; culture often demonstrates anaerobic organ-

	Clinical features	Age	Radiographic appearance	Treatment	Comments
Garré's osteomyelitis (chronic osteomyelitis with proliferative periostitis)	Pain, tenderness, enlargement, and drainage of long duration; symptoms may vary in intensity, but course is progressive	Usually younger than 30; uncommon	Heterogeneous admixture of radiolucency and radiopacity with peripheral cortical expansion exhibiting a laminar or "onion skin" appearance	Resolution in most cases following removal of the source of infection and extended course of antibiotic therapy	isms; often follows a chronic course of inadequate treatment of the infection Represents diffuse extent and chronic duration of bone infection secondary to dental infection; history often reveals a chronic course of inadequate control therapy or poor patient compliance
Osteoradionecrosis	Gradual progression of pain and delayed healing following tooth extraction, superficial infection, or minor injury of the alveolar mucosa	Usually older than 50; uncommon	Heterogeneous admixture of radiolucency and radiopacity with poorly delineated peripheral borders	Symptoms may be controlled by a combination of antibiotics, debridement, and hyperbaric oxygen therapy of extended duration	History of radiotherapy with direct exposure of the jaw exceeding 50 grays; mandible is much more likely to be infected than maxilla

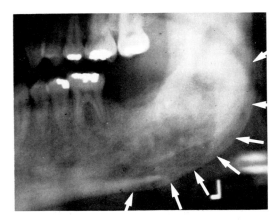

Fig. 19-25 Garré's osteomyelitis. Note the diffuse cortical enlargement of the inferior cortical surface near the angle that exhibits a laminar or "onion skin" appearance (*arrows*) of proliferative periostitis. (Courtesy of Dr Gilbert Lilly, University of Iowa College of Dentistry, Iowa City, Iowa.)

the same heterogeneous radiographic appearance as diffuse sclerosing osteomyelitis with the additional observation of fusiform expansion consisting of laminar bands of cortical bone often described as an "onion skin" appearance (Fig. 19-25). This is typically located along the inferior border of the mandible, although occlusal radiographs may reveal similar lamination of the buccal and lingual surfaces.

Clinical features. The pain of chronic osteomyelitis is often described as deep, constant, and boring or burning with episodes of increased severity corresponding to acute exacerbations. Swelling, jaw enlargement, erythema, a draining sinus, and other indications of bacterial infection are present. The patient history frequently includes episodes of ineffective treatment for localized dental infections such as noncompliance with antibiotic regimens, inadequate empiric antibiotic treatment, and incomplete endodontic procedures. Anemia, diabetes, and other causes of diminished host resistance are often associated with chronic osteomyelitis.

Osteoradionecrosis is associated with a history of radiotherapy exceeding a dosage of 50 Gy to the mandible. Months or years later an extraction site, minor infection, or mucosal wound fails to heal, and the features of chronic osteomyelitis subsequently develop.

Differential diagnosis. The combination of an initial bacterial infection followed by a chronic course of pain that affects the region of a mixed radiolucent-radiopaque lesion is strong evidence of chronic osteomyelitis. Malignant neoplastic lesions of bone can produce pain, enlargement, and similar radiographic features and must be considered in the differential diagnosis. However, central jaw malignancies progress with consistent increase in severity in contrast to the episodic acute exacerbations of chronic osteomyelitis. Several fibro-osseous lesions can produce similar radiographic findings, but pain, tenderness, and other signs of infection are absent. Increased vulnerability to chronic osteomyelitis is suggested by conditions that cause decreased vascularity of bone or diminished host resistance.

Management. Chronic focal sclerosing osteomyelitis responds favorably to elimination of the causative infection by appropriate dental care in concert with a therapeutic antibiotic regimen of several weeks duration. Garré's osteomyelitis can also be eliminated by similar treatment, although a longer duration of antibiotic therapy is generally required.

Diffuse sclerosing osteomyelitis and osteoradionecrosis are difficult infections to treat because the infection is deeply ingrained within a large volume of relatively avascular bone. Therefore the infection often persists following removal of the cause and antibiotic therapy. In many cases the therapeutic goal becomes control of pain and progression rather than elimination of the infection. High-dose antibiotic therapy for many months in addition to removal of the original infection, surgical debridement, and hyperbaric oxygen therapy may be necessary to achieve control. Partial mandibulectomy may become necessary in severe cases.

Effective treatment of chronic osteomyelitis relies on microbial culture and antibiotic sensitivity studies, which will be adversely affected by initial empiric antibiotic therapy. Therefore culture specimens should be obtained before treatment is initiated, and anaerobic culture techniques should be included. Any systemic condition that adversely affects host resistance requires medical referral and treatment as a part of effectively managing chronic osteomyelitis.

Malignant Neoplasms of the Jaws

Definition. A mixed radiolucent-radiopaque appearance can be produced by malignant neoplasms in three ways. First, osteosarcoma and chondrosarcoma can produce calcified malignant tissues in addition to areas of nonmineralized tumor. Second, prostatic carcinoma metastatic to the jaws and Ewing's sarcoma often stimulate bone formation adjacent to the tumor. This produces an intermixture of tumor radiolucency and induced radiopacity. Third, malignant neoplasms classified as radiolucencies can exhibit rapid, multifocal growth that isolates areas of bone and yields a mixed appearance.

Radiographic features. The proportions of radiolucent and radiopaque components within malignant neoplasms of the jaws vary considerably, but a heterogeneous appearance or admixture of components is the typical pattern. Osteosarcomas occasionally produce a radial striated pattern that is described as a "sunburst" appearance. Poorly delineated borders make the determination of the lesion extent difficult. Alterations of adjacent structures can include extrusion of teeth, external resorption, and the absence of typical anatomic structures. The general impression is destructive replacement of normal anatomy by the lesion.

Clinical features. The steady enlargement of most jaw malignancies within weeks to months produces relatively constant pain that gradually increases in severity. Paresthesia and anesthesia may develop. Clinical examination may reveal ulceration, lobulated contours, or other alterations of the superficial mucosa. History of a distant primary malignant tumor raises the possibility of a metastatic lesion within the jaws.

Differential diagnosis. A history of painful enlargement noted within a period of months and heterogeneous radiographic features suggestive of destruction limit the differential diagnosis to chronic osteomyelitis and central malignancies. Episodic variation in the severity of pain and purulence suggest osteomyelitis. Also, the source of infection is usually apparent. Malignancy usually produces steady progression and increasing severity of pain with the eventual development of paresthesia.

Management. The suspicion of malignant neoplasia requires referral for definitive diagnosis, staging, and treatment.

RADIOPAQUE LESIONS OF THE JAWS

Relatively few jaw lesions are totally radiopaque. Many abnormalities, the odontoma for example, that are included with radiopaque lesions in some differential diagnosis schemes actually exhibit a distinct but proportionally small radiolucent component. Therefore these abnormalities are more appropriately considered with mixed radiolucent-radiopaque lesions. The radiograph of any grossly radiopaque jaw lesion should be carefully examined, particularly near the borders, for evidence of radiolucency. The differential diagnostic strategy for totally radiopaque jaw lesions is illustrated in Fig. 19-26.

Focal Sclerosis

Definition. Focal sclerosis is a descriptive term for the most common radiopaque lesion of the jaws. Focal sclerosis is the final, static manifestation of three different processes. The radiopaque component of *condensing osteitis* in most cases does not remodel to normal trabecular morphology following resolution of

Fig. 19-26 Differential diagnosis of radiopaque jaw lesions.

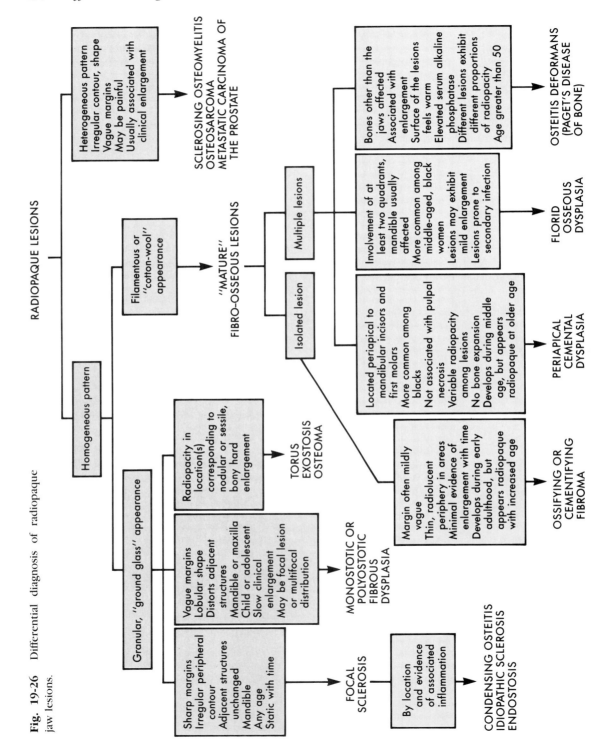

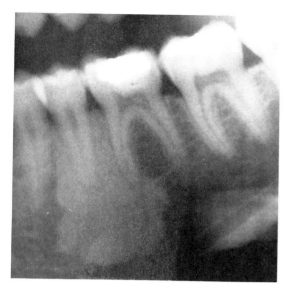

Fig. 19-27 Focal sclerosis of the mandibular premolar area. This segment of a panoramic radiograph demonstrates the homogeneous radiopacity with sharp delineation and irregular contour of the lesional margins.

the inflammation. This leaves a permanent focal radiopacity often referred to as a *bone scar*. Identical lesions are occasionally discovered without evidence of an inflammatory process and are referred to as *idiopathic osteosclerosis*. Many examples of idiopathic sclerosis are located in the mandibular premolar region (Fig. 19-27), which suggests inflammation related to the deciduous molars as a possible cause. A similar radiographic appearance results from *endostosis*, which is an idiopathic replacement of trabecular bone by medullary thickening of cortical bone analogous to the outward cortical thickening of tori. Speculation about possible causes is usually of little clinical significance when the focal sclerosis is identified.

Radiographic features. Focal sclerosis consists of a homogeneous, granular radiopacity with sharply delineated margins that often exhibit a slightly irregular or "jagged" contour (Fig. 19-27). Trabeculae of normal bone adja-

cent to the radiopacity appear to blend or fuse with the lesion without peripheral radiolucency. The periapical region of the mandible is the typical location, and maxillary lesions are unusual. Lesion size is typically 1 cm or less, but larger lesions occasionally develop. Comparison of radiographs representing a duration of months or years reveals no changes. Multiple lesions may be aligned at the periapical level of the mandible of patients who have suffered numerous dental infections.

Clinical features. No pain, enlargement, or other significant findings are associated with focal sclerosis.

Differential diagnosis. A definitive diagnosis based on the radiographic features and the absence of symptoms is possible in most cases. Similar radiopacities can result from metastatic prostatic carcinoma and renal osteodystrophy, but the patient history, additional radiographic abnormalities, and serum chemistry studies serve to distinguish these diseases. Superimposition of soft tissue calcifications, tori, or normal anatomic structures can be confused with focal sclerosis. Tori are easily identified as clinical enlargements. Additional radiographs exposed with different beam angulation reveal changes in the relative positions of jaw structures and the radiopaque images of soft tissue calcifications.

Management. No treatment or additional reevaluation is necessary.

Torus, Exostosis, and Osteoma

Definition. Exostosis is nodular or sessile enlargement of the cortical surface of a bone. This enlargement may be a chronic response to functional stress or a developmental abnormality, but it is definitely not neoplastic. Most examples of the jaws develop on the lingual alveolar surface in the mandibular canine-premolar region or are centered at the midline of the palatal vault. Exostosis at these sites is so common that the specific designations *mandibular torus* and *palatal torus* are used. The osteoma is a roughly spherical enlargement of bone tissue that is considered to be a hamartoma with limited potential for growth. The formation of multiple osteomas is a diagnostic feature of Gardner syndrome, as described in Chapter 20.

Radiographic features. These lesions produce homogeneous radiopacity with variable delineation of the borders depending on the size and shape of the enlargement and its alignment with the x-ray beam and the film.

Clinical features. These nodular or broad-based enlargements are painless and bony hard to palpation. Tori and exostoses of the alveolar processes are common among adults and generally are more prominent with increased age. Bilateral occurrence of mandibular tori is typical and a symmetric distribution of large exostoses affecting multiple alveolar surfaces is not unusual. The patient may be aware of the gradual increase in size and long duration of these lesions. Enlargement in areas such the buccal aspect of the maxilla can limit jaw movement.

Differential diagnosis. The bony hardness, absence of pain, long duration, characteristic locations, and homogeneous radiopacity are an adequate basis for a definitive diagnosis in most instances. Jaw expansion caused by central jaw lesions can usually be distinguished by more fusiform shape of the enlargement and the radiographic features of the central lesion.

Management. No treatment is necessary in most cases. Surgical removal may be indicated to facilitate the adaptation of dentures or to eliminate functional interference.

Advanced Fibro-Osseous Lesions

Definition. The mineralization of most fibro-osseous lesions progresses until eventually the overwhelming majority of the lesion is calcified. The predominant radiopacity of these "mature" fibro-osseous lesions can obscure the radiolucent fibrous connective tissue component that is apparent early in development. Therefore fibro-osseous lesions such as the ossifying fibroma, periapical cemental dysplasia, florid osseous dysplasia, osteitis deformans, and fibrous dysplasia must be included in the differential diagnosis of lesions that appear totally radiopaque.

Radiographic features. The totally radiopaque appearance of advanced fibrous dysplasia consists of a characteristic homogeneous, "ground glass" radiopacity with poorly delineated borders. The "cotton-wool" appearance that is typical of the multiple lesions of Paget's disease of bone and florid osseous dysplasia also indicates a long duration of the condition. Periapical cemental dysplasia and ossifying fibromas of long duration may exhibit either homogeneous, granular radiopacity or a more filamentous, cotton-wool appearance with relatively well-delineated borders.

Careful examination of all of these lesions except fibrous dysplasia usually reveals a thin radiolucent zone peripheral to the radiopacity, which demonstrates the mixed nature of these lesions. The superior resolution of intraoral radiographs may be necessary to appreciate this feature.

Clinical features. Clinical findings for the various fibro-osseous conditions are described in the previous section of this chapter and are summarized in Fig. 19-26.

Differential diagnosis. The differential diagnosis of radiopacities including fibro-osseous lesions is shown in Fig. 19-26. A definitive radiographic diagnosis of fibrous dysplasia is usually possible based on occurrence during adolescence, slow enlargement for several years, absence of pain, and the granular radiopaque appearance. Osteosarcoma may produce radiopacity in approximately the same age group, but the radiopacity is more heterogeneous, pain is present, and enlargement usually is apparent within months. Ossifying fibromas are distinguished from fibrous dysplasia and osteosarcoma by their relatively well-delineated borders. Metastatic prostatic carcinoma and some other glandular malignancies can produce radiopacity of the jaws. This possibility is usually revealed by the history of the primary tumor.

Periapical cemental dysplasia, florid osseous dysplasia, and osteitis deformans all produce multiple lesions among middle-aged and older adults. Osteitis deformans is distinguished by lesions affecting other bones in addition to the jaws and elevated serum alkaline phosphatase. Florid osseous dysplasia is distinguished from periapical cemental dysplasia by larger individual lesions, jaw enlargement, and development of lesions in the maxilla.

Management. Management for each condition is described in the radiolucent-radiopaque lesion section of this chapter.

Osteosarcoma

Definition. Osteosarcoma, also called *osteogenic sarcoma,* is a malignant neoplasm originating from bone tissue. The disease most commonly affects long bones of adolescents, and jaw occurrence is rare. The disease may also affect older adults in association with Paget's disease of bone and secondary to tumoricidal radiotherapy after a latent period of several decades.

Radiographic features. Osteosarcomas of the jaws produce a mixed radiolucent-radiopaque appearance more frequently than a totally radiopaque appearance. However, the heterogeneous pattern and multifocal growth of the lesion may obscure areas of radiolucency. A radial arrangement of radiopaque striations referred to as a "sunburst" pattern is a characteristic feature of long bone osteosarcomas, but this feature is less frequently observed in the jaws. The most consistent radiographic features of jaw osteosarcomas are heterogeneous x-ray attenuation, poorly delineated borders, and a general impression of anatomic destruction (Fig. 19-28). An additional feature of osteosarcoma illustrated by this example is the ragged, uniform widening of the periodontal ligament spaces of adjacent teeth.

Clinical features. Most osteosarcomas of the jaws affect late adolescents or young adults. Older adults with a history of Paget's disease of bone or radiotherapy are also at risk.

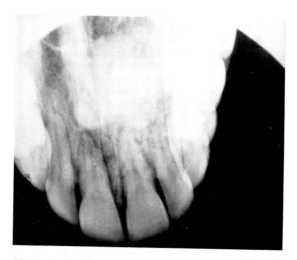

Fig. 19-28 Osteosarcoma of the anterior maxilla. Note predominant radiopacity of the lesion and the ragged widening of the periodontal ligament spaces of the central incisors. (Courtesy Dr Ed Menton, Arlington, Texas.)

Progressive swelling of several months duration and constant dull pain of gradually increasing severity are often described by the patient. Paresthesia may develop with neural invasion. Examination reveals diffuse enlargement and ulceration or other alteration of the superficial mucosa in some cases. Shifting or extrusion of teeth, trismus, or limitation of opening may be present depending on the location of the tumor.

Differential diagnosis. Symptoms of osteosarcoma such as relatively rapid swelling and pain often misdirect the clinician's differential diagnosis to inflammatory disease. The absence of a dental infection to explain an osseous infection is often the first indication of this error. Also, the pain and other symptoms are less episodic than with most infections. Radiographic features are compatible with chronic sclerosing osteomyelitis, but the lesion is generally too extensive to be explained by the duration of the symptoms. The radiographic features of osteosarcoma can also be

Table 19-6 Summary of conditions that can cause generalized radiolucency of bone

Condition	Factors	Mechanism(s)
LIMITED SYNTHESIS OF BONE MATRIX		
Osteoporosis	Advanced age	Multifactorial: combination of poor diet, hormonal deficiency (menopause), compromised circulation, inflammation (osteoarthritis), and other consitutional conditions limit osteoid formation and potential for physiologic remodeling
	Idiopathic	Affects children and young adults, no underlying condition can be identified
	Malnutrition (malabsorption)	Deficiency of vitamin D, protein, calcium, and other nutrients causes limited formation of osteoid and physiologic remodeling
	Endocrine dysfunction	Menopausal decrease of estrogens, birth control medication, adrenal excess (Cushing's syndrome), and chronic hyperthyroidism can all interfere with bone metabolism
	Heritable connective tissue disorders	Osteogenesis imperfecta, Ehlers-Danlos syndrome, Marfan syndrome
	Other conditions	Mechanisms are poorly understood, but osteoporosis is commonly associated with rheumatoid arthritis, alcoholism, epilepsy, diabetes mellitus, and chronic obstructive pulmonary disease
LIMITED CALCIFICATION OF BONE MATRIX		
Rickets (children)	Limited calcium availability	Lack of calcium during development produces hypomineralization of bone and limitation of growth and development; deformity of weight-bearing bones and malformation of teeth are common and proportional to the severity of the deficiency; underlying conditions are similar to those listed below for osteomalacia affecting adults
Vitamin D resistant rickets	Limited phosphate availability	Genetic condition of impaired renal tubule reabsorption of phosphate leads to limited phosphate availability; mineralization defects are similar to those of rickets
Hypophosphatasia	Alkaline phosphate deficiency	This genetically determined condition produces features similar to those of rickets in many respects; an important diagnostic feature of hypophosphatasia is premature loss of teeth caused by defective cementum formation and the resulting deficiency of the attachment apparatus
Osteomalacia (adults)	Limited calcium availability	Numerous conditions can cause defective calcium metabolism in adults; dietary deficiency, malabsorption, acidosis, chronic renal disease, and abnormal vitamin D metabolism are common examples

Data from Wilson JD and others, editors: Harrison's principles of internal medicine, ed 12, New York, 1991, McGraw-Hill.

Table 19-6 Summary of conditions that can cause generalized radiolucency of bone—cont'd

Condition	Factors	Mechanism(s)
LIMITED CALCIFICATION OF BONE MATRIX—cont'd		
Renal osteodystrophy	Chronic renal failure	A form of osteomalacia resulting from excessive renal loss of calcium, which stimulates parathyroid hormone release (secondary hyperparathyroidism), and gradual, progressive loss of calcium from bone tissue
Hypophosphatemia	Limited phosphate availability	Altered mineralization of bone is unusual unless hypophosphatemia is severe; insufficient dietary intake or malabsorption in concert with ingestion of phosphate-binding antacids can cause features similar to osteomalacia
REPLACEMENT OF TRABECULAR BONE		
Hemolytic anemias	Sickle cell disease and thalassemia	Short average life span of red blood cells stimulates hyperplasia of hemopoietic marrow, which replaces trabecular bone

suggestive of fibrous dysplasia, but the clinically rapid enlargement and pain provide an adequate basis for distinction.

Management. Referral to a tertiary oncology care center is appropriate if osteosarcoma of the jaws is suspected.

GENERALIZED RADIOGRAPHIC ABNORMALITIES OF BONE

Generalized alteration of bone morphology can be caused by a variety of systemic conditions. These alterations include generalized abnormality of trabecular size, density, and arrangement as well as alterations in the radiopacity and thickness of cortical bone. Observation of these radiographic features seldom contributes to the diagnosis of the disease. More obvious clinical aspects of the condition have led to the diagnosis before generalized bone changes become adequately apparent to be identified. Generalized alteration of bone morphology should not be confused with the manifestations of diseases that cause *multifocal lesions* within normal bone.

Generalized Radiolucency of Bone

Definition. Conditions that can cause generalized radiolucency of bone are listed in Table 19-6. *Osteoporosis* is a condition caused by several diseases that is characterized by a decreased amount of bone tissue and normal calcification of the bone that is present. *Rickets* and *osteomalacia* are conditions of a normal amount of bone tissue, but the bone is hypocalcified as a consequence of inadequate calcium and/or phosphate availability. Rickets is calcium deficiency during development, which produces hypomineralization and secondary developmental defects. *Vitamin D–resistant rickets* produces similar hypocalcification and dental malformations but the cause is a genetic defect in phosphate resorption in the kidneys. Osteomalacia is the hypocalcification of bone tissue after growth and development are complete.

Radiographic features. Osteoporosis and osteomalacia produce identical radiographic manifestations in the jaws. Trabeculae are generally small and indistinct, which results in a generalized granular radiolucency of medullary spaces suggestive of a "ground glass" appearance. Cortical bone generally appears thinner, less radiopaque, and less distinct than normal. This may be observed by the dentist as decreased radiopacity of the lamina dura. Development of these radiographic features is usually a relative severe manifestation of both osteoporosis and osteomalacia.

Similar radiographic findings are expected in rickets along with the additional observation of development abnormalities. The width of dentin from the dentinoenamel junction (DEJ) to the pulp chamber is often abnormally narrow and pulp horns are exceptionally prominent. Dental development and eruption are often delayed.

Clinical features. The patient history and clinical findings often reveal contributory conditions from among those listed in Table 19-6. In addition, the patient may describe fractures resulting from relatively minor injuries. The child with rickets characteristically exhibits bowed legs and abnormal gait caused by inability of the hypocalcified bone to withstand the child's weight. Enamel hypocalcification is also commonly observed.

Differential diagnosis. The radiographic features are inadequate to distinguish most acquired metabolic mineral disorders. Laboratory tests useful in evaluating mineral metabolism and contributory systemic diseases are essential to the differential diagnosis.

Management. Referral for medical evaluation and management is indicated if the condition has not been previously diagnosed. The treatment goals are to control, if possible, contributory conditions and to promote calcium absorption.

Renal Osteodystrophy

Definition. Renal osteodystrophy is the combination of pathophysiologic effects involving bone that develop when chronic renal failure causes excessive calcium loss in the urine. The compensatory response to maintain the physiologically vital serum calcium con-

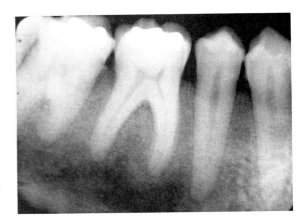

Fig. 19-29 Renal osteodystrophy of a 44-year-old woman undergoing hemodialysis treatment for chronic renal failure. The medullary bone appears abnormally granular and radiolucent. In addition, the lamina dura is not radiographically apparent. These features were present in all areas of the maxilla and mandible.

centration is increased parathyroid hormone secretion that mobilizes calcium from bone. This mechanism explains the synonym *secondary hyperparathyroidism* for the condition. This loss of calcium content from bone tissue is a form of osteomalacia and is commonly observed among renal dialysis and transplant patients. *Primary hyperparathyroidism* results from functional neoplasms of parathyroid origin and is a rare cause of similar radiographic abnormalities.

Radiographic features. The generalized radiolucency of medullary bone exhibits the same granular, "ground glass" appearance described for osteomalacia and osteoporosis. The exceptional feature is that the disappearance of cortical bone (Fig. 19-29) is more dramatic in renal osteodystrophy and primary hyperparathyroidism than in more gradually progressive forms of osteomalacia. Intraoral radiographs often reveal little or no lamina dura associated with the teeth in the chronic renal failure patient. Panoramic radiographs may demonstrate that the normally prominent inferior cortex of the mandible is thin or unapparent. Totally radiolucent lesions may develop in severe cases and are referred to as *brown tumors* or *osteitis fibrosa cystica.* In addition, the abnormal calcium metabolism of the patient with chronic renal failure may cause metastatic calcification of soft tissues and focal radiopaque lesions of bone identical to those described as focal sclerosis.

Clinical features. The patient with features of renal osteodystrophy has generally progressed to chronic renal failure and is either undergoing renal dialysis or has received a renal transplant. The radiographic features of renal osteodystrophy persist for years after renal transplantation, suggesting that aspects of abnormal calcium metabolism persist despite the restoration of renal function.

Differential diagnosis. The combination of granular radiolucency of medullary bone, absence of cortical bone such as the lamina dura, and the history of severe renal disease is adequate to make a definitive diagnosis of renal osteodystrophy. Similar radiographic findings without evidence of renal disease must be considered to be osteomalacia or osteoporosis. The differential diagnosis includes primary hyperparathyroidism, as well as other conditions listed in Table 19-6.

Management. No specific treatment is available for renal osteodystrophy beyond treatment of the primary renal disease. Ablation of the parathyroid glands in primary hyperparathyroidism may be accomplished surgically.

Anemias

Definition. Several forms of anemia can produce generalized alterations of bone as a consequence of extensive hemopoietic hyperplasia. The prominence of the radiographic abnormalities generally reflects the severity and duration of the anemia. Therefore, mild anemias caused by dietary deficiency of iron or folic acid seldom stimulate significant hemopoietic hyperplasia in contrast to severe anemias related to genetic defects.

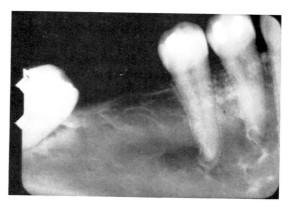

Fig. 19-30 The radiographic appearance of the alveolar bone of a 28-year-old man with sickle cell disease. Abnormal features include the generalized radiolucency of the alveolar bone, scarcity of trabeculae, and the prominence of the trabeculae that are present. Compare these features with those of Fig. 19-29.

Sickle cell anemia and thalassemia are two of the more common genetic defects that in their most severe forms cause significant alterations of bone. Both conditions are characterized by structurally abnormal hemoglobin that results in a tendency for excessive hemolysis leading to anemia. Sickle cell anemia is either clinically mild in the heterozygous form known as *sickle cell trait* or severe in the homozygous form known as *sickle cell disease.* The clinical manifestations of thalassemia also vary in severity among patients. *Thalassemia minor* is clinically asymptomatic in most respects and *thalassemia major* causes severe anemia first identified during infancy.

Radiographic features. The replacement of fatty marrow with hemopoietic marrow in the jaws results in fewer trabeculae in the medullary spaces, but the individual trabeculae tend to be longer and more prominent. Large medullary spaces of severely affected individuals may show little trabecular bone (Fig. 19-30). This can yield a "honeycomb" pattern of the trabeculae or a "stair-step" appearance between the roots of teeth. Although these tra-

Table 19-7   Summary of maxillary sinus lesions

Condition	Cause	Occurrence	X-ray attenuation	Extent or shape	Sinus wall	Clinical features	Course
Acute sinusitis	Aperture obstruction, spread of dental infection	Common	Homogeneous soft tissue radiopacity	Entire sinus or air-fluid level, unilateral	Unaffected, intact	Pain, tenderness, purulent drainage, discomfort changes with postural changes	Acute onset, rapid resolution with treatment
Chronic sinusitis	Chronic inflammation (e.g., asthma and seasonal allergies)	Common	Homogeneous soft tissue radiopacity	Bandlike, parallel to sinus floor, bilateral	Intact, may show sclerotic cortical thickening	Congestion, serous drainage, and mild discomfort; may be currently asymptomatic	Episodic, especially "in season"; may progress to acute sinusitis
Mucous retention phenomenon	Inflammation, specific cause usually not apparent	Common	Homogeneous soft tissue radiopacity	Dome-shaped enlargement, base on sinus floor	Unaffected, intact	Patient unaware of any abnormality	Static
Mucocele	Inflammation, specific cause usually not apparent	Rare	Homogeneous soft tissue radiopacity	Entire sinus	Distended, distorted contours	Constant pressure, pain, expansion	Gradual onset, progresses until removed
Dental inflam-	Usually peri-	Common	Homogeneous	Focal, near	Interruption of	Tenderness of	Acute epi-

matory lesions	apical abscess caused by to pulpal necrosis or periodontal abscess		soft tissue radiopacity	apices, floor of the sinus	sinus wall or superior distortion of contour	teeth, evidence of pulpal necrosis/periodontitis, may be asymptomatic	sodes, usually asymptomatic
Oroantral defect	Passage between oral cavity and sinus following extraction of maxillary tooth	Uncommon	Homogeneous soft tissue radiopacity	Focal thickening near extraction site	Discontinuity of sinus floor may or may not be apparent	Recent extraction, oral mucosal defect, passage of air, may cause chronic sinusitis	Episodes of congestion, may progress to acute sinusitis
Enlargement of maxillary lesion into the sinus	Cysts or benign neoplasms originating from maxillary bone or teeth	Uncommon	Varies, usually a homogeneous soft tissue radiopacity	Dome-shaped enlargement	Intact, but the sinus floor follows the superior edge of the lesion	Usually asymptomatic, may be associated with enlargement or sensation of fullness	Slow progression
Antrolith	Dystrophic calcification of chronic inflammatory lesion	Uncommon	Homogeneous mineralized radiopacity	Focal lesion, round or ovoid shape	Unaffected, intact	Patient unaware of any abnormality	Static
Squamous cell carcinoma of the maxillary sinus	Nonspecific, exposure to aerosol carcinogens	Rare	Heterogeneous soft tissue radiopacity	Usually entire sinus	Perforation, bone destruction	Pressure, pain, expansion, neck node enlargement	Gradual onset of weeks or months, progressive

becular patterns may be observed focally among healthy patients, the anemic patient is distinguished by the generalized distribution of the abnormal trabecular pattern and excessive radiolucency.

Clinical features. Sickle cell anemia and thalassemia can both be suspected on the basis of familial occurrence and manifestations such as fatigue and weakness. Severe forms of both diseases produce obvious clinical abnormalities that lead to diagnosis during infancy.

Differential diagnosis. The definitive diagnosis of anemia relies on clinical laboratory studies as described in Chapter 11. Observation of these radiographic features in the patient without a history of a genetic hemolytic anemia raises the possibility of an acquired hemolytic anemia.

Management. The radiographic abnormalities of the jaws are of no particular consequence other than as an indication of the severity of the hemolytic anemia.

Generalized Increase in Radiopacity

Definition. Generalized increased radiopacity of bone tissue can reflect replacement of normal medullary trabecular bone with either cortical bone or a compact arrangement of trabecular bone. Several rare, genetic conditions can cause this abnormal morphology including *osteopetrosis,* also known as *Albers-Schönberg disease* and *marble bone disease.*

Radiographic features. Normal bone morphology is replaced by a homogeneous granular, sclerotic, or "milky" radiopaque appearance. The uniform radiopacity and the generalized distribution often leave the unsuspecting clinician with the impression that the appearance has been caused by underexposure of the radiograph or a film processing error.

Clinical features. Two forms of osteopetrosis are recognized. The benign form is usually first observed radiographically among young adults as an incidental finding because clinical symptoms are unusual. The malignant form of osteopetrosis is appreciated during infancy because the abnormal bone architecture

results in pathologic fractures, hematologic abnormalities from displacement of hematopoietic tissue, and neuropathies such as deafness from neural compression.

Differential diagnosis. The generalized radiopacity and the relatively characteristic clinical features of such diseases allow a definitive diagnosis.

Management. Supportive care is the only available treatment for these conditions.

MAXILLARY SINUS ABNORMALITIES

Most maxillary sinus abnormalities are inflammatory in origin and produce homogeneous radiopaque replacement of some portion of the sinus air space with fluid or soft tissue. The differential diagnosis of these conditions relies on the clinical symptoms, the shape of the radiopacity, and the cortical integrity of sinus walls. These conditions are summarized in Table 19-7.

Acute Sinusitis

Definition. Acute inflammation of the maxillary sinus is a common sequela of progressive odontogenic infections, secondary infection of allergic sinusitis, and obstruction of the sinus aperture.

Radiographic features. Homogeneous, soft tissue radiopacity of the entire sinus reflects unilateral air space replacement by purulent fluid (Fig. 19-31). This is effectively demonstrated by Water's skull view, panoramic images, and other projections that include the entire sinus and the contralateral sinus for comparison. Acute sinusitis can also produce partial filling of the sinus, which yields a radiographic appearance known as an *air-fluid level.* This appearance is characterized by a straight, sharp interface between homogeneous radiopacity in the inferior portion of the sinus and normal radiolucency superiorly. The contours of the sinus and the continuity of the cortical walls appear normal.

Clinical features. Symptoms include acute onset of pain with increasing severity, tenderness to palpation, and purulent nasal drainage.

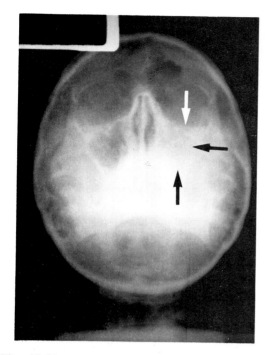

Fig. 19-31 Water's skull projection demonstrating unilateral maxillary sinus radiopacity caused by acute sinusitis. The normal contours and integrity of the cortical borders of the maxilla are dependable features to exclude the possibility of malignant neoplasia of the sinus.

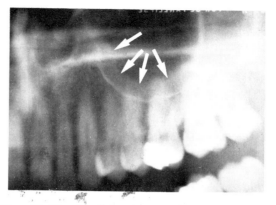

Fig. 19-32 Chronic sinusitis (*arrows*) demonstrated by this segment of a panoramic radiograph. The abnormality was bilateral.

Postural changes often alter the discomfort and the associated maxillary teeth may also be tender. Severe pain or sensitivity to percussion of a single tooth suggests that the sinusitis may have originated from a dental infection.

Differential diagnosis. A definitive diagnosis of acute maxillary sinusitis can be confidently made on the basis of acute onset of pain and homogeneous radiopacity of the entire sinus. The diagnostic problem for the dentist is to determine whether acute sinusitis or a dental abscess is the primary infection. An intraoral radiograph generally demonstrates the radicular radiolucency produced by a progressive odontogenic infection.

Management. The combination of a decongestant and an antibiotic effectively controls most episodes of acute maxillary sinusitis. Treatment to eliminate a dental infection as the cause of the sinusitis may also be necessary.

Chronic Sinusitis

Definition. Chronic sinusitis is generalized inflammation of the sinus mucosa in response to various airborne allergens and irritants. The typical radiographic feature of this common condition is thickening of the sinus mucosa. Focal soft tissue enlargements called *nasal polyps* may also result from chronic sinusitis, but their radiographic demonstration is unusual.

Chronic periapical lesions and periodontitis adjacent to the sinus can also produce thickening of the sinus lining, but it is focal rather than generalized. Focal inflammation can be associated with an *oroantral defect* or *fistula*, which is an epithelial lined passage between the sinus and oral cavity that is caused by sinus perforation during the extraction of a maxillary posterior tooth.

Radiographic features. The sinus mucosa appears radiographically as a homogeneous radiopaque band of relatively uniform width between the cortical sinus wall and the radiolucency of the central air space (Fig. 19-32). This is most apparent along the inferior sinus wall, and the condition is usually bilateral. The degree of radiopacity corresponds to soft tissue attenuation, and the cortical bone of the sinus wall appears unaffected or sclerotic.

Chronic dental inflammatory lesions and oroantral defects can produce similar radiopaque thickening of the sinus mucosa, but the radiopacity is limited to the immediate vicinity of the lesion. In addition, radiographic features of chronic dental infections affect a tooth near the mucosal thickening. The sinus wall discontinuity of oroantral defects may be revealed by intraoral radiographs.

Clinical features. Patients with chronic sinusitis are likely to be asymptomatic when the radiographic abnormality is identified, but they describe a chronic, episodic course of serous sinus drainage, congestion, and related symptoms. Patients often refer to this as seasonal "asthma" or a "sinus problem." Isolated occurrences of superimposed acute sinusitis may also be described.

Chronic dental infections that have produced focal sinus mucosal thickening are usually asymptomatic, but acute exacerbation of the infection may draw attention to the lesion. Clinical findings associated with an oroantral defect include a previous extraction site in the region and a mucosal defect that allows passage of air between the oral and sinus cavities.

Differential diagnosis. The generalized, bandlike thickening of the sinus mucosa caused by chronic sinusitis is easily distinguished from the focal lesions caused by chronic dental infections, oroantral defects, and the mucous retention phenomenon. Acute sinusitis is distinguished by abrupt onset of pain and more extensive radiopacity of the sinus.

Management. Chronic sinusitis unrelated to dental lesions requires no treatment other than symptomatic care during bouts of drainage and discomfort. Treatment of chronic dental inflammation and surgical repair of oroantral fistulas promotes resolution of focal inflammation, but the mucosal thickening usually persists.

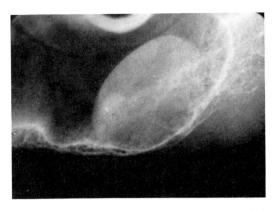

Fig. 19-33 Mucous retention phenomenon of the maxillary sinus. The normal contour and integrity of the inferior sinus wall is an important feature to distinguish mucous retention phenomena from lesions of maxillary bone that have enlarged into the sinus (see Fig. 19-6).

Mucous Retention Phenomenon of the Maxillary Sinus

Definition. The mucous retention phenomenon of the nasal sinuses is caused by accumulation of secretions from the accessory mucosal glands within the fibrous connective tissue. A specific cause of this common lesion cannot be identified in most instances, although chronic inflammation is presumed to be contributory. After initial enlargement, the mucous retention phenomenon of the maxillary sinus becomes static without progression, discomfort, or other adverse effects. This contrasts with the progressive enlargement, pain, and bone remodeling produced by a *mucocele.* This lesion usually affects the frontal sinuses, and maxillary sinus occurrence is rare.

Radiographic features. The mucous retention phenomenon is characterized by dome-shaped, homogeneous radiopaque enlargement within the maxillary sinus. Fig. 19-33 demonstrates the typical sharp delineation and curved border that is present between the soft tissue of the enlargement and the sinus air space. The base of the soft tissue radiopacity is located along the inferior or posterior sinus wall, which exhibits normal contour and integrity.

Clinical features. The patient is generally unaware of the abnormality.

Differential diagnosis. The radiographic features of mucous retention phenomena allow a definitive diagnosis in most instances. Maxillary sinus mucoceles produce chronic discomfort and homogeneous radiopacity of the entire sinus space similar to acute sinusitis. The differential diagnosis should include the possibility of a benign enlargement from the maxillary alveolus into the sinus. This is indicated by continuity of the cortical sinus wall along the superior border of the enlargement.

Management. No treatment is indicated.

Carcinoma of the Maxillary Sinus

Definition. Development of a malignant neoplasm within the maxillary sinus is rare. Most are squamous cell carcinomas and occupational exposure to irritating particulate material or chemical fumes has been suggested as a significant causative factor.

Radiographic features. Generalized radiopacity of the sinus is usually present at the time of discovery. Splotchy variation in the degree of x-ray attenuation yields a vaguely heterogeneous consistency of the radiopacity. Erosion or destruction of the cortical sinus walls in one or more areas is the most distinctive radiographic feature.

Clinical features. The patient is usually middle-aged or older and may report dull pain and nasal obstruction. Enlargement into the oral cavity, the orbit, or superficial tissues eventually develops. Identification of regional lymph node enlargement of the anterior superficial cervical group may be the initial clinical sign of carcinoma within the maxillary sinus.

Differential diagnosis. The heterogeneous radiopacity and the destruction of the sinus walls are the most reliable radiographic features in distinguishing malignant neoplasia from the much more common inflammatory sinus lesions. Intraoral radiographs are often the most sensitive method of demonstrating corti-

cal destruction of the inferior maxillary sinus wall.

Management. Referral to a tertiary oncology care center is justified if maxillary sinus carcinoma is suspected.

SOFT TISSUE CALCIFICATIONS

The diagnosis of most soft tissue calcifications is suggested by the location. Many soft tissue calcifications such as *calcified atherosclerotic plaques* of the carotid arteries demonstrate interesting manifestations of common degenerative conditions but are of little clinical significance. However, soft tissue radiopacities may present a diagnostic question because the lesions are related to discomfort or they appear superimposed over the image of the jaws. Sialolithiasis, dystrophic calcification of lymphoid tissues, and stylohyoid ligament ossification are all common examples.

Sialolithiasis

Definition. Sialoliths are calcified bodies formed by mineralization of congealed, proteinaceous bodies called *mucus plugs* within the excretory ducts of the major salivary glands. Mucus plugs may form during periods of limited saliva flow, but the mechanism is not well understood. Total obstruction of salivary flow is unusual because the duct gradually distends as the mucus plug and sialolith form. Obstruction may develop if the sialolith or mucus plug becomes lodged in a narrower duct segment.

Radiographic features. Mucus plugs are totally radiolucent and can only be demonstrated by injection of a radiopaque contrast medium into the duct. Sialoliths are ovoid or elongated radiopacities located along the course of the excretory ducts of the major salivary glands. Occlusal radiographs demonstrate the most common location in the floor of the mouth as shown in Fig. 19-34. Panoramic radiographs occasionally reveal sialoliths near the angle of the mandible corresponding to the most proximal segment of Wharton's duct and in the maxillary molar region representing the

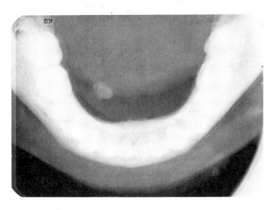

Fig. 19-34 Sialolith of Wharton's duct demonstrated by a mandibular occlusal projection. Note the laminated appearance of the stone.

distal segment of Stensen's duct. Careful examination of intraoral radiographs often demonstrates a "target" or laminar appearance consisting of concentric radiolucent and radiopaque rings. Sialoliths are usually solitary, but multiple calcifications may develop. Superimposition of sialoliths on the image of the jaw and teeth in periapical and panoramic projections can yield the appearance typical of focal sclerosis.

Clinical Features. Most patients are unaware of the abnormality. Obstruction of salivary flow is indicated by diffuse, unilateral pain in the body of the blocked salivary gland during salivary stimulation. The discomfort is usually episodic and varies in intensity. Palpation or "milking" the gland may produce a little saliva, an abnormally viscous or cloudy fluid, or a sudden outflow. Limited salivary flow contributes to retrograde bacterial infection, *sialodochitis,* that produces tenderness, erythema of the duct orifice, foul taste, and purulence.

Differential diagnosis. Calcified lymph nodes may appear similar to sialoliths, and lymph nodes are located in regions where sialoliths commonly form. Most sialoliths are associated with some symptoms of intermittent salivary obstruction, laminar appearance of the radiopacity, and elongated shape. Calcified lymph nodes are associated with a history of granulomatous or other severe infection and calcification of other nodes in the regional group is likely.

Management. No treatment is necessary if the patient is asymptomatic. Symptoms of obstruction may be relieved by injection of the excretory duct with a lipid-soluble radiographic contrast material. This dilates the duct and provides lubrication that occasionally promotes passage of the obstruction. The only other alternative is surgical removal.

Dystrophic Calcification of Lymphoid Tissue

Definition. Dystrophic calcification is a nonspecific degenerative response of tissues following severe inflammation, and lymphoid tissues are often affected. Chronic granulomatous infections such as tuberculosis characteristically cause dystrophic calcification of lymph nodes.

Radiographic features. Calcified lymph nodes are usually ovoid in shape and approximately 1 cm in diameter. The radiopacity often exhibits a patchy pattern with a reticular arrangement of radiolucent lines or gaps. Dystrophic calcification of the tonsils can produce a "speckled" appearance of multiple radiopaque foci superimposed bilaterally on the images of the mandibular rami in a panoramic radiograph.

Clinical features. The patient with calcified lymph nodes or tonsillar tissues is asymptomatic but may recall a severe infection that could explain degeneration of lymphoid tissues. Superficial calcified lymph nodes are usually firm, nontender, and mobile during palpation.

Differential diagnosis. Calcified lymph nodes can often be distinguished from sialoliths on the basis of history, clinical findings, and radiographic features as described in the differential diagnosis section for sialoliths.

Management. No treatment is indicated.

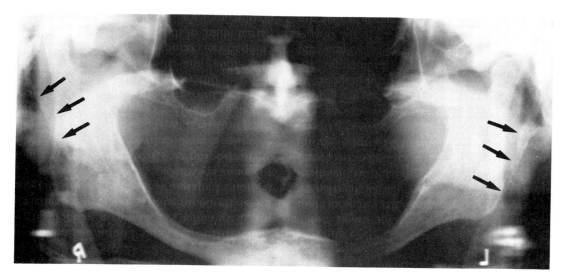

Fig. 19-35   Bilateral ossification of the stylohyoid ligaments (*arrows*). The degree of ossification of the right ligament is a rather routine panoramic finding, whereas the ossification on the left side with pseudoarticular formation is unusually prominent.

Stylohyoid Ligament Ossification

Definition. Stylohyoid ligament ossification is a common developmental abnormality in which bone tissue forms within segments of the stylohyoid ligament. Other ligaments of the styloid complex such as the stylomandibular ligament can also undergo this ossification.

Radiographic features. Elongation of the styloid process is most apparent in panoramic and lateral skull projections. The styloid process projects inferior to the level of the mandibular foramen on the panoramic view and bilateral occurrence is typical. Ossification of the ligament roughly parallels the posterior border of the ramus and may be discontinuous with gaps or a rudimentary jointlike formation called *pseudoarthrosis* as shown by the example in Fig. 19-35. The ossification of the ligament may extend the entire distance to the lesser horn of the hyoid bone.

Clinical features. Most patients are asymptomatic and unaware of the abnormality. However, swallowing and extreme movements can produce pain or the sensation of a foreign object caught in the throat. This results from fibrosis following tonsillectomy or severe tonsillitis that entraps the stylohyoid ligament. Rigidity and pain results years later when the entrapped ligament ossifies within the scarred tissue lateral to the throat. This condition is referred to as *Eagle's syndrome.*

Differential diagnosis. The radiographic features of stylohyoid ossification are distinctive and are unlikely to be confused with other abnormalities.

Management. No treatment is indicated for the asymptomatic individual. Surgical removal is the only treatment option for the pain of Eagle's syndrome.

ABNORMALITIES OF THE TEMPOROMANDIBULAR JOINT AND JAW FRACTURES

Clinical examination usually provides the most definitive diagnostic information concerning temporomandibular joint (TMJ) conditions. Most radiographic techniques produce either relatively poor resolution, or the TMJ is obscured by superimposed cranial structures. Advanced degenerative joint changes may be demonstrated but early, subtle alterations are usually unapparent. In addition, displacement of the meniscus known as *internal derangement* (see Chapter 9) contributes to osseous deterioration in most cases and can only be demonstrated by complex techniques such as arthrotomography and magnetic resonance imaging. Nevertheless, radiographs provide valuable confirmation of clinical impressions and may reveal unusual conditions.

Arthritis of the Temporomandibular Joint

Definition. Arthritis is a nonspecific term for joint inflammation. The most clinically significant forms of arthritis are those that produce chronic joint inflammation leading to gradual degeneration of articular tissues. *Osteoarthritis* results from traumatic injury or repetitious, functional stress to the joint and can be thought of as "wear and tear" arthritis. This is the most common degenerative joint disease, and its cumulative effects are most apparent in weight-bearing joints of older adults. *Rheumatoid arthritis* is immune-mediated joint inflammation as described in Chapter 7. The symmetric distribution of joint degeneration progresses more rapidly than osteoarthritis and affects younger individuals.

Radiographic features. Sclerotic cortical thickening called *eburnation* of the opposing surfaces of the head of the condyle and the glenoid fossa is the earliest osseous feature of TMJ osteoarthritis. This may be associated with a decrease in subcortical trabecular density. More advanced degeneration is indicated by flattening of the articular surfaces of the condylar and eminence. A combination of condylar flattening and osteophyte formation of the anterior surface of the condyle yields a "bird beak" contour (Fig. 19-36) in severe cases. High resolution tomographs may reveal rough-

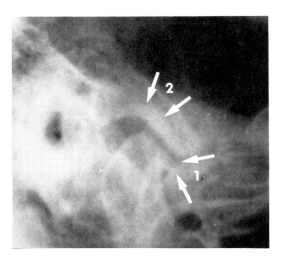

Fig. 19-36   Advanced osteoarthritis of the temporomandibular joint demonstrated by a transcranial projection. Characteristic radiographic features of degenerative joint disease include flattening of the anterior-superior surface of the condylar head, "bird beak" contour of the anterior surface (1), and sclerotic cortical thickening that is most apparent within the bone of the glenoid fossa (2).

ness or more extensive erosion of articular surfaces. The radiographic features of rheumatoid arthritis affecting the TMJ are similar but the osseous degeneration tends to be more severe as shown by the example in Fig. 19-37.

Clinical features. Clinical features associated with degenerative joint disease of the TMJ are described in Chapter 9.

Differential diagnosis. Rheumatoid arthritis can usually be distinguished from osteoarthritis by onset before age 40, symmetric joint degeneration, and laboratory findings such as elevated erythrocyte sedimentation rate and demonstration of rheumatoid factor. Other lesions that affect the TMJ such as neoplasms produce enlargement rather than degeneration.

Management. Symptomatic treatment of mild osteoarthritis relies on aspirin and nonsteroidal antiinflammatory medications. Bite splint therapy may be beneficial in some cases

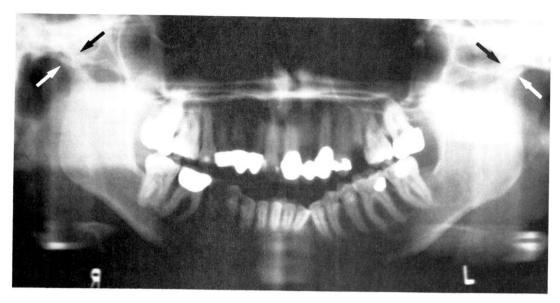

Fig. 19-37 Severe malformation of the condylar heads (*arrows*) caused by rheumatoid arthritis. Note the resulting acquired anterior open bite.

by minimizing dysfunctional habits. Rheumatoid arthritis of the TMJ must be managed in concert with the patient's physician and with consideration of the generalized manifestations of the disease.

Jaw Fractures

Definition. Fractures of the facial bones represent a diagnostic and therapeutic challenge for several reasons. Radiographic demonstration of the complex facial structures may be compromised by management problems immediately after an injury. Head trauma often produces altered patient responsiveness, which limits the clinician's examination and the selection of optimal radiographic projections for suspected fracture sites. Also, facial trauma commonly causes multiple fractures, which increases the chances that subtle breaks may be overlooked after more obvious fractures are identified.

Radiographic features. Fractures without significant displacement of the bone appear as

a radiolucent line of relatively uniform width and a jagged course. Fig. 19-38 illustrates that fracture lines are often continuous with a wid-

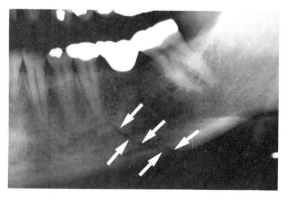

Fig. 19-38 Fracture (*arrows*) of the body of the mandible that involves the socket of the mandibular second premolar. Note the uniform widening of the periodontal ligament space along the mesial surface of the tooth root. (Courtesy of Dr Marvin Vore, Hudson, Iowa.)

ened periodontal ligament space if the fracture involves a tooth socket. A network of interconnected radiolucent lines indicates the multiple fragments of a comminuted fracture. Displacement of bone fragments can produce either a wide radiolucent gap or a radiopaque zone caused by overlapping of the fragments. This is most likely with subcondylar and angle fractures of the mandible as a consequence of spastic contraction of the masseter and pterygoid muscles. Most displaced fractures also exhibit an abrupt "step" defect in the peripheral cortical contour. Fracture or displacement of teeth as well as homogeneous radiopacity of the maxillary sinuses caused by hemorrhage or edema are additional radiographic features associated with jaw fractures.

Clinical features. The possibility of jaw fracture is implied by a recent history of significant facial injury. However, the traumatic event can be surprisingly minor or it may be denied in cases of abuse. Facial swelling, facial asymmetry, pain, ecchymosis, dramatic occlusal discrepancy, trismus, and point tenderness at suspected fracture sites are typical features associated with jaw fractures. Midface mobility indicates separation of the maxillary alveolus from the cranial base by a continuous, bilateral discontinuity known as a *Le Fort fracture*. Fractures of multiple bones and at multiple sites of a single bone are common with facial injury. Patients occasionally describe past treatment of jaw fractures and exhibit limited opening as a consequence of undetected fractures that have healed without reduction (Fig. 19-39).

Differential diagnosis. Few radiographic abnormalities are likely to be confused with jaw fractures. Occasionally, thin radiolucent lines in the ramus region of panoramic radiographs that represent the oropharyngeal air space may be mistaken for a fracture line. Any diagnostic uncertainty justifies the exposure of additional radiographs.

Management. Consultation with specialists experienced in the assessment of facial injuries is essential in cases of suspected jaw fracture. Methods of repositioning of displaced bone fragments, *reduction,* and stabilizing the bone during healing, *fixation,* are determined by the nature and extent of the injury.

SUMMARY

Radiographs provide essential information concerning the composition, rate of growth, relationship to anatomic structures, and other differential diagnostic characteristics of central jaw lesions. The differential diagnostic strategy is to classify a radiographic abnormality by x-ray attenuation as radiolucent, mixed radiolucent-radiopaque, or radiopaque. Within the radiolucent lesion category, the lesion shape, location, and delineation of the borders allow determination of the most likely diagnostic possibilities. The proportion and arrangement of the radiolucent and radiopaque components within mixed lesions in addition to the delineation of the lesion borders provide a dependable basis for narrowing the diagnostic possibilities. The pattern, location, and marginal delineation of totally radiopaque jaw lesions provide an effective assessment of the relatively few lesions in this category. The combination of clinical findings, symptoms, patient age, and other information with the radiographic interpretation of a lesion yields a basis for a realistic working diagnosis and for management decisions. This is also true for other radiographic abnormalities of the jaws and associated structures.

BIBLIOGRAPHY

Ariyan S: Cancer of the head and neck, St Louis, 1987, Mosby–Year Book.

Barr JH, Stephens RG: Dental radiology: pertinent basic concepts and their applications in clinical practice, Philadelphia, 1980, Saunders.

Batsakis JG: Tumors of the head and neck: clinical and pathological considerations, ed 2, Baltimore, 1979, Williams & Wilkins.

Eversole LR: Clinical outline of oral pathology: diagnosis and treatment, ed 2, Philadelphia, 1984, Lea & Febiger.

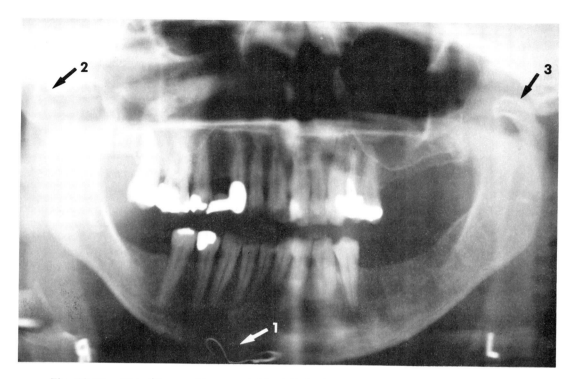

Fig. 19-39   This 42-year-old man exhibited limited opening and reported repair of a jaw fracture caused by a car accident 5 years previously. The panoramic radiograph reveals the radiopaque ligature wire (1) of the reduced and fixated fracture near the midline. The posterior inclination of the right condyle (2) and the anterior-inferior position of the left condyle (3) suggest that bilateral subcondylar fractures were unappreciated at the time of injury. They eventually healed without reduction, which explains the functional limitation.

Goaz PW, White SC: Oral radiology: principles and interpretation, ed 2, St Louis, 1987, Mosby–Year Book.

Keller EE, Gunderson LL: Lesions of the jaw. In Sim FH, editor: Diagnosis and management of metastatic bone disease: a multidisciplinary approach, New York, 1988, Raven.

Langlais RP and others: Oral diagnosis, oral medicine and treatment planning, Philadelphia, 1984, Saunders.

Langland OE and others: Panoramic radiology, ed 2, Philadelphia, 1989, Lea & Febiger.

Lilly GE: Differential diagnosis of lesions of the jawbones, Oral Surg Oral Med Oral Path 28:65, 1970.

Lynch MA, Brightman VJ, Greenberg MS, editors: Burket's oral medicine: diagnosis and treatment, ed 8, Philadelphia, 1984, Lippincott.

Regezi JA and Sciubba JJ: Oral pathology: clinical-pathologic correlations, Philadelphia, 1989, Saunders.

Shafer WG, Hine MK, Levy BM: A textbook of oral pathology, ed 4, Philadelphia, 1983, Saunders.

Valvassori GE and others: Radiology of the ear, nose and throat, Philadelphia, 1984, Saunders.

Wilson JD and others, editors: Harrison's principles of internal medicine, ed 12, New York, 1991, McGraw-Hill, Health Professions Division.

Wood NK, Goaz PW: Differential diagnosis of oral lesions, ed 4, St Louis, 1991, Mosby–Year Book.

Worth HM: Principles and practice of oral radiologic interpretation, St Louis, 1963, Mosby–Year Book.

CHAPTER 20

Differential Diagnosis of Syndromes with Orofacial Features

GARY C. COLEMAN

The term *syndrome* is defined as the aggregate of signs and symptoms associated with any morbid process that together constitute the picture of the disease. Clinical use of the term generally implies that several outwardly diverse clinical features are actually manifestations of a common cause. *Acquired* syndromes develop entirely after birth as a consequence of many pathologic mechanisms. *Congenital syndromes* are caused either by genetic defects or adverse influences during gestation. Some manifestations of congenital syndromes may not become clinically apparent until later in life, but the essential abnormality is present at birth.

Hundreds of acquired and congenital syndromes have been described and many include orofacial manifestations. A complete and detailed discussion in this context is not practical. However, certain syndromes warrant discussion because they are relatively common, present particularly significant dental abnormalities, or illustrate important diagnostic considerations. Fig. 20-1 illustrates a general differential diagnosis approach to syndromes with orofacial features based on predominant clinical findings.

SYNDROMES OF DEFICIENT MANDIBULAR DEVELOPMENT

Mandibular hypoplasia and the resulting retrognathic, convex facial profile can be recognized in most cases at birth or within the first year of life. Malformations of the mandible are often associated with malformations of the ears as well as cleft lip and palate deformities. Treacher Collins syndrome and the Pierre Robin syndrome are well recognized and relatively common examples of the syndromes that produce mandibular deficiency.

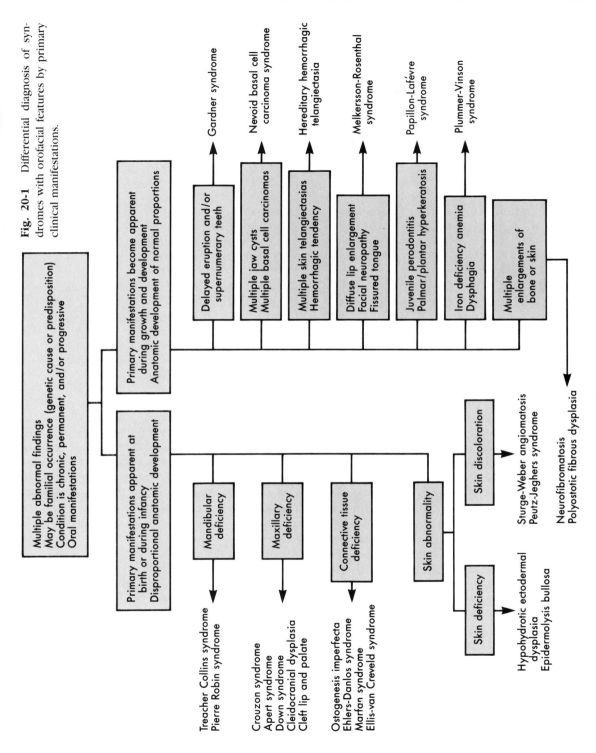

Fig. 20-1 Differential diagnosis of syndromes with orofacial features by primary clinical manifestations.

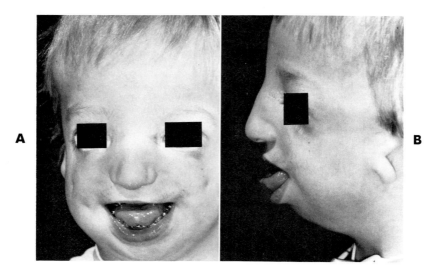

Fig. 20-2   Treacher Collins syndrome affecting a 4-year-old boy. **A,** Frontal view reveals characteristic deficiency of the zygomatic arches. **B,** Profile demonstrates the convex facial contour resulting from deficient development of the mandible. Note the malformation of the external ear. (Courtesy of Dr Edward Genecov, Dallas, Texas.)

Treacher Collins Syndrome

Synonyms. Mandibulofacial dysostosis, Collins syndrome, Treacher Collins-Franceschetti syndrome.

Definition. The characteristic facial appearance produced by symmetric malar and mandibular hypoplasia defines Treacher Collins syndrome for all practical purposes. This is an autosomal dominant genetic condition with high penetrance and variable expressivity, although most cases result from new mutations.

Clinical features. The most prominent and consistent malformations of Treacher Collins syndrome are hypoplasia of the mandible and zygomatic arches as shown in Fig. 20-2. Mandibular hypoplasia produces a retrognathic appearance in profile (Fig. 20-2, *B*) and the mandibular angle is obtuse. The depression in the malar region contributes to the appearance of a downward lateral slant of the palpebral fissures that is referred to as *antimongoloid obliquity* (Fig. 20-3). This combination yields a characteristic facial appearance that has been referred to as "fishlike"; this appearance is diagnostic of the condition. The cranial structures are unaffected and intelligence is usually within the normal range.

Numerous other anatomic defects may also be present. Most patients have a gap or coloboma in the lower eyelid and additional ophthalmic abnormalities may also be identified. Both external and internal ear malformations (Fig. 20-2) with hearing loss or deafness

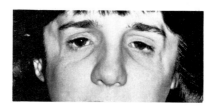

Fig. 20-3   Treacher Collins syndrome affecting a 20-year-old woman. The midface appearance is characterized by symmetrical depression of the malar region, a sunken appearance of the lateral wall of the orbit, and antimongoloid obliquity of the palpebral fissures. (Courtesy of Dr Edward Genecov, Dallas, Texas.)

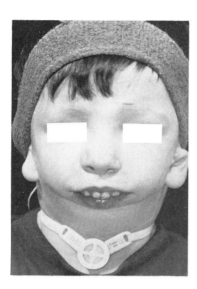

Fig. 20-4 Pierre Robin syndrome. Severe retrognathic appearance of the mandible and malformation of auricles are shown by this 3-year-old boy. The white, plastic device on the boy's neck is a screen for the tracheostomy stoma that is required for breathing because of the severe glossoptosis. (Courtesy of Dr Edward Genecov, Dallas, Texas.)

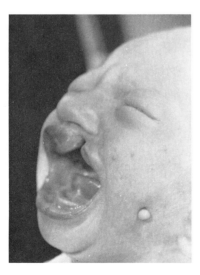

Fig. 20-5 Pierre Robin syndrome affecting a neonate. Unilateral alveolar and lip cleft as well as the nodular "ear tag" deformity of the cheek are present. (Courtesy of Dr Edward Genecov, Dallas, Texas.)

are common associated features. The paranasal sinuses and mastoid air spaces are often small or unapparent radiographically. Approximately one third of patients with Treacher Collins syndrome are affected by palatal clefts. Mental retardation, parotid aplasia, malformations of other bones, and cardiac anomalies are occasionally observed.

Clinical considerations. Longevity is normal except in patients whose cardiac abnormalities cause complications. Esthetics can be corrected by reconstructive surgery. However, multiple procedures are required for significant improvement. Severe malocclusion requires orthognathic surgery in concert with orthodontic treatment. Surgical closure of clefts may also be necessary.

Pierre Robin Syndrome

Synonyms. Robin sequence; Robin anomalad; and cleft palate, micrognathia, and glossoptosis.

Definition. The condition consists of micrognathia, cleft palate, and glossoptosis. The congenital malformations of this relatively common condition result from arrested development, but a number of specific genetic conditions and environmental influences appear capable of producing the clinical features. Identification of the three definitional features raises the expectation that additional anomalies are probably present.

Clinical features. The anatomic malformations of variably severe palatal clefting and symmetric mandibular hypoplasia yield a retrognathic appearance (Fig. 20-4). Glossoptosis is the functional consequence of the hypoplastic mandible failing to adequately support the tongue. This produces labored inspirational breathing and cyanotic episodes because the airway space becomes occluded, particularly in the supine position. Additional developmental abnormalities may be present including cardiac defects, ocular abnormalities, anomalies of bone formation, mental retardation, and ear malformations (Fig. 20-5).

Clinical considerations. Breathing sup-

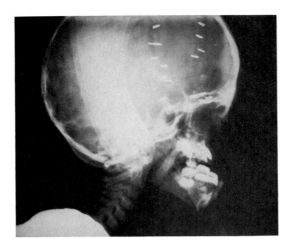

Fig. 20-6 Lateral skull projection of a child with Crouzon syndrome. Hypoplasia of the maxilla has resulted in the concave contour of the facial structures. The "digital impressions" appearance is most obvious in the posterior occipital and parietal regions. The metallic bodies are vascular clips from a previous surgical procedure. (Courtesy of Dr Edward Genecov, Dallas, Texas.)

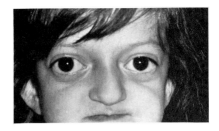

Fig. 20-7 The midface region of a 5-year-old girl with Crouzon syndrome illustrates ocular hypertelorism and protrusion of the eyes that are typical features of the condition. (Courtesy of Dr Edward Genecov, Dallas, Texas.)

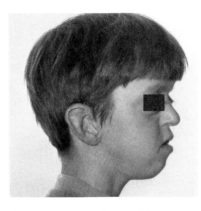

Fig. 20-8 Crouzon syndrome. This 8-year-old boy exhibits concave facial contour and "parrot-shaped" nose associated with midface hypoplasia. (Courtesy of Dr Edward Genecov, Dallas, Texas.)

port and feeding assistance are necessary during infancy. Mandibular growth will eventually produce improvement in the relationship of the jaws later in childhood, although a short ramus and obtuse mandibular angle will still be apparent. Surgical cleft closure and orthodontic treatment are indicated. Cardiac defects may require infective endocarditis prophylaxis during most dental procedures.

CONDITIONS OF DEFICIENT MAXILLARY DEVELOPMENT

Hypoplasia of the midface region is recognized by a concave facial profile and a relative prognathic relationship with the normal mandible. Also, the relative size and position of the eyes and nose are frequently altered. This produces the appearance of abnormal width of the bridge of the nose and excessive separation of the eyes referred to as *ocular hypertelorism*. In addition, midface deficiency is often associated with abnormal closure of cranial sutures, which produces abnormal cranial shape as an additional associated finding. Developmental conditions with these features include Crouzon syndrome, Apert syndrome, Down syndrome, and cleidocranial dysplasia.

Crouzon Syndrome

Synonyms. Craniofacial dysostosis, Crouzon's disease, Apert-Crouzon's syndrome.

Definition. This relatively common syndrome is characterized by cranial malformation, midface hypoplasia, and ocular proptosis resulting from shallow orbits. The cranial deformities are explained by premature closure or *synostosis* of cranial sutures, which usually occurs by age 3. Autosomal dominant transmission with complete penetrance is the mode of inheritance, although approximately one half of cases result from spontaneous mutations.

Clinical features. Cranial shape varies depending on which cranial sutures close prematurely, but brachycephaly is most common. Thinned cranial bone relative to convoluted cerebral contours produces radiographic features described as "digital impressions" or a "beaten silver" appearance (Fig. 20-6). Shallow, hypoplastic formation of orbital bones produces protrusion of the eyes and ocular hypertelorism (Fig. 20-7). Relative prognathism, short upper lip, and "parrot-shaped" prominence of the nose (Fig. 20-8) are attributable to the hypoplasia of midface bones. This also causes crowding of the maxillary teeth, a narrow maxillary arch, and malocclusion (Fig. 20-9). Occasional findings include ocular malformations, cleft palate, and hearing loss. Mental retardation is unusual.

Clinical considerations. Surgical correction of midfacial deficiency in concert with orthodontic treatment to improve esthetics and masticatory efficiency may be beneficial in selected cases.

Apert Syndrome

Synonyms. Acrocephalosyndactyly, syndactylic oxycephaly.

Definition. Apert syndrome is defined clinically as cranial malformation caused by synostosis, midface hypoplasia, and bilateral *syndactyly* or fusion of the digits. This rare condition is usually a sporadic genetic mutation, although autosomal dominant transmission has been suggested in some cases.

Clinical features. The fusion of coronal sutures at birth produces frontal flattening. In addition, occipital flattening and midface hypoplasia produces a high, conical cranial shape. The nasal bridge is dramatically depressed with ocular hypertelorism as shown in Fig. 20-10. The eyes are mildly exophthalmic with antimongoloid obliquity of palpebral fissures. Hypoplasia of the maxillae causes a constricted palate, narrow arch shape, crowding of teeth,

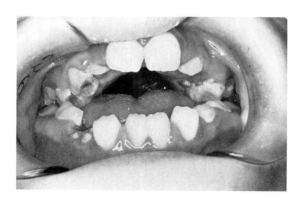

Fig. 20-9 Crouzon syndrome. The severe malocclusion and anterior open bite are associated with the maxillary hypoplasia. (Courtesy of Dr Edward Genecov, Dallas, Texas.)

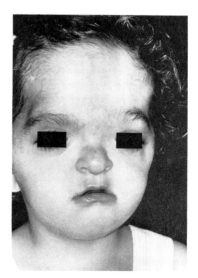

Fig. 20-10 Apert syndrome. Characteristic features include ocular hypertelorism, depressed nasal bridge, and high, conical cranial shape. (Courtesy of Dr Edward Genecov, Dallas, Texas.)

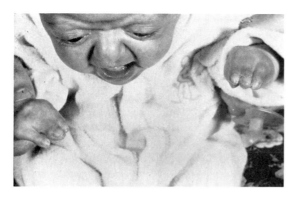

Fig. 20-11 A neonate with Apert syndrome exhibits the combination of syndactyly and exophthalmos that are characteristic of the condition. (Courtesy of Dr Edward Genecov, Dallas, Texas.)

and relative prognathic malocclusion. Symmetric syndactyly of the middle digits (Fig. 20-11), short stature, and mental retardation are the other consistent features of the syndrome. Clefts of the soft palate, abnormalities of long bone growth, cardiovascular malformations, delayed eruption of teeth, and other findings are occasionally observed.

Clinical considerations. Longevity is normal unless cardiac abnormalities are present. Surgical correction of digital and craniofacial deformities should be considered in addition to orthodontic treatment.

Down Syndrome

Synonyms. Trisomy 21 syndrome, chromosome 21 trisomy syndrome, mongolism.

Definition. Down syndrome is a widely recognized developmental syndrome both because of its common occurrence and because of the characteristic facial appearance and mental deficiency that accompany it. The malformations characteristic of the syndrome result from excessive chromosomal material involving all or a portion of chromosome 21. The incidence of Down syndrome increases with advanced maternal age at conception. Advanced paternal age also increases risk, but to a lesser degree.

Clinical features. The combination of mental retardation, round face, and brachycephalic skull shape with frontal prominence and occipital flattening is diagnostic of Down syndrome. The palpebral fissures are almond-shaped with superior-lateral or mongolian obliquity. Midface deficiency with relative prognathism, flattened nasal bridge, and ocular hypertelorism contribute to the impression of a flattened facial profile. Hypoplasia and aplasia of paranasal sinuses and persistence of open cranial sutures may be identified radiographically. More than one third of patients with Down syndrome exhibit cardiac malformations. Numerous other morphologic and functional abnormalities have also been identified.

Possible dental features of Down syndrome include malocclusion attributable to small maxillary arch size relative to the mandibular arch, congenitally missing teeth, microdontia, and delayed eruption. Severe periodontitis frequently develops and may be explained by a combination of immune system dysfunction as a syndrome feature and the limited oral hygiene effectiveness attainable by these patients. Interestingly, dental caries resistance is comparatively normal. Additional findings often include mouth breathing, macroglossia, and fissured tongue.

Clinical considerations. Shortened life span is most directly explained by cardiovascular and other internal malformations. However, advances in the detection and treatment of these abnormalities offer improved prognosis. Vulnerability to periodontitis necessitates concerted preventive efforts and a comparatively short recall interval. The presence of a cardiac malformation may require antibiotic prophylactic coverage during dental treatment. Orthognathic surgery and orthodontic treatment of the prognathic malocclusion may be justified in some cases.

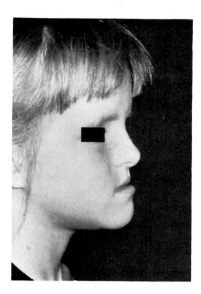

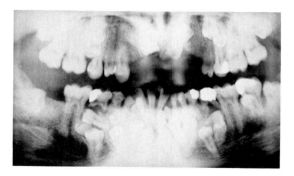

Fig. 20-13 This panoramic radiograph of a 26-year-old man with cleidocranial dysplasia reveals numerous impacted supernumerary teeth of the anterior segments and premolar regions.

Fig. 20-12 Cleidocranial dysplasia. The condition is characterized by midface deficiency and frontal prominence referred to as bossing, which combine to yield a concave facial profile. However, the contour of the nose is relatively normal in contrast to Apert (Fig. 20-10) and Crouzon (Fig. 20-8) syndromes. This 9-year-old girl also exhibited short stature and delayed eruption of teeth. (Courtesy of Dr Edward Genecov, Dallas, Texas.)

Cleidocranial Dysplasia

Synonyms. Cleidocranial dysostosis, Marie-Sainton syndrome.

Definition. The primary features of cleidocranial dysplasia are hypoplasia of the clavicles and malformation of craniofacial bones caused by delayed closure of sutures and fontanels. Numerous additional anomalies associated with the condition indicate an extremely diverse potential impact of the genetic defect, but the mechanism has not been clarified. An autosomal dominant mode of transmission with high penetrance and variable expression is observed for cleidocranial dysplasia, although a significant proportion of cases represent new mutations.

Clinical features. The skull is brachycephalic with bossing of the frontal, parietal, and occipital regions. Wormian bones are usually present in the open suture areas. The midface is hypoplastic, which produces a small facial appearance compared with the cranial prominence (Fig. 20-12). Paranasal sinuses are often absent or small. Hypoplasia or aplasia of one or both clavicles may allow dramatic hypermobility anteriomedially and produces the appearance of drooping shoulders and a long neck. Other skeletal abnormalities are often present. The patient exhibits normal intelligence and short stature.

Maxillary hypoplasia yields a high palatal arch and relative prognathism. Submucosal and palatal clefts are occasionally observed. Eruption of deciduous teeth is normal or somewhat delayed, but exfoliation of the deciduous teeth is dramatically delayed by failure of most succedaneous teeth to erupt. Radiographic examination reveals numerous impacted teeth, as well as supernumerary teeth (Fig. 20-13), particularly in the anterior and premolar regions. The combination of maxillary retrusion and failure of teeth to erupt causes severe malocclusion. Other dental malformations and para-

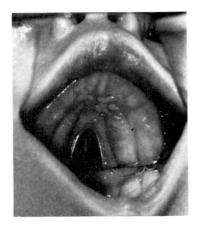

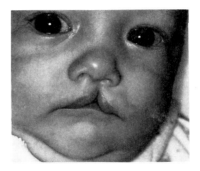

Fig. 20-15 Unilateral cleft lip. (Courtesy of Dr Edward Genecov, Dallas, Texas.)

Fig. 20-14 Palatal cleft of a neonate. (Courtesy of Dr Edward Genecov, Dallas, Texas.)

coronal cystic radiolucencies may also be present.

Clinical considerations. Eruption of the succedaneous teeth may be facilitated by surgical exposure and orthodontic guidance after removal of the deciduous and supernumerary teeth. Optimal correction of the severe malocclusion may require orthognathic surgery in combination with orthodontic treatment.

Cleft Palate and Lip

Synonyms. None.

Definition. Clefts of the lip and palate are isolated developmental anomalies rather than a legitimate syndrome with multiple features. However, the congenital nature of the defect and the observation of clefts as one element of many developmental syndromes warrants inclusion in this section with other maxillary malformations.

Maxillary clefts result from the failure of mesodermal tissues to penetrate the ectodermal grooves at the posterior palatal midline and lateral to the premaxilla during the first trimester of gestation. This causes failure of the medial and lateral nasal processes or the lateral palatal processes to completely fuse. Both genetic predisposition and adverse environmental influences contribute in a multifactorial manner to these malformations. Other deformities related to cleft lip and palate include lip pits, submucosal clefts of the palatal bone, bifid tongue, bifid uvula, and a variety of rare facial and midline clefts. Cleft lip and palate are among the most common congenital malformations. The factors capable of exerting the adverse influence necessary to cause clefts often produce other developmental abnormalities.

Clinical features. Considerable variation in the severity and extent of facial clefts can be observed among affected infants. Submucosal palatal clefts are often clinically subtle because the mucosa is continuous and the superficial appearance is relatively normal. This defect of deep tissues is indicated by bifid uvula and a palpable midline depression of the palate. Abnormal breathing or nursing difficulties such as passage of milk through the nose are often the initial indication of palatal clefts (Fig. 20-14).

Cleft lips are visually apparent at birth and prompt examination will determine the extent of the cleft—as limited to the lip, involving the alveolus, or continuous with a cleft palate. Cleft lip may be unilateral, as shown in Fig. 20-15, or bilateral. Severe bilateral clefting can yield a lateral discontinuity with the premaxilla segment, which is then attached only to the midline nasal structures as demonstrated in

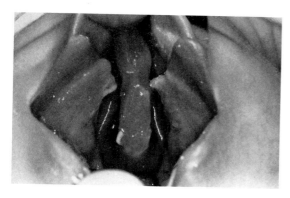

Fig. 20-16 Severe bilateral alveolar clefts and cleft palate. (Courtesy of Dr Edward Genecov, Dallas, Texas.)

Fig. 20-16. The maxillary lateral incisor teeth are usually missing in patients with alveolar clefts, and adjacent teeth may eventually fail to erupt or become malaligned. Other dental abnormalities may also be present. Functional complications related to cleft lip and palate include nursing, swallowing, and speaking difficulties. Aspiration of food and fluids can cause pulmonary obstruction and infection.

Clinical considerations. The treatment for clefts is dictated by the extent and severity of the defect. Immediate treatment considerations include preventing food and fluid aspiration and establishing effective feeding. If feasible, to improve eating and to foster normal speech development, soft tissue clefts are surgically repaired and an obturator is fabricated for extensive palatal defects during infancy. Surgical repair of osseous defects is generally delayed until later in development. Additional surgical procedures to improve esthetics, orthodontic treatment, prosthodontic treatment, and speech therapy may eventually be indicated.

SYNDROMES OF CONNECTIVE TISSUE DEFICIENCY

Conditions of connective tissue deficiency are generally attributable to genetic defects in the metabolism of collagen or another primary connective tissue component. One consequence of this is that the clinical manifestations may appear relatively diverse and apparently unrelated until the underlying cause is appreciated. The tissue abnormality will be generalized, which means that if bone tissue is abnormal, then all bones will be affected. An obvious clinical feature of many of these conditions is a malformation of the sclera that is identified by a light blue appearance. Also, these conditions tend to produce alterations in body size or relative size of different parts. Therefore short stature, disproportional dwarfism, or disproportional size of extremities will often be a feature of these syndromes. Osteogenesis imperfecta, Marfan syndrome, Ehlers-Danlos syndrome, and Ellis-van Creveld syndrome are examples of such conditions with associated dental features.

Osteogenesis Imperfecta

Synonyms. Osteogenesis imperfecta tarda and osteogenesis imperfecta congenita.

Definition. Osteogenesis imperfecta is a designation that includes several distinct, genetic conditions that result in the malformation of bone and other mesenchymal tissues as a consequence of abnormal collagen synthesis. The differences among the types of osteogenesis imperfecta are related to mode of inheritance, radiographic features, the presence of blue sclera, and the severity of the malformation relative to life expectancy. The form of osteogenesis imperfecta described below (type I) provides a general indication of the clinical consequences of these related conditions. Transmission of most types of osteogenesis imperfecta is autosomal dominant with variable penetrance and expressivity. Some cases of subtle expression may not be identified unless suspected because of an affected family member.

Clinical features. Vulnerability of bones to fracture with mild or incidental trauma is the most dramatic clinical feature of osteogen-

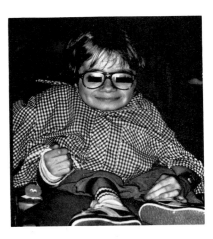

Fig. 20-17 Osteogenesis imperfecta. This 4-year-old boy had suffered numerous bone fractures since birth. The cranial size is relatively large compared with the short stature and small face. Additional features included blue sclera, dentinogenesis imperfecta, and a bleeding tendency. (Courtesy of Dr Catherine Flaitz, University of Texas Dental Branch at Houston, Houston, Texas.)

esis imperfecta (Fig. 20-17), although the degree of fracture diathesis varies considerably. The fracture tendency is generally greater during infancy, childhood, and old age, and fractures are less likely during adolescence and adulthood. Short stature, spinal deformities, exuberant callus formation of healed fractures, hypermobility of joints, and hearing loss are additional findings. Cranial size is often comparatively large relative to the stature and the face. Blue scleras are present as with other conditions of deficient collagen formation. The skin is often thin and transparent with abnormal capillary fragility and an associated bleeding tendency. Malformation of teeth described as *dentinogenesis imperfecta* in Chapter 8 is frequently observed. However, the generalized malformation of teeth may also be more typical of dentin dysplasia in some cases or the teeth may be unaffected.

Clinical considerations. Fracture preven-

tion, management, and rehabilitation can be challenging in severe cases. This, in addition to the bleeding tendency, requires that dental procedures should be performed with particular care. If dentinogenesis imperfecta is present, coronal restoration of all teeth is usually required to protect against excessive attrition and to improve esthetics.

Ehlers-Danlos Syndrome

Synonyms. Cutis hyperelastica, dermatorrhexis.

Definition. The designation refers to patients who exhibit extreme stretchability of the skin and hypermobility of joints. Ehlers-Danlos syndrome is similar to osteogenesis imperfecta in that the term encompasses a number of distinct forms of the condition and the features are related to abnormalities of collagen or other connective tissue components. The distinction of Ehlers-Danlos conditions from osteogenesis imperfecta is that the skin and joints are primarily affected rather than bone. Most forms demonstrate autosomal dominant inheritance.

Clinical features. The diagnostic features are hyperelastic skin, fragility of the skin, and hypermobility of joints. The skin draws back to normal position after being stretched to an abnormally great degree. The skin has a thin, velvety texture and may be torn or bruised by relatively minor lateral pressure or abrasion. Healing in severe forms of the disease produces "cigarette paper" scars. Joint hypermobility can be demonstrated by extreme range of movement of the digits or the "limber" ability to accomplish extreme movements of the limbs. Joint instability may predispose to luxation and the early onset of arthritis. Blue sclera is observed in some cases. Mitral valve prolapse and other cardiac abnormalities are frequently present. The oral mucosa is unusually vulnerable to injury, and healing after surgical procedures is somewhat delayed. Various dental abnormalities such as conical incisor shape, short tooth root malformation (Fig. 20-

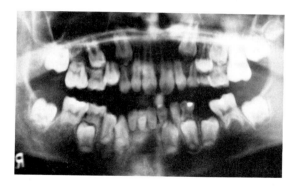

Fig. 20-18 Ehlers-Danlos syndrome. Dental malformations include abnormally short root formation of numerous teeth and conical incisor shape as illustrated by this panoramic radiograph of a 10-year-old boy. (Courtesy of Dr Edward Genecov, Dallas, Texas.)

18), and prominent pulpal calcification may be present.

Clinical considerations. Life span is normal for the most common forms of Ehlers-Danlos syndrome. Incidental injury to the mucosa and skin should be avoided during dental procedures. Infective endocarditis prophylaxis is indicated because of the likelihood of valvular dysfunction. Surgical procedures should be planned to maximize healing by achieving primary closure of surgical wounds and leaving sutures in place longer than for unaffected patients.

Marfan Syndrome

Synonyms. Arachnodactyly.

Definition. Abnormally long, slender extremities and digits, dislocation of the lens of the eyes, and aortic aneurysms are the most consistently observed features of Marfan syndrome. The genetic abnormality directly affects elastic fibers probably by alteration of collagen metabolism, but the specific mechanism has not been clarified. Autosomal dominant inheritance with complete penetrance and variable expressivity has been determined for this condition, and advanced maternal age at conception has been associated with isolated cases.

Clinical features. Abnormalities of the syndrome may be present in infancy, but the condition is often not appreciated until adolescence. Tall stature, slender habitus, arm span exceeding height, and arachnodactyly (long, thin digits) are consistent features. Fig. 20-19

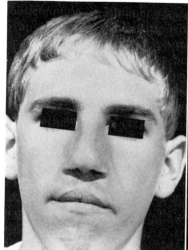
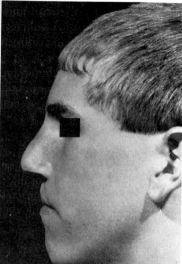

A

B

Fig. 20-19 Marfan syndrome. Frontal (**A**) and profile (**B**) views of a 17-year-old boy demonstrate the long, narrow facial appearance and skull shape described as dolichocephaly. (Courtesy of Dr Edward Genecov, Dallas, Texas.)

demonstrates the typical dolichocephalic skull shape, prognathic mandible, and long, narrow facial appearance with frontal bossing. Malocclusion is a frequent consequence of the mandibular prognathism. Lens dislocation resulting from weak suspensory ligaments affects most patients. Blue sclera and other abnormalities of the eyes are also commonly observed. Aortic distention, aortic aneurysm, and valvular defects attributable to degeneration of elastic fibers are the most serious alterations for patients with Marfan syndrome. Additional observations include hypermobility of joints, kyphoscoliosis, and sunken or prominent sternum.

Clinical considerations. Life span is shortened primarily as a consequence of aortic and cardiac abnormalities. The presence of these malformations also warrants infective endocarditis prophylaxis in most cases during dental procedures expected to cause a transient bacteremia. Orthognathic surgery and orthodontic correction of malocclusion may be indicated.

Ellis-van Creveld Syndrome

Synonyms. Chondroectodermal dysplasia and mesoectodermal dysplasia

Definition. This autosomal recessive condition is a form of dwarfism related to chondrodysplasia of the long bones as well as dysplasia of the nails and teeth.

Clinical features. The short stature is attributable to shortness of the limbs, which in combination with thoracic constriction makes the trunk appear elongated. The nails are consistently small, recessed in surrounding tissue, and poorly formed. Bilateral *polydactyly* of the hands is frequently observed. The upper lip is attached or confluent with the anterior maxillary alveolus, which results in absence of the mucolabial sulcus in this area. Cardiac malformations affect more than one half of the patients. Microdontic, conical tooth form is characteristic and several teeth are congenitally missing, particularly in the anterior mandibular segment.

Clinical considerations. Surgical correction of the oral soft tissue malformation may be beneficial. Prosthodontic and orthodontic procedures are usually necessary. The presence of cardiac defects may require antibiotic prophylaxis during dental procedures expected to cause a bacteremia.

SYNDROMES OF CONGENITAL SKIN ABNORMALITY

The diagnosis of the conditions in this group is usually uncomplicated because the characteristic diagnostic features of the superficial skin surface are visually apparent. Hypohidrotic ectodermal dysplasia and epidermolysis bullosa illustrate defective formation of skin and adnexal structures. Ellis-van Creveld syndrome could have been included with these two conditions on the basis of malformation of the nails. The skin discolorations of Sturge-Weber syndrome, Peutz-Jeghers syndrome, neurofibromatosis, and polyostotic fibrous dysplasia result from an excessive proportion of normal vascular and melanocytic tissue components. Such abnormalities are referred to as *hamartomas*. The discolorations are clinically inconsequential except as diagnostic indicators that the patient will develop other hamartomatous enlargements that are of clinical significance.

Hypohidrotic Ectodermal Dysplasia

Synonyms. Anhidrotic ectodermal dysplasia, Crist-Siemens-Touraine syndrome

Definition. The genetic defect produces hypoplasia or aplasia of ectodermal structures including hair, teeth, and superficial glands. Most examples have x-linked recessive inheritance with the heterozygous female carrier exhibiting mild expression of the features.

Clinical features. The initial symptom during infancy is often a persistent fever caused by ineffective body heat regulation in the absence of significant sweat production. The skin is thin and dry. Hair appears fine, thin, sparse, and blond in color as shown in Fig. 20-

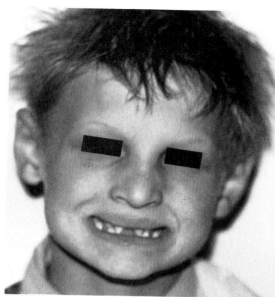

A

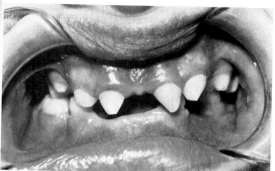

B

Fig. 20-20 Hypohidrotic ectodermal dysplasia. **A,** The typical appearance of the hair. **B,** The intraoral photograph demonstrates that many teeth are absent, and those present are microdontic and conical in shape. (Courtesy of Dr Catherine Flaitz, University of Texas Dental Branch at Houston, Houston, Texas.)

20, *A*, but the nails are relatively normal. Salivary, lacrimal, and mucosal gland function is diminished in varying degrees. Most of the deciduous and permanent teeth do not form and the teeth that do form are conical and somewhat microdontic (Fig. 20-20, *B*). The frontal region is prominent and the bridge of the nose is depressed. This combined with mandibular overclosure caused by the absence of teeth produces a concave facial profile.

Clinical considerations. The teeth that are present must be removed in many cases and a series of dentures must be fabricated during growth.

Epidermolysis Bullosa

Synonyms. None

Definition. Epidermolysis bullosa is the designation for a group of hereditary disorders with the common feature of vesicle and bulla formation affecting the skin and mucous membranes after mild frictional trauma. The separation tendency results from deficiency in the intercellular attachment apparatus of the epithe-

lial cells, basement membrane defects, or excessive secretion of collagenase. Classification of the different forms of the disease is based on the microscopic site of epithelial separation, the anatomic locations of lesions, whether lesions heal with scarring, and the inheritance pattern.

Clinical features. The extensive, hemorrhagic blisters of severe forms of epidermolysis bullosa are apparent at birth and can be life threatening. Milder types of the disease may not become apparent until later in infancy. Blister formation is most typically located on the hands (Fig. 20-21, *A*) and feet, but blisters may develop in any sites subjected to recurring, frictional pressure. The frequency and severity of oral bullae (Fig. 20-21, *B*) formation is roughly proportional to the tendency to develop skin lesions, although no oral lesions occur in some forms of epidermolysis bullosa.

Clinical considerations. The only available management techniques are prevention of blistering by minimizing friction pressure and supportive treatment of bullae that do form.

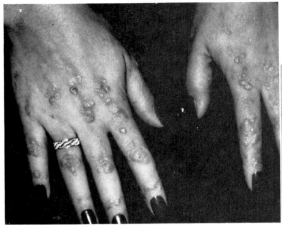

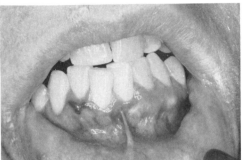

Fig. 20-21   Epidermolysis bullosa. Bullae affecting the hands (**A**) and gingiva (**B**) have been experienced by this 26-year-old woman since infancy.

Sturge-Weber Angiomatosis

Synonyms. Sturge-Weber disease, encephalofacial angiomatosis, encephalotrigeminal angiomatosis.

Definition. Sturge-Weber angiomatosis is characterized by intracranial vascular malformations and ipsilateral vascular discoloration of facial skin. Although the skin discoloration does not represent an epidermal malformation in the strictest sense, the condition is included with other skin discolorations on the basis of clinical appearance. The angiomatosis apparently results from a developmental defect during early gestation, and all cases have been isolated.

Clinical features. The sharply delineated, pink to purple skin discoloration is referred to as *nevus flammeus* or "port wine stain" (Fig. 20-22, *A*), and it is usually located unilaterally in the distribution of the ophthalmic branch of the trigeminal nerve. The discoloration is usually flat but it can be slightly elevated, and it extends beyond the distribution of the trigeminal nerve in some cases. The other early diagnostic feature is the development during infancy of focal seizures on the opposite side from the skin discoloration. Generalized seizures, mental retardation, and other neurologic disorders develop less frequently. The central

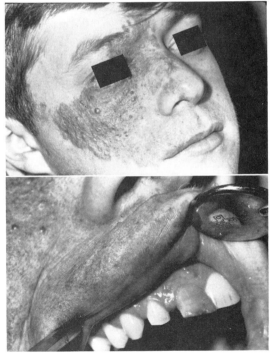

Fig. 20-22   Sturge-Weber angiomatosis. **A,** The unilateral "port wine stain" discoloration of the face is limited to the distribution of the second division of the trigeminal nerve. **B,** The vascular malformation has also produced mild enlargement and discoloration of the ipsilateral lip and gingiva.

nervous system dysfunction is associated with angiomatosis of the leptomeninges, which also produces abnormal calcification of associated tissues that can be demonstrated radiographically.

Intraoral angiomatosis is occasionally present if the second or third division of the trigeminal nerve is affected. The buccal mucosa and lips are the sites most often affected. Involvement of the alveolus can produce vascular gingival enlargement (Fig. 20-22, *B*). Abnormal dental development including delayed eruption, accelerated eruption, and malalignment may also be present. Vascular malformations of other tissues are also identified in some instances.

Clinical considerations. The primary treatment goal is to control the seizures and other neurologic complications. Removal of oral tissue enlargements and correction of malocclusion are necessary in some instances.

Peutz-Jeghers Syndrome

Synonyms. Mucocutaneous melanotic pigmentation and gastrointestinal polyposis, familial polyposis coli, intestinal polyposis I and II.

Definition. The features of Peutz-Jeghers syndrome include macular hyperpigmentation of the face near the lips and formation of multiple intestinal polyps. This hamartomatous condition exhibits autosomal dominant inheritance with high penetrance, although many cases are isolated.

Clinical features. The numerous pigmented macules are flat and brown to bluish-black in color, and they are located on skin and oral mucosa near the lips. The appearance suggests an abnormal cluster of large "freckles." Approximately one half of affected individuals also exhibit similar pigmentations of the hands and near mucocutaneous junctions in the region of the eyes, anus, or genitalia. Hamartomatous polyposis of the gastrointestinal tract may involve any mucous-secreting gastrointestinal segment, or it may be limited to the large bowel. Features such as cramping,

gastrointestinal bleeding, and anemia generally become apparent during adulthood. Complications such as intussusception and significant blood loss occasionally develop. An increase in the risk of gastrointestinal malignancy and cancer of other tissues approaching 50% occurrence is associated with Peutz-Jeghers syndrome.

Clinical considerations. The perioral pigmentations are insignificant except as an indication of the condition. Management of the gastrointestinal symptoms and periodic evaluation for evidence of malignancy are the treatment priorities.

Neurofibromatosis

Synonyms. Von Recklinghausen syndrome I, von Recklinghausen disease of skin.

Definition. Neurofibromatosis is characterized by cutaneous pigmentation and the formation of multiple *neurofibromas*. The neurofibroma of neurofibromatosis is indistinguishable microscopically from the isolated neurofibroma that develops in a unaffected patient. Although several forms of neurofibromatosis are recognized, approximately 90% of cases are consistent with the classic, or type I, neurofibromatosis, which is described below. Autosomal dominant inheritance is demonstrated and approximately one half of cases represent new mutations.

Clinical findings. Macular pigmentations of the skin are usually apparent at birth and are referred to as *café-au-lait* spots. These pigmentations as illustrated in Fig. 20-23 are flat with a smooth peripheral contour, sharply delineated borders, and a homogeneous, light brown color. The presence of more than five café-au-lait spots that are all more than 1.5 cm in greatest dimension fulfills the diagnostic criteria for neurofibromatosis. Axillary freckling referred to as *Crowe's sign* is also present in approximately one half of affected patients. Melanotic discoloration of the iris referred to as Lisch nodules may also be observed.

Neurofibromas are identified in some cases

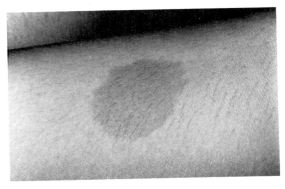

Fig. 20-23 Café-au-lait spot of an 8-year-old girl. These macular pigmentations are nonpalpable, homogeneous, and light brown in color with a sharply delineated peripheral border.

during infancy, but the enlargements usually becomes obvious in early adolescence. Nearly any tissue can be affected and wide variation in lesion size is possible. The lesions appear nodular or as a diffuse, hanging mass of tissue referred to as a *plexiform neurofibroma.* Skin lesions are most obvious, and hundreds of individual enlargements can occur (Fig. 20-24). Individual lesions gradually increase in size, and the appearance of new neurofibromas continues throughout adulthood. A variety of other tumors and malformations are occasionally associated with the condition. Sarcomatous transformation of neurofibromas is a possible complication observed among older neurofibromatosis patients.

The most commonly affect oral site is the tongue. Occasionally, enlargement of the inferior alveolar canal demonstrated radiographically indicates the presence of a neurofibroma within bone.

Clinical considerations. No effective treatment is available. The onset of relatively rapid enlargement of a neurofibroma strongly suggests the development of a neurofibrosarcoma.

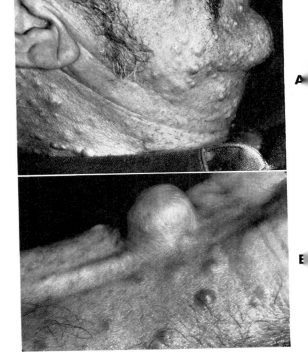

Fig. 20-24 Neurofibromatosis. This condition has produced numerous papular and nodular enlargements of the face and neck (**A**), wrist (**B**), and most other skin surfaces of this 56-year-old man.

Polyostotic Fibrous Dysplasia

Synonyms. Includes Jaffe-Lichtenstein syndrome, craniofacial fibrous dysplasia, Albright's syndrome, McCune-Albright syndrome.

Definition. The presence of café-au-lait skin pigmentations and fibrous dysplasia affecting more than one bone are required for the diagnosis of polyostotic fibrous dysplasia. Polyostotic fibrous dysplasia is much less common than monostotic fibrous dysplasia and several polyostotic forms are recognized. The combination of skin pigmentations and several bones affected by fibrous dysplasia has been referred to as *Jaffe's type of polyostotic fibrous dysplasia* or *Jaffe-Lichtenstein syndrome. Craniofacial* *polyostotic fibrous dysplasia* refers to this condition if the affected bones are grouped in the head. *McCune-Albright syndrome* or *Albright syndrome* refers to the combination of skin pigmentation, fibrous dysplasia affecting several bones, and manifestations of endocrine hyperfunction, which is usually precocious onset of puberty of a female. A genetic influence is suspected with these conditions, but definitive conclusions about the etiology and pathogenesis are difficult because all cases have been isolated.

Clinical features. The radiographic features and clinical course of fibrous dysplasia is described in Chapter 19. Pathologic fractures often result if long bones are affected. The café-au-lait pigmentations are similar to those described above for neurofibromatosis except that the peripheral borders frequently exhibit a "jagged" or irregular peripheral contour. The endocrine hyperfunction of McCune-Albright syndrome is demonstrated by premature development of secondary sexual characteristics and menarche, often before 5 years of age. Hyperthyroidism, hyperadrenal function with cushingoid features, and hyperparathyroidism are among the other possible endocrine abnormalities.

Clinical considerations. The clinical approach to fibrous dysplasia of facial bones is discussed in Chapter 19.

SYNDROMES THAT BECOME APPARENT AFTER INFANCY

A number of syndromes with significant dental features are not apparent at birth or during early infancy. Gardner syndrome, nevoid basal cell carcinoma syndrome, and hereditary hemorrhagic telangiectasia are genetically determined conditions of hamartoma or neoplasm formation in which the lesions become obvious during puberty or later. Melkersson-Rosenthal and Papillon-Lefévre syndromes illustrate manifestations of abnormal inflammatory responses. Plummer-Vinson syndrome is an acquired syndrome without significant genetic contribution that is of clinical concern because it is associated with an increased incidence of oropharyngeal carcinoma. Numerous other acquired syndromes that could be included in this section, such as AIDS and a variety of autoimmune syndromes, have been adequately discussed in the chapters concerned with the primary clinical manifestations.

Gardner Syndrome

Synonyms. Intestinal polyposis III, osteomatosis—intestinal polyposis syndrome.

Definition. Diagnostic features include osteomas of the facial bones, polyposis of the large bowel, cutaneous epidermoid cysts, and dental abnormalities. Complete penetrance of autosomal dominant inheritance is observed, but the expressivity is highly variable.

Clinical features. Osteomas are the most consistent feature of Gardner syndrome other than the intestinal polyps. Any bone may be affected, but the facial bones are the typical location, and several osteomas are usually present. A wide range of lesion size is possible, and enlargement eventually ceases, indicating limited growth potential. Uniform radiopacities with an ovoid or "lumpy" contour within or adjacent to the facial bones is the typical radiographic appearance. Clinically apparent enlargement or interference with jaw movements may be associated with the enlargement of exostoses, whereas endostoses are usually asymptomatic. Approximately one half of patients develop multiple epidermoid cysts during puberty. These compressible enlargements most often affect the skin of the head and extremities.

The most consistent but clinically unapparent feature of the syndrome is intestinal polyposis, which usually develops during puberty. The lesions may be suggested by gastrointestinal bleeding or cramping abdominal pain. The tendency for carcinomatous transformation of the intestinal polyps is believed to approach 100%, and evidence of intestinal cancer is expected by the end of the third decade in approximately one half of affected patients. A variety of other benign and malignant neoplasms such as abdominal and extraabdominal desmoid tumors occasionally develop.

Less than one third to one half of patients with Gardner syndrome exhibit dental abnormalities. The most commonly described anomalies include supernumerary teeth, generalized failure of teeth to erupt, and formation of multiple odontomas.

Clinical considerations. Surgical removal of the large bowel is indicated after definitive diagnosis of intestinal polyposis. Polyps of the small bowel and gastric mucosa may also develop, but the likelihood of malignant transformation is much less than that of colonic polyps. Surgical removal of supernumerary and impacted teeth may be necessary. Removal of osteomas for both cosmetic and functional reasons is often beneficial.

Nevoid Basal Cell Carcinoma Syndrome

Synonyms. Gorlin-Goltz syndrome, Gorlin syndrome, basal cell nevus syndrome, jaw cyst–basal cell nevus–bifid rib syndrome.

Definition. The diagnostic abnormalities of the syndrome are the formation of multiple basal cell carcinomas of the skin, the development of multiple jaw cysts, and skeletal malformations. Inheritance is autosomal dominant with complete penetrance and widely variable expressivity. The complexity of this hamarto-neoplastic, malformation syndrome is indicated by the numerous additional abnormalities that have been identified affecting the skin, the central nervous system, and the skeleton.

Clinical features. The basal cell carcinomas of this syndrome are different from the common, isolated lesions of the general population in that multiple lesions develop before middle-age, and the lesions are not limited to sun-exposed skin. Also, an unusual association

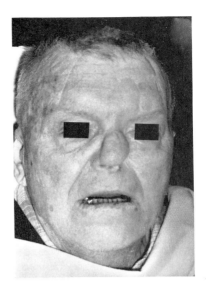

Fig. 20-25 Nevoid basal cell carcinoma syndrome. The facial scars are the consequence of the removal of numerous basal cell carcinomas. This patient also experienced several jaw cysts that microscopic examination revealed to be odontogenic keratocysts.

of melanotic pigmentation and focal calcification with the lesions and less aggressive progression are observed in nevoid basal cell carcinoma syndrome. The number of lesions varies from several to hundreds, and the face is the most frequently affected region (Fig. 20-25). The multiple jaw cysts are identical microscopically to the common, isolated odontogenic keratocyst. The cysts usually develop during late childhood, adolescence, or early adulthood, which is significantly earlier than the occurrence of most isolated odontogenic keratocysts. The unilocular or multilocular cystic radiolucencies develop more often in the mandible and may produce malocclusion by causing ectopic eruption or displacement of permanent teeth.

An extensive assortment of additional abnormalities have been identified among patients affected by nevoid basal cell carcinoma syndrome. Relatively large cranial size attributable to frontal and parietal prominence affects more than one half of patients. Excessive contour of the supraorbital ridges and mandibular prognathism yield a concave facial profile. Radiographs may reveal calcification of the falx cerebri, large paranasal sinuses, and rib abnormalities such as fusion, hypoplasia, and bifid malformations. Ocular abnormalities, other skeletal malformations, and neoplasms other than basal cell carcinomas are less frequent observations.

Clinical considerations. Surgical removal of the basal cell carcinomas and jaw cysts is indicated to avoid the complications of unchecked progression. Orthodontic and surgical management of malocclusion may be necessary.

Hereditary Hemorrhagic Telangiectasia

Synonyms. Osler-Rendu-Weber syndrome, Rendu-Osler-Weber syndrome, familial hemorrhagic telangiectasia.

Definition. When several family members are affected by numerous hemorrhagic vascular lesions, hereditary hemorrhagic telangiectasia should be suspected. Transmission of the condition is autosomal dominant with nearly complete penetrance. The lesions consist of dilated vessels rather than an abnormally dense concentration of vessels.

Clinical features. Most patients with hereditary hemorrhagic telangiectasia develop numerous papular to nodular elevations of superficial surfaces during adolescence or early adulthood (Fig. 16-8) and the lesions become more prominent with increasing age. The clinically apparent sites of involvement include nasal mucosa, facial skin, skin of the digits, and oral mucosa, although the distribution is variable and nearly any organ system may be affected. The enlargements are compressible, blanching, and red or bluish-red in color.

Hemorrhage results from mild, incidental abrasion of lesions, and it can be difficult to control. Persistent epistaxis is a frequent initial complaint that often precedes the appearance of skin or oral lesions. Spontaneous and recurring hemorrhage results in anemia that increases in severity with age. This is a particular problem if gastrointestinal lesions develop. Other vascular abnormalities are also present in some cases; such as pulmonary arteriovenus malformations, which increase the risk of brain abscess and embolic infarction.

Clinical considerations. The diagnosis is suspected in most cases because of the familial occurrence. Care to avoid incidental injury to the vascular lesions during routine dental treatment is necessary. Severe anemia may lead to reduced host resistance to infection. This and the increased risk of brain abscess may justify antibiotic prophylaxis during dental procedures likely to cause bacteremia.

Papillon-Lafévre Syndrome

Synonyms. Hyperkeratosis palmoplantaris and periodontoclasia in childhood.

Definition. The two clinical features of the condition are juvenile periodontitis and skin thickening of the palms and soles. Autosomal recessive inheritance is indicated by the relatively frequent association with consanguinity. A deficiency of neutrophil function has been suggested.

Clinical features. Between the ages of 2 and 4 the plantar and palmar skin becomes erythematous, scaly, rough, and thickened in a somewhat patchy distribution. Simultaneously, the gingiva near recently erupted deciduous teeth becomes erythematous, edematous, and hemorrhagic. The deciduous teeth are all soon lost to periodontal destruction, and the alveolar mucosa heals to a normal appearance. Progressive periodontitis then develops around each succedaneous tooth in sequence as they erupt, which soon leads to the loss of all teeth as well as destruction of a large proportion of the alveolar bone.

Clinical considerations. Treatment of the periodontal condition is described in Chapter 8, however, the periodontal prognosis is poor.

Plummer-Vinson Syndrome

Synonyms. Sideropenic dysphagia, Paterson's syndrome, Kelly-Paterson syndrome.

Definition. The diagnostic features of this acquired syndrome are iron deficiency anemia and dysphagia. Iron deficiency caused by inadequate dietary intake or a malabsorption condition leads to iron deficiency anemia, which results in secondary degeneration of esophageal muscles and atrophy of oropharyngeal epithelium.

Clinical features. Middle-aged women are affected in most cases, and laboratory studies typically reveal a hypochromic, microcytic anemia. Weakness, fatigue, facial pallor, and brittle, spoon shaped nails (koilonychia) are often present. Oral consequences of the anemia include atrophic oral mucosa, atrophic glossitis, a burning sensation of the tongue, and angular cheilitis.

Clinical considerations. Referral for evaluation and treatment of the anemia should be the initial priority. Symptomatic treatment includes a nonabrasive diet and the use of bland, coating suspensions or anesthetic preparations as described in Chapter 13 for mucositis caused by radiation and chemotherapy. The patient should be reexamined at frequent recall intervals if the condition persists because a predisposition to oropharyngeal carcinoma is associated with Plummer-Vinson syndrome.

SUMMARY

Syndromes of interest to the dentist can be categorized by the stage of development in which they become clinically identifiable: either soon after birth or later in life. Syndromes that are identifiable soon after birth result from either genetic defects or adverse influences during gestation. They can be further classified by a clinically obvious feature within one of the following groups:

1. Deficient mandibular development
2. Deficient maxillary development
3. Generalized connective tissue deficiency
4. Defective skin formation or discoloration of skin

Syndromes that become apparent later in life can be either genetically determined or acquired by various other pathologic mechanisms such as autoimmune conditions, degenerative diseases, or infections. Several examples of late onset syndromes of genetic origin are characterized by the development of multiple hamartomatous or neoplastic enlargements, while others are manifest by unusual inflammatory lesions. Many acquired syndromes consist of multiple clinical findings that are diverse pathophysiologic consequences of an underlying abnormality such as anemia.

Developmental syndromes with oral features present a diagnostic challenge because most examples occur relatively rarely, which limits the clinician's opportunity to gain direct familiarity with many examples. Also, the diverse manifestations that characterize many syndromes can become confused with the coincidental occurrence of several abnormalities caused by unrelated conditions. The diagnosis of patients with multiple abnormalities requires correlation of the pattern of observed abnormalities with features of recognized syndromes. This frequently involves anatomic and functional abnormalities not directly related to oral structures.

BIBLIOGRAPHY

Buyse ML, editor: Birth defects encyclopedia, Dover, 1990, Center for Birth Defects Information Services.

Gorlin RJ, Cohen MM, Levin LS: Syndromes of the head and neck, ed 3, New York, 1990, Oxford University Press.

Magalini SI, Magalini SC, de Francisci G: Dictionary of medical syndromes, ed 3, Philadelphia, 1990, Lippincott.

Index